OAT®

DATE DUE

07-21			
			PRINTED IN U.S.A.

© 2012 Kaplan, Inc.

Published by Kaplan Publishing, a division of Kaplan, Inc.
395 Hudson Street
New York, NY 10014

Printed in the United States of America

10 9 8 7 6 5 4

ISBN: 978-1-60978-109-5

Kaplan Publishing books are available at special quantity discounts to use for sales promotions, employee premiums, or educational purposes. For more information or to purchase books, please call the Simon & Schuster special sales department at 866-506-1949.

Contents

OAT Study Sheets

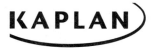

AVAILABLE ONLINE

Free Additional Practice
kaptest.com/booksonline

As owner of this book, you are entitled to get even **more** OAT practice. Additional online materials include an entire **OAT Practice Test** in the most test-like computerized format.

To access these resources, simply go to **kaptest.com/booksonline**

Follow the on-screen instructions. Please have a copy of your book available.

Access to the online companion is limited to the original owner of this book and is nontransferable. Kaplan is not responsible for providing access to the online companion for customers who purchase or borrow used copies of this book. Access to the online companion expires one year after you register.

For Any Test Changes or Late-Breaking Developments
kaptest.com/publishing

The material in this book is up-to-date at the time of publication. However, the testmaker may have instituted changes in the test after this book was published. Be sure to read carefully the materials you receive when you register for the test. If there are any important late-breaking developments—or any changes or corrections to the Kaplan test preparation materials in this book—we will post that information online at **kaptest.com/publishing**.

Feedback and Comments
booksupport@kaplan.com

We'd love to hear your comments and suggestions about this book. Please provide any additional suggestions or feedback you have for improvement of the book to **booksupport@kaplan.com**. Your feedback is extremely helpful as we continue to develop high-quality resources to meet your needs.

Periodic Table of the Elements

Group	1	2	3	4	5	6	7	8	9	10	11	12	13	14	15	16	17	18
Period																		
1	1 H																	2 He
2	3 Li	4 Be											5 B	6 C	7 N	8 O	9 F	10 Ne
3	11 Na	12 Mg											13 Al	14 Si	15 P	16 S	17 Cl	18 Ar
4	19 K	20 Ca	21 Sc	22 Ti	23 V	24 Cr	26 Mn	26 Fe	27 Co	28 Ni	29 Cu	30 Zn	31 Ga	32 Ge	33 Ss	34 Se	35 Br	36 Kr
5	37 Rb	38 Sr	39 Y	40 Zr	41 Nb	42 Mo	42 Tc	44 Ru	45 Rh	46 Pd	47 Ag	48 Cd	49 In	50 Sn	51 Sb	52 Te	53 I	54 Xe
6	55 Cs	56 Ba	71 Lu *	72 Hf	73 Ta	74 W	75 Re	76 Os	77 Ir	78 Pt	79 Au	80 Hg	81 Ti	82 Pb	83 Bi	84 Po	85 At	86 Rn
7	87 Fr	88 Ra	103 Lr **	104 Rf	105 Db	106 Sg	107 Bh	108 Hs	109 Mt	110 Ds	111 Rg	112 Cn	113 Uut	114 Fl	115 Uup	116 Lv	117 Uus	118 Uuo

*Lanthanoids	57 La	58 Ce	59 Pr	60 Nd	61 Pm	62 Sm	63 Eu	64 Gd	65 Tb	66 Dy	67 Ho	68 Er	69 Tm	70 Yb
**Actinoids	89 Ac	90 Th	91 Pa	92 U	93 Np	94 Pu	95 Am	96 Cm	97 Bk	98 Cf	99 Es	100 Fm	101 Md	102 No

Introduction

ABOUT THE OAT

The Optometry Admission Test, affectionately known as the OAT, is different from any other test you've encountered in your academic career. It's not like the knowledge-based exams from high school and college, whose emphasis was on memorizing and regurgitating information. Optometry schools can assess your academic prowess by looking at your transcript. The OAT isn't even like other standardized tests you may have taken, where the focus was on proving your general skills.

The Optometry Admission Test (OAT) was developed by the American Optometry Association and is sponsored by the Association of Schools and Colleges of Optometry (www. opted.org). All schools and colleges of optometry require candidates to submit OAT scores for admission. The OAT is designed to predict general academic ability and measure the two skills needed by future optometrists: scientific knowledge and analytical ability. It does this by testing your knowledge of physics, chemistry, and biology; your reading comprehension ability; and your quantitative reasoning skills.

Optometry schools use OAT scores to assess whether you possess the foundation upon which to build a successful career in optometry. Though you certainly need to know the content to do well, the stress is on thought process, because the OAT is above all else a thinking test. That's why it emphasizes reasoning, critical and analytical thinking, reading comprehension, data analysis, and problem-solving skills.

The OAT's power comes from its use as an indicator of your abilities. Good scores can open doors. Your power comes from preparation and mindset, because the key to OAT success is knowing what you're up against. And that's where this section of this book comes in. We'll explain the philosophy behind the test, review the sections one by one, share some of Kaplan's proven methods, and clue you in to what the test makers are really after. You'll get a handle on the process, find a confident new perspective, and achieve your highest possible scores.

The Computer-Based OAT

Now that a computer-based version of the Optometry Admission Test is available, the paper-based OAT has been phased out. Now instead of being restricted to two testing dates a year, testing is available year round and an examinee can select the date, time, and place.

A summary of the test changes is as follows:

- Students must wait 90 days between test administrations.
- The computer-based test (CBT) will be offered year round.
- Students may take the test an unlimited number of times, but only scores from the four most recent attempts will be reported.
- OAT CBT test-takers will get their scores on the day of their test. Schools will have a three-week period after the test to receive the scores.
- Once students begin any section of the test, they cannot void or cancel it.
- An extra 10 minutes have been added to the computer OAT Reading Comprehension section, to provide time for scrolling the passages on the computer.
- There is a set fee for the OAT exam.

Registration

To apply for the OAT, you can submit an electronic application at www.opted.org using a credit card. It is possible to request a paper application form by submitting a written request to oatexam@ada.org or by fax (312.587.4105). Examinees submitting a paper application must pay the required fee by money order/certified check.

The OAT™ Program will assign you an OATPIN when you apply. The OATPIN is a unique personal identifier that helps ensure confidential, secure reporting of test scores and related academic data.

Upon completion of your application processing, Prometric will receive notification of your eligibility for testing and you will receive instructions by e-mail (or letter if no e-mail address is on file) to contact the Prometric Contact Center. Please wait 24 hours after notification before scheduling a testing appointment to allow adequate time for processing of the eligibility file. An application may be submitted no more than six (6) months before the test date

Anatomy of the OAT

Before mastering strategies, you need to know exactly what you're dealing with on the OAT. Let's start with the basics: The OAT is, among other things, an endurance test. It consists of close to four hours of stand-alone multiple-choice questions. Add in the administrative details at both ends of the testing experience, plus breaks, and you can count on being in the test room for well over five hours. It's a grueling experience, to say the least. If you can't approach it with confidence and stamina, you'll quickly lose your composure. That's why it's so important that you take control of the test.

The OAT consists of four timed sections: Survey of the Natural Sciences, Reading Comprehension, Physics, and Quantitative Reasoning. Later in this book you will get an in-depth review of each section. For now, you'll find a general overview in the table below.

Section	Time	Number of Questions	Topics Tested
1. Survey of Natural Sciences	90 minutes	100 questions	Biology (40) Inorganic Chemistry (30) Organic Chemistry (30)
2. Reading Comprehension	50 minutes	40 questions	Ability to find main idea Ability to process information Ability to read and understand dense passages
3. Physics	50 minutes	40 questions	Vectors Energy and Momentum Thermodynamics Magnetism Optics
4. Quantitative Reasoning	45 minutes	40 questions	Arithmetic Algebra Geometry Trigonometry

The sections of the test always appear in the same order as above. There is a 15-minute introductory tutorial and a 10-minute post-test survey. Examinees may request scratch work materials from the administrator. All scratch work must be returned to the administrator before leaving the testing center. A basic function computer-based calculator can be used on the Quantitative Reasoning section only.

Scoring

The OAT is given a scaled score of 200–400, 300 being the median representing the 40th–52nd percentile. Separate subscores are reported for biology, general chemistry, organic chemistry, reading comprehension, and quantitative reasoning.

Each question within a section is worth the same amount, and *there's no penalty for guessing. That means that you should always answer every question whether you get to that question or not!* This is an important piece of advice, so pay it heed. Never let time run out on any section without filling in an answer for every question.

Your score report will tell you (and optometry schools) not only your scaled scores but also your percentile ranking. Students often ask: what's a good score? Much depends on the strength of the rest of your application (if your transcript is first-rate, the pressure to strut your stuff on the OAT isn't as intense) and on where you want to go to school (different schools have different score expectations).

Take Control: The OAT Mindset

In addition to being a thinking test, as we've stressed, the OAT is a standardized test. As such, it has its own consistent patterns and idiosyncrasies that can actually work in your favor. This is the key to why test preparation works. You have the opportunity to familiarize yourself with those consistent peculiarities, to adopt the proper test-taking mindset.

The OAT Mindset is something you want to bring to every question and section you encounter. Being in the OAT Mindset means reshaping the test-taking experience so that you are in the driver's seat:

- Answer questions when you want to—feel free to skip tough but doable passages and questions, coming back to them only after you've racked up points on easy ones.
- Answer questions how you want to—use our shortcuts and methods to get points quickly and confidently, even if those methods aren't exactly what the test makers had in mind when they wrote the test.

The following are some overriding principles of the OAT Mindset that are covered in depth in the chapters to come:

- Read actively and critically.
- Translate prose into your own words.
- Save the toughest questions for last.
- Know the test and its components inside and out.
- Do OAT-style problems in each topic area after you've reviewed it.
- Allow your confidence to build on itself.
- Take full-length practice tests a week or two before the test to break down the mystique of the real experience.
- Learn from your mistakes—get the most out of your practice tests.
- Look at the OAT as a challenge, the first step in your optometry career, rather than as an arbitrary obstacle.

And that's what the OAT Mindset boils down to: taking control, being proactive, being on top of the testing experience so that you can get as many points as you can as quickly and as easily as possible. Keep this in mind as you read and work through the material in this book and, of course, as you face the challenge on Test Day.

KAPLAN'S OAT STRATEGIES

The first year of optometry school is a frenzied experience for most students. In order to meet the requirements of a rigorous work schedule, they either learn to prioritize and budget their time or else fall hopelessly behind. It's no surprise, then, that the OAT, the test specifically designed to predict success in the first year of optometry school, is a high-speed, time-intensive test.

It's one thing to answer a Reading Comprehension question correctly; it's quite another to answer 40 of them correctly in 50 minutes. And the same goes for Natural Sciences, Physics, and Quantitative Reasoning. It's a whole new ball game once you move from doing an individual passage at your leisure to handling a full section under actual timed conditions. When it comes to the multiple-choice sections, time pressure is a factor that affects virtually every test taker.

So when you are comfortable with the content of the test, your next challenge will be to take it to the next level, test expertise, which will enable you to manage the all-important time element of the test.

Kaplan's Five Basic Principles of Test Expertise

On some tests, if a question seems particularly difficult, you spend significantly more time on it, since you'll probably be given more points for correctly answering a hard question. Not so on the OAT. Remember, every OAT question, no matter how hard, is worth a single point. There's no partial credit or "A" for effort. And since there are so many questions to do in so little time, it wouldn't make sense to spend ten minutes getting a point for a hard question and then not have time to get a couple of quick points from three easy questions later in the section.

Given this combination—limited time, all questions equal in weight—you have to develop a way of handling the test sections to make sure you get as many points as you can as quickly and easily as you can. Here are the principles that will help you do that:

1. **FEEL FREE TO SKIP AROUND**

   One of the most valuable strategies to help you finish the sections in time is to learn to recognize and deal first with the questions that are easier and more familiar to you. That means temporarily skipping those that promise to be difficult and time-consuming, if you feel comfortable doing so. You can always come back to these at the end, and if you run out of time, you're much better off not getting to questions you may have had difficulty with, rather than missing out on potentially score-raising material. Of course, since there's no guessing penalty, always fill in an answer to every question on the test, whether you get to it or not.

   This strategy is difficult for most test takers; we're conditioned to do things in order. But give it a try when you practice. Remember, if you do the test in the exact order given, you're letting the test makers control you. But *you* control how you take this test. On the other hand, if skipping around goes against your moral fiber and makes you a nervous wreck—don't do it. Just be mindful of the clock and don't get bogged down with the tough questions.

2. **LEARN TO RECOGNIZE AND SEEK OUT QUESTIONS YOU CAN DO**

   Another thing to remember about managing the test sections is that OAT questions and passages, unlike items on the SAT and other standardized tests, are not presented in order of difficulty. There's no rule that says you have to work through the sections in any particular order; in fact, the test makers scatter the easy and difficult questions throughout the section, in effect rewarding those who actually get to the end. Don't lose sight of what you're being tested for along with your reading and thinking skills: efficiency and cleverness. If organic chemistry questions are your thing, head straight for them when you first turn to the Natural Sciences section.

   Don't waste time on questions you can't do. We know that skipping a possibly tough question is easier said than done; we all have the natural instinct to plow through test sections in their given order. But it just doesn't pay off on the OAT. The computer won't be impressed if you get the toughest question right. If you dig in your heels on a tough question, refusing to move on until you've cracked it, well, you're letting your ego get in the way of your test score. A test section (not to mention life itself) is too short to waste on lost causes.

3. USE A PROCESS OF ANSWER ELIMINATION

Using a process of elimination is another way to answer questions both quickly and effectively. There are two ways to get all the answers right on the OAT. You either know all the right answers, or you know all the wrong answers. Since there are three times as many wrong answer choices, you should be able to eliminate some if not all of them. By doing so, you either get to the correct response or increase your chances of guessing the correct response. You start out with a 25 percent chance of picking the right answer, and with each eliminated answer, your odds go up. Eliminate one, and you'll have a 33 1/3 percent chance of picking the right one; eliminate two, and you'll have a 50 percent chance; and, of course, eliminate three, and you'll have a 100 percent chance. Increase your efficiency by actually crossing out the wrong choices in your test booklet. Remember to look for wrong-answer traps when you're eliminating. Some answers are designed to seduce you by distorting the correct answer.

4. REMAIN CALM

It's imperative that you remain calm and composed while working through a section. You can't allow yourself to become so rattled by one hard reading passage that it throws off your performance on the rest of the section. Expect to find at least a few killer questions in every section, but remember, you won't be the only one to have trouble with it. The test is curved to take the tough material into account. Having trouble with a difficult question isn't going to ruin your score—but getting upset about it and letting it throw you off track will. When you understand that part of the test-maker's goal is to reward those who keep their composure, you'll recognize the importance of not panicking when you run into challenging material.

5. KEEP TRACK OF TIME

Of course, the last thing you want to happen is to have time called on a particular section before you've gotten to half the questions. Therefore, it's essential that you pace yourself, keeping in mind the general guidelines for how long to spend on any individual question. Have a sense of how long you have to do each question, so you know when you're exceeding the limit and should start to move faster.

When working on a section, always remember to keep track of time. Don't spend a wildly disproportionate amount of time on any one question or group of questions. Also, give yourself 30 seconds or so at the end of each section to fill in answers for any questions you haven't gotten to.

OAT Section-Specific Pacing

NATURAL SCIENCES

You have 90 minutes to answer 40 questions on Biology, 30 questions on General Chemistry, and 30 questions on Organic Chemistry for a total of 100 stand-alone multiple-choice questions. Essentially, you have a little under a minute per question (52 seconds, to be exact). The key to remember is that some questions require more time whereas others don't take as much time. Begin with your strengths and answer all questions that you are comfortable with. Mark the tough questions and come back to them at the end.

READING COMPREHENSION

You have 50 minutes to do a total of 40 questions. Do the easiest passages first. Within a section, if you're deciding which passage to do based on time alone, do the one with the most questions. That way you maximize your reading efficiency. However, keep in mind that some passages are longer than others.

PHYSICS AND QUANTITATIVE REASONING

You have 50 minutes to answer 40 stand-alone multiple-choice questions in Physics (a little over a minute per question) and 45 minutes to answer 40 stand-alone multiple-choice questions in Quantitative Reasoning (a little under a minute per question). The same strategy that is useful in Natural Sciences applies here. Go with your strengths and answer the questions that are easiest for you. Mark the tough questions so you can come back to them at the end.

Comptuter-Based OAT Strategies

Since the OAT is only given in the CBT format, it is important to keep the following strategies in mind:

TUTORIAL

Don't ignore this section of your test experience. Even if you are a computer whiz, this is a source of important information. Be as prepared and comfortable with your test station as possible.

MARKING FUNCTION

On the computer-based OAT, it is a bit less easy to jump around the testing sections and go back and forth between questions than it was on the paper-and-pencil test. You can go back and forth within a section, but this takes time. However, you have a function available to you called "Mark" that you can use to mark the tough questions with. You can get back to these after you've answered all the easy questions. At the end of the section, the screen will prompt you to review marked questions, and you can go back to answer these then. There is no penalty for guessing, so answer them all.

KAPLAN'S OAT MASTERY GUIDE

In this section, we first glanced at the content that makes up each specific section of the OAT, focusing on the strategies and techniques you'll need to tackle individual questions and passages. Then we discussed the test expertise involved in moving from individual items to working through full-length sections. Now we're ready to turn our attention to the often-overlooked attitudinal aspects of the test, to put the finishing touches on your comprehensive OAT approach.

Kaplan's Four Basic Principles of Good Test Mentality

Knowing the test content arms you with the weapons you need to do well on the OAT. But you must wield those weapons with the right frame of mind and in the right spirit. Otherwise, you could end up shooting yourself in the foot. This involves taking a certain stance toward the entire test. Here's what's involved:

1. TEST AWARENESS

To do your best on the OAT, you must always keep in mind that the test is like no other test you've taken before, both in terms of content and in terms of the scoring system. If you took a test in high school or college and got a number of the questions wrong, you wouldn't receive a perfect grade. But on the OAT, you can get a handful of questions wrong and still get a "perfect" score. The test is geared so that only the very best test takers are able to finish every section. But even these people rarely get every question right.

What does this mean for you? Well, just as you shouldn't let one bad question ruin an entire section, you shouldn't let what you consider to be a subpar performance on one section ruin your performance on the entire test. If you allow that subpar performance to rattle you, it can have a cumulative negative effect, setting in motion a downward spiral. It's that kind of thing that could potentially do serious damage to your score. Losing a few extra points won't do you in, but losing your cool will.

Remember, if you feel you've done poorly on a section, don't sweat it. Chances are it's just a difficult section, and that factor will already be figured into the scoring curve. The point is, remain calm and collected. Simply do your best on each section, and once a section is over, forget about it and move on.

2. STAMINA

You must work on your test-taking stamina. Overall, the OAT is a fairly grueling experience, and some test takers simply run out of gas on the last section. To avoid this, you must prepare by taking a few full-length Practice Tests in the weeks before the test, so that on Test Day, all four sections will seem like a breeze. (Well, maybe not a breeze, but at least not a hurricane.)

Take the full-length practice tests included in this book. You'll be able to review answer explanations and assess your performance. You should, of course, keep in mind that every OAT administration differs; you can't assume that your actual score will be predicted by your score on a Practice Test. The score you'll get on any Practice Test is less important than the practice itself.

For those students who want more intensive preparation, Kaplan offers a wide range of OAT prep options, including classroom-based courses, private tutoring, and online courses. Visit kaptest.com for more information or to enroll in these courses. Your best option, if you have time, would be to take the live Kaplan course. We'll give you access to all the released material plus loads of additional material, so you can really build up your OAT stamina. You'll also have the benefit of our expert live instruction on every aspect of the OAT. To go this route, call 800-KAP-TEST or visit kaptest.com for a Kaplan center location near you.

Reading this chapter is a great start in your preparation for the test, but it won't get you your best score. That can happen only after lots of practice and skill-building. You've got to train your brain to be test-smart! Kaplan has been helping people do that for over 60 years, so giving us a call would be a great way to move your test prep into high gear!

3. CONFIDENCE

Confidence feeds on itself, and unfortunately, so does the opposite of confidence—self-doubt. Confidence in your ability leads to quick, sure answers and a sense of well-being that translates into more points. If you lack confidence, you end up reading the sentences and answer choices two, three, or four times, until you confuse yourself and get off track. This leads to timing difficulties, which only perpetuate the downward spiral, causing anxiety and a tendency to rush in order to finish sections.

If you subscribe to the OAT Mindset we've described, however, you'll gear all of your practice toward the major goal of taking control of the test. When you've achieved that goal—armed with the principles, techniques, strategies, and approaches set forth in this book—you'll be ready to face the OAT with supreme confidence. And that's the one sure way to score your best on Test Day.

4 THE RIGHT ATTITUDE

Those who approach the OAT as an obstacle, who rail against the necessity of taking it, who make light of its importance, who spend more time making fun of the OAT than studying for the test, usually don't fare as well as those who see the OAT as an opportunity to show off the reading and reasoning skills that the optometry schools are looking for. Don't waste time making value judgments about the OAT. It is not going to go away, so deal with it. Those who look forward to doing battle with the OAT—or, at least, who enjoy the opportunity to distinguish themselves from the rest of the applicant pack—tend to score better than do those who resent or dread it.

It may sound a little dubious, but take our word for it: attitude adjustment is a proven test-taking technique. Here are a few steps you can take to make sure you develop the right OAT attitude:

- Look at the OAT as a challenge, but try not to obsess over it; you certainly don't want to psyche yourself out of the game.
- Remember that, yes, the OAT is obviously important, but contrary to what some students think, this one test will not single-handedly determine the outcome of your life.
- Try to have fun with the test. Learning how to match your wits against the test makers can be a very satisfying experience, and the reading and thinking skills you'll acquire will benefit you in optometry school as well as in your future optometry career.
- Remember that you're more prepared than most people. You've trained with Kaplan. You have the tools you need, plus the know-how to use those tools.

Quick Tips for the Days Just Before the Exam

- The best test takers do less and less as the test approaches. Taper off your study schedule and take it easy on yourself. Give yourself time off, especially the evening before the exam. By that time, if you've studied well, everything you need to know is firmly stored in your memory bank.
- Positive self-talk can be extremely liberating and invigorating, especially as the test looms closer. Tell yourself things such as "I will do well," rather than "I hope things go well"; "I can," rather than "I cannot." Replace any negative thoughts with affirming statements that boost your self-esteem.
- Get your act together sooner rather than later. Have everything (including choice of clothing) laid out in advance. Most important, make sure you know where the test will be held and the

easiest, quickest way to get there. You'll have great peace of mind by knowing that all the little details—gas in the car, directions, etc.—are set before the day of the test.

- Go to the test site a few days in advance, particularly if you are especially anxious. Better yet, bring some practice material and do at least a section or two.

- Forego any practice on the day before the test. It's in your best interest to marshal your physical and psychological resources for 24 hours or so. Even horses are kept in the paddock and treated like princes the day before a race. Keep the upcoming test out of your consciousness; go to a movie, take a pleasant hike, or just relax. Don't eat junk food or tons of sugar. And, of course, get plenty of rest the night before—just don't go to bed too early. It's hard to fall asleep earlier than you're used to, and you don't want to lie there worrying about the test.

Handling Stress During the Test

The biggest stress monster will be the test itself. Fear not; there are methods of quelling your stress during the test.

- Keep moving forward instead of getting bogged down in a difficult question. You don't have to get everything right to achieve a fine score. So don't linger out of desperation on a question that is going nowhere even after you've spent considerable time on it. The best test takers skip difficult material temporarily in search of the easier stuff. They mark and return to the questions that require extra time and thought.

- Don't be thrown if other test takers seem to be working more busily and furiously than you are. Don't mistake the other people's sheer activity as signs of progress and higher scores.

- Keep breathing! Weak test takers tend to share one major trait: they don't breathe properly as the test proceeds. They might hold their breath without realizing it or breathe erratically or arrhythmically. Improper breathing hurts confidence and accuracy. Just as importantly, it interferes with clear thinking.

- Some quick isometrics during the test—especially if concentration is wandering or energy is waning—can help. Try this: Put your palms together and press intensely for a few seconds. Concentrate on the tension you feel through your palms, wrists, forearms, and up into your biceps and shoulders. Then quickly release the pressure. Feel the difference as you let go. Focus on the warm relaxation that floods through the muscles. Now you're ready to return to the task.

- Here's another isometric that will relieve tension in both your neck and eye muscles. Slowly rotate your head from side to side, turning your head and eyes to look as far back over each shoulder as you can. Feel the muscles stretch on one side of your neck as they contract on the other. Repeat five times in each direction.

With what you've just learned here, you're armed and ready to do battle with the test. This book and your studies have given you the information you'll need to answer the questions. It's all firmly planted in your mind. You also know how to deal with any excess tension that might come along, both when you're studying for and taking the exam. You've experienced everything you need to tame your test anxiety and stress. You're going to get a great score.

Kaplan's Top Ten OAT Tips

1. Relax!

2. Remember: It's primarily a thinking test. Never forget the purpose of the OAT: it's designed to test your powers of analytical reasoning. You need to know the content, as each section has its own particular "language," but the underlying OAT intention is consistent throughout the test.

3. Feel free to skip around within each section. Attack each section confidently. You're in charge. Move around if you feel comfortable doing so. Work your best areas first to maximize your opportunity for OAT points. Choose the order in which to complete questions. Don't be a passive victim of the test structure!

4. Avoid wrong-answer traps. Try to anticipate answers before you read the answer choices. This helps boost your confidence and protects you from persuasive or tricky incorrect choices. Most wrong answer choices are logical twists on the correct choice.

5. Think, think, think! We said it before, but it's important enough to say again: think. Don't compute.

6. Don't look back. Don't spend time worrying about questions you had to guess on. Keep moving forward. Don't let your spirit start to flag, or your attitude will slow you down. You can recheck answers within a section if you have time left, but don't worry about a section after time has been called.

7. Be sure to take the computer tutorial. Learn how to mark questions so you can return to review them at the end of each section. There is no penalty for wrong answers, so be sure to answer every question.

8. Don't leave any questions unanswered. There are no points taken off for wrong answers, so if you're unsure of an answer, guess.

9. Take advantage of the "Mark" feature on the computer for questions you may want to revisit. At the end, you can review all your marked answers before you submit them as final.

10. Call us! We're here to help! 800-KAP-TEST. Or visit us on the Web at kaptest.com.

HOW TO USE THIS BOOK

Congratulations on buying the best Optometry Admissions Test (OAT) test-prep book available. Kaplan's OAT provides you with key test strategies, content review for each of the four OAT sections, and two full-length OAT practice tests (one in the book and one online). All the questions in this book are followed by thorough, detailed explanations.

This book will test your understanding of college-level biology, general chemistry, organic chemistry, and physics, as well as your reading comprehension ability. In addition, you will become familiar with the format and style of the OAT. Here's how to use the various components of Kaplan's OAT.

Step One: Read the OAT Strategies Section

In this section, we've distilled the main techniques and approaches from our popular live OAT course in a clear, easy-to-grasp format. We'll introduce you to the idiosyncrasies of the OAT and show you how to take control of the test-taking experience on all levels, including:

- Test strategies
- Specific methods and strategies for tackling OAT passages and questions
- Test expertise
- Test mentality

You'll review item-specific techniques, and get advice on how to pace yourself on each section and how to decide when to answer questions and when to guess. We'll teach you how the peculiarities of a standardized test can be used to your advantage. Plus, you'll learn the winning attitude for executing all you've learned and for facing the OAT with confidence.

Step Two: Review Content

This book provides a detailed content review of each of the sections tested on the OAT. Shore up your knowledge-base so you can be confident on test day!

Step Three: Take Kaplan's Full-Length Practice OATs

After you've learned valuable test strategies and content, take the full-length practice tests—two timed, simulated OATs—as a test run for the real thing. The explanations for every question on the test are included so you can understand your mistakes. Try not to confine your review to the explanations for the questions you've gotten wrong. Instead, read all the explanations to reinforce key concepts and sharpen your skills. Note that one practice test is accessible in this book, and the other online for CBT practice.

Step Four: Review to Shore Up Weak Points

If you find your performance was weak in any area, go back to the section in which that material was tested and review the explanations.

After you're finished, relax! You've prepared with the best and are ready for Test Day!

READING COMPREHENSION

Reading Comprehension Practice Test

50 minutes—40 questions

DIRECTIONS: The following test consists of several reading passages and questions that test your comprehension of the passages. Read each passage carefully, and when you believe you have sufficient comprehension of the passage, go on to the questions. You may look back at a passage as often as you wish. Each question item consists of a question or an unfinished sentence followed by possible answers or completions. After reading a question, decide which choice is best and mark your answer.

The growth and development of mammalian teeth is the result of a complex series of tissue interactions that occurs during the embryonic and post-natal periods. The permanent tooth and its associated structures are composed of a wide variety of tissue types, including bone, epithelium, connective tissue, nerves, and blood vessels. Its anatomic structure is based upon a central pulp cavity containing the neural and vascular supply. This is surrounded by a layer of dentin, a yellowish material that is somewhat harder than bone. Finally, the dentin is covered by a layer of mineralized enamel, the hardest substance in the body. The dentin and enamel are each produced by highly specialized cells known as odontoblasts and ameloblasts, respectively.

The nerves responsible for pain sensation in the teeth are the superior and inferior alveolar nerves, which are derived from the fifth cranial (trigeminal) nerve. These are the sole sensory nerves for the teeth. The autonomic nervous system also innervates the teeth through the parasympathetic vasodilator fibers of the otic ganglion of the ninth cranial (glossopharyngeal) nerve and the fibers of the cervical sympathetic chain.

The blood supply to the upper jaw is provided by the superior alveolar arteries, which arise from the infraorbital and maxillary arteries. Blood to the lower jaw is carried by the inferior alveolar artery, another branch of the maxillary artery. These arteries are controlled by the vasoconstrictor fibers of the cervical sympathetic system, which stimulates contraction of the arterial smooth muscle fibers. All of the blood to the teeth comes originally from the right and left common carotid arteries, which supply the entire head and face.

The rate of tooth eruption in mammals has been studied for over 150 years. Early observations in 1823 led Oudet to conclude that rat incisors were capable of persistent growth, even in mature animals. Although it was long suspected that innervation might be responsible for control of this growth, it was not until 1919 that Moral and Hosemann were the first to measure tooth growth after cutting the inferior alveolar nerve. In 1927, Leist reported increased growth of guinea pig incisors after cutting the inferior alveolar nerve and the cervical sympathetic chain. However, he believed that the observed increase may have been due to secondary hyperemia of the pulp following the cervical sympathectomy.

This belief shifted attention, at least temporarily, away from the nervous system and toward the circulatory system. Despite the wide range of possible explanations for the control of tooth growth, the most commonly accepted theory was that first proposed by Leist—that blood supply was the important regulatory influence. it was not until the work of Butcher and Taylor in 1951 that any significant change in thought evolved.

The two investigators, working at New York University, studied five factors—blood supply, innervation, the shape of the tooth, physical stress, and the consistency of the diet—and their influence upon tooth growth rates. They explained that rat incisors were capable of two processes, eruption and attrition. The former refers to extrusion of a tooth into the oral cavity, while the latter results in a shortening of the tooth due to breakage or grinding, usually the result of normal feeding activity. Changes in tooth length were measured by initially cutting a notch in the tooth at the gingival crest. Eruption was quantified by measuring the distance between the notch and the gingival crest after a period of a few days, during which the tooth was allowed to grow. Attrition was measured as the decrease in distance from the notch to the incisal edge after breaking or grinding had occurred.

Studying the blood supply, Butcher and Taylor found that unilateral ligation of the common carotid artery decreased blood supply to teeth on the corresponding side but also produced bilateral fluctuation in eruption rate, although there was no clear decrease in tooth growth. Further, they showed that ligation of the inferior alveolar artery, while decreasing blood flow considerably, had no effect on rate of eruption. However, when all blood flow to a tooth was stopped by applying retroactive tension to the tooth, eruption ceased. Thus, the demonstration that only complete ischemia, or total lack of blood, would drastically reduce tooth growth led Butcher and Taylor to conclude that circulation was not the most important regulatory factor.

Considering innervation, they discovered that cutting the inferior alveolar nerve resulted in an average increase in growth rate of 26 to 30 percent. Teeth so denervated appeared microscopically normal, except for a decrease in nerve fibers in the periodontal tissue and pulp cavity. Sympathetic denervation in the rats had no effect on tooth growth, despite contrary results observed in guinea pigs. Likewise, removal of the rat's otic ganglion had no effect upon the rate of growth. Thus, Butcher and Taylor surmised that the role of the inferior alveolar nerve was due to its sensory fibers, since the autonomic system had no apparent influence. They hypothesized that the phenomenon was due to sensory impulses conducted from the tooth by the inferior alveolar nerve whenever the tooth met its antagonist in occlusion. This suggested the presence of a feedback system where lack of sensory impulse served as a stimulus to additional growth and presence of sensory impulse served to inhibit additional growth. A loss of the sensory nerve, then, would

render the animal unable to detect normal occlusion of the tooth or injury to the tooth.

This hypothesis was tested by artificially altering the physical stress upon a tooth by adjusting its shape. When all occlusal stress was relieved by repeated fracture of the incisor, eruption rate was accelerated. Extrusion rate was increased in every case of relieved functional pressure, and the increase reached a maximum of 200 percent above normal with prolonged repeated fracture. This was considered to be the maximum growth potential of the tooth. When the tooth was allowed to resume normal contact with its antagonist, there was an immediate return of growth rate to the normal levels. Rapidly erupting teeth were found to be abnormal in cross-sectional appearance, with decreased content of dentin and enamel and a widely dilated pulp cavity. Individual odontoblasts and ameloblasts, however, were found to be normal.

Finally, the consistency of the diet and its relation to functional stress were considered, and the results further supported the sensory feedback hypothesis. The standard consistency diet of all experiments was Purina Dog Chow. To prevent fracture and grinding, a soft consistency diet of cornmeal was used; to promote fracture and grinding, a hard consistency diet of whole kernel corn was used. When animals were placed on the soft consistency diet, eruption rate decreased 20 percent from the normal value of 0.5 mm/day. The rate gradually returned to normal when the animals were returned to the dog chow.

Similarly, eruption rate increased when the rats were fed whole kernel corn, a food that caused increased fracture and grinding. The overall difference in eruption rate from the hard to soft consistency diets was 35 percent.

Thus, the work of Butcher and Taylor shifted the focus of attention from the circulatory system to the nervous system and was largely responsible for the direction and emphasis of future research. To date, no major evidence in opposition to the theory of Butcher and Taylor has been found.

1. Vasodilator nerve fibers that innervate teeth in mammals are found in

   A. the trigeminal nerve.
   B. the otic ganglion.
   C. the cervical sympathetic chain.
   D. the inferior alveolar nerve.
   E. the superior alveolar nerves.

2. Since the work of Butcher and Taylor, the accepted theory for control of tooth eruption rate has been based upon

   A. sensory nerve feedback.
   B. blood supply.
   C. the role of odontoblasts.
   D. the role of ameloblasts.
   E. None of the above

3. In the experiment described in the passage, when a rat on a soft diet was returned to the standard consistency diet, its tooth growth rate

   A. remained depressed.
   B. immediately returned to normal.
   C. gradually returned to normal.
   D. remained elevated.
   E. decreased even further.

4. Which of the following statements correctly summarizes the sensory feedback hypothesis of Butcher and Taylor?

   A. Lack of sensory impulse causes increased blood flow to the tooth.
   B. Lack of sensory impulse causes decreased tooth growth rate.
   C. Lack of sensory impulse causes gradual pulp ischemia.
   D. Lack of sensory impulse causes increased tooth growth rate.
   E. The absence of a feedback system allows for an increased tooth growth rate.

5. Before 1951, tooth growth was commonly thought to be regulated by

   A. diet.
   B. physical stress.
   C. blood supply.
   D. innervation.
   E. both (C) and (D).

6. Which of the following would be most likely to cause the greatest increase in blood supply to the teeth in mammals?

   A. A cervical sympathectomy
   B. Ligation of the common carotid artery
   C. Cutting the inferior alveolar nerve
   D. Removal of the otic ganglion
   E. Ligation of the inferior alveolar nerve

7. Based on information in the passage, which of the following statements best defines the term *antagonistic teeth*?

   A. Two adjacent teeth on the upper jaw
   B. Two adjacent teeth on the lower jaw
   C. Two teeth with opposite functional properties
   D. One tooth on the upper jaw, one on the lower
   E. Upper and lower teeth that meet in normal biting

8. According to the author, odontoblasts are responsible for the production of

   A. enamel.
   B. dentin.
   C. pulp.
   D. gingival tissue.
   E. dentin and enamel.

9. In the experiments on normal adult rats, significant incisor growth could be measured within

   A. 24 hours.
   B. 48 hours.
   C. 72 hours.
   D. 1 week.
   E. 2 weeks.

10. The greatest increase in eruption rate was achieved by

    A. altering the consistency of the diet.
    B. relieving the tooth of all functional stress.
    C. ligating the common carotid artery.
    D. removing the otic ganglion.
    E. returning the tooth to normal contact with its antagonist.

11. To destroy pain sensation in the teeth, which of the following nerves must be cut?

    A. The ninth cranial nerve
    B. The cervical sympathetic fibers
    C. The otic ganglion
    D. The glossopharyngeal nerve
    E. The inferior alveolar nerve

12. What observation was made about rat teeth that were permitted to grow at their maximum potential rate?

    A. They were more prone to fracture.
    B. They were lacking in nerve fibers.
    C. They had decreased amounts of dentin and enamel.
    D. They had unusually small pulp cavities.
    E. They appeared normal at the microscopic level.

13. Which of the following may be concluded from the observation of Butcher and Taylor?

    A. Teeth are more likely to fracture in older mammals.
    B. Occlusal stress may account for suppression of the maximum tooth growth rate.
    C. Mammals fed a "soft" diet will exhibit an increased number of ameloblasts.
    D. Occlusion involves only antagonistic teeth.
    E. Circulation plays a critical role in the regulation of tooth growth.

14. Butcher and Taylor's findings on the effects of dietary consistency upon tooth growth rate

    A. are inconsistent with the hypothesis of a sensory feedback system.
    B. show that consistency of the diet has little effect on rate of tooth eruption in rats, even if the diet consists solely of Purina Dog Chow.
    C. suggest that a mechanism other than sensory feedback affects tooth growth rate.
    D. are irrelevant, since rats would never duplicate the experimental diet under normal circumstances.
    E. indicate that tooth growth rate is affected by more than one factor.

Since estimates of future population growth are based on projections regarding complex and changeable social factors, it is not surprising to find that the estimates are often markedly inaccurate. For several decades following World War II, unprecedented population growth in the United States exceeded all projections. A 1947 Census Bureau prediction of the U.S. population in 1970, for example, underestimated the actual 1970 population by 65 million, falling far short of the count of 205 million that year. Today, predicting population growth is still an inexact science, but discrepancies often stem from overestimation rather than underestimation. Only a few years ago, demographers projected that our national population would reach the 300 million mark in the year 2000, but even after the turn of the century, the nation's population has not reached that mark. Such discrepancies stem from the fact that population predictions involve a certain amount of guesswork. The complexity and variability of social and economic factors involved in predicting population make the enterprise one of educated speculation.

Population predictions are based primarily upon studies of the "total fertility rate" of a country, defined as the average number of births a woman is expected to have over the course of her reproductive life. This rate is related to the "replacement level," a constant that describes the fertility rate at which a population neither grows nor declines. Today, the U.S. fertility rate is 1.7, considerably less than the replacement level of 2.1, so our population is expected to decrease. While demographers differ on exactly why and to what extent this diminution will occur, many agree that the decline in fertility is related to changes in the status and expectations of women.

Radical and rapid changes in attitudes toward marriage and family partly explain recent unanticipated declines in the rate of U.S. population growth. In the past few decades, there has been a considerable decline in the number of women who marry young. In 1960, only 29 percent of women under 24 had never married; by 1978,

that percentage had jumped to 48 percent. This seems related to the tendency for unmarried couples to postpone marriage and live together, an arrangement that has become increasingly popular in recent years. Whether cohabitation is a likely prelude to marriage or an indication of a basic change in attitudes toward that institution, it is clear that cohabitation results in lower fertility than does marriage. Growing instability of marital relationships also affects fertility rates: As marriage rates have declined, divorce rates have increased, with half of all American marriages ending in divorce.

The shifting economic role that women play in society also effects childbearing. The relationship between fertility and the growing participation of women in the workplace is complex. A few demographers actually suggest that there is a positive correlation between women's working and fertility; this school of thought speculates that because increased prosperity positively affects fertility, women's economic gains will result in boosted fertility rates. But most demographers agree that work and fertility are negatively correlated in women. Some believe that women will have fewer children in order to facilitate their ability to join the workforce and gain financial stability. Others claim that, at the same time as increasingly effective methods of contraception have given women greater control over their own childbearing, the growing financial independence of women has weakened the economic rationale for marriage. This theory suggests that marriage offers women financial security in return for their childbearing and housekeeping services. Thus, if women no longer need to "barter" for economic support, childbearing becomes less of an automatic and expected social response.

In addition to the changing attitudes and status of women, even larger, more sweeping processes are at work in declining birthrates. Broad societal trends, including increasing urbanization and decreasing religiosity, are playing a significant role in lowering fertility rates. Migration to urban areas, for instance, has stripped away a powerful economic incentive for childbearing. In agrarian economies, there is a need for large families, as children play an important role in agricultural production. But in industrial economies, children are—in an economic sense—burdens, as they consume limited resources without producing much in return.

Similarly, declining subscription to traditional religious values weakens the emphasis formerly placed upon and reduces attachment to family and childbearing. Some demographers have argued that the spread of evangelical religious movements, with their strong emphasis on traditional values, may eventually reverse this trend, but this seems doubtful. While these movements are certainly attracting an increasing number of followers, they appeal mainly to rural elements of the population. Put differently, evangelical movements tend to attract people who are already very religious, so it is unlikely that their ultimate impact on demographic trends will be significant.

Hence, most demographers now agree that a declining birthrate is a long-term feature of U.S. society, especially since there does not appear to be any sense of urgency about altering the status quo. Indeed, the general belief about desirable population levels in this country was best summed up by the Commission on Population Growth and the American Future, which concluded that declining fertility was a positive development, since it may—in sheer terms of numbers—help to alleviate many of our most pressing social and economic problems.

Consequently, the United States has expressed no interest in pronatalist policies. In contrast, many nations in both Eastern and Western Europe have instituted a wide variety of pronatalist measures. In most instances, national security was cited as the reason for their introduction—demographic projections for many of these nations predicted rapid falls in population by the 21st century. Whatever the case, pronatalist polices led to an almost immediate rise in European birthrates. In former East Germany, for example, the birthrate went from 10.6 per 1,000 inhabitants in 1975 to 13.3 in 1977. Most of these countries have thus far restricted themselves mainly to liberal economic measures, such as family cash allowances, generous tax relief, subsidized child care services, and improved housing.

Should the U.S. government ever decide that the declining birthrate has become a threat to the nation's well-being, it may very well take steps to encourage population growth similar to those adopted by European countries. If that were to occur, once again demographers would have to drastically revise today's population predictions.

15. Which of the following statements best expresses the author's opinion about the relationship between marriage and the economic status of women?

A. Lower economic status generally results in reduced fertility.

B. Working women give birth to fewer children than do nonworking women.

C. The effect of women's economic position on fertility has not yet been determined.

D. Women who receive economic support tend to exhibit lower fertility rates.

E. Urban women of lower economic status have higher birth rates than do rural women of lower economic status.

16. The "replacement level" is defined as

    A. the number of births the average woman has over her lifetime.

    B. the difference between a nation's birth and death rates.

    C. the birthrate necessary to ensure population growth.

    D. the number of deaths that must occur in order to keep the population from increasing.

    E. the birthrate at which a nation's population will remain stable.

17. Which of the following "total fertility rates" would most probably signal an increase in U.S. population?

    A. 2.0

    B. 1.7

    C. 1.8

    D. 2.1

    E. 2.4

18. The author mentions the increasingly popular trend of cohabitation in order to

    A. make a generalization about shifting moral values.

    B. support the claim that marriage is losing its economic rationale.

    C. provide an example of a social factor that contributes to lower fertility rates.

    D. underscore the relationship between cohabitation and increased divorce rates.

    E. recommend it as a guarantor of increased fertility.

19. Which of the following would most demographers probably NOT consider a factor in decreasing fertility rates?

    A. Increasingly effective methods of birth control

    B. Greater societal acceptance of childless marriages

    C. Growing demand for women in the workplace

    D. Liberalized attitudes toward unwed motherhood

    E. An increasing divorce rate

20. It can be inferred from the author's discussion of the economic rationale for marriage that

    A. the institution of marriage has generally lost its romantic veneer.

    B. women seek financial security when choosing husbands.

    C. romantic illusions often mask exploitive financial relationships.

    D. marriage is an idyllic state of shared responsibility.

    E. some demographers consider marriage primarily an economic relationship.

21. Which of the following is the most appropriate title for the passage?

    A. Decline in Birthrate Illustrates New Social Realities

    B. Growth Rate Falls as Women's Economic Status Improves

    C. Demographers Admit Futility of Population Prediction

    D. Shifting Social Values Lessen Nation's Social and Economic Ills

    E. New Women's Attitudes and National Birthrate Trends

22. Which of the following is NOT mentioned in the passage as a pronatalist measure?

    A. Tax relief

    B. Cash allowances

    C. Subsidized child care

    D. Land grants

    E. Improved housing

23. According to most demographers, the U.S. birthrate will

    A. decline for a few more years but then increase.

    B. decline steadily for the indefinite future.

    C. increase over the next decade but then decline.

    D. increase drastically over the next couple of centuries.

    E. remain stable, without decline or increase.

24. The primary purpose of the first paragraph is to

    A. suggest that demographers are poor statisticians.

    B. argue that predicting population is difficult.

    C. prove that Census Bureau figures are highly accurate.

    D. discuss the social and economic factors that affect population estimates.

    E. analyze the Census Bureau's prediction of the U.S. population in 1970.

25. Rural families tend to be larger than their urban counterparts. The passage implies that this is because

    A. children are important as productive members of agrarian economies.

    B. rural couples are more likely to be traditional and religious.

    C. women are less likely to pursue careers in an agrarian environment.

    D. rural couples experience less difficulty conceiving than urban couples.

    E. urban couples are better educated about the use of contraception.

26. The author believes that the growth of evangelical religious movements will

    A. eventually lead to an upswing in the U.S. birthrate.

    B. cause an immediate drop in the U.S. birthrate.

    C. have no real impact on the U.S. birthrate.

    D. cause an upswing in the U.S. birthrate initially but a drop in the long run.

    E. cause an eventual decline in the U.S. birthrate.

27. The passage suggests that, in the future, young women will become

    A. more interested in marrying at a young age.

    B. less likely to give birth out of wedlock.

    C. more interested in pursuing a career.

    D. less interested in being financially independent.

    E. uninterested in maintaining a long-term career.

28. The author suggests that current population predictions

    A. are extremely accurate.

    B. overestimate the actual population.

    C. underestimate the actual population.

    D. ignore the growth of illegal immigrant populations.

    E. are anomalous in their inaccuracy.

Adequate nutrition is essential to the development, growth, and sustenance of the human organism. A good diet must supply the body with sufficient energy to power all life support activities. Amino acids play an important role in this dietary process.

The amino acid molecule is composed of an amino group (-NH$_2$), a carboxyl group (-COOH), a hydrogen atom (-H), and a unique R group (or side chain), all bonded to a central alpha carbon atom (C). Although amino acids occur in two stereoisomeric forms, D- (dextrorotary) and L- (levorotary), only the L-form is nutritionally active in the human body. There are twenty L-amino acids in total, each identifiable by its side chains, which differ in terms of size, shape, charge, hydrogen-bonding capacity, and chemical reactivity.

The primary role of L-amino acids is to provide the biologically active building blocks for proteins. Proteins are formed when groups of amino acids become linked in polypeptide chains. Peptide bonds are formed between the alpha-carboxyl group of one amino acid and the alpha-amino group of the next. These polypeptide chains link in turn to become proteins—in certain cells, they become the precursors of neurotransmitters, skin pigments, or hormones. All twenty amino acids must be present for the complete range of body proteins to be synthesized. The human body is capable of synthesizing several amino acids, such as alanine, glutamate, and proline, and these are classified as nonessential in dietary terms. Others, however, designated essential amino acids, must be supplied in the diet. The absence of any single amino acid disrupts protein synthesis and can result in a negative nitrogen balance within the body. When this occurs, protein degradation exceeds protein synthesis, and the body excretes a greater quantity of nitrogen than it ingests to replace it.

The body obtains essential amino acids by extracting them from food proteins in the digestive process, which begins in the stomach. Firstly, the oxyntic (parietal) cells of the fundic gastric glands lower the pH level of the stomach by secreting 0.15 M HCl into the stomach. Zymogenic (chief) cells secrete quantities of pepsin, the first proteolytic enzyme to break down the ingested proteins, as well as rennin, an enzyme that curdles milk. The pepsin is secreted in an inactive form (pepsinogen) and is converted to the active enzymatic form by the HCl acid. In this state, it catalyzes the hydrolysis of the peptide bonds between amino acids within the proteins.

The majority of protein degradation and absorption occurs in the small intestine. The two primary proteolytic enzymes of the small intestine are trypsin and chymotrypsin. Trypsin breaks polypeptide chains on the carboxyl side of arginine and lysine residues. Chymotrypsin, on the other hand, cleaves preferentially on the carboxyl side of aromatic and other bulky, nonpolar amino acids.

The major end products of digestion are L-amino acids, which are absorbed by the intestinal mucosa cells through a complex transport mechanism. First, a basolateral membrane Na$^+$-K$^+$-ATPase pump (powered by cellular ATP) sets up a favorable concentration gradient, where the concentration of sodium ions is greater outside the cell than inside. Then, as sodium ions diffuse into the cell, L-amino acids are transported simultaneously with sodium ions across the cell membrane.

The intestinal mucosal cells are also capable of absorbing dipeptides and tripeptides; their microvillus membranes contain enzymes that specifically split off dipeptides from the amino terminal end of protein polypeptide chains prior to absorption. All of the amino acids absorbed from the lumen of the intestine are then transported by the mucosal cells into the blood, where they proceed to the liver via the hepatic portal system. Any excess of absorbed amino acids, above that required for protein synthesis, is not stored in the body and is much too valuable to be excreted. Instead, surplus amino acids are degraded in the liver and utilized as metabolic fuel.

Amino acid degradation primarily involves conversion of the alpha-amino group to urea. This group is transferred to the molecule alpha-ketoglutarate to form glutamate, which is subsequently oxidatively deaminated to the ammonium ion (NH_4^+) by the enzyme glutamate dehydrogenase, then converted via the enzymes of the urea cycle into the excretion product.

A special class of enzymes called transaminases catalyzes the transfer of the amino group from an alpha-amino acid to an alpha-keto acid, such as alpha-ketoglutarate. These transaminases require a prosthetic group (or coenzyme) called pyridoxal phosphate, which is derived from pyridoxine (vitamin B_6) to become active. The transaminase enzyme has a terminal lysine residue at its active site that combines with the aldehyde group of pyridoxal phosphate in a covalent Schiff-base linkage prior to the binding of the amino acid substrate. The transaminases form a new covalent Schiff-base intermediate with the alpha-amino group of the amino acid, which displaces an epsilon-amino group of the enzyme's active site lysine. As a result of this reaction, the pyridoxal phosphate is converted to pyridoxamine phosphate, and the alpha-amino becomes an alpha-keto acid. The pyridoxamine phosphate-enzyme complex subsequently combines with alpha-ketoglutarate to yield glutamates and a regenerated pyridoxal phosphate enzyme. Other pyridoxal phosphate enzymes can catalyze decarboxylations, deaminations, racemizations, and aldol cleavages of amino acid substrates.

The main benefits of the transamination process are that it enables the glutamate formed to be oxidatively deaminated by glutamate dehydrogenase to regenerate alpha-ketoglutarate and thus form ammonium ions for the urea cycle. In this particular process, either NAD^+ or $NADP^+$ are energized with electrons to form NADH or NADPH respectively, and both can be used as electron carriers. NADH is an active electron carrier in oxidative phosphorylation, which generates cellular ATP, whereas NADPH is more active in reductive biosynthesis.

The process of energy production is controlled by the enzyme glutamate dehydrogenase and pre-existing cellular energy levels. It is an allosterically regulated enzyme (i.e., it is only active when low-energy precursors are present, such as ADP and GDP). Conversely, it is inhibited when high-energy molecules are in abundance, such as ATP and GTP. Thus, under low-energy states, surplus amino acids can generate high-energy molecules and raise the caloric content in the body. In contrast, amino acid carbon skeletons are transformed into acetyl-CoA, pyruvate, or one of the intermediates of the citric acid cycle. The citric acid cycle is the final common route of oxidation of fuel molecules such as carbohydrates, fatty acids, and amino acids. The reactions of this cycle occur within the cells' mitochondria, and most fuel molecules enter as acetyl-CoA. However, some amino acids enter the cycle in the form of intermediates. Phenylalanine (derived from phenylpyruvate) is degraded to tyrosine by phenylalanine hydroxylase, and tyrosine is further transaminated back to *p*-hydroxyphenylpyruvate (the precursor of tyrosine), which is in turn oxidized to homogentisate. Homogentisate oxidase then converts homogentisate to 4-maleylacetoacetate, which is subsequently isomerized and hydrolyzed to become acetoacetate and fumarate, a cycle intermediate.

Those amino acids that are degraded to acetyl-CoA or acetoacetyl-CoA are called ketogenic and ultimately may also give rise to the ketone bodies acetone, *D*-3-hydroxybutyrate, and acetoacetate, which is a preferred fuel of heart muscle and renal cortex cells. Other amino acids are called glucogenic because they are degraded to pyruvate and fumarate or oxaloacetate. Of all the twenty acids, only leucine is purely ketogenic, while isoleucine, lysine, phenylalanine, tryptophan, and tyrosine are both ketogenic and glucogenic. The remaining fourteen amino acids are purely glucogenic.

29. Negative nitrogen balance is a state in the body in which

    A. essential amino acids are absent.
    B. protein synthesis exceeds protein degradation.
    C. protein degradation exceeds protein synthesis.
    D. the body ingests too much nitrogen.
    E. both (A) and (C) are correct.

30. In the process of absorption, an *L*-amino acid is cotransported with

    A. a K^+ ion.
    B. a Cl^- ion.
    C. a Na^+ ion.
    D. a Na^+ and a Cl^- ion simultaneously.
    E. a glucose molecule.

31. Which of the following amino acids is purely ketogenic?

    A. Tyrosine
    B. Phenylalanine
    C. Leucine
    D. Isoleucine
    E. Tryptophan

32. Ketone bodies are

    A. *D*-3-hydroxybutyrate molecules.
    B. acetone molecules.
    C. used by renal and heart cells as fuel.
    D. products of degradation.
    E. All of the above

33. Pyridoxal phosphate enzymes

    A. can only catalyze transaminations.
    B. catalyze aldol cleavages of amino acids.
    C. catalyze carboxylations of amino acids.
    D. All of the above
    E. None of the above

34. The bond formed by a transaminase and its coenzyme

    A. is a covalent Schiff-base reaction.
    B. is a noncovalent Schiff-base reaction.
    C. occurs between a lysine residue of the enzyme and an aldehyde group of the coenzyme.
    D. occurs between a tyrosine residue of the enzyme and a carboxyl group of the coenzyme.
    E. both (A) and (C) are correct.

35. The main benefit of transamination is the

    A. conversion of coenzyme to NH_4^+.
    B. decrease in the caloric content of the body.
    C. generation of GDP and ADP.
    D. generation of NADH to participate in oxidative phosphorylation.
    E. catabolism of ammonium ions.

36. Side chains of amino acids differ in regard to which of the following?

    A. Size
    B. Hydrogen-binding capacity
    C. Shape
    D. Charge
    E. All of the above

37. The enzyme glutamate dehydrogenase is allosterically regulated, such that

    A. an increase in GTP and ATP levels activates the enzyme.
    B. an increase in UTP and GTP levels activates the enzyme.
    C. an increase in GDP and ADP levels activates the enzyme.
    D. only an increase in UTP activates the enzyme.
    E. only a decrease in UTP activates the enzyme.

38. Trypsin and chymotrypsin cleave protein polypeptide chains at or between

    A. the same site.
    B. different sites.
    C. arginine and lysine residues for trypsin and aromatic residues for chymotrypsin.
    D. (A), (B), and (C) are correct.
    E. both (B) and (C) are correct.

39. Amino acid degradation involves

    A. transamination.
    B. change of amino acids to acetyl-CoA and acetoacetyl-CoA.
    C. change of amino acids to pyruvate and fumarate.
    D. conversion of the alpha-amino group to urea.
    E. All of the above

40. Which of the following compounds can act as electron carriers in oxidative phosphorylation?

    A. $NADP^+$
    B. NAD^+
    C. Both NADPH and NADH
    D. ATP
    E. None of the above

STOP! END OF TEST.

Reading Comprehension Practice Test: Answers and Explanations

ANSWER KEY

1.	B	21.	A
2.	A	22.	D
3.	C	23.	B
4.	D	24.	B
5.	C	25.	A
6.	A	26.	C
7.	E	27.	C
8.	B	28.	B
9.	C	29.	E
10.	B	30.	C
11.	E	31.	C
12.	C	32.	E
13.	B	33.	B
14.	E	34.	E
15.	B	35.	D
16.	E	36.	E
17.	E	37.	C
18.	C	38.	E
19.	D	39.	E
20.	E	40.	C

EXPLANATIONS

1. B

The passage states that the vasodilator nerve fibers are parasympathetic fibers found in the otic ganglion of the glossopharyngeal nerve, making choice (B) correct. They are not found in the inferior alveolar nerve, the superior alveolar nerve, a branch of the trigeminal nerve, or the cervical sympathetic chain. Thus, answer choices (A), (C), (D), and (E) are all incorrect.

2. A

Each of the five factors (blood supply, innervation, shape of the tooth, physical stress, and the consistency of the diet) that Butcher and Taylor examined pointed to sensory nerve feedback, choice (A), as the predominant controller of the rate of tooth growth. While the blood supply was thought at one point in time to be important in tooth eruption, Taylor and Butcher concluded that it was not the most important regulatory factor. In addition, the accepted theory for control of tooth eruption rate since Butcher and Taylor has not been based in the roles of odontoblasts or of ameloblasts.

3. C

Although animals which were placed on a soft consistency diet experienced decreases of tooth eruption rate of up to 20 percent from the normal value of 0.5 mm/day, the passage states that the animals' eruption rates gradually returned to normal when the animals returned to the dog chow (the standard consistency diet).

4. D

The passage states that Butcher and Taylor surmised that the sensory fibers of the inferior alveolar nerve would provide a feedback system where a lack of sensory impulse would serve as a stimulus for a tooth to grow—choice (D)—and, conversely, the presence of a sensory impulse would serve to inhibit a tooth's growth. The sensory feedback hypothesis did not address the lack of sensory impulses and their relation to blood flow or ischemia.

5. C

The passage states that prior to 1951 and subsequent to 1927, the most commonly accepted theory of tooth growth was the one proposed by Leist—that blood supply was the important regulatory influence. Although innervation was considered at one time, it is not the optimal answer because in the years pursuant to 1951, blood supply was more highly considered. Physical stress and diet were never thought to be extremely important regulators of tooth growth.

6. A

The passage states that following cervical sympa-thectomy, a secondary hyperemia (increase in blood flow to the site of innervation) occurs. Therefore, choice (A) would be most correct. Ligation of the common carotid artery would decrease the amount of blood flow to teeth, and the denervation of the inferior alveolar nerve would have little to do with blood supply. Finally, the removal of the otic gan-glion may actually decrease the amount of blood to the teeth due to the presence of parasympathetic autonomic nerve fibers in the otic ganglion.

7. E

The use of the word *antagonist* in the passage refers to a tooth that makes normal contact with another. Therefore, answer choice (E) is most correct. While the word *antagonists* might conjure up images of teeth with opposite functional properties—choice (C), it was not used in this context in the passage. Clearly, answer choices (A) and (B) are incorrect; they are not mentioned as valid choices in the pas-sage. Finally, answer choice (D) is too vague—choice (E) is far more accurate.

8. B

The author states that odontoblasts are responsible for the production of dentin and that ameloblasts are responsible for the production of enamel. The pulp is littered with neural and vascular supply, and the author does not mention the origin of gingival tissue.

9. C

The passage states that eruption (the extrusion of a tooth into the oral cavity) was measured by exam-ining the distance between the notch (cut initially at the gingival crest) and the gingival crest after a period of a few days (during which time the tooth was allowed to grow). Three days, or 72 hours, is the best choice.

10. B

The passage states that ligating the common carotid artery or removing the otic ganglion did nothing to affect the eruption rate. Altering the consistency of the diet, while affecting the eruption rate slightly, could not compare to relieving the tooth of all func-tional stress (which was shown to increase eruption

by 200 percent). Finally, returning the tooth to nor-mal contact with its antagonist reinstituted normal growth rates.

11. E

The inferior alveolar nerve carries sensory nerve fibers that the cervical sympathetic fibers and the otic ganglion do not. While the glossopharyngeal nerve does have sensory fibers, this nerve does not innervate the teeth. Therefore, the inferior alveolar nerve is the most correct answer.

12. C

The passage states that Butcher and Taylor found that rapidly erupting teeth were abnormal in cross-sectional appearance (thus, answer choice (E) is not correct). They possessed decreased contents of den-tin and enamel—choice (C)—and a widely dilated pulp cavity (therefore, choice (D) is not correct). No mention was made of their propensity for fracture or their abundance of nerve fibers; therefore, these answers—choices (A) and (B)—are incorrect.

13. B

According to the sensory feedback hypothesis pro-posed by Butcher and Taylor, it is the absence of sensory influences that causes an increase in the growth rate of teeth. No mention is made of tooth fracture and older mammals or of the occlusive ability of nonantagonistic teeth. Mammals fed on a "soft" diet exhibit a decrease in the eruption rate, indicating—if anything—a decrease in the number of ameloblasts.

14. E

Butcher and Taylor's experiments revealed that both occlusal stress and diet consistency affected tooth eruption. This corresponds to many other findings in science, namely that they are multifactorial. The fact that dietary consistency affected tooth growth rate does not obviate the hypothesis of a sensory feedback system, nor does it suggest that a sole mechanism other than sensory feedback affects tooth growth rate. These diet consistency experi-ment results are relevant and should be examined from a multifactorial perspective.

15. B

Although the author concedes that some demographers believe that there is a positive correlation between women's working and fertility, he argues that most demographers agree that work and fertility are negatively correlated in women. He also believes that higher economic status of women generally results in reduced fertility and that women who receive economic support (i.e., are dependent upon it) tend to exhibit higher fertility rates. Finally, although the author states that higher economic status is associated with lower fertility, he never compares the fertility rates of women of lower economic status in rural and urban areas. One factor that immediately undermines this supposition is the indication that urbanization provides fewer incentives for childbearing and has thus played a role in lowering fertility rates.

16. E

The passage defines "replacement level" as a birthrate at which a nation's population will remain stable (will neither decline nor grow). Note that the question stem refers to "replacement," which implies a need for production to fill a void (or births to fill the population void caused by deaths). Thus, one could automatically eliminate choice (D), which only focuses on deaths, and choice (C), which refers to actual growth, not just replacement. Choice (A) is incorrect, as well, as it refers to "total fertility rate" as defined in the passage, and choice (B) is incorrect as it refers to a measurement of a status quo, not of a determined "level."

17. E

The total fertility rate of a country is defined as the average number of births a woman is expected to have over the course of her reproductive life. This rate is related to the replacement level (the fertility rate at which population remains stable), which is defined as 2.1 in the passage. As the total fertility rate must exceed the replacement rate for population growth to occur, the answer choice must be greater than 2.1. Choice (E) satisfies this requirement.

18. C

The author cites cohabitation as an example of a social factor that contributes to lower fertility rates. She makes little judgment about shifting moral values; she does not support the claim that marriage is losing its economic rationale. In addition, the author never correlates cohabitation with increased divorce rates. Finally, cohabitation is anything but a guarantor of fertility, as the author indicates that it is more clearly associated with lower fertility rates than is marriage.

19. D

The author cites several factors that demographers believe to be important in decreasing fertility rates. They include contraception, more women working, increased societal acceptance of childless marriages, and increased divorce rates. However, the author does not address the role of liberalized attitudes toward unwed motherhood, implying that it is not a factor.

20. E

The passage discusses the rationale behind marriage in strictly economic terms and indicates that many demographers regard marriage in this way. While it might be argued that choice (B) is also correct, it is not, since it makes an assumption about all women's reasons for marriage—an inference that is too drastic. Note that choice (E) makes a less inclusive conclusion by referring to "some demographers." Finally, answers (A), (C), and (D) are poor choices because they are not addressed in the passage.

21. A

Whether the author talks about urbanization, contraception, or cohabitation, it is clear that she is referring to the relationship of new social realities and decline in birthrate. While answer choice (B) is factually correct, it is a limited title because it does not include other causes of declining birthrates. The author does not deem population prediction futile; she only admits that it is an "enterprise of educated speculation." In addition, the author never correlates shifting social values with a lessening of the nation's social and economic ills. Finally, national birthrate trends are related not just to women's new attitudes but to other issues such as divorce, cohabitation, and contraception (all of which might involve men's attitudes, as well).

22. D

The passage mentions that European pronatalist policies included family cash allowances, generous tax relief, subsidized child-care services, and improved housing. There is no mention in the passage of land grants, choice (D).

23. B

The passage states that most demographers now agree that the present declining birthrate is a long-term feature of U.S. society, especially since there does not appear to be any sense of urgency about altering the status quo.

24. B

The purpose of the first paragraph can be identified in its last sentence, which states, "The complexity and variability of social and economic factors involved in predicting population make the enterprise one of educated speculation." In other words, it is difficult. The paragraph never states that demographers are poor statisticians. Rather, it says population growth prediction is an inexact science. And, on the contrary, it reveals the inaccuracy of Census Bureau figures. Finally, while the paragraph mentions social and economic factors, as well as the Census Bureau's prediction of the 1970 U.S. population, it does not focus on any of these points as its central purpose.

25. A

The author states that rural families have higher fertility rates than urban families. This is, she argues, because in agrarian (i.e., more rural) economies, children play an important role in agricultural production and are thus necessities of life. While it may be that rural couples are more likely to be traditional and religious, this cannot be argued from the passage. Further, the passage provides no indication that women are less likely to pursue careers in rural areas, that rural couples experience less difficulty conceiving than urban couples, or that urban couples are better educated about contraception.

26. C

The author does correlate a decline in subscription to religious values with a reduced attachment to childbearing, which would imply that an extension of religious values through evangelism would potentially increase birthrates. However, the author specifically indicates that "evangelical movements tend to attract people who are already very religious," or who already embrace values of family and childbearing. Thus, evangelism, according to the passage, causes neither an increase nor decline in the birthrate.

27. C

The author claims that there is a growing financial independence of women owing to an increased number of women in the workplace. Therefore, it follows that women will be less interested in marrying at a young age, more likely to give birth out of wedlock, more interested in remaining financially independent, and more interested in maintaining a long-term career. These are opposite to the responses seen in choice (A), (B), (D), and (E), respectively.

28. B

The first paragraph of the passage states that discrepancies in current population predictions for the year 2000 reflect an overestimation rather than an underestimation. Thus, choices (A) and (C) are automatically eliminated as possibilities. In terms of choice (D), the author never indicates that current population predictions fail to account for the growth of illegal immigrant populations. Finally, the author's description of the 1947 underestimation of the population for 1970 indicates that present inaccuracies in prediction are not anomalous.

29. E

The passage defines negative nitrogen balance as a process in which protein degradation exceeds protein synthesis, so the body excretes a greater quantity of nitrogen than it ingests to replace it. In this state, essential amino acids are absent, making choice (E) the most correct one.

30. C

The passage states that end products of digestion— L-amino acids—are absorbed by the intestinal mucosal cells via a complex transport mechanism that involves cotransport of sodium ion. It makes no mention of the simultaneous transport of chloride ions, making choice (C) optimal.

31.   C
The last few sentences of the passage categorize amino acids, which are either gluconeogenic, keto-genic, or both. Leucine is the only ketogenic amino acid; therefore, choice (C) is the correct answer.

32.   E
All of the answer choices work. Amino acids that are degraded to acetyl-CoA or acetoacetyl-CoA are considered ketogenic. They may give rise to *D*-3-hydroxybutyrate, acetone molecules, and acetoac-etate. They are the preferred fuel of cardiac muscle and renal cortical cells; thus, choice (E) is correct.

33.   B
Pyridoxal phosphate enzymes may cause transami-nation, decarboxylation deamination, racemization, and aldol cleavage of amino acids. Therefore, choice (B) is correct.

34.   E
The bond between pyridoxal phosphate and a trans-aminase occurs at a terminal lysine residue. The bond is a Schiff-base linkage, which is covalent in property. Therefore, choice (E) correct.

35.   D
According to the passage, the main benefit of the transamination process is that it enables the glu-tamate formed to be oxidatively deaminated (by glutamate dehydrogenase) to regenerate alpha-ketoglutarate. This results in the formation of ammonium ions (from the glutamate, not the coen-zyme pyridoxal phosphate) for the urea cycle and the regeneration of NADH and NADPH (involved in oxidative phosphorylation and reductive biosyn-thesis, respectively). Therefore, answer choice (D) is correct.

36.   E
The passage states the differences in amino acids are in their side chains, which themselves differ in size, shape, charge, hydrogen bonding capacity, and chemical reactivity. The passage does not indicate

that side chains differ in carbon-binding capacity or number. Therefore, choice (E) is correct.

37.   C
The passage states that glutamate dehydrogenase is an allosterically regulated enzyme that is active only when low-energy precursors are present, such as ADP and GDP. In contrast, the activity of gluta-mate dehydrogenase is low when ATP and GTP are present. Therefore, choice (C) is correct.

38.   E
The passage states that trypsin breaks poly-peptide chains on the carboxyl side of arginine and lysine residues, while chymotrypsin cleaves preferentially on the carboxyl side of aromatic and other bulky, nonpolar amino acids. There-fore, choice (E) is correct.

39.   E
The passage states that amino acid degradation involves primarily the conversion of an alpha-amino group to urea. The alpha-amino group is initially transferred to the molecule alpha-ketoglutarate to form glutamate, which is oxidatively deaminated to form NH4+. The ammonium ion is then converted to an excretion product and launched into the urea cycle. Amino acid skeletons may be converted to acetyl-CoA, pyruvate, or one of the intermediates of the citric acid cycle (e.g., fumarate). Alternatively, for ketogenic amino acids, degradation may involve the formation of acetyl-CoA or acetoacetyl-Coa and may give rise to ketone bodies, such as acetone, D-3-hydroxybutyrate, and acetoacetate. Therefore, choice (E) is correct.

40.   C
The passage states that while NADH is an active electron carrier in the oxidative phosphorylation that generates cellular ATP, NADPH is more active in reductive biosynthesis. However, this implies that NADPH has some activity in oxidative phosphoryla-tion. Therefore, choice (C) is correct.

II

QUANTITATIVE REASONING

1

Arithmetic

FRACTIONS

A. Fast Fractions Overview

Multiplying fractions: Multiply numerators by each other and denominators by each other.

$$\frac{3}{4} \times \frac{9}{7} = \frac{3 \times 9}{4 \times 7} = \frac{27}{28}$$

Dividing fractions: Flip the numerator and denominator of the fraction that you're dividing by, then multiply.

$$\frac{1}{5} \div \frac{4}{11} = \frac{1}{5} \times \frac{11}{4} = \frac{1 \times 11}{5 \times 4} = \frac{11}{20}$$

Adding fractions: You can add fractions only when they have the same denominator. When you add, add only the numerators, NOT the denominators.

$$\frac{2}{3} + \frac{5}{3} = \frac{2+5}{3} = \frac{7}{3}$$

If you don't have a common denominator, you have to find one. The fastest way to get a common denominator is to multiply each fraction by a fraction whose numerator and denominator are the same as the denominator of the other fraction (cross multiply). (You can do this because any fraction with the same numerator and denominator is equal to 1, and multiplying any number by 1 doesn't change the value of the number.)

$$\frac{1}{3} + \frac{2}{5} = \left(\frac{1}{3} \times \frac{5}{5}\right) + \left(\frac{2}{5} \times \frac{3}{3}\right) = \frac{5}{15} + \frac{6}{15} = \frac{11}{15}$$

Subtracting fractions: This works the same way as adding fractions, except you subtract the numerators instead of adding them.

$$\frac{6}{7} - \frac{1}{2} = \left(\frac{6}{7}\right)\left(\frac{2}{2}\right) - \left(\frac{1}{2}\right)\left(\frac{7}{7}\right) = \frac{12}{14} - \frac{7}{14} = \frac{5}{14}$$

Remember, parentheses can be used to indicate multiplication instead of the "×" sign.

Reducing fractions: Whenever there is a common **factor** in the numerator and denominator, you can reduce the fraction by removing the factor from both parts of the fraction. You can do this because dividing the numerator and denominator by the same number doesn't change the value of the fraction as a whole. This will often make working with the fraction much easier, because you'll be using smaller numbers.

$$\frac{4}{12} = \frac{1 \times 4}{3 \times 4} = \frac{1}{3} \times \frac{4}{4} = \frac{1}{3} \times 1 = \frac{1}{3}$$

Obviously, you don't have to write out all this math. We're just doing it to show you exactly what's going on. On the test, you should do easy fractions like these in one step, like in the next example.

You can reduce $\frac{42}{28}$ by canceling like this:

$$\frac{\overset{6}{\cancel{42}}}{\underset{4}{\cancel{28}}} = \frac{\overset{3}{\cancel{6}}}{\underset{2}{\cancel{4}}} = \frac{3}{2}$$

Let's look more closely at how we reduced $\frac{42}{28}$. Since both 42 and 28 are divisible by 7, we can divide both the numerator (42) and the denominator (28) by 7. Thus $\frac{42}{28}$ was reduced to $\frac{6}{4}$. Since both 6 and 4 are divisible by 2, we can divide both the numerator (6) and the denominator (4) by 2. Thus $\frac{6}{4}$ was reduced to $\frac{3}{2}$.

Canceling: Whenever you have to multiply two or more fractions, you should cancel common factors before you multiply. This is a lot like reducing and has the same advantages. $\frac{1}{7} \times \frac{7}{3}$ can be cancelled like this:

$$\frac{1}{\cancel{7}} \times \frac{\overset{1}{\cancel{7}}}{3} = \frac{1}{1} \times \frac{1}{3} = \frac{1}{3}$$

$\frac{4}{5} \times \frac{15}{12}$ can be cancelled like this:

$$\frac{\overset{1}{\cancel{4}}}{\underset{1}{\cancel{5}}} \times \frac{\overset{3}{\cancel{15}}}{\underset{3}{\cancel{12}}} = \frac{1}{1} \times \frac{3}{3} = 1$$

Notice that we divided both the 5 in the denominator of the first fraction and the 15 in the numerator of the second fraction by 5. We also divided the 4 in the numerator of the first fraction and the 12 in the denominator of the second fraction by 4.

B. Comparing Fractions

One way to compare fractions is to re-express them with a common denominator: $\frac{3}{4} = \frac{21}{28}$ and $\frac{5}{7} = \frac{20}{28}$ because $\frac{21}{28}$ is greater than $\frac{20}{28}$, $\frac{3}{4}$ is greater than $\frac{5}{7}$. Another way to compare fractions is to convert them both to decimals: $\frac{3}{4}$ converts to 0.75, and $\frac{5}{7}$ converts to approximately 0.714.

C. Mixed Numbers and Improper Fractions

A **mixed number** consists of an integer and a fraction. For example, $3\frac{1}{4}$, $12\frac{2}{5}$, and $5\frac{7}{8}$ are all mixed numbers.

To convert an **improper fraction** (a fraction whose numerator is greater than its denominator) to a mixed number, divide the numerator by the denominator. The number of "whole" times that the denominator goes into the numerator will be the integer portion of the improper fraction; the remainder will be the numerator of the fractional portion.

Example: Convert $\frac{23}{4}$ to a mixed number.

Dividing 23 by 4 gives you 5 with a remainder of 3, so $\frac{23}{4} = 5\frac{3}{4}$.

To change a mixed number to a fraction, keep the denominator of the fraction. To figure out the numerator, multiply the integer portion of the mixed number by the number in the denominator. Then add this result to the numerator of the mixed number.

Example: Convert $2\frac{3}{7}$ to a fraction.

$$2\frac{3}{7} = \frac{(2 \times 7) + 3}{7} = \frac{17}{7}$$

Example: Convert $5\frac{8}{9}$ to a fraction.

$$5\frac{8}{9} = \frac{(5 \times 9) + 8}{9} = \frac{53}{9}$$

D. Adding and Subtracting Mixed Numbers

Adding or subtracting mixed numbers whose fractional parts have the same denominator will probably be on the test.

Example: $3\frac{12}{17} + 4\frac{10}{17} = ?$

First, add the integer parts: $3 + 4 = 7$.

Next, add the fractional parts: $\frac{12}{17} + \frac{10}{17} = \frac{22}{17}$.

Now, $\frac{22}{17} = 1\frac{5}{17}$.

Therefore, $3\frac{12}{17} + 4\frac{10}{17} = 7 + 1\frac{5}{17} = 8\frac{5}{17}$.

Example: $4\frac{5}{8} - 2\frac{7}{8} = ?$

The wrinkle here is that the fractional part of the first number is smaller than the fractional part of the second number (i.e., $\frac{5}{8}$ is smaller then $\frac{7}{8}$). What we need to do, therefore, is to borrow from the integer part of the first number to make the fractional part of the first number bigger. We'll borrow 1 from the integer part and add it to the fractional part (remembering that 1 can be rewritten as $\frac{8}{8}$).

So $4\frac{5}{8} = 3 + \frac{8}{8} + \frac{5}{8} = 3\frac{13}{8}$. So the problem of finding $4\frac{5}{8} - 2\frac{7}{8}$ has been replaced with the problem of finding $3\frac{13}{8} - 2\frac{7}{8}$, which is easier, because the fractional part of the first number is greater than the fractional part of the second number.

Notice that all we've done is replace $4\frac{5}{8}$ with $3\frac{13}{8}$, which is equal to $4\frac{5}{8}$. To find $3\frac{13}{8} - 2\frac{7}{8}$, first subtract the integer parts: $3 - 2 = 1$. Next subtract the fractional parts: $\frac{13}{8} - \frac{7}{8} = \frac{6}{8} = \frac{3}{4}$. So $4\frac{5}{8} - 2\frac{7}{8} = 1\frac{3}{4}$.

Example: $5\frac{1}{4} - 1\frac{3}{4} = ?$

$$5\frac{1}{4} - 1\frac{3}{4} = 5 + \frac{1}{4} - 1\frac{3}{4} =$$

$$\left(4 + \frac{4}{4}\right) + \frac{1}{4} - 1\frac{3}{4} = 4\frac{5}{4} - 1\frac{3}{4} = 3\frac{2}{4} = 3\frac{1}{2}$$

When you gain experience with this, you'll be able to skip some of the steps and do this type of problem more quickly.

Example: $8\frac{3}{25} - 4\frac{12}{25} = ?$

$$8\frac{3}{25} - 4\frac{12}{25} = 7 + \frac{25}{25} + \frac{3}{25} - 4\frac{12}{25} = 7\frac{28}{25} - 4\frac{12}{25} = 3\frac{16}{25}$$

RATIOS

A. Setting Up a Ratio

To find a ratio, put the number associated with the word *of* **on top** and the quantity associated with the word *to* **on the bottom** and reduce. The ratio *of* 20 oranges *to* 12 apples is $\frac{20}{12}$, which reduces to $\frac{5}{3}$.

B. Part-to-Part Ratios and Part-to-Whole Ratios

If the parts add up to the whole, a part-to-part ratio can be turned into two part-to-whole ratios by putting each number in the original ratio over the sum of the numbers. If the ratio of males to females is 1 to 2, then the males-to-people ratio is $\frac{1}{1+2} = \frac{1}{3}$ and the females-to-people ratio is $\frac{2}{1+2} = \frac{2}{3}$. In other words, $\frac{2}{3}$ of all the people are female.

C. Solving a Proportion

To solve a proportion, **cross multiply**:

$$\frac{x}{5} = \frac{3}{4}$$

$$4x = 5 \times 3$$

$$x = \frac{15}{4} = 3.75$$

DECIMALS

There are two different ways to express numbers that are not integers: as fractions and as decimals. Fractions we've already discussed; now it's time to talk about decimals.

A. Changing Fractions to Decimals

It's easy to change a fraction into a decimal—all you do is divide the denominator of the fraction into the numerator.

Example: Change $\frac{415}{3,220}$ into a decimal.

First write the fraction as long division.

$$3,220\overline{)4\,15}$$

Since 3,220 is much bigger than 415, what we do is add a zero to the 415 to make the division work out. The only way we can do this without changing the value of 415 is if we add a decimal point after the 5. Then we're just changing 415 to 415.00—and those zeros don't change the value of anything. We divide normally, but we put a decimal point in the **quotient** (the answer) directly above the decimal point in 415.

$$
\begin{array}{r}
.12 \\
3{,}220\overline{)415.000} \\
4150 \\
\underline{3220} \\
9330 \\
\underline{6440} \\
28600
\end{array}
$$

How far we should go depends on how much accuracy we need, but at this point, we can tell that the answer is going to be close to 0.13.

B. Changing Decimals to Fractions

How do you express 0.5 as a fraction? Well, 0.1 represents $\frac{1}{10}$, and 0.5 is five times as much as 0.1, so 0.5 must represent 5 times $\frac{1}{10}$ or $\frac{5}{10}$. Of course, we can reduce $\frac{5}{10}$ to $\frac{1}{2}$.

How do you express 0.55 as a fraction? Well—let's think of it in terms of dollars and cents. We know that $0.01 is one cent, and that's $\frac{1}{100}$ of a dollar. Then $0.55 is 55 cents, and that's 55 times as much, so $0.55 must be $\frac{55}{100}$ of a dollar. We can reduce this by dividing the top and bottom by 5, giving us $\frac{11}{20}$. That's the fractional equivalent of 0.55.

Hopefully by this point you recognize a pattern:

$$0.1 = 1 \times \frac{1}{10} \text{ or } \frac{1}{10}$$

$$0.11 = 11 \times \frac{1}{100} \text{ or } \frac{11}{100}$$

$$0.111 = 111 \times \frac{1}{1{,}000} \text{ or } \frac{111}{1{,}000}$$

$$0.1111 = 1{,}111 \times \frac{1}{10{,}000} \text{ or } \frac{1{,}111}{10{,}000}$$

and so on.

What we did on the previous page to change these decimals to fractions was to put the digits to the right of the decimal point in the numerator. To figure out the denominator, we put a 1 in the denominator and followed it with as many zeros as there were digits to the right of the decimal point.

Example: Change 0.564 to a fraction.

There are three digits to the right of the decimal point, so the denominator of our fraction will be 1,000 (a 1 followed by three zeros). The numerator of the fraction is 564.

$$0.564 = \frac{564}{1,000}$$

But notice that $\frac{564}{1,000}$ can be reduced. Since both 564 and 1,000 are divisible by 4, we can divide both the numerator and the denominator by 4; therefore, $\frac{564}{1,000} = \frac{564 \div 4}{1,000 \div 4} = \frac{141}{250}$.

C. Addition and Subtraction of Decimals

You add and subtract decimals the same way you add and subtract whole numbers. Just make sure the decimal points are lined up, then add. In the answer, put the decimal point directly below the other decimal points.

$$
\begin{array}{r}
0.456 + 1.234 = 0.456 \\
+ 1.234 \\
\hline
1.690 = 1.69
\end{array}
$$

If one of the terms you are adding or subtracting is longer than another (has more digits to the right of the decimal), it helps to add zeros to the shorter number.

$$
\begin{array}{r}
6.97 - 3.567 = 6.970 \\
- 3.567 \\
\hline
3.403
\end{array}
$$

D. Multiplication of Decimals

As with addition and subtraction, you multiply decimals as if they were whole numbers and worry about the decimal points later. You don't need to add zeros to make the numbers the same length when you multiply, however.

$$4.5 \times 3.2 = \begin{array}{r} 4.5 \\ \times\ 3.2 \\ \hline 9\ 0 \\ 13\ 5 \\ \hline 14.4\ 0 \end{array}$$

To place the decimal point in the answer, count the number of digits to the right of the decimal point in each number. Here we have one decimal place in 4.5 and one in 3.2 for a total of 1 + 1 or 2 places. Put the decimal point two places from the right in the answer: 14.40.

It's a good idea when you get the answer to check that you put the decimal point in the right place by seeing if the answer makes sense. Here the answer should be a little bigger than 4 × 3, or 12. So 14.40 should be about right. If you had placed the decimal point incorrectly and ended up with 144, you would know that was wrong.

E. Division of Decimals

It's easiest to discuss division of decimals if we express the division in fractional form.

Example: $4.15 \div 32.2 = \dfrac{4.15}{32.2}$

Make both the numerator and the denominator of the fraction whole numbers; to do this, multiply both top and bottom by a sufficient power of 10. In our example, we need to multiply by 100; this will make the denominator 3,220 and the numerator 415. We're left with

$$\frac{4.15}{32.2} = \frac{415}{3,220}$$

Now divide 3,220 into 415.

F. Rounding Decimals to the Nearest Place

To round a decimal to the nearest place, look at the digit immediately to the right of that place. If that digit is 5, 6, 7, 8, or 9, then round up the place you are rounding to. If the digit immediately to the right of the place you are rounding to is 0, 1, 2, 3, or 4, then don't change the digit at the place you are rounding to. In either case, in the rounded-off number, there will be no digits to the right of the place you are rounding off to.

Example: Round 0.12763 to the nearest thousandth.

The digit in the thousandths place is 7. The digit immediately to the right of the 7 is a 6. Since 6 is among the digits that are 5 or more, we round up the thousandths digits from 7 to 8. So 0.12763 rounded to the nearest thousandth is 0.128.

Example: Round 0.5827 to the nearest hundredth.

The digit in the hundredths place is 8. Immediately to the right of the 8 is a 2. Since 2 is among the digits 0 through 4, we keep the digit in the hundredths place the same. So 0.5827 rounded to the nearest hundredth is 0.58.

Example: Round $\frac{5}{37}$ to the nearest hundredth.

$$
\begin{array}{r}
0.135 \\
37\overline{)5.000} \\
50 \\
\underline{37} \\
130 \\
\underline{111} \\
190 \\
\underline{185} \\
5
\end{array}
$$

Since the digit in the thousandths place is a 5, which is among the digits 5 through 9, the hundredths digit is rounded up from 3 to 4. So $\frac{5}{37}$ rounded to the nearest hundredth is 0.14.

PERCENTS

Percents are a special kind of ratio. Any percent can be expressed as a fraction with a denominator of 100 (*cent* means "one hundred," so *percent* means "*per* one hundred"). Because of this, it is very easy to convert percents into decimals as well as fractions.

To convert a percent to a fraction or decimal, just drop the percent symbol and divide the number by 100. (To convert to decimals, the shortcut is simply to drop the percent symbol and move the decimal point two places to the left.)

Percent to fraction: $78\% = \frac{78}{100}$

Percent to decimal: $78\% = 0.78$

$$\frac{78}{100} = 0.78$$

To convert any fraction or decimal to a percent, just multiply by 100 and add a percent sign. (For decimals, just move the decimal point two places to the right and add a percent sign. For fractions, remember to reduce if you can before you multiply.)

Decimal to percent: 0.29 = 29%
0.3 = 30%
1.45 = 145%

Fraction to percent: $\dfrac{3}{5} = \dfrac{3}{5} \times 100\% = \dfrac{3(100)}{5}\% = 3(20)\% = 60\%$

Know these common conversions. They come up frequently on the test, and you can avoid errors and save time by memorizing them instead of having to calculate them on the test.

In general, a digit with a bar over it means that the digit repeats indefinitely. In the table below, $0.3\overline{3}$ means that the 3 with the bar over it repeats indefinitely. Thus, $0.3\overline{3} = 0.3333...$

Fraction	Decimal	Percent
$\dfrac{1}{1}$	1.0	100%
$\dfrac{3}{4}$	0.75	75%
$\dfrac{2}{3}$	$0.6\overline{6}$	$66\dfrac{2}{3}\%$
$\dfrac{1}{2}$	0.5	50%
$\dfrac{1}{3}$	$0.3\overline{3}$	$33\dfrac{1}{3}\%$
$\dfrac{1}{4}$	0.25	25%
$\dfrac{1}{5}$	0.2	20%
$\dfrac{1}{8}$	0.125	$12\dfrac{1}{2}\%$
$\dfrac{1}{10}$	0.1	10%
$\dfrac{1}{20}$	0.05	5%

A. The Percent Formula

The percent formula is commonly expressed in two different ways that are mathematically identical. Memorize and use whichever version of the formula you prefer. Notice how easy it is to get from one formula to the other—just multiply or divide both sides of the equation by the Whole.

$$\text{Percent} = \frac{\text{Part}}{\text{Whole}}$$

or

$$\text{Percent} \times \text{Whole} = \text{Part}$$

If the Part is 3 and the Whole is 4, then the Percent $= \dfrac{3}{4} = 0.75 = 75\%$.

If the Percent is 20% and the Whole is 8, then the Part $= 20\%(8) = (0.2)(8) = 1.6$

If the Percent is 60% and the Part is 12, then 60% (Whole) $= 12$. Thus,

$$\text{Whole} = \frac{12}{60\%} = \frac{12}{\left(\dfrac{6}{10}\right)} = 12\left(\frac{10}{6}\right) = 20.$$

B. Percent Increase/Decrease

Once you understand percents, calculating percent increase and decrease is not as difficult as it may seem.

$$\% \text{ increase} = \frac{\text{Amount of increase}}{\text{Original whole}}\ (100\%)$$

$$\% \text{ decrease} = \frac{\text{Amount of decrease}}{\text{Original whole}}\ (100\%)$$

New Whole = Original whole ± Amount of change

Look at the first equation above. To find a percent increase, divide the amount of increase by the original whole. Then multiply this fraction by 100%.

Example: If a number increases from 50 to 70, what is the percent increase?

The amount of increase is $70 - 50$, or 20. The original whole is 50. So the percent increase is $\dfrac{20}{50} \times 100\% = \dfrac{2}{5} \times 100\%$. What you learned reducing fractions can help here.

$$\frac{2}{5} \times 100\% = 2 \times 20\% = 40\%$$

If the new price of an item is 130% of its previous price, then it has increased in price by 30%. If an item goes on sale at 60% of its previous price, then it has decreased in price by 40%.

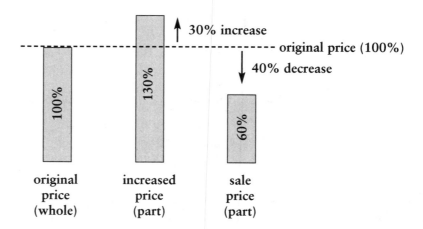

original price (100%)

30% increase

40% decrease

| original price (whole) | increased price (part) | sale price (part) |

The percent increase or decrease is just the difference in percent from the whole (which is always equal to 100%).

When you come across the following phrases, use the percent increase/decrease formula:

If *X* is 10% greater than *Y*, then *X* is 110% of *Y*.

If *X* is 70% less than *Y*, then *X* is 30% of *Y*.

Example: If the value of a certain piece of property now is 350% of its original value when Kim purchased it, by what percent has the value of the property increased since Kim purchased it?

The percent increase is the difference from 100%. So 350% − 100% = 250% increase.

AVERAGES

A. Formula for Computing Averages

To find the average of a set of numbers, add them up and divide by the number of terms (the number of numbers).

$$\text{Average} = \frac{\text{Sum of the terms}}{\text{Number of terms}}$$

To find the average of the five numbers 12, 15, 23, 40, and 40, first add them: 12 + 15 + 23 + 40 + 40 = 130. Then divide the sum by 5: 130 ÷ 5 = 26.

B. Using the Average to Find the Sum

Sum = (Average) × (Number of terms)

If the average of 10 numbers is 50, then they add up to 10 × 50, or 500.

C. Finding the Missing Number

To find a missing number when you're given the average, **use the sum**. If the average of four numbers is 7, then the sum of those four numbers is 4 × 7, or 28. Suppose that three of the numbers are 3, 5, and 8. These three numbers add up to 16 of that 28, which leaves 12 for the fourth number.

PROBABILITY

The probability of an event is the possible number of **desired outcomes** divided by the total number of **possible outcomes**. Its numerical value is always less than or equal to 1. The probability of two independent events both occurring is the product of the individual probabilities.

Example: If we rolled two dice, what is the probability that we would make a total of 4?

There are six possible outcomes for each roll of a die, so with two dice, there are 6 × 6 = 36 possible outcomes. There are three outcomes that will lead to a total of 4: rolling 1 and 3, 3 and 1, or 2 and 2. The probability is therefore $\frac{3}{36} = \frac{1}{12}$.

2

Algebra

EXPONENTS—KEY OPERATIONS

You can't be adept at algebra unless you're completely at ease with exponents. Here's what you need to know.

Multiplying powers with the same base: To multiply powers with the same base, keep the base and add the exponents:

$$x^3 \times x^4 = x^{3+4} = x^7$$

Dividing powers with the same base: To divide powers with the same base, keep the base and subtract the exponents:

$$y^{13} \div y^8 = y^{13-8} = y^5$$

Raising a power to an exponent: To raise a power to an exponent, keep the base and multiply the exponents:

$$(x^3)^4 = x^{3 \times 4} = x^{12}$$

Multiplying powers with the same exponent: To multiply powers with the same exponent, multiply the bases and keep the exponent:

$$(3x)(4x) = 12x^2$$

Dividing powers with the same exponent: To divide powers with the same exponent, divide the bases and keep the exponent:

$$\frac{6^x}{2^x} = 3^x$$

Example: For all $xyz \neq 0$, $\dfrac{6x^2y^{12}z^6}{(2x^2yz)^3} =$

There's nothing tricky about this question if you know how to work with exponents. The first step is to eliminate the parentheses. Everything inside gets cubed:

$$\frac{6x^2y^{12}z^6}{(2x^2yz)^3} = \frac{6x^2y^{12}z^6}{8x^6y^3z^3}$$

KEY CONCEPT

1. $(x^m)(x^n) = x^{m+n}$
2. $\dfrac{x^m}{x^n} = x^{m-n}$
3. $(x^m)^n = x^{mn}$
4. $(x^n)(y^n) = (xy)^n$
5. $\dfrac{x^n}{y^n} = \left(\dfrac{x}{y}\right)^n$

The next step is to look for factors common to the numerator and denominator. The 6 on top and the 8 on bottom reduce to 3 over 4. The x^2 on top cancels with the x^6 on bottom, leaving x^4 on bottom. You're actually subtracting the exponents of x: $2 - 6 = -4$; x^{-4} is the same as $\frac{1}{x^4}$. The y^{12} on top cancels with the y^3 on bottom, leaving y^9 on top. And the z^6 on top cancels with the z^3 on bottom, leaving z^3 on top:

$$\frac{6x^2y^{12}z^6}{8x^6y^3z^3} = \frac{3y^9z^3}{4x^4}$$

ADDING, SUBTRACTING, AND MULTIPLYING POLYNOMIALS

Algebra is the basic language of mathematics, and you will want to be fluent in that language. You might not get a whole lot of questions that ask explicitly about such basic algebra procedures as combining like terms, multiplying binomials, or factoring algebraic expressions, but you will do all of those things in the course of working out the answers to more advanced questions. So it's essential that you be at ease with the mechanics of algebraic manipulations.

Combining like terms: To combine like terms, keep the variable part unchanged while adding or subtracting the coefficients:

$$2a + 3a = (2 + 3)a = 5a$$

Adding or subtracting polynomials: To add or subtract polynomials, combine like terms:

$$(3x^2 + 5x - 7) - (x^2 + 12) =$$
$$(3x^2 - x^2) + 5x + (-7 - 12) =$$
$$2x^2 + 5x - 19$$

Multiplying monomials: To multiply monomials, multiply the coefficients and the variables separately:

$$2x \times 3x = (2 \times 3)(x \times x) = 6x^2$$

Multiplying binomials: To multiply binomials, use **FOIL**. To multiply $(x + 3)$ by $(x + 4)$, first multiply the **First** terms: $x \times x = x^2$. Next the **Outer** terms: $x \times 4 = 4x$. Then the **Inner** terms: $3 \times x = 3x$. And finally the **Last** terms: $3 \times 4 = 12$. Then add and combine like terms:

$$x^2 + 4x + 3x + 12 = x^2 + 7x + 12$$

Multiplying polynomials: To multiply polynomials with more than two terms, make sure you multiply each term in the first polynomial by each term in the second. (FOIL works only when you want to multiply two binomials.)

$$(x^2 + 3x + 4)(x + 5) = x^2(x + 5) + 3x(x + 5) + 4(x + 5)$$

$$= x^3 + 5x^2 + 3x^2 + 15x + 4x + 20$$

$$= x^3 + 8x^2 + 19x + 20$$

After multiplying two polynomials together, the number of terms in your expression before simplifying should equal the number of terms in one polynomial multiplied by the number of terms in the second. In the example above, you should have $3 \times 2 = 6$ terms in the product before you simplify like terms.

DIVIDING POLYNOMIALS

To divide polynomials, you can use long division. For example, divide $2x^3 + 13x^2 + 11x - 16$ by $x + 5$:

$$x + 5 \overline{)2x^3 + 13x^2 + 11x - 16}$$

KEY CONCEPT
$(a + b)(c + d) = ?$
First $= ac$
Outer $= ad$
Inner $= bc$
Last $= bd$
Product $= ac + ad + bc + bd$

The first term of the quotient is $2x^2$, because that's what will give you a $2x^3$ as a first term when you multiply it by $x + 5$:

$$
\begin{array}{r}
2x^2 \\
x + 5 \overline{)2x^3 + 13x^2 + 11x - 16} \\
\underline{2x^3 + 10x^2}
\end{array}
$$

Subtract and continue in the same way as when dividing numbers:

$$
\begin{array}{r}
2x^2 + 3x - 4 \\
x + 5 \overline{)2x^3 + 13x^2 + 11x - 16} \\
\underline{2x^3 + 10x^2} \\
3x^2 + 11x \\
\underline{3x^2 + 15x} \\
-4x - 16 \\
\underline{-4x - 20} \\
4
\end{array}
$$

The result is $2x^2 + 3x - 4$ with a remainder of 4.

Long division is the way to do the following:

Example: When $2x^3 + 3x^2 - 4x + k$ is divided by $x + 2$, the remainder is 3. What is the value of k ?

To answer this question, start by cranking out the long division:

$$
\require{enclose}
\begin{array}{r}
2x^2 - x - 2 \\
x + 2 \enclose{longdiv}{2x^3 + 3x^2 - 4x + k} \\
\underline{2x^3 + 4x^2} \\
-x^2 - 4x \\
\underline{-x^2 - 2x} \\
-2x + k \\
\underline{-2x - 4}
\end{array}
$$

The question says that the remainder is 3, so, whatever k is, when you subtract -4 from it, you get 3:

$$k - (-4) = 3$$
$$k + 4 = 3$$
$$k = -1$$

FACTORING

Performing operations on polynomials is largely a matter of cranking it out. Once you know the rules, adding, subtracting, multiplying, and even dividing is automatic. Factoring algebraic expressions is a different matter. To factor successfully you have to do more thinking and less cranking. You have to try to figure out what expressions multiplied will give you the polynomial you're looking at. Sometimes that means having a good eye for the test makers' favorite factorables:

- Factor common to all terms
- Difference of squares
- Square of a binomial

A. Factor Common to All Terms

A factor common to all the terms of a polynomial can be factored out. This is essentially the distributive property in reverse. For example, all three terms in the polynomial $3x^3 + 12x^2 - 6x$ contain a factor of $3x$. Pulling out the common factor yields $3x(x^2 + 4x - 2)$.

B. Difference of Squares

You will want to be especially keen at spotting polynomials in the form of the difference of squares. Whenever you have two identifiable squares with a minus sign between them, you can factor the expression like this:

$$a^2 - b^2 = (a + b)(a - b)$$

$4x^2 - 9$, for example, factors to $(2x + 3)(2x - 3)$.

C. Squares of Binomials

Learn to recognize polynomials that are squares of binomials:

$$a^2 + 2ab + b^2 = (a + b)^2$$
$$a^2 - 2ab + b^2 = (a - b)^2$$

For example, $4x^2 + 12x + 9$ factors to $(2x + 3)^2$, and $a^2 - 10a + 25$ factors to $(a - 5)^2$.

D. Factoring Other Expressions

Sometimes you'll want to factor a polynomial that's not in any of these classic factorable forms. When that happens, factoring becomes a kind of logic exercise, with some trial and error thrown in. To factor a **quadratic expression**, think about what binomials you could use FOIL to get that quadratic expression. For example, to factor $x^2 - 5x + 6$, think about what **First** terms will produce x^2, what **Last** terms will produce +6, and what **Outer** and **Inner** terms will produce $-5x$. Some common sense—and a little trial and error—will lead you to $(x - 2)(x - 3)$.

Example: For all $x \neq \pm 3$, $\dfrac{3x^2 - 11x + 6}{9 - x^2} =$

(A) $\dfrac{2 - 3x}{x - 3}$ (B) $\dfrac{2 - 3x}{x + 3}$ (C) $\dfrac{2x - 3}{x - 3}$ (D) $\dfrac{3x - 2}{x + 3}$ (E) $\dfrac{3x - 2}{x - 3}$

To reduce a fraction, you eliminate factors common to the top and bottom. So the first step in reducing an algebraic fraction is to factor the numerator and denominator. Here the denominator is easy since it's the difference of squares: $9 - x^2 = (3 - x)(3 + x)$. The numerator takes some thought and some trial and error. For the first term to be $3x^2$, the first terms of the factors must be $3x$ and x. For the last term to be +6, the last terms must be either +2 and +3, or -2 and -3, or +1 and +6, or -1 and -6. After a few tries, you should come up with $3x^2 - 11x + 6 = (3x - 2)(x - 3)$. Now the fraction looks like this:

$$\frac{3x^2 - 11x + 6}{9 - x^2} = \frac{(3x - 2)(x - 3)}{(3 - x)(3 + x)}$$

In this form, there are no precisely common factors, but there is a factor in the numerator that's the opposite (negative) of a factor in the denomina- tor: $x - 3$ and $3 - x$ are opposites. Factor -1 out of the numerator and get this:

$$\frac{(3x - 2)(x - 3)}{(3 - x)(3 + x)} = \frac{(-1)(3x - 2)(3 - x)}{(3 - x)(3 + x)}$$

Now $(3 - x)$ can be eliminated from both the top and the bottom:

$$\frac{(-1)(3x - 2)(3 - x)}{(3 - x)(3 + x)} = \frac{-(3x - 2)}{3 + x} = \frac{-3x + 2}{3 + x}$$

That's the same as choice (B):

$$\frac{-3x + 2}{3 + x} = \frac{2 - 3x}{x + 3}$$

Alternative method: Here's another way to answer this question. *Pick a number for x and see what happens.* One of the answer choices will give you the same value as the original fraction will, no matter what you plug in for *x*. Pick a number that's easy to work with—like 0.

When you plug $x = 0$ into the original expression, any term with an *x* drops out, and you end up with $\frac{6}{9}$, or $\frac{2}{3}$. Plug $x = 0$ into each answer choice to see which ones equal $\frac{2}{3}$.

When you get to (B), it works, but you can't stop there. It might be just a coincidence. When you pick numbers, *look at every answer choice.* Choice (E) also works for $x = 0$. At least you know one of those is the correct answer, and you can decide between them by picking another value for *x*.

This is not a sophisticated approach, but who cares? You don't get points for elegance. You get points for right answers.

THE GOLDEN RULE OF EQUATIONS

You probably remember the basic procedure for solving algebraic equations: *Do the same thing to both sides.* You can do almost anything you want to one side of an equation as long as you preserve the equality by doing the same thing to the other side. Your aim in whatever you do to both sides is to get the variable (or expression) you're solving for all by itself on one side.

Example: If $\sqrt[3]{8x + 6} = -3$, what is the value of *x* ?

To solve this equation for *x* means to do whatever is needed to both sides of the equation to get *x* all by itself on one side. Layer by layer, you want to peel away all those extra symbols and numbers around the *x*. First you want to get rid of that cube-root symbol. The way to undo a cube root is to cube both sides:

$$\sqrt[3]{8x + 6} = -3$$
$$\left(\sqrt[3]{8x + 6}\right)^3 = (-3)^3$$
$$8x + 6 = -27$$

The rest is easy. Subtract 6 from both sides and divide both sides by 8:

$$8x + 6 = -27$$
$$8x = -27 - 6$$
$$8x = -33$$
$$x = -\frac{33}{8} = -4.125$$

The test makers have a couple of favorite equation types that you should be prepared to solve. Solving **linear equations** is usually pretty straightforward. Generally it's obvious what to do to isolate the unknown. But when the unknown is in a denominator or an exponent, it might not be so obvious how to proceed.

UNKNOWN IN A DENOMINATOR

The basic procedure for solving an equation is the same even when the unknown is in a denominator: Do the same thing to both sides. In this case you multiply in order to undo division.

If you wanted to solve $1 + \dfrac{1}{x} = 2 - \dfrac{1}{x}$, you would multiply both sides by x:

$$1 + \frac{1}{x} = 2 - \frac{1}{x}$$
$$x\left(1 + \frac{1}{x}\right) = x\left(2 - \frac{1}{x}\right)$$
$$x + 1 = 2x - 1$$

Now you have an equation with no denominators, which is easy to solve:

$$x + 1 = 2x - 1$$
$$x - 2x = -1 - 1$$
$$-x = -2$$
$$x = 2$$

Another good way to solve an equation with the unknown in the denominator is to *cross multiply*. That's the best way to do the following example.

Example: If $\dfrac{5}{x+3} = \dfrac{1}{x} + \dfrac{1}{2x}$, what is the value of x?

Before you can cross multiply, you need to re-express the right side of the equation as a single fraction. That means giving the two fractions a common denominator and adding them. The common denominator is $2x$:

$$\frac{5}{x+3} = \frac{1}{x} + \frac{1}{2x}$$

$$\frac{5}{x+3} = \frac{2}{2x} + \frac{1}{2x}$$

$$\frac{5}{x+3} = \frac{3}{2x}$$

Now you can cross multiply:

$$\frac{5}{x+3} = \frac{3}{2x}$$

$$(5)(2x) = (x+3)(3)$$

$$10x = 3x + 9$$

$$10x - 3x = 9$$

$$7x = 9$$

$$x = \frac{9}{7}$$

UNKNOWN IN AN EXPONENT

The procedure for solving an equation when the unknown is in an exponent is a little different. What you want to do in this situation is to re-express one or both sides of the equation so that the two sides have the same base.

Example: If $8^x = 16^{x-1}$, then $x =$

(A) $\dfrac{1}{8}$ (B) $\dfrac{1}{2}$ (C) 2   (D) 4   (E) 8

In this case, the base on the left is 8 and the base on the right is 16. They're both powers of 2, so you can reexpress both sides as powers of 2:

$$(2^3)^x = (2^4)^{x-1}$$
$$2^{3x} = 2^{4x-4}$$

Now that both sides have the same base, you can simply set the exponent expressions equal and solve for x:

$$3x = 4x - 4$$
$$3x - 4x = -4$$
$$-x = -4$$
$$x = 4$$

Alternative method: Here's another way to answer this question. Nobody says you have to figure out the answer to the question and then look for your solution among the answer choices. If you don't see how to do it the front way, *try working backwards*. Try plugging the answer choices back into the problem until you find the one that works. Here, if you start with (C) and $x = 2$, you get $8x = 8^2 = 64$ on the left side of the equation and $16x^{-1} = 16^1 = 16$ on the right side. It's not clear whether (C) was too small or too large, so you should probably try (D) next—it's easier to work with than (B), which is a fraction. If $x = 4$, then $8x = 8^4 = 4,096$ on the left, and $16x^{-1} = 16^3 = 4,096$. No need to do any more. (D) works, so it's the answer.

REMEMBER

You don't have to try all the answer choices when back-solving. As soon as you find a choice that works, you're finished.

Don't depend on backsolving too much. There are lots of math questions that can't be backsolved at all. And most that *can* be backsolved are almost certainly more *quickly* solved by a more direct approach.

QUADRATIC EQUATIONS

To solve a quadratic equation, put it in the $ax^2 + bx + c = 0$ form, factor the left side (if you can), and set each factor equal to 0 separately to get the two solutions. For example, to solve $x^2 + 12 = 7x$, first rewrite it as $x^2 - 7x + 12 = 0$. Then factor the left side:

$$x^2 - 7x + 12 = 0$$
$$(x - 3)(x - 4) = 0$$
$$x - 3 = 0 \text{ or } x - 4 = 0$$
$$x = 3 \text{ or } 4$$

Sometimes the left side may not be obviously factorable. You can always use the *quadratic formula*. Just plug in the coefficients a, b, and c from $ax^2 + bx + c = 0$ into the formula:

$$x = \frac{-b \pm \sqrt{b^2 - 4ac}}{2a}$$

For example, to solve $x^2 + 4x + 2 = 0$, plug $a = 1$, $b = 4$, and $c = 2$ into the formula:

$$x = \frac{-4 \pm \sqrt{4^2 - 4 \times 1 \times 2}}{2 \times 1}$$

$$= \frac{-4 \pm \sqrt{8}}{2} = -2 \pm \sqrt{2}$$

"IN TERMS OF"

So far in this chapter, solving an equation has meant finding a numerical value for the unknown. When there's more than one variable, it's generally impossible to get numerical solutions. Instead, what you do is solve for the unknown *in terms of* the other variables.

To solve an equation for one variable in terms of another means to isolate the one variable on one side of the equation, leaving an expression containing the other variable on the other side of the equation.

For example, to solve the equation $3x - 10y = -5x + 6y$ for x in terms of y, isolate x:

$$3x - 10y = -5x + 6y$$
$$3x + 5x = 6y + 10y$$
$$8x = 16y$$
$$x = 2y$$

Example: If $a = \frac{b + x}{c + x}$, what is the value of x in terms of a, b, and c?

You want to get x on one side by itself. First thing to do is eliminate the denominator by multiplying both sides by $c + x$:

$$a = \frac{b + x}{c + x}$$

$$a(c + x) = \left(\frac{b + x}{c + x}\right)(c + x)$$

$$ac + ax = b + x$$

Next move all terms with x to one side and all terms without to the other:

$$ac + ax = b + x$$
$$ax - x = b - ac$$

Now factor x out of the left side and divide both sides by the other factor to isolate x:

$$ax - x = b - ac$$
$$x(a - 1) = b - ac$$
$$x = \frac{b - ac}{a - 1}$$

SIMULTANEOUS EQUATIONS

You can get numerical solutions for more than one unknown if you are given more than one equation. Simultaneous equations questions take a little thought to answer. Solving simultaneous equations almost always involves combining equations, but you have to figure out what's the best way to combine the equations.

You can solve for two variables only if you have two distinct equations. Two forms of the same equation will not be adequate. Combine the equations in such a way that one of the variables cancels out. For example, to solve the two equations $4x + 3y = 8$ and $x + y = 3$, multiply both sides of the second equation by -3 to get $-3x - 3y = -9$. Now add the two equations; the $3y$ and the $-3y$ cancel out, leaving $x = -1$. Plug that back into either one of the original equations, and you'll find that $y = 4$.

Example: If $2x - 9y = 11$ and $x + 12y = -8$, what is the value of $x + y$?

If you just plow ahead without thinking, you might try to answer this question by solving for one variable at a time. That would work, but it would take a lot more time than this question needs. As usual, the key to this simultaneous equations question is to combine the equations, but combining the equations doesn't necessarily mean losing a variable. Look what happens here if you just add the equations as presented:

$$\begin{array}{r} 2x - 9y = 11 \\ +[x + 12y = -8] \\ \hline 3x + 3y = 3 \end{array}$$

Suddenly you're almost there! Just divide both sides by 3, and you get $x + y = 1$.

ABSOLUTE VALUE AND INEQUALITIES

To solve an equation that includes absolute value signs, think about the two different cases. For example, to solve the equation $|x - 12| = 3$, think of it as two equations:

$$x - 12 = 3 \text{ or } x - 12 = -3$$
$$x = 15 \text{ or } 9$$

To solve an inequality, do whatever is necessary to both sides to isolate the variable. Just remember that when you multiply or divide both sides by a negative number, you must reverse the sign. To solve $-5x + 7 < -3$, subtract 7 from both sides to get $-5x < -10$. Now divide both sides by -5, remembering to reverse the sign: $x > 2$.

Example: What is the solution set of $|2x - 3| < 7$?

(A) {x: $-5 < x < 2$}
(B) {x: $-5 < x < 5$}
(C) {x: $-2 < x < 5$}
(D) {x: $x < -5$ or $x > 2$}
(E) {x: $x < -2$ or $x > 5$}

What does it mean if $|2x - 3| < 7$? It means that if the expression between the absolute value bars is positive, it's less than $+7$, or if the expression between the bars is negative, it's greater than -7. In other words, $2x - 3$ is between -7 and $+7$:

$$-7 < 2x - 3 < 7$$
$$-4 < 2x < 10$$
$$-2 < x < 5$$

KEY CONCEPT

If $n > 0$,

$|$whatever$| < n$

⇓

$-n <$ whatever $< n$

$|$whatever$| > n$

⇓

whatever $< -n$ OR whatever $> n$

In fact, there's a general rule that applies here: To solve an inequality in the form $|$whatever$| < p$, where $p > 0$, just put that "whatever" inside the range $-p$ to p:

$$|\text{whatever}| < p \text{ means } -p < \text{whatever} < p$$

For example, $|x - 5| < 14$ becomes $-14 < x - 5 < 14$.

And here's another general rule: To solve an inequality in the form $|$whatever$| > p$, where $p > 0$, just put that "whatever" outside the range $-p$ to p :

$$|\text{whatever}| > p \text{ means whatever} < -p \text{ OR whatever} > p$$

For example, $\left|\dfrac{3x + 9}{2}\right| > 7$ becomes $\dfrac{3x + 9}{2} < -7$ OR $\dfrac{3x + 9}{2} > 7$.

3

Plane Geometry

ADDING AND SUBTRACTING SEGMENT LENGTHS

Example:

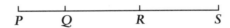

In the figure above, the length of segment *PS* is $2x + 12$, and the length of segment *PQ* is $6x - 10$. If *R* is the midpoint of segment *QS*, what is the length of segment *PR*?

Usually the best thing to do to start on a plane geometry question is to mark up the figure. Put as much of the information into the figure as you can. That's a good way to organize your thoughts. And that way, you don't have to go back and forth between the figure and the question.

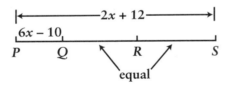

Now you can plan your attack. First subtract *PQ* from the whole length *PS* to get *QS*:

$$QS = PS - PQ = (2x + 12) - (6x - 10) = 2x + 12 - 6x + 10 = -4x + 22$$

Then, because *R* is the midpoint of *QS*, you can divide *QS* by 2 to get *QR* and *RS*:

$$QR = RS = \frac{QS}{2} = \frac{-4x + 22}{2} = -2x + 11$$

What you're looking for is *PR*, so you have to add:

$$PR = PQ + QR = (6x - 10) + (-2x + 11) = 4x + 1$$

BASIC TRAITS OF TRIANGLES

Most plane geometry questions are about **closed figures**: polygons and circles. And the test makers' favorite closed figure by far is the three-sided polygon; that is, the **triangle**. All three-sided polygons are interesting because they share so many characteristics, and certain special three-sided polygons—*equilateral*, *isosceles*, and *right triangles*—are interesting because of their special characteristics.

Let's look at the traits that all triangles share.

Sum of the interior angles: The three interior angles of any triangle add up to 180°.

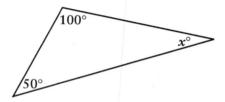

In the figure above, $x + 50 + 100 = 180$, so $x = 30$.

Measure of an exterior angle: The measure of an exterior angle of a triangle is equal to the sum of the measures of the remote interior angles.

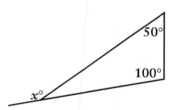

In the figure above, the measure of the exterior angle labeled $x°$ is equal to the sum of the measures of the remote interior angles: $x = 50 + 100 = 150$.

Sum of the exterior angles: The measures of the three exterior angles of any triangle add up to 360°.

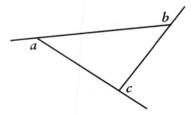

In the figure above, $a + b + c = 360°$. (Note: In fact, the measures of the exterior angles of any polygon add up to 360°.)

Area formula: The general formula for the area of a triangle is always the same:

$$\text{Area of Triangle} = \frac{1}{2}(\text{base})(\text{height})$$

The height is the perpendicular distance between the side that's chosen as the base and the opposite vertex.

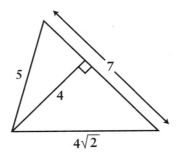

In the triangle above, 4 is the height when the 7 side is chosen as the base.

$$\text{Area of Triangle} = \frac{1}{2}(\text{base})(\text{height})$$

$$= \frac{1}{2}(7)(4) = 14$$

Triangle inequality theorem: The length of any one side of a triangle must be greater than the positive difference and less than the sum of the lengths of the other two sides. For example, if it is given that the length of one side is 3 and the length of another side is 7, then the length of the third side must be greater than $7 - 3 = 4$ and less than $7 + 3 = 10$.

SIMILAR TRIANGLES

Example:

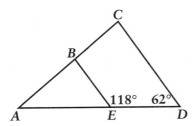

In the figure above, $AB = BC$. If the area of $\triangle ABE$ is x, what is the area of $\triangle ACD$?

You might wonder here how you're supposed to find the area of $DACD$ when you're given no lengths you can use for a base or an altitude. The only numbers you have are the angle measures. They must be there for some reason—the test makers rarely provide superfluous information. In fact, because the two angle measures provided add up to 180°, they tell you that *BE* and *CD* are parallel. And that, in turn, tells you that D*ABE* is similar to D*ACD*—because they have the same three angles.

Similar triangles are triangles that have the same shape: Corresponding angles are equal, and corresponding sides are proportional. In this case, because it's given that *AB* = *BC*, you know that *AC* is twice *AB* and that corresponding sides are in a ratio of 2:1. Each side of the larger triangle is twice the length of the corresponding side of the smaller triangle. That doesn't mean, however, that the ratio of the areas is also 2:1. In fact, the area ratio is the square of the side ratio, and the larger triangle has four times the area of the smaller triangle, so the answer is 4*x*.

THREE SPECIAL TRIANGLE TYPES

Three special triangle types deserve extra attention:

- Isosceles triangles
- Equilateral triangles
- Right triangles

Be sure you know not just the definitions of these triangle types but, more importantly, their special characteristics: side relationships, angle relationships, and area formulas.

Isosceles triangle: An isosceles triangle is a triangle that has two equal sides. Not only are two sides equal, but the angles opposite the equal sides, called *base angles*, are also equal.

Equilateral triangle: An equilateral triangle is a triangle that has three equal sides. Since all the sides are equal, all the angles are also equal. All three angles in an equilateral triangle measure 60 degrees, regardless of the lengths of the sides. You can find the area of an equilateral triangle by dividing it into two 30°-60°-90° triangles, or you can use this formula in terms of the length of one side *s*:

$$\textbf{Area of Equilateral Triangle} = \frac{s^2\sqrt{3}}{4}$$

Right triangle: A right triangle is a triangle with a right angle. The two sides that form the right angle are called *legs*, and you can use them as the base and height to find the area of a right triangle.

$$\textbf{Area of Right Triangle} = \frac{1}{2}(\text{leg}_1)(\text{leg}_2)$$

Pythagorean theorem: If you know any two sides of a right triangle, you can find the third side by using the Pythagorean theorem:

$$(\text{leg}_1)^2 + (\text{leg}_2)^2 = (\text{hypotenuse})^2$$

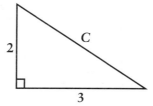

For example, if one leg is 2 and the other leg is 3, then

$$2^2 + 3^2 = c^2$$
$$c^2 = 4 + 9$$
$$c = \sqrt{13}$$

Pythagorean triplet: A Pythagorean triplet is a set of integers that fits the Pythagorean theorem. The simplest Pythagorean triplet is (3, 4, 5). In fact, any integers in a 3:4:5 ratio make up a Pythagorean triplet. And there are many other Pythagorean triplets: (5, 12, 13); (7, 24, 25); (8, 15, 17); (9, 40, 41); all their multiples; and infinitely many more.

3-4-5 triangle: If a right triangle's leg-to-leg ratio is 3:4, or if the leg-to-hypotenuse ratio is 3:5 or 4:5, then it's a 3-4-5 triangle, and you don't need to use the Pythagorean theorem to find the third side. Just figure out what multiple of 3-4-5 it is.

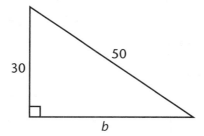

In the right triangle shown, one leg is 30 and the hypotenuse is 50. This is 10 times 3-4-5. The other leg b is 40.

5-12-13 triangles: If a right triangle's leg-to-leg ratio is 5:12, or if the leg-to-hypotenuse ratio is 5:13 or 12:13, then it's a 5-12-13 triangle and you don't need to use the Pythagorean theorem to find the third side. Just figure out what multiple of 5-12-13 it is.

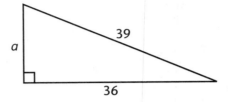

Here one leg is 36 and the hypotenuse is 39. This is 3 times 5-12-13. The other leg a is 3×5 or 15.

45°-45°-90° triangles: The sides of a 45°-45°-90° triangle are in a ratio of $1:1:\sqrt{2}$

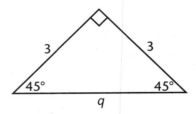

If one leg is 3, then the other leg is also 3, and the hypotenuse q is equal to a leg times $\sqrt{2}$, or $3\sqrt{2}$.

30°-60°-90° triangles: The sides of a 30°-60°-90° triangle are in a ratio of $1:\sqrt{3}:2$. You don't need to use the Pythagorean theorem.

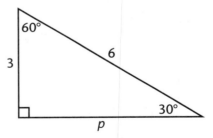

If the hypotenuse is 6, then the shorter leg is half that, or 3; and then the longer leg p is equal to the short leg times $\sqrt{3}$, or $3\sqrt{3}$.

Example:

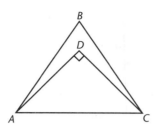

In the above figure, △*ABC* is equilateral and △*ADC* is isosceles. If *AC* = 1, what is the distance from *B* to *D*?

To get the answer to this question, you need to know about equilateral, 45°-45°-90°, and 30°-60°-90° triangles. If you drop an altitude from *B* through *D*, you will divide the equilateral triangle into two 30°-60°-90° triangles, and you will divide the right isosceles (or 45°-45°-90°) triangle into two smaller right isosceles triangles:

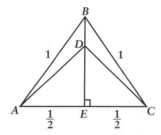

Using the side ratios for 30°-60°-90° and 45°-45°-90° triangles, you know that $BE = \dfrac{\sqrt{3}}{2}$ and that $DE = \dfrac{1}{2}$.

Therefore, $BD = BE - DE = \dfrac{\sqrt{3}}{2} - \dfrac{1}{2} = \dfrac{\sqrt{3}-1}{2}$.

HIDDEN SPECIAL TRIANGLES

It happens a lot that the key to solving a geometry problem is to add a line segment or two to the figure. Often what results is one or more special triangles.

KEY CONCEPT

Perpendiculars can be especially useful. They can function as rectangle sides or triangle altitudes or right triangle legs.

Example:

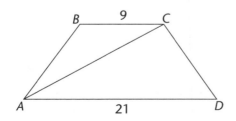

In the above figure, the perimeter of isosceles trapezoid *ABCD* is 50. If *BC* = 9 and *AD* = 21, what is the length of diagonal *AC*?

As you read the stem, you might wonder what an *isosceles trapezoid* is. If you'd never heard the term before, you still might have been able to extrapolate its meaning from what you know of isosceles triangles. *Isosceles* means "having two equal sides." When applied to a trapezoid, it tells you that the two nonparallel sides—the legs—are equal. In this case, that's *AB* and *CD*. If the total perimeter is 50, and the two marked sides add up to 21 + 9 = 30, then the two unmarked sides split the difference of 50 − 30 = 20. In other words, *AB* = *CD* = 10.

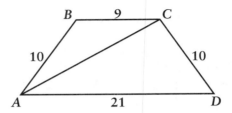

There aren't any special triangles yet. As so often happens, though, you can get some by constructing altitudes. Drop perpendiculars from points *B* and *C*, and you make two right triangles. The length 21 of side *AD* then gets split into 6, 9, and 6.

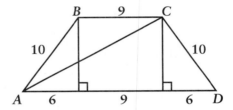

Now you can see that those right triangles are 3-4-5s (times 2) and that the height of the trapezoid is 8. Now look at the right triangle of which *AC* is the hypotenuse.

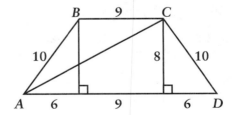

One leg is 6 + 9 = 15, and the other leg is 8; therefore, the hypotenuse *AC* is as follows:

$$\text{hypotenuse} = \sqrt{(\text{leg}_1)^2 + (\text{leg}_2)^2}$$
$$= \sqrt{15^2 + 8^2}$$
$$= \sqrt{225 + 64} = \sqrt{289} = 17$$

SPECIAL QUADRILATERALS

The trapezoid is just one of five special quadrilaterals you need to be familiar with. As with triangles, there is some overlap among these categories, and some figures fit into none of these categories. Just as a 45°-45°-90° triangle is both right and isosceles, a quadrilateral with four equal sides and four right angles is not only a square but also a rhombus, a rectangle, and a parallelogram. It is wise to have a solid grasp of the definitions and special characteristics of these five quadrilateral types.

A. Trapezoids

A trapezoid is a four-sided figure with one pair of parallel sides and one pair of nonparallel sides.

$$\text{Area of Trapezoid} = \left(\frac{\text{base}_1 + \text{base}_2}{2}\right) \times \text{height}$$

Think of this formula as the average of the bases (the two parallel sides) times the height (the length of the perpendicular altitude).

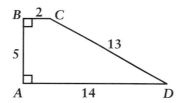

In the trapezoid *ABCD* above, you can use side *AB* for the height. The average of the bases is $\frac{2 + 14}{2} = 8$, so the area is 8 × 5, or 40.

B. Parallelograms

A parallelogram is a four-sided figure with two pairs of parallel sides. Opposite sides are equal. Opposite angles are equal. Consecutive angles add up to 180°.

Area of Parallelogram = base × height

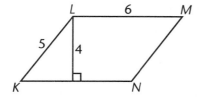

In parallelogram *KLMN* above, 4 is the height when *LM* or *KN* is used as the base. Base × height = 6 × 4 = 24.

Remember that to find the area of a parallelogram you need the height, which is the perpendicular distance from the base to the opposite side.

You can use a side of a parallelogram for the height only when the side is perpendicular to the base, in which case you have a rectangle.

C. Rectangles

A rectangle is a four-sided figure with four right angles. Opposite sides are equal. Diagonals are equal. The perimeter of a rectangle is equal to the sum of the lengths of the four sides, which is equal to 2(length + width).

Area of Rectangle = length × width

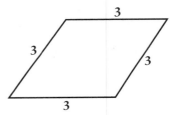

The area of a 7-by-3 rectangle is 7 × 3 = 21.

D. Rhombus

A rhombus is a four-sided figure with four equal sides.

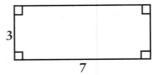

All four sides of the quadrilateral above have the same length, so it's a rhombus. A rhombus is also a parallelogram, so to find the area of a rhombus, you need its height. The more a rhombus "leans over," the smaller the height and, therefore, the smaller the area. The maximum area for a rhombus of a certain perimeter is a rhombus that has each pair of adjacent sides perpendicular, in which case you have a square.

E. Square

A square is a four-sided figure with four right angles and four equal sides. A square is also a rectangle, a parallelogram, and a rhombus. The perimeter of a square is equal to 4 times the length of one side.

$$\text{Area of Square} = (\text{side})^2$$

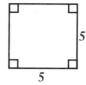

The square above, with sides of length 5, has an area of $5^2 = 25$.

POLYGONS—PERIMETER AND AREA

The test makers like to write problems that combine the concepts of perimeter and area. What you need to remember is that perimeter and area are not directly related. In the following example, for instance, you have two figures with the same perimeter, but that doesn't mean they have the same area.

Example: A square and a regular hexagon have the same perimeter. If the area of the square is 2.25, what is the area of the hexagon?

The way to get started with this question is to sketch what's described in the question. A square of area 2.25 has sides each of length $\sqrt{2.25} = 1.5$. So the perimeter of the square is $4(1.5) = 6$. Since that's also the perimeter of the regular hexagon, and a regular hexagon has six equal sides, the length of each side of the hexagon is 1.

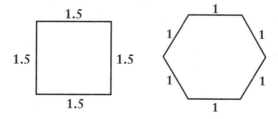

> **REMEMBER**
>
> The best way to get a handle on a figureless geometry problem is usually to sketch a figure of your own. You don't have to be an artist. Just be neat and clear enough to get the picture.

Now the problem is one of finding the area of a regular hexagon of side length 1. The fastest way to do that would be to use the formula, if you know it. If the length of one side is s,

$$\textbf{Area of Hexagon} = \frac{3s^2\sqrt{3}}{2}$$

This formula is not one the test makers expect you to know—there's always a way around it—but if you like formulas and you're good at memorizing them, it can only help. Let's proceed, however, as if we didn't know the formula. Another way to go about finding this area is to add a line segment or two to the figure and divide it up into more familiar shapes. You could, for example, draw in three diagonals and turn the hexagon into six equilateral triangles of side 1:

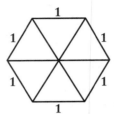

Each of those six triangles has base 1 and height $\dfrac{\sqrt{3}}{2}$, and therefore,

$$\textbf{Area of one triangle} = \frac{1}{2}(\text{base})(\text{height}) = \frac{1}{2}(1)\left(\frac{\sqrt{3}}{2}\right) = \frac{\sqrt{3}}{4}$$

The area of the hexagon is 6 times that.

$$\textbf{Area of Hexagon} = 6\left(\frac{\sqrt{3}}{4}\right) = \frac{3\sqrt{3}}{2} \approx 2.598.$$

CIRCLES—FOUR FORMULAS

After the triangle, the test makers' favorite plane geometry figure is the circle. Circles don't come in as many varieties as triangles do. In fact, all circles are similar—they're all the same shape. The only difference among them is size. So you don't have to learn to recognize types or remember names. All you have to know about circles is how to find four things:

- Circumference
- Length of an arc
- Area
- Area of a sector

You could think of the task as one of memorizing four formulas, but you'll be better off in the end if you have some idea of where the arc and sector formulas come from and how they are related to the circumference and area formulas.

A. Circumference

Circumference is a measurement of length. You could think of it as the perimeter: It's the total distance around the circle. If the radius of the circle is r,

$$\text{Circumference} = 2\pi r$$

Since the diameter is twice the radius, you can easily express the formula in terms of the diameter d:

$$\text{Circumference} = \pi d$$

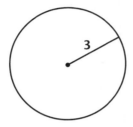

In the circle above, the radius is 3, so the circumference is $2\pi(3) = 6\pi$.

B. Length of an Arc

An **arc** is a piece of the circumference. If n is the degree measure of the arc's central angle, then the formula is

$$\text{Length of an Arc} = \left(\frac{n}{360}\right)(2\pi r)$$

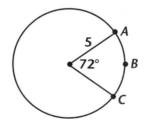

In the figure above, the radius is 5 and the measure of the central angle is 72°. The arc length is $\frac{72}{360}$ or $\frac{1}{5}$ of the circumference:

$$\left(\frac{72}{360}\right)(2\pi)(5) = \left(\frac{1}{5}\right)(10\pi) = 2\pi$$

C. Area

The area of a circle is usually found using this formula in terms of the radius r:

$$\text{Area of a Circle} = \pi r^2$$

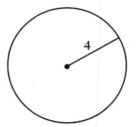

The area of the circle above is $\pi(4)^2 = 16\pi$.

D. Area of a Sector

A **sector** is a piece of the area of a circle. If n is the degree measure of the sector's central angle, then the area formula is

$$\textbf{Area of a Sector} = \left(\frac{n}{360}\right)(\pi r^2)$$

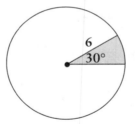

In the figure above, the radius is 6 and the measure of the sector's central angle is 30°. The sector has $\dfrac{30}{360}$ or $\dfrac{1}{12}$ of the area of the circle:

$$\left(\frac{30}{360}\right)(\pi)(6^2) = \left(\frac{1}{12}\right)(36\pi) = 3\pi$$

CIRCLES COMBINED WITH OTHER FIGURES

Some of the most challenging plane geometry questions are those that combine circles with other figures.

Example:

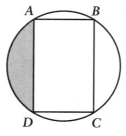

In the figure above, rectangle *ABCD* is inscribed in a circle. If the radius of the circle is 1 and *AB* = 1, what is the area of the shaded region?

Once again, the key here is to add to the figure. And in this case, as is so often the case when there's a circle, what you should add is radii. The equilateral triangles tell you that the central angles are 60° and 120°.

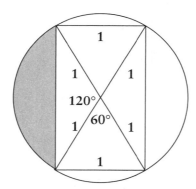

The shaded region is what's left of the 120° sector after you subtract the area of the triangle with the 120° vertex angle.

To find the area of the shaded region, you want to find the areas of the sector and triangle, then subtract. The sector is exactly one-third of the circle (because 120° is one-third of 360°), so

$$\text{Area of sector} = \frac{1}{3}\pi r^2 = \frac{1}{3}\pi(1)^2 = \frac{\pi}{3}$$

You can divide the triangle into two 30°-60°-90° triangles:

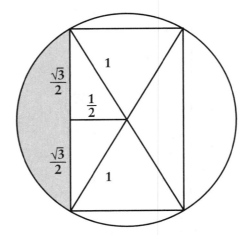

The area of each 30°-60°-90° triangle is $\frac{1}{2}\left(\frac{1}{2}\right)\left(\frac{\sqrt{3}}{2}\right) = \frac{\sqrt{3}}{8}$, so the area of the triangle with the 120° vertex is twice that, or $\frac{\sqrt{3}}{4}$.

The area of the shaded region is, therefore,

$$\frac{\pi}{3} - \frac{\sqrt{3}}{4}$$

4

Solid Geometry

FIVE FORMULAS

A. Lateral Area of a Cone

Given base circumference c and slant height ℓ,

$$\textbf{Lateral Area of Cone} = \frac{1}{2}c\ell$$

The **lateral area** of a cone is the area of the part that extends from the vertex to the circular base. It does not include the circular base.

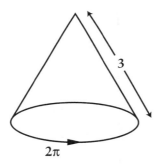

For example, in the figure above, $c = 2\pi$ and $\ell = 3$, so

$$\text{Lateral Area} = \frac{1}{2}(2\pi)(3) = 3\pi$$

B. Volume of a Cone

Given base radius r and height h,

$$\textbf{Volume of Cone} = \frac{1}{3}\pi r^2 h$$

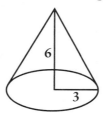

For example, in the figure on the previous page, $r = 3$ and $h = 6$, so

$$\text{Volume} = \frac{1}{3}\pi(3^2)(6) = 18\pi$$

C. Surface Area of a Sphere

Given radius r,

Surface Area of Sphere $= 4\pi r^2$

For example, if the radius of a sphere is 2, then

$$\text{Surface Area} = 4\pi(2^2) = 16\pi$$

D. Volume of a Sphere

Given radius r,

Volume of Sphere $= \dfrac{4}{3}\pi r^3$

For example, if the radius of a sphere is 2, then

$$\text{Volume} = \frac{4}{3}\pi(2)^3 = \frac{32\pi}{3}$$

E. Volume of a Pyramid

Given base area B and height h,

Volume of Pyramid $= \dfrac{1}{3}Bh$

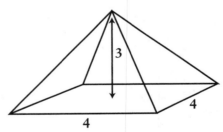

For example, in the figure above, $h = 3$, and if the base is a square, $B = 16$. Thus,

$$\text{Volume} = \frac{1}{3}(16)(3) = 16$$

Here's a question that uses some of these formulas.

Example: A right circular cone and a sphere have equal volumes. If the radius of the base of the cone is $2x$ and the radius of the sphere is $3x$, what is the height of the cone in terms of x?

As you can see, this question is hard enough even with the formulas provided. This is no mere matter of plugging values into a formula and cranking out the answer. This question is more algebraic than that and takes a little thought. It's really a word problem. It describes in words a mathematical situation (in this case, geometric) that can be translated into algebra. The pivot in this situation is that the cone and sphere have equal volumes. You're looking for the height h in terms of x, and fortunately you can express both volumes in terms of those two variables. Be careful. Both formulas include r, but they're not the same r's. In the case of the cone, $r = 2x$, but in the case of the sphere, $r = 3x$:

$$\text{Volume of cone} = \frac{1}{3}\pi r^2 h = \frac{1}{3}\pi(2x)^2 h = \frac{4}{3}\pi x^2 h$$

$$\text{Volume of sphere} = \frac{4}{3}\pi r^3 = \frac{4}{3}\pi(3x)^3 = 36\pi x^3$$

Now write an equation that says that the expressions for the two volumes are equal to each other and solve for h:

$$\frac{4}{3}\pi x^2 h = 36\pi x^3$$

$$\pi x^2 h = \frac{3}{4}(36\pi x^3)$$

$$\pi x^2 h = 27\pi x^3$$

$$h = \frac{27\pi x^3}{x^2\pi}$$

$$h = 27x$$

THE RECTANGULAR SOLID

The rectangular solid is the official geometric term for a *box*, which has 6 rectangular faces and 12 edges that meet at right angles at 8 vertices.

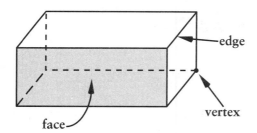

The surface area of a rectangular solid is simply the sum of the areas of the faces. That's what the formula **Surface Area = 2ℓw + 2wh + 2ℓh** says. If the length is ℓ, the width is w, and the height is h, then two rectangular faces have area ℓw, two have area wh, and two have area ℓh. The total surface area is the sum of those three pairs of areas.

Instead of the surface area, you may be asked to find the distance between opposite vertices of a rectangular solid.

Example:

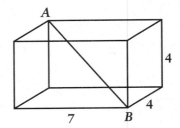

In the rectangular solid in the above figure, what is the distance from vertex *A* to vertex *B*?

One way to find this distance is to apply the Pythagorean theorem twice. First plug the dimensions of the base into the Pythagorean theorem to find the diagonal of the base:

$$\text{Diagonal of base} = \sqrt{4^2 + 7^2} = \sqrt{16 + 49} = \sqrt{65}$$

Notice that the base diagonal combines with an edge and with the segment *AB* you're looking for to form a right triangle:

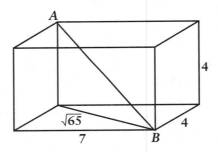

So you can plug the base diagonal and the height into the Pythagorean theorem to find *AB*:

$$AB = \sqrt{(\sqrt{65})^2 + 4^2} = \sqrt{65 + 16} = \sqrt{81} = 9$$

Another way to find this distance is to use the formula, which you could say is just the Pythagorean theorem taken to another dimension. If the length is ℓ, the width is w, and the height is h, the formula is

$$\text{Distance} = \sqrt{\ell^2 + w^2 + h^2}$$

UNIFORM SOLIDS

A rectangular solid is one type of *uniform solid*. A uniform solid is what you get when you take a plane and move it, without tilting it, through space. Here are some uniform solids.

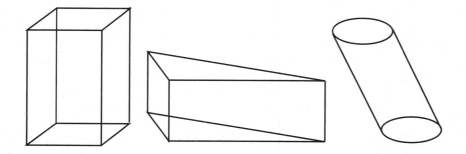

The way these solids are drawn, the top and bottom faces are parallel and congruent. These faces are called the *bases*. You can think of each of these solids as the result of sliding the base through space. The perpendicular distance through which the base slides is called the *height*.

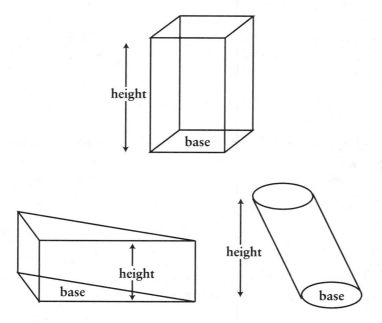

In every one of the above cases—indeed, in the case of *any* uniform solid—the volume is equal to the area of the base times the height. So you can say that for any uniform solid, given the area of the base *B* and the height *h*,

Volume of a Uniform Solid = *Bh*

Example:

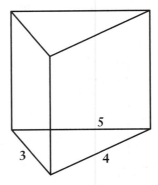

In the figure above, the bases of the right uniform solid are triangles with sides of lengths 3, 4, and 5. If the volume of the solid is 30, what is the total surface area?

The **surface area** is the sum of the areas of the faces. To find the areas of the faces, you need to figure out what kinds of polygons they are so that you'll know what formulas to use. Start with the bases, which are said to be "triangles with sides of lengths 3, 4, and 5." If side lengths don't ring a bell in your head, then you'd better go back and bone up on your special triangles. This is a 3-4-5 triangle, which means that it's a right triangle, which means that you can use the legs as the base and height to find the area:

$$\textbf{Area of Right Triangle} = \frac{1}{2}(\text{leg}_1)(\text{leg}_2) = \frac{1}{2}(3)(4) = 6$$

That's the area of each of the bases. The other three faces are rectangles. To find their areas, you need first to determine the height of the solid. If the area of the base is 6, and the volume is 30, then

$$\text{Volume} = Bh$$
$$30 = 6h$$
$$h = 5$$

So the areas of the three rectangular faces are $3 \times 5 = 15$, $4 \times 5 = 20$, and $5 \times 5 = 25$. The total surface area, then, is $6 + 6 + 15 + 20 + 25 = 72$.

A. Volume of a Rectangular Solid

A rectangular solid is a uniform solid whose base is a rectangle and whose height is perpendicular to its base. Given the length ℓ, width w, and height h, the area of the base is ℓw, so the volume formula is

Volume of a Rectangular Solid = ℓwh

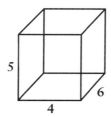

The volume of a 4-by-5-by-6 box is

$$4 \times 5 \times 6 = 120$$

B. Volume of a Cube

A cube is a rectangular solid with length, width, and height all equal. If e is the length of an edge of a cube, the volume formula is

Volume of a Cube = e^3

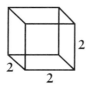

The volume of this cube is $2^3 = 8$.

C. Volume of a Cylinder

A cylinder is a uniform solid whose base is a circle. Given base radius r and height h, the area of the base is πr^2, so the volume formula is

Volume of a Cylinder = $\pi r^2 h$

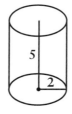

In the cylinder above, $r = 2$ and $h = 5$, so

$$\text{Volume} = \pi(2^2)(5) = 20\pi$$

5

Coordinate Geometry

MIDPOINTS AND DISTANCES

Some of the more basic coordinate geometry questions concern themselves with the layout of the grid, the location of points, distances between them, midpoints, and so on.

Example:

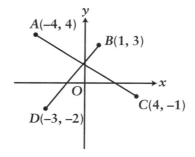

In the above figure, what is the distance from the midpoint of segment *AC* to the midpoint of segment *BD*?

To find the **midpoint** of a segment, average the *x-coordinates* and average the *y-coordinates* of the endpoints:

$$\text{midpoint of } AC = \left(\frac{-4 + 4}{2}, \frac{4 - 1}{2} \right) = (0, 1.5)$$

$$\text{midpoint of } BD = \left(\frac{-3 + 1}{2}, \frac{-2 + 3}{2} \right) = (-1, 0.5)$$

To find the distance between two points, use the distance formula:

$$\text{Distance} = \sqrt{(x_1 - x_2)^2 + (y_1 - y_2)^2}$$

The distance from (0, 1.5) to (–1, 0.5) is calculated as follows:

$$\text{Distance} = \sqrt{(-1 - 0)^2 + (0.5 - 1.5)^2}$$
$$= \sqrt{1 + 1}$$
$$= \sqrt{2}$$

SLOPE-INTERCEPT FORM

Slopes and intercepts are descriptions of lines and points on the grid, but the processes of finding and/or using slopes and/or intercepts are generally algebraic processes.

KEY CONCEPT

For any equation in the form
$y = mx + b$:

  m = slope
  b = y-intercept

Example: Which of the following lines has no point of intersection with the line $y = 4x + 5$?

(A) $y = \dfrac{1}{4}x - 5$

(B) $y = -\dfrac{1}{4}x - 5$

(C) $y = 4x + \dfrac{1}{5}$

(D) $y = -4x + \dfrac{1}{5}$

(E) $y = -4x - \dfrac{1}{5}$

What does *has no intersection with* mean? It means that the lines are parallel, which in turn means that the lines have the same slope. If you know the slope-intercept form, you're able to spot the correct answer instantly.

When an equation is in the form $y = mx + b$, the letter m represents the slope, and the letter b represents the y-intercept. The equation in the stem is $y = 4x + 5$. That's in slope-intercept form, so the coefficient of x is the slope.

$$y = \textcircled{4}x + 5$$
$$\text{slope} = 4$$

Now look for the answer choice with the same slope. Conveniently, all the answer choices are presented in slope-intercept form, so spotting the one with $m = 4$ is a snap. It's (C):

$$y = \textcircled{4}x + \dfrac{1}{5}$$
$$\text{slope} = 4$$

People who are good at memorizing methods and formulas are not necessarily the ones who get the best scores; instead it's the people who have a deeper understanding of mathematics. If you really want to ace coordinate geometry questions, it's not enough to memorize the midpoint formula, the distance formula, the slope definition, the slope-intercept equation form, and so on. What you want is to have a real grasp of what slope is and what perpendicular, parallel, positive, negative, zero, and undefined slopes tell you.

Slope is a description of the "steepness" of a line. Lines that go uphill (from left to right) have positive slopes:

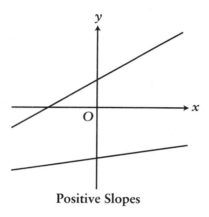

Positive Slopes

Lines that go downhill have negative slopes:

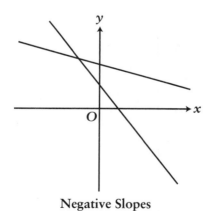

Negative Slopes

KEY CONCEPT

Lines that go uphill from left to right have positive slopes. The steeper the uphill grade, the greater the slope.

Lines that go downhill from left to right have negative slopes. The steeper the downhill grade, the less the slope.

Lines parallel to the *x*-axis have slope = 0, and lines parallel to the *y*-axis have *undefined slope.*

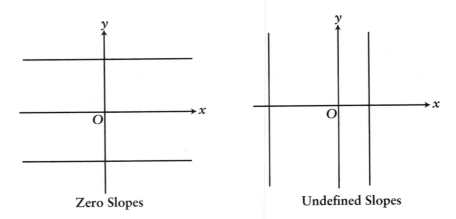

Zero Slopes   Undefined Slopes

Lines that are parallel to each other have the same slope, and lines that are perpendicular to each other have *negative-reciprocal slopes.*

In the figure below, the two parallel lines both have slope = 2, and the line that's perpendicular to them has slope = $-\frac{1}{2}$:

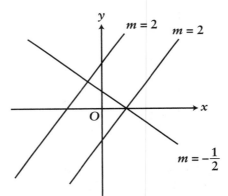

Parallel and Perpendicular Lines

ABSOLUTE VALUE AND INEQUALITIES

Example: Which of the following shaded regions shows the graph of the inequality $y \leq |x + 2|$?

(A)

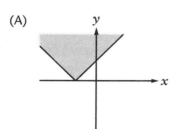

(B)

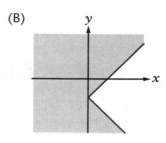

(C)

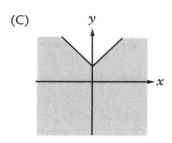

(D)

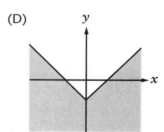

(E)

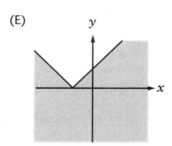

The way to handle an inequality is to think of it as an equation first, plot the line, and then figure out which side of the line to shade. This inequality is extra complicated because of the absolute value. When you graph an equation with an absolute value, you generally get a line with a bend, as in all of the answer choices above. To find the graph of an absolute value equation, figure out where that bend is. In this case, $|x + 2|$ has a turning-point value of 0, which happens when $x = -2$. So the bend is at the point $(-2, 0)$. That narrows the choices down to (A) and (E).

Next, figure out which side gets shaded. Pick a convenient point on either side and see if that point's coordinates fit the given inequality. The point $(0, 0)$ is an easy one to work with. Do those coordinates satisfy the inequality?

$$y \le x + 2$$

$$0 \overset{?}{\le} 0 + 2$$

$$0 \overset{?}{\le} 2 \quad \text{Yes.}$$

The point (0, 0) must be on the shady side of the bent line. The answer is (E).

6

Trigonometry

RIGHT TRIANGLES AND SOH-CAH-TOA

Trigonometry is really all about right triangles—and we're concerned not with the right angle, per se, but with one of the *other angles*, denoted by the θ in the figure below. The **sine** of angle θ is simply the length of the side opposite the angle divided by the length of the hypotenuse (the **hypotenuse** is the side opposite the right angle). The mathematical abbreviation for sine is "sin," and in mathematics, the sine of the angle θ is written sin θ.

The **cosine** is simply the length of the side adjacent to angle θ (actually, there will be two sides adjacent to the angle, but one of those sides will be the hypotenuse, so by *adjacent*, we really mean the side adjacent to angle that is NOT the hypotenuse) divided by the length of the hypotenuse. The mathematical abbreviation for cosine is "cos," and in mathematics, the cosine of the angle θ is written cos θ.

Finally, the **tangent** of angle is the length of the opposite side over the length of the adjacent side. The mathematical abbreviation for tangent is "tan," and in mathematics, the tangent of the angle is written tan θ.

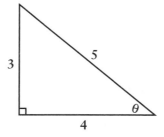

So for instance, in the figure above, the sine of angle θ, sin θ, is the length of the side opposite angle θ (3) divided by the length of the hypotenuse (5). So the sine is 0.60. That is, sin θ = 0.60.

The cosine of angle θ is the length of the side adjacent to angle θ (4) divided by the length of the hypotenuse (5). So the cosine of angle θ is 0.80, or cos θ = 0.80.

Finally, the tangent is the length of the side opposite angle θ (3) divided by the length of the side adjacent to angle θ (4). So the tangent of angle θ is 0.75, or tan θ = 0.75. To help you remember the definitions of sine, cosine, and tangent as they apply to right triangles, use the mnemonic **SOHCAHTOA** (the first letters of each of the words below).

$$\text{Sine} = \frac{\text{Opposite}}{\text{Hypotenuse}} \qquad \text{Cosine} = \frac{\text{Adjacent}}{\text{Hypotenuse}} \qquad \text{Tangent} = \frac{\text{Opposite}}{\text{Adjacent}}$$

We can also use this information to help us figure out the lengths of sides of triangles.

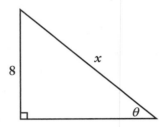

Example: In the right triangle above, if the sine of angle θ = 0.5, what is the value of x?

The angle is opposite the given side, and the side you're looking for is the hypotenuse, so you can use the sine formula to find x:

$$\sin \theta = \frac{\text{Opposite}}{\text{Hypotenuse}}$$

$$0.5 = \frac{8}{x}$$

$$x = \frac{8}{0.5}$$

$$x = 16$$

There are three other trig functions you should be aware of—and each is the *reciprocal* of one of the trig functions introduced above. They are called **cotangent**, **secant**, and **cosecant**.

$$\text{Cotangent} = \frac{\text{Adjacent}}{\text{Opposite}} \qquad \text{Secant} = \frac{\text{Hypotenuse}}{\text{Adjacent}} \qquad \text{Cosecant} = \frac{\text{Hypotenuse}}{\text{Opposite}}$$

The mathematical abbreviation for cotangent is "cot," and in mathematics, the cotangent of the angle θ is written cot θ. The mathematical abbreviation for secant is "sec," and in math, the secant of the angle θ is written sec θ. The mathematical abbreviation for cosecant is "csc," and in math, the cosecant of the angle θ is written csc θ.

There are also three identities that you should probably be aware of:

$$\sin^2 x + \cos^2 x = 1$$
$$\tan^2 x + 1 = \sec^2 x$$
$$1 + \cot^2 x = \csc^2 x$$

So for any angle x, you could take the sine and cosine, square them both, and the squares will add up to 1. These relationships are really just restatements of the Pythagorean theorem. To make it easier for you to remember them, the proof of the first identity is presented below, but you certainly don't need to know the proof.

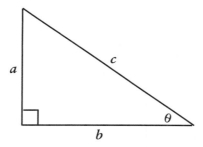

The Pythagorean theorem says that in a right triangle, the square of the hypotenuse is equal to the sum of the squares of the legs. In the right triangle in the figure above, $c^2 = a^2 + b^2$. Let's write this as $a^2 + b^2 = c^2$. Now divide both sides of this equation by c^2. Then $\dfrac{a^2 + b^2}{c^2} = \dfrac{c^2}{c^2}$, $\dfrac{a^2}{c^2} + \dfrac{b^2}{c^2} = 1$, and $\left(\dfrac{a}{c}\right)^2 + \left(\dfrac{b}{c}\right)^2 = 1$. Now $\dfrac{a}{c} = \sin\theta$ and $\dfrac{b}{c} = \cos\theta$. So $\sin^2\theta + \cos^2\theta = 1$.

The identity $\tan^2 x + 1 = \sec^2 x$ is proved by dividing both sides of the equation $a^2 + b^2 = c^2$ by b^2, and the identity $1 + \cot^2 x = \csc^2 x$ is proved by dividing both sides of the equation $a^2 + b^2 = c^2$ by a^2.

Example: Simplify $5\sin^2 x + 5\cos^2 x$.

When you spot a trigonometric expression where quantities are being squared, as in $5\sin^2 x + 5\cos^2 x$, you should think immediately about how to extract $\sin^2 x + \cos^2 x$ from it. You do that by factoring out a 5:

$$5\sin^2 x + 5\cos^2 x = 5(\sin^2 x + \cos x)$$
$$= 5(1)$$
$$= 5$$

DEGREE MEASURE AND RADIAN MEASURE

By definition, if you go all the way around a circle, you have traveled 360 degrees. The **degree** is a unit of measure for describing angles. An angle that is 1 degree is $\dfrac{1}{360}$ of a complete circle.

The **radian** is another measure used to describe an angle and is often used in trigonometry.

The word *radian* is related to the word *radius*. Before we define *radian*, let's repeat the definition of a central angle of a circle. In a circle, a **central angle** is the angle formed by two radii of the circle.

If a central angle of a circle intercepts an arc of a circle with length ℓ, then the number of radians in the central angle that contains this arc is $\frac{\ell}{r}$.

If a central angle in a circle intercepts an arc equal in length to 1 radius of a circle, that central angle has a radian measure of 1. So an angle can be described by its degree measure or by its radian measure. The circumference C of a circle is related to its radius r by the formula $C = 2\pi r$. So the number of radians in the circumference of any circle is 2π because there are precisely 2π radii in the length of the circumference of any circle. However, there are also 360 degrees in any full circle, so 2π radians is equal to 360 degrees.

Therefore 1 radian is equal to $\frac{360}{2\pi} = \frac{180}{\pi}$ degrees. $\frac{180}{\pi}$ is approximately 57.3.

So 1 radian is approximately 57.3 degrees. You are probably best off if you remember that 2π radians is equal to 360 degrees. Then you can work with this to convert from some other given number of degrees to the corresponding number of radians, or you can convert from the number of radians to the corresponding number of degrees. (You may also remember that π radians is equal to 180 degrees and do your converting based on this, if you are more comfortable doing so.)

Example: How many degrees are there in $\frac{5\pi}{6}$ radians?

Let x be the number of degrees. Then $\dfrac{x}{\left(\frac{5\pi}{6}\right)} = \dfrac{360}{2\pi}$.

So $x = \dfrac{5\pi}{6} \times \dfrac{360}{2\pi} = \dfrac{5}{6} \times \dfrac{360}{2} = \dfrac{5}{1} \times \dfrac{60}{2} = 5 \times 30 = 150$.

So there are 150 degrees in $\frac{5\pi}{6}$ radians.

Example: How many radians are there in 270 degrees?

Let y be the number of radians. Then $\dfrac{y}{270} = \dfrac{2\pi}{360}$. So $y = 270 \times \dfrac{2\pi}{360} = \dfrac{\pi}{2} = \dfrac{3\pi}{2}$. There are $\frac{3\pi}{2}$ radians in 270 degrees.

Notice that in the first example, we set up our equation so that we had the number of degrees in the numerator and the number of radians in the denominator, while in the second example, our equation had the number of radians in the numerator and the number of degrees in the denominator.

This is just a matter of setting up an equation so that might be a little easier to work with. It seemed easier to begin with the unknown in the numerator in each case. What's really important is that you set up your equation correctly. Then if you can, try to work with an equation that's a little easier.

TRIGONOMETRIC FUNCTIONS OF OTHER ANGLES

To find a trigonometric function of an angle greater than or equal to 90°, sketch a circle of radius *r* and centered at the origin of the coordinate grid. Start from the point (*r*, 0) and rotate the appropriate number of degrees *θ* counterclockwise.

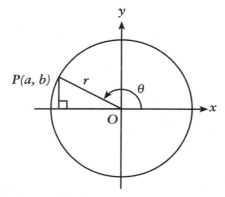

In this "circle setup," the basic trigonometric functions are defined in terms of the coordinates *a* and *b*:

$$\sin \theta = \frac{b}{r}$$

$$\cos \theta = \frac{a}{r}$$

$$\tan \theta = \frac{b}{a}$$

$$\cot \theta = \frac{a}{b}$$

$$\sec \theta = \frac{r}{a}$$

$$\csc \theta = \frac{r}{b}$$

Notice that tan and sec are undefined if *a* = 0 and cot and csc are undefined if *b* = 0. Notice also that you are working with a right triangle whose hypotenuse is a radius of the circle. One of the legs of this right triangle is on the part of the *x*-axis that is closest to the hypotenuse (which is the rotated radius).

Example: sin 210° = ?

Setup: Sketch a 210° angle in the coordinate plane:

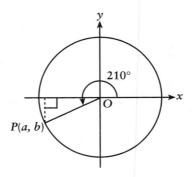

Because the triangle shown in the figure above is a 30°-60°-90° right triangle whose side lengths are in the ratio of 1:$\sqrt{3}$:2, it is convenient to use a radius of 2. The coordinates of point P are (–$\sqrt{3}$, –1).

Therefore $b = -1$, $r = 2$, and $\sin 210° = \dfrac{b}{r} = \dfrac{-1}{2} = -\dfrac{1}{2}$.

THE GRAPHS OF $Y = \text{SIN } X$, $Y = \text{COS } X$, AND $Y = \text{TAN } X$

The graph of $y = \sin x$ repeats itself every interval of length 360 degrees (or 2π radians). When $0 \le x \le 90°$, sin x increases from 0 (when $x = 0°$) to 1 (when $x = 90°$). When $90 \le x \le 180°$, sin x decreases from 1 (when $x = 90°$) to 0 (when $x = 180°$). When $180 \le x \le 270°$, sin x decreases from 0 (when $x = 180°$) to –1 (when $x = 270°$). When $270 \le x \le 360°$, sin x increases from –1 (when $x = 270°$) to 0 (when $x = 360°$). Right after 360°, sin x begins another cycle. Sin x increases from 0 to 1 (in the interval $360° \le x \le 450°$), then decreases from 1 to 0 (in the interval $450° \le x \le 540°$), then continues to decrease from 0 to –1 (interval $540° \le x \le 630°$), and then increases from –1 to 0 (in the interval $630° \le x \le 720°$). This graph also repeats its cycle for values of x less than 0°.

This is the graph of $y = \sin x$.

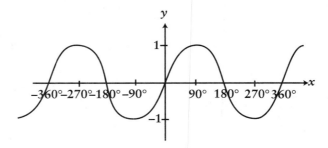

The graph of $y = \cos x$ also repeats itself every 360 degrees or 2π radians. It begins at 1 when $x = 0°$, and in the interval $0 \le x \le 90°$, it decreases from 1 to 0. When $90° \le x \le 180°$, $\cos x$ continues its decrease from 0 when $x = 90°$ to -1 when $x = 180°$. When $180 \le x \le 270°$, $\cos x$ increases from -1 when $x = 180°$ to 0 when $x = 270°$. When $270 \le x \le 360°$, $\cos x$ increases from 0 when $x = 270°$ to 1 when $x = 360°$. Then, for $360° \le x \le 720°$, the graph repeats itself again with one more complete cycle in the interval $360° \le x \le 720°$.

This is the graph of $y = \cos x$.

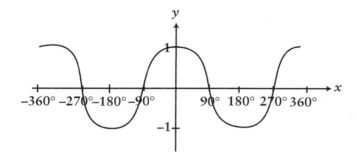

The graph of $y = \tan x$ repeats itself every $180°$, which is unlike the graphs of $y = \sin x$ and $y = \cos x$, which repeat themselves every $360°$. This is because $\tan x$ is positive for $0° < x < 90°$, $\tan x$ is negative for $90° < x < 180°$, $\tan x$ is positive again for $180° < x < 270°$, and $\tan x$ is negative again for $270° < x < 360°$.

Notice that $\tan x$ is undefined for every odd multiple of $90°$ or $\frac{\pi}{2}$. Thus, $\tan x$ is undefined when x is any of..., $-630°$, $-450°$, $-270°$, $-90°$, $90°$, $270°$, $450°$, $630°$, ..., or in terms of radians, $\tan x$ is undefined when x is any of..., $-\frac{7\pi}{2}$, $-\frac{5\pi}{2}$, $\frac{-3\pi}{2}$, $\frac{-\pi}{2}$, $\frac{\pi}{2}$, $\frac{3\pi}{2}$, $\frac{5\pi}{2}$, $\frac{7\pi}{2}$,....

When $-90° < x < 0°$, $\tan x$ is negative, and $\tan x$ increases from negative numbers with very large absolute values when x is near but greater than $-90°$ to negative values with small absolute values when x is near but less than $0°$. So in the interval $-90° < x < 0°$, $\tan x$ is increasing. When $x = 0°$, $\tan x = 0$. When $0 < x < 90°$, $\tan x$ continues to increase from positive values that have a small absolute value for values of x that are near but greater than $0°$ to positive values that have a large absolute value for values of x that are close to but less than $90°$. The graph of $y = \tan x$ in the interval $-90° < x < 90°$ is repeated in the interval $90° < x < 270°$.

In trigonometry, scales are often given in terms of radians. The x-axis of the graph of $y = \tan x$ will be labeled with radians, unlike the graphs of $y = \sin x$ and $y = \cos x$, which had their x-axes labeled with degrees.

This is the graph of $y = \tan x$.

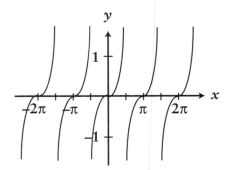

It can be seen from the graph above that when x approaches $\frac{\pi}{2}$ through values of x that are greater than $\frac{\pi}{2}$, $y = \tan x$ approaches negative infinity. When x approaches $\frac{\pi}{2}$ through values of x that are less than $\frac{\pi}{2}$, $y = \tan x$ approaches positive infinity. This can be seen on the graph of $y = \tan x$ above.

PERIODIC FUNCTIONS

A **function** f is a set of instructions that associates each number of a set A (which is called the **domain**) with a number in a set B (which is called the **range**). Often the domain and/or the range are not specified. What is important is that you just follow the instructions: For each given number, use the function to find the number associated with it.

If x is a point of the domain, then $f(x)$ is the number associated with x by the function f. Notice the difference between f and $f(x)$. f refers to the entire process of using the instructions to associate numbers with other numbers, while $f(x)$ means the exact number that the function f associates with the number x. So $f(x)$ is a number for any specified x. (While f is probably the most common, other letters such as g, h, and r may all be used to denote functions.)

The trigonometric function $\sin x$ repeats itself every 360°. For example, $\sin 30°$ equals $\sin 390°$; both of these equal $\frac{1}{2}$.

Let R be a positive constant. If f is a function such that $f(x) = f(x + R)$ for all x, and R is the smallest positive number for which this is true, then the function is said to be periodic with period R. Notice that for the function f defined by $f(x) = \sin x$, $\sin (x + 2\pi) = \sin x$ for all x. Because 2π is the smallest possible positive value for R for which $\sin (x + R) = \sin x$ for all x, 2π is the period of $\sin x$. While it is also true that $\sin (x + 4\pi) = \sin x$ for all x, 4π is not the smallest possible positive value for R such that $\sin (x + R) = \sin x$ for all x. So even though for any x, $\sin x$ does have the same value at $x + 4\pi$ that is has at x, we would not say that the period of $f(x) = \sin x$ is 4π. Again, the period of $\sin x$ is 2π.

THE INVERSE SINE FUNCTION AND THE INVERSE TANGENT FUNCTION

By the inverse sine function of x, which is denoted by arcsin x, or $\sin^{-1}x$, it is meant that angle y is such that $\sin y = x$ and $-90° \le y \le 90°$. Because $-1 \le \sin y \le 1$, the inverse sine function cannot be defined for values of x such that $x < -1$ or $x > 1$. Therefore, the inverse sine function of x is defined only for x such that $-1 \le x \le 1$.

For example, $\arcsin\left(\dfrac{1}{2}\right) = \sin^{-1}\left(\dfrac{1}{2}\right) = 30°$ because $\sin 30° = \dfrac{1}{2}$ and $30°$ is in the interval $-90° \le y \le 90°$.

The reason that for a given x, the value of $\sin^{-1} x$ is defined to be in the interval $-90° \le y \le 90°$ is that for a given x, there are infinitely many y such that $\sin y = x$, and a function must associate exactly one number with each number in the domain.

For example, look at $\sin^{-1}\left(\dfrac{1}{2}\right)$ again. It is true that..., $\sin(-570°) = \dfrac{1}{2}$, $\sin(-330°) = \dfrac{1}{2}$, $\sin(-210°) = \dfrac{1}{2}$, $\sin 30° = \dfrac{1}{2}$, $\sin 150° = \dfrac{1}{2}$, $\sin 390° = \dfrac{1}{2}$, $\sin 510° = \dfrac{1}{2}$, $\sin 750° = \dfrac{1}{2}$,.... To be able to assign a unique value to $\sin^{-1}\left(\dfrac{1}{2}\right)$, the requirement that the angle be in the interval $-90° \le y \le 90°$ is included.

By the inverse tangent function of x, which is denoted by arctan x, or $\tan^{-1} x$, it is meant that angle y is such that $-90° < y < 90°$ and $\tan y = x$. The inverse tangent function is defined for all real x. For example, $\arctan(-1) = \tan^{-1}(-1) = -45°$ because $-45°$ is in the interval $-90° < y < 90°$ and $\tan(-45°) = -1$.

The reason that for a given x the value of $\tan^{-1} x$ is defined to be in the interval $-90° < y < 90°$ is that for any given real number x, there are infinitely many values of y such that $\tan y = x$ and a function must associate exactly one number with each number in the domain. For example, look at $\tan^{-1}(-1)$ again. It is true that $\tan(-765°) = -1$, $\tan(-585°) = -1$, $\tan(-405°) = -1$, $\tan(-225°) = -1$, $\tan(-45°) = -1$, $\tan(135°) = -1$, $\tan 315° = -1$, $\tan 495° = -1$, $\tan 675° = -1$,.... To be able to assign a unique value to $\tan^{-1}(-1)$, the requirement that the angle be in the interval $-90° < y < 90°$ is included.

Notice that the possible values of the inverse sine function are in the interval $-90° \le y \le 90°$, while the possible values of the inverse tangent function are in the interval $-90° < y < 90°$. The values of $-90°$ and $90°$ are not possible values of the inverse tangent function because $\tan 90°$ and $\tan(-90°)$ are both undefined.

Example: Which of the following is equal to $\tan\left(\sin^{-1}\left(\dfrac{7}{\sqrt{74}}\right)\right)$?

(A) $\dfrac{\sqrt{74}}{7}$ (B) $\dfrac{5}{\sqrt{74}}$ (C) $\dfrac{5}{7}$ (D) $\dfrac{7}{\sqrt{74}}$ (E) $\dfrac{7}{5}$

We want to find the tangent of a certain angle. That angle is $\sin^{-1}\left(\dfrac{7}{\sqrt{74}}\right)$. Call $\sin^{-1}\left(\dfrac{7}{\sqrt{74}}\right)$ the angle y. Then $\sin y = \dfrac{7}{\sqrt{74}}$. Remember that in a right triangle, the sine of an angle is equal to the length of the leg opposite that angle divided by the length of the hypotenuse. So draw yourself a picture of a right triangle with an angle y whose sine is $\dfrac{7}{\sqrt{74}}$:

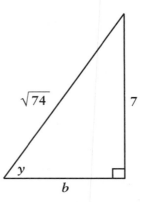

If we can find the length of b, we can find $\tan\left(\sin^{-1}\left(\dfrac{7}{\sqrt{74}}\right)\right) = \tan y$ by remembering that in a right triangle, the tangent of an angle is equal to the length of the leg opposite that angle divided by the length of the leg adjacent to that angle. The length b of the other leg can be found by using the Pythagorean theorem, which says that in a right triangle, the square of the hypotenuse is equal to the sum of the squares of the legs. Here,

$$7^2 + b^2 = (\sqrt{74})^2$$
$$49 + b^2 = 74$$
$$b^2 = 25$$
$$b = 5$$

(By the way, $b = -5$ is also a solution of the equation $b^2 = 25$, but here we're concerned with lengths and you can't have a negative length, so $b = -5$ is a solution of the equation $b^2 = 25$ that does not apply here.)

So $b = 5$, and now we can find $\tan y$: $\tan y = \tan\left(\sin^{-1}\left(\dfrac{7}{\sqrt{74}}\right)\right) = \dfrac{7}{5}$, and choice (E) is correct.

BIOLOGY

The Basis of Life

ORIGIN OF LIFE

A. The Heterotroph Hypothesis

The first forms of life lacked the ability to synthesize their own nutrients; they required preformed molecules for sustenance. These "organisms" were **heterotrophs**, which means they depended upon outside sources for food. The primitive seas contained **simple inorganic** and **organic** compounds such as salts, methane, ammonia, hydrogen, and water. **Energy** was present in the form of **heat, electricity, solar radiation** (including **X-rays** and **ultraviolet light**), **cosmic rays**, and **radioactivity**.

The presence of these building blocks and energy may have led to the synthesis of simple organic molecules such as sugars, amino acids, and nucleotides like purines and pyrimidines. These molecules dissolved in the "**primordial soup**," and after many years, the simple monomeric molecules combined to form a supply of macromolecules.

1. EVIDENCE OF ORGANIC SYNTHESIS

In 1953, **Stanley L. Miller** set out to demonstrate that the application of ultraviolet radiation, heat, or a combination of these to a mixture of methane, hydrogen, ammonia, and water could result in the formation of complex organic compounds. Miller set up an apparatus in which the four gases were continuously circulated past electrical discharges from tungsten electrodes.

After circulation of the gases for one week, Miller analyzed the liquid in the apparatus and found that an amazing variety of organic compounds, including **urea, hydrogen cyanide, acetic acid,** and **lactic acid**, had been synthesized.

2. FORMATION OF PRIMITIVE CELLS

Colloidal protein molecules tend to clump together to form **coacervate droplets** (a cluster of colloidal molecules surrounded by a shell of water). These droplets tend to **absorb** and incorporate substances from the surrounding environment. In addition, the droplets tend to possess a definite internal structure. It is highly likely that such droplets developed on the early earth. Although these coacervate droplets were not living, they did possess some properties normally associated with living organisms, such as the ability to selectively metabolize material.

Most of these systems were **unstable**; however, a few systems may have arisen that were **stable** enough to survive. A small percentage of the droplets possessing favorable characteristics eventually developed into the first primitive cells. These first primitive cells probably possessed **nucleic acid polymers** and became capable of reproduction.

B. Development of Autotrophs

The primitive heterotrophs slowly evolved complex **biochemical pathways**, which enabled them to use a wider variety of nutrients. They evolved **anaerobic respiratory processes** to convert these nutrients into energy. However, these organisms required nutrients at a faster rate than they were being synthesized. Life would have ceased to exist if **autotrophic nutrition** had not developed. The pioneer autotrophs (organisms capable of producing some of their own nutrients) developed primitive **photosynthetic** pathways, capturing solar energy and using it to synthesize carbohydrates from carbon dioxide and water.

C. Development of Aerobic Respiration

The primitive autotrophs fixed **carbon dioxide** during the synthesis of carbohydrates and released molecular oxygen as a waste product. The addition of molecular oxygen to the atmosphere converted the atmosphere from a **reducing** to an **oxidizing** one. Some molecular oxygen was converted to ozone, which functions in the atmosphere to block high-energy radiation. In this way, living organisms **destroyed** the conditions that made their development possible. Once molecular oxygen became a major component of the earth's atmosphere, both heterotrophs and autotrophs evolved the biochemical pathways of aerobic respiration necessary to convert nutrients into energy using oxygen.

D. General Categories of Living Organisms

All living organisms can be divided into four basic categories. The **autotrophic anaerobes** include chemosynthetic bacteria. The **autotrophic aerobes** include the green plants and photoplankton. The **heterotrophic anaerobes** include yeasts. The **heterotrophic aerobes** include amoebas, earthworms, and humans.

BIOCHEMISTRY

Despite the uncertainties concerning the origin of life, it is well known that all living organisms share important characteristics. All living things are composed primarily of the elements carbon, hydrogen, oxygen, nitrogen, sulfur, and phosphorus. Traces of magnesium, iodine, iron, calcium, and other minerals are also components of **protoplasm**, the substance of life.

The unit of an element is the atom. The unit of a compound is the **molecule**. **Atoms** are joined by chemical bonds to form **molecules**. Water (H_2O), carbon dioxide (CO_2), and glucose ($C_6H_{12}O_6$) are some familiar molecules.

The chemical compounds in living matter can be divided into inorganic and organic compounds. **Inorganic compounds** are compounds that do not contain the element carbon, including salts and HCl. **Organic compounds** are made by living systems and contain carbon. They include carbohydrates, lipids, proteins, and nucleic acids.

In addition, various processes are required to maintain an organism's internal environment and regulate the basic activities of life. In this chapter and beyond, you will see how heredity, cellular organization, growth, development, reproduction, regulation, and homeostasis control the acquisition, conversion, and some of the uses of energy by a living organism.

A. Carbohydrates

Carbohydrates are composed of the elements carbon, hydrogen, and oxygen in a 1:2:1 ratio, respectively. They are used as storage forms of energy or as structural molecules. For example, glucose and glycogen store energy in animals while starch stores energy in plants. The test may require you to recognize the following types of carbohydrates but you do not need to memorize their structure.

1. MONOSACCHARIDE

Monosaccharides like glucose and fructose are single sugar subunits.

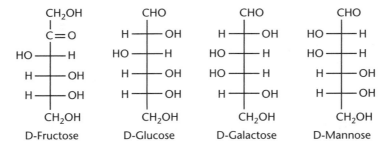

Figure 1.1

You should also recognize glucose, $C_6H_{12}O_6$, as a hexagonal structure with a 6 carbon ring and with an H and OH bonded to each carbon.

2. DISACCHARIDE

Disaccharides like maltose and sucrose are composed of two mono-saccharide subunits joined by **dehydration synthesis**, a reaction that involves the loss of a water molecule.

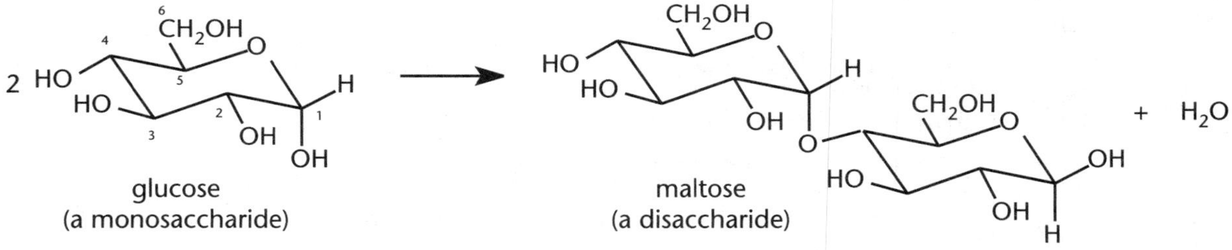

glucose
(a monosaccharide)

maltose
(a disaccharide)

$+ \quad H_2O$

Figure 1.2

3. POLYSACCHARIDE

Polysaccharides are **polymers** or chains of repeating monosaccharide subunits. Both glycogen and starch are polysaccharides. Cellulose is a polysaccharide that serves a structural role in plants. These poly-saccharides are insoluble in water.

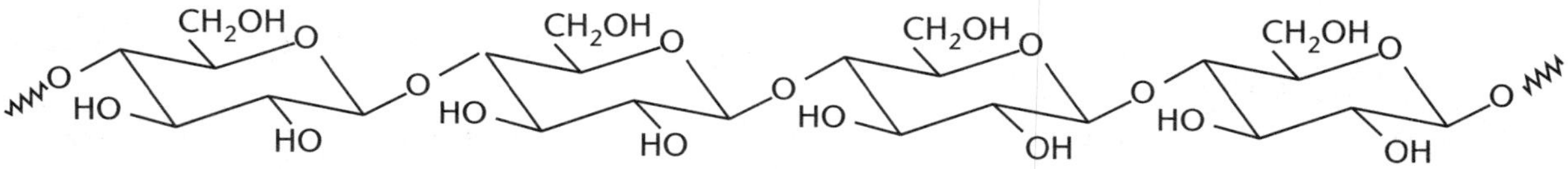

Cellulose, a 1,4´-β-D-Glucose polymer

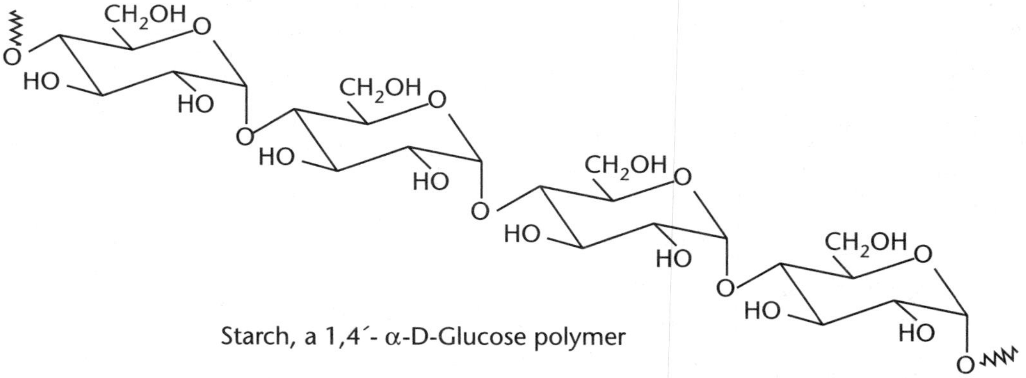

Starch, a 1,4´- α-D-Glucose polymer

Figure 1.3

4. DEHYDRATION AND HYDROLYSIS

Polysaccharides are formed by removing water (**dehydration**) from the molecule. By contrast, adding water to large polymers breaks them down into smaller subunits in a process called **hydrolysis**.

B. Lipids (Fats and Oils)

Like carbohydrates, lipids are also composed of C,H, and O but their H:O ratio is much greater than 2:1 as they have much more H than O. A lipid consists of **three fatty acid** molecules bonded to a single **glycerol** backbone. Fatty acids have long carbon side chains (–R groups) that give them their hydrophobic (fatty) character, and carboxylic acid groups that make them acidic. Three dehydration reactions are needed to form one fat molecule. Lipids do not form polymers.

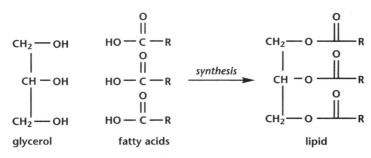

Figure 1.4

1. LIPID DERIVATIVES

Lipids are the chief means of food storage in animals. They release more energy per gram weight than any other class of biological compounds. They also provide insulation and protection against injury since they are a major component of fatty (**adipose**) tissue. Lipid derivatives are:

a. Phospholipids

Phospholipids contain glycerol, two fatty acids, a phosphate group, and a nitrogen containing alcohol, e.g., lecithin (a major constituent of cell membranes) and cephalin (found in brain, nerves, and neural tissue).

b. Waxes

Waxes are esters of fatty acids and monohydroxylic alcohols. They are found as protective coatings on skin, fur, leaves of higher plants, and on the exoskeleton of many insects (e.g., lanolin).

c. Steroids

All steroids have three fused cyclochexane rings and one fused cyclopentane ring. They include **cholesterol**, the **sex hormones** testosterone and estrogen, and **corticosteroids**.

d. Carotenoids

These are fatty acid-like carbon chains containing conjugated double bonds and carrying six-membered carbon rings at each end. These compounds are the **pigments** that produce red, yellow, orange, and brown colors in plants and animals. Two subgroups are the **carotenes** and the **xanthophylls**.

e. Porphyrins

Porphyrins, also called tetrapyrroles, contain four joined **pyrrole** rings. They are often complexed with a metal. For example, the porphyrin **heme** complexes with Fe in hemoglobin and chlorophyll is complexed with Mg.

C. Proteins

Proteins are composed primarily of the elements C, H, O, and N but may also contain phosphorus (P) and sulfur (S). They are polymers of **amino acids**.

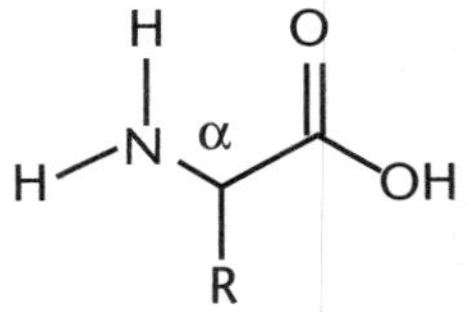

Figure 1.5

Amino acids are connected by **peptide bonds** through dehydration reactions. Chains of such bonds produce a polymer called a **polypeptide**, or simply a peptide, which is another term for protein. The sequence of amino acids in a protein is referred to as the 1° (primary) structure. Proteins can also coil or fold to form α-helices and β-pleated sheets. These are considered part of the protein's 2° (secondary) structure.

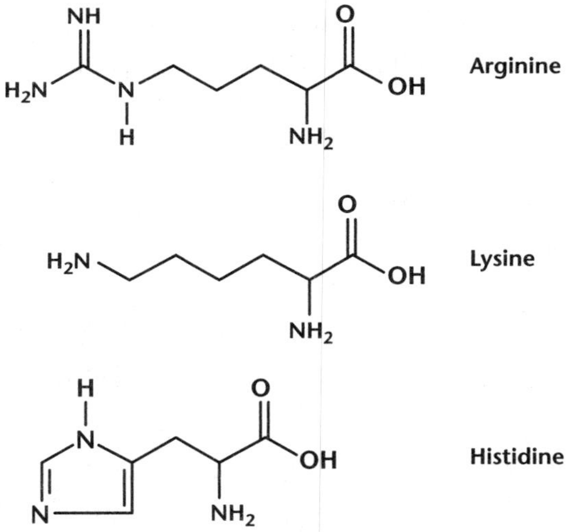

Figure 1.6

1. PROTEIN STRUCTURE

Proteins can be classified on the basis of structure:

- **Simple proteins** – these are composed entirely of amino acids.
- **Albumins and globulins** – these are primarily globular in nature. They are functional proteins that act as carriers or enzymes and are usually found in the serum.
- **Scleroproteins** – these are fibrous in nature and act as structural proteins. Collagen is a scleroprotein.
- **Conjugated proteins** – these contain a simple protein portion, plus at least one nonprotein fraction.
- **Lipoproteins** – protein bound to **lipid**
- **Mucoproteins** – protein bound to **carbohydrate**
- **Chromoproteins** – protein bound to pigmented molecules
- **Metalloproteins** – protein complexed around a **metal ion**
- **Nucleoproteins** – protein bound to **nucleic acids**, either DNA or RNA. In the case of DNA the protein is combined with either histone or protamine.

2. PROTEIN FUNCTION

- **Hormones** – these are proteins that function as chemical messengers secreted into the circulation. Insulin and ACTH are protein hormones.
- **Enzymes** – these are biological catalysts that act by increasing the rate of chemical reactions important for biological functions. For example: amylase, lipase, ATPase.
- **Structural proteins** – these contribute to the physical support of a cell or tissue. They may be extracellular (e.g., collagen in cartilage bone and tendons) or intracellular (e.g., proteins in cell membranes).
- **Transport proteins** – these are carriers of important materials. For example, hemoglobin carries oxygen in the circulation and cytochromes carry electrons during cellular respiration.
- **Antibodies** – these bind to foreign particles (antigens), including disease-causing organisms, that have entered the body and start the chain of events to protect against them.

D. Enzymes

Enzymes are organic catalysts. A catalyst is any substance that affects the rate of a chemical reaction without itself being changed. Enzymes are crucial to living things because all living systems must have **continuous controlled** chemical activity. Enzymes regulate metabolism by speeding up or slowing down certain chemical reactions. They affect the reaction rate by decreasing the activation energy.

Enzymes are **proteins** and thus thousands of different enzymes can conceivably be formed. Many enzymes are conjugated proteins and have a non-protein **co-enzyme**. In these cases, both components must be present for the enzyme to function.

KEY CONCEPTS

Enzymes:
- Lower activation energy of a reaction
- Increase the rate of the reaction
- Do not affect the overall ΔG of the reaction ·
- Are not changed or consumed in the course of the reaction

1. ENZYME SPECIFICITY

Enzymes are very selective; they may catalyze only one reaction, or one specific class of closely related reactions. The molecule upon which an enzyme acts is called the **substrate**. There is an area on each enzyme to which the substrate binds called the **active site**. There are two models describing the binding of the enzyme to the substrate:

a. Lock and Key Theory

This theory holds that the spatial structure of an enzyme's active site is exactly complementary to the spatial structure of its substrate. The two fit together like a lock and key. This theory has been largely discounted.

b. Induced Fit Theory

This more widely accepted theory describes the active site as having flexibility of shape. When the appropriate substrate comes in contact with the active site, the conformation of the active site changes to fit the substrate.

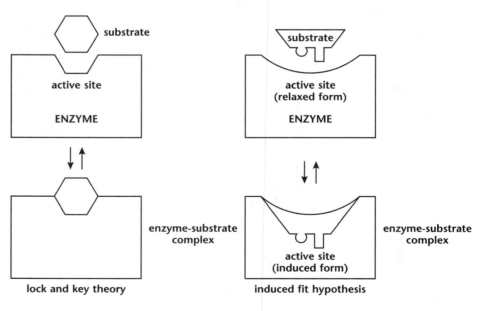

Figure 1.7. Models for Enzyme-Substrate Interactions

2. ENZYME REVERSIBILITY

Most enzyme reactions are reversible. The product synthesized by an enzyme can be decomposed by the same enzyme. For example, an enzyme that synthesizes maltose from glucose can also hydrolyze maltose back to glucose.

3. ENZYME ACTION

Enzyme action and the reaction rate depend on several environmental factors including temperature, pH, and the concentration of the enzyme and the substrate.

a. Effects of Temperature

In general, as the temperature increases, the rate of enzyme action increases, until an optimal temperature is reached (usually around 40°C). Beyond optimal temperature, heat alters the shape of the active site of the enzyme molecule and deactivates it, leading to a rapid drop in reaction rate.

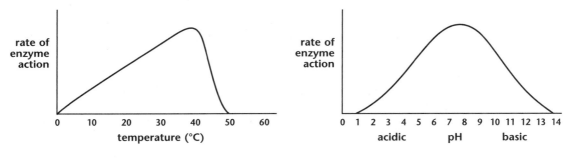

Figure 1.8

b. Effects of pH

For each enzyme there is an optimal pH above and below which enzymatic activity declines. Maximal activity of many human enzymes occurs around pH 7.2, which is the pH of most body fluids. Exceptions include **pepsin**, which works best in the highly acidic conditions of the stomach (pH = 2), and pancreatic enzymes, which work optimally in the alkaline conditions of the small intestine (pH = 8.5). In most cases, the optimal pH matches the conditions under which the enzyme operates.

c. Effects of Concentration

The concentrations of substrate and enzyme greatly affect the reaction rate. When the concentrations of both enzyme and substrate are low, many of the active sites on the enzyme are unoccupied and the reaction rate is low. Increasing the substrate concentration will increase the reaction rate until all of the active sites are occupied. After this point, further increase in substrate concentration will not increase the reaction rate because the reaction has reached its V_{max} or maximum velocity.

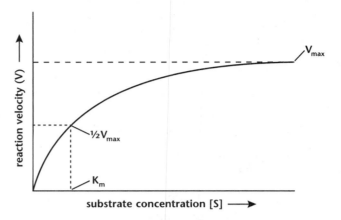

Figure 1.9. Michaelis-Menten Model

4. EXAMPLES OF ENZYME ACTIVITY

Every reaction in the body is regulated by enzymes. Some of the basic reaction types are listed here:

a. Hydrolysis

Hydrolysis reactions function to digest large molecules into smaller components. **Lactase** hydrolyzes lactose to the monosaccharides glucose and galactose. **Proteases** degrade proteins to amino acids and **lipases** break down lipids to fatty acids and glycerol. Other hydrolytic reactions occur within cells.

b. Synthesis

Synthesis reactions (including dehydrations) can be catalyzed by the same enzymes as hydrolysis reactions, but the direction of the reaction is reversed.

These reactions occur in various parts of the cell. For example, protein synthesis occurs in the ribosomes, and involves dehydration synthesis between amino acids. Synthesis is required for growth, repair, regulation, protection, and production of food reserves (such as fat and glycogen) by the cell.

The survival of an organism depends on its ability to ingest substances that it needs but cannot synthesize. Once ingested, these substances are converted into useful products. Certain vitamin cofactors and essential amino acids cannot be synthesized by humans. If they are not available in the diet, deficiency diseases will occur.

5. COFACTORS

Many enzymes require the incorporation of a nonprotein molecule to become active. These molecules, called **cofactors**, can be metal cations like Zn^{2+} or Fe^{2+}, or small organic groups called coenzymes. Most coenzymes cannot be synthesized by the body and are obtained from the diet as vitamin derivatives. Cofactors that bind to the enzyme by strong covalent bonds are called **prosthetic groups**.

E. Nucleic Acids

Nucleic acids are another type of organic molecule (distinct from proteins and carbohydrates) that contain the elements C,H,O,N, and P. They are polymers of subunits called **nucleotides**. Nucleic acids (DNA and RNA) code all of the information required by an organism to produce proteins and replicate.

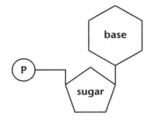

Figure 1.10. Nucleotide

THE CELL

The cell is the fundamental unit of all living things. Every function in biology involves a process that occurs within cells or at the interface between cells. Therefore, to understand biology, you need to appreciate the structure and function of different parts of the cell.

A. Cell Theory

The cell was not discovered or studied in detail until the development of the microscope in the 17th century. Since then, much more has been uncovered, and a unifying theory known as the Cell Theory has been proposed.

Cell Theory is summarized as follows:

• All living things are composed of cells.

• The cell is the basic functional unit of life.

• Cells arise only from pre-existing cells.

• Cells carry genetic information in the form of **DNA**. This genetic material is passed from parent cell to daughter cell during cell division.

• Energy flow (metabolism and biochemistry) occurs within cells.

B. Studying the Cell

Various tools are used to study the cell and its structure.

1. MICROSCOPY

Of the many tools used by scientists to study cells, the microscope is the most basic. **Magnification** is the increase in apparent size of an object. **Resolution** is the differentiation of two closely situated objects.

a. Compound Light Microscope

A compound light microscope uses two lenses or lens systems to magnify an object. The total magnification is the product of the magnification of the eyepiece and the magnification of the objective:

Total magnification =
   Magnification of eyepiece × Magnification of objective

- The **diaphragm** controls the amount of light passing through the specimen.
- The **coarse adjustment** knob roughly focuses the image.
- The **fine adjustment** knob sharply focuses the image.

In general, light microscopy is used to observe nonliving specimens. Light microscopy requires contrast between cells and cell structures. Such contrast is obtained through staining techniques, which cause cell death.

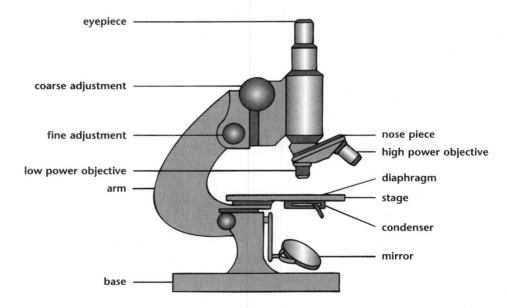

Figure 1.11. Compound Light Microscope

b. Phase Contrast Microscopy

A phase contrast microscope is a special type of light microscope that permits the study of living cells. Differences in refractive index are used to produce contrast between cellular structures. Therefore, this technique does not kill the specimen.

c. Electron Microscopy

An electron microscope uses a beam of electrons to allow a thousandfold higher magnification than is possible with light microscopy. Unfortunately, examination of living specimens is not possible because of the preparations necessary for electron microscopy; tissues must be fixed and sectioned and, sometimes, stained with solutions of heavy metals.

2. CENTRIFUGATION

Differential centrifugation can be used to separate cells or mixtures of cells without destroying them in the process. Spinning fragmented cells at high speeds in the centrifuge will cause their components to sediment at different levels in the test tube on the basis of their respective densities. Denser parts, such as nuclei, endoplasmic reticulum, and mitochondria, will sink to the bottom, while less dense material will remain at the top.

CELL BIOLOGY

The components of the cell are specialized in their structure and function. These components are referred to as **organelles** and include the nucleus, ribosomes, endoplasmic reticulum, Golgi apparatus, vesicles, vacuoles, lysosomes, mitochondria, chloroplasts, and centrioles.

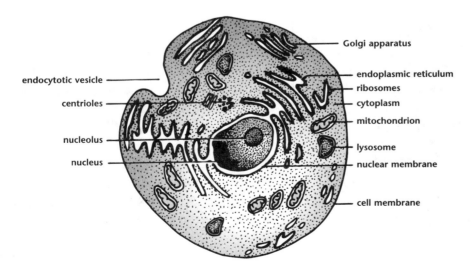

Figure 1.12. Eukaryotic Cell

A. Cell Membrane

The cell membrane (plasma membrane) encloses the cell and exhibits selective permeability, which means it regulates the passage of materials into and out of the cell. According to the generally accepted **fluid mosaic model**, the cell membrane consists of a phospholipid bilayer with proteins embedded throughout. The lipids and many of the proteins can move freely within the membrane.

As a result of its lipid bilayer structure, the plasma membrane is readily permeable to both small, nonpolar molecules, such as oxygen, and small, polar molecules, such as water. Small charged particles are usually able to cross the membrane through protein channels. Some larger, charged molecules cross the membrane with the assistance of **carrier proteins**.

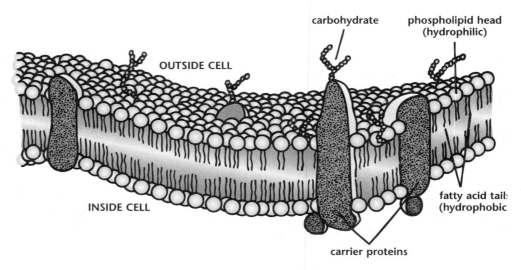

Figure 1.13. Fluid Mosaic Model

B. Nucleus

The nucleus controls the activities of the cell, including cell division. It is surrounded by a nuclear membrane. The nucleus contains the DNA, which is complexed with structural proteins called **histones** to form **chromosomes**. The **nucleolus** is a dense structure in the nucleus where **ribosomal RNA** (rRNA) synthesis occurs.

C. Ribosome

Ribosomes are the sites of protein production and are synthesized by the nucleolus. Free ribosomes are found in the cytoplasm, while bound ribosomes line the outer membrane of the endoplasmic reticulum.

D. Endoplasmic Reticulum

The endoplasmic reticulum (ER) is a network of membrane-enclosed spaces involved in the transport of materials throughout the cell, particularly those materials destined to be secreted by the cell.

E. Golgi Apparatus

The Golgi apparatus receives vesicles and their contents from the smooth ER, modifies them (e.g., glycosylation), repackages them into vesicles, and distributes them to the cell surface by exocytosis.

F. Mitochondria

Mitochondria are the sites of aerobic respiration within the cell and, hence, the suppliers of energy. Each mitochondrion is bounded by an outer and inner phospholipid bilayer.

G. Cytoplasm

Most of the cell's metabolic activity occurs in the cytoplasm. Transport within the cytoplasm occurs by **cyclosis** (streaming movement of the cytoplasm within the cell).

H. Vacuole

Vacuoles and vesicles are membrane-bound sacs involved in the transport and storage of materials that are ingested, secreted, processed, or digested by the cell. Vacuoles are larger than vesicles and are more likely to be found in plant than in animal cells.

I. Centrioles

Centrioles are a specialized **microtubule** involved in spindle organization during cell division and are not bound by a membrane. Animal cells usually have a pair of centrioles that are oriented at right angles to each other and lie in a region called the centrosome. Plant cells do not contain centrioles.

J. Lysosome

Lysosomes are membrane-bound vesicles that contain **hydrolytic enzymes** involved in intracellular digestion. Lysosomes break down material ingested by the cell. An injured or dying tissue may "commit suicide" by rupturing the lysosome membrane and releasing its hydrolytic enzymes; this process is called **autolysis**.

K. Cytoskeleton

The cytoskeleton, composed of microtubules and microfilaments, gives the cell mechanical support, maintains its shape, and functions in cell motility.

Note that not all cells have the same relative distribution of organelles. Form follows function: Cells that require a lot of energy for locomotion (e.g., sperm cells) have lots of mitochondria; cells involved in secretion (e.g., pancreatic islet cells) have lots of Golgi bodies; and cells such as red blood cells, which primarily serve a transport function, have no organelles at all!

TRANSPORT ACROSS THE CELL MEMBRANE

Substances can move into and out of cells in various ways. Some methods occur passively, without energy, while others are active and require energy expenditure (ATP).

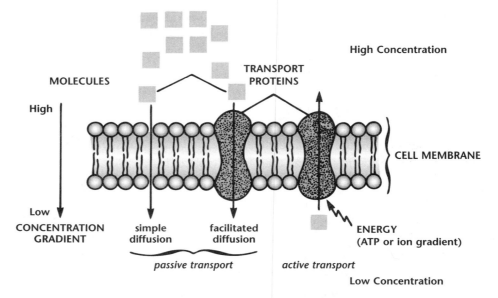

Figure 1.14. Movement Across Membranes

A. Simple Diffusion

Simple diffusion is the net movement of dissolved particles down their concentration gradients—from a region of higher concentration to a region of lower concentration. This is a passive process that requires no external source of energy.

1. OSMOSIS

Osmosis is the simple diffusion of water from a region of lower solute (higher water) concentration to a region of higher solute (lower water) concentration. When the cytoplasm of a cell has a lower concentration of nonpenetrating solutes than the extracellular medium, the extracellular medium is said to be **hypertonic** to the cell, and water will flow out of the cell. This process, also called **plasmolysis**, will cause the cell to shrivel.

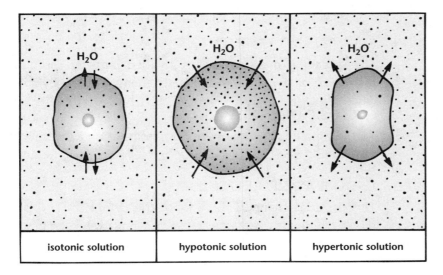

Figure 1.15. Osmosis

If the extracellular environment is less concentrated than the cytoplasm of the cell, the extracellular medium is said to be **hypotonic**, and water will flow into the cell, causing it to swell and **lyse** (burst). For example, red blood cells will burst if placed in distilled water. Some organisms, like freshwater protozoa, have contractile vacuoles to pump out excess water and prevent bursting.

B. Facilitated Diffusion

Facilitated diffusion (another type of passive transport) is the net movement of dissolved particles down their concentration gradient through special channels or via carrier proteins in the cell membrane. This process, like simple diffusion, does not require energy.

C. Active Transport

Active transport is the net movement of dissolved particles *against* their concentration gradient with the help of transport proteins. Unlike diffusion, active transport requires energy, either in chemical form (ATP) or via an electrochemical gradient.

KEY CONCEPT

Types of transport:

Passive diffusion
- Down gradient
- No carrier
- No energy required

Facilitated diffusion
- Down gradient
- Carrier
- No energy required

Active transport
- Against gradient
- Carrier
- Energy required

CIRCULATION

Circulation is the transportation of material within cells and throughout the body of a multicellular organism.

A. Intracellular Circulation

Materials move about within a cell in a number of ways:

1. BROWNIAN MOVEMENT

The spreading movement of suspended particles throughout the cytoplasm of the cell via the kinetic energy created by collisions.

2. CYCLOSIS OR STREAMING

This is the circular motion of cytoplasm around the cell transport molecules.

3. ENDOPLASMIC RETICULUM

This provides channels throughout the cytoplasm and provides a direct continuous passageway from the plasma membrane to the nuclear membrane.

B. Extracellular Circulation

A number of systems have been devised to deal with the movement of materials on a larger scale, through the body of an organism:

1. DIFFUSION

If cells are in direct or close contact with the external environment, diffusion can serve as a sufficient means of transport for food and oxygen from the environment to the cells. In larger, more complex animals, diffusion is important for the transport of materials between cells and the interstitial fluid that bathes the cells.

2. CIRCULATORY SYSTEM

Complex animals, whose cells are too far from the external environment to transport materials by diffusion, require a circulatory system. This generally includes vessels to transport fluid and a pump to drive the circulation.

Reproduction

Reproduction is the process by which an organism perpetuates itself and its species. It's hard to believe, but all the nucleated cells of your body, regardless of their structure and function, have the *exact* same chromosomes (including two sex chromosomes inside their nuclei). The only exceptions are the sex cells, which have only half the number of chromosomes as somatic cells. This is all possible because of cell division.

CELL DIVISION

Cell division is the process by which a cell doubles its organelles and cytoplasm, replicates its DNA, and then divides in two. For **unicellular organisms**, cell division is a means of reproduction, while for **multicellular organisms**, it is a method of growth, development, and replacement of worn-out cells. Cell division can follow two different courses, mitosis and meiosis, depending on the type of cell.

A. Mitosis

Mitosis is the division and distribution of the somatic cell's DNA to its two daughter cells such that each cell receives a complete copy of the original genome. Nuclear division **(karyokinesis)** is followed by cell division **(cytokinesis)**. Prior to the initiation of mitosis, the cell undergoes a period of growth and replication of genetic material called interphase.

1. INTERPHASE

A cell normally spends at least 90 percent of its life in interphase. During this period, each chromosome is replicated so that during division, a complete copy of the genome can be distributed to both daughter cells. After replication, the chromosomes consist of two identical **sister chromatids** held together at a central region called the **centromere**. During interphase, the individual chromosomes are not visible. The DNA is uncoiled and is called **chromatin**. The term **chromosome** may be used to refer to either a single chromatid *or* the pair of chromatids attached at the centromere. However, this naming convention should not be confused with the designation of the chromosome number within the cells, which is known as **ploidy**.

All human somatic cells have a characteristic number of chromosomes in their cells, referred to as **diploid** (or 2N). This number in a single cell is due to the presence of homologous pairs of chromosomes made up of two sets of **haploid** (or N) chromosomes that originate from the gamete cells of each parent. Essentially, the two haploid chromosome complements unite to make an offspring with the diploid complement of chromosomes.

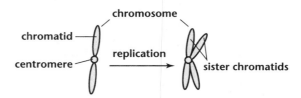

Figure 2.1. Chromosome Replication

2. **PROPHASE**

During prophase, the initiation phase of mitosis, the chromosomes condense and the centriole pairs (in animals) separate and move towards the opposite poles of the cell. The spindle apparatus forms between them, and the nuclear membrane dissolves, allowing the spindle fibers to interact with the chromosomes.

3. **METAPHASE**

During this phase of mitosis, the centriole pairs are now at opposite poles of the cell. The fibers of the spindle apparatus attach to each chromatid at the centromere to align the chromosomes at the center of the cell (equator), forming the **metaphase plate**.

4. **ANAPHASE**

In this next phase of mitosis, the centromeres split so that each chromatid has its own distinct centromere, thus allowing sister chromatids to separate. The sister chromatids are pulled towards the opposite poles of the cell by the shortening of the spindle fibers which are composed of microtubules.

5. **TELOPHASE**

During this last phase of mitosis, the spindle apparatus disappears and a nuclear membrane forms around each set of newly formed chromosomes. Thus, each nucleus contains the same number of chromosomes as the original or parent nucleus. The chromosomes uncoil, resuming their interphase form.

6. CYTOKINESIS

Near the end of telophase, the cytoplasm divides into two daughter cells, each with a complete nucleus and its own set of organelles. In animal cells, a **cleavage furrow** forms, and the cell membrane indents along the equator of the cell and finally pinches through the cell, separating the two nuclei.

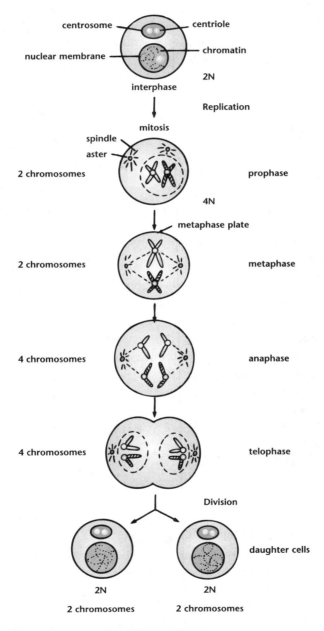

Figure 2.2. Mitosis

7. ANIMAL CELLS VS. PLANT CELLS

There are two major differences between cell division in animal cells and plant cells. One is that plant cells lack centrioles. The spindle apparatus is synthesized by microtubule organizing centers, which are not visible.

The second difference is that while cytokinesis in animal cells proceeds through production of a cleavage furrow, plant cells are rigid and cannot form a cleavage furrow. Thus, they divide by the formation of a **cell plate**, an expanding partition that grows outward from the interior of the cell until it reaches the cell membrane (see Figure 2.3).

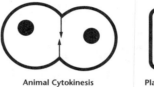 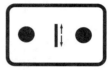

Animal Cytokinesis Plant Formation of Cell Plate

Figure 2.3. Comparison of Animal and Plant Cell Division

B. Meiosis

Sexual reproduction differs from asexual reproduction in that two parents are involved. Sexual reproduction occurs via the fusion of two **gametes**—specialized sex cells produced by each parent. **Meiosis** is the process by which these sex cells are produced. Meiosis is similar to mitosis in that a cell duplicates its chromosomes before undergoing the process. However, while mitosis preserves the diploid (2N) number of the cell, meiosis produces the **haploid** (1N) number, halving the number of chromosomes. To accomplish this, meiosis involves two divisions of **primary sex cells** (whereas mitosis only involves one division), resulting in four haploid cells known as **gametes**.

1. INTERPHASE

As in mitosis, the parent cell's chromosomes are replicated during interphase, resulting in the 4N number of chromosomes.

2. FIRST MEIOTIC DIVISION

The first division produces two intermediate daughter cells with 2N chromosomes with sister chromatids.

a. Prophase I

The chromatin condenses into chromosomes, the spindle apparatus forms, and the nucleoli and nuclear membrane disappear. **Homologous chromosomes** (chromosomes that code for the same traits, one inherited from each parent), come together and intertwine in a process called **synapsis** (see Figure 2.4). Since at this stage, each chromosome consists of two sister chromatids, each synaptic pair of homologous chromosomes contains four chromatids and is, therefore, often called a **tetrad**. Sometimes chromatids of homologous chromosomes connect and then break at corresponding points called **chiasmata** where they exchange equivalent pieces of DNA; this process is called **crossing over**. Note that crossing over occurs between homologous chromosomes and not between sister chromatids of the same chromosomes (the latter are identical, so crossing over would not produce any genetic variation). Once the chromosomes have recombined, the chromatids involved are left with an altered but complete set of genes. Recombination among chromosomes results in increased genetic diversity within a species. Note that sister chromatids are no longer identical after recombination has occurred.

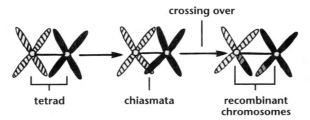

Figuare 2.4. Synapsis

b. **Metaphase I**

Homologous pairs (tetrads) align at the equatorial plate, and each pair attaches to a separate spindle fiber by its kinetochore.

c. **Anaphase I**

The homologous pairs separate and are pulled to opposite poles of the cell. This process is called **disjunction**, and it accounts for a fundamental Mendelian law. During disjunction, each chromosome of paternal origin separates (or disjoins) from its homologue of maternal origin, and either chromosome can end up in either daughter cell. Thus, the distribution of homologous chromosomes to the two intermediate daughter cells is random with respect to parental origin. Each daughter cell will have a unique pool of genes from a random mixture of maternal and paternal origin.

d. **Telophase I**

A nuclear membrane forms around each new nucleus. At this point, each chromosome still consists of sister chromatids joined at the centromere.

3. SECOND MEIOTIC DIVISION

This second division is very similar to mitosis, except that meiosis II is *not* preceded by chromosomal replication. The chromosomes consisting of sister chromatids align at the equator. Then the sister chromatids separate, move to opposite poles, and are surrounded by a re-formed nuclear membrane. The new cells will have the haploid number of chromosomes due to this second division with no replication. Note that in human females, only one of these daughter cells becomes a functional gamete.

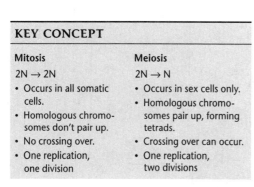

KEY CONCEPT

Mitosis	Meiosis
2N → 2N	2N → N
• Occurs in all somatic cells.	• Occurs in sex cells only.
• Homologous chromosomes don't pair up.	• Homologous chromosomes pair up, forming tetrads.
• No crossing over.	• Crossing over can occur.
• One replication, one division	• One replication, two divisions

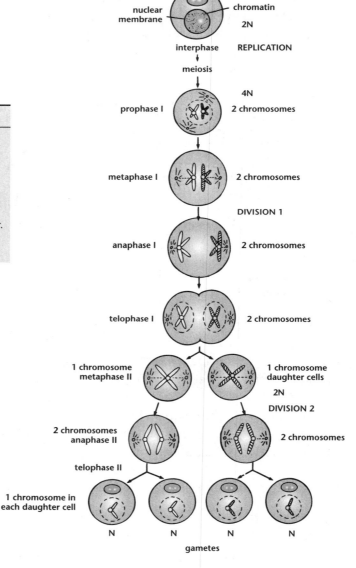

Figure 2.5. Meiosis

SEXUAL REPRODUCTIVE MECHANISMS

Recall that sexual reproduction differs from asexual reproduction in that two parents are involved and the end result is a genetically unique offspring. Sexual reproduction occurs via the fusion of two gametes and requires the following:

- The production of **functional sex cells** or **gametes** by adult organisms
- The union of these cells (**fertilization** or **conjugation**) to form a zygote
- The development of the zygote into another adult, completing the cycle

A. Sexual Reproduction In Animals

Sexual reproduction in animals is a complex process involving the formation and fertilization of gametes and regulation of these processes by both parents.

1. GONADS

The gametes are produced in specialized organs called the gonads. The male gonads, called **testes**, produce sperm in the tightly coiled seminiferous tubules. The female gonads, called **ovaries**, produce **oocytes** (eggs). Some species are **hermaphrodites**, which have both functional male and female gonads. These include the hydra and the earthworm.

2. SPERMATOGENESIS

Spermatogenesis, or sperm production, occurs in the seminiferous tubules. Diploid cells called **spermatogonia** undergo meiosis to produce four haploid sperm of equal size. The mature sperm is an elongated cell with a head, tail, neck, and body. The **head** consists almost entirely of the nucleus, which contains the paternal genome. The tail (**flagellum**) propels the sperm, while mitochondria in the neck and body provide energy for locomotion.

3. OOGENESIS

Oogenesis, the production of female gametes, occurs in the ovaries. One diploid primary female sex cell undergoes meiosis in the ovaries to produce a **single mature egg**. Each meiotic division produces a **polar body**, which is a small cell that contains little more than the nucleus. The mature ovum is a large cell containing most of the cytoplasm, RNA, organelles, and nutrients needed by a developing embryo. The polar bodies rapidly degenerate.

In addition to the presence of polar bodies, oogenesis differs from spermatogenesis in that it is a discontinuous process. For example, a female is born with a given number of eggs arrested in prophase of meiosis I. The first meiotic division is not complete until ovulation, and the second meiotic division is not complete until fertilization!

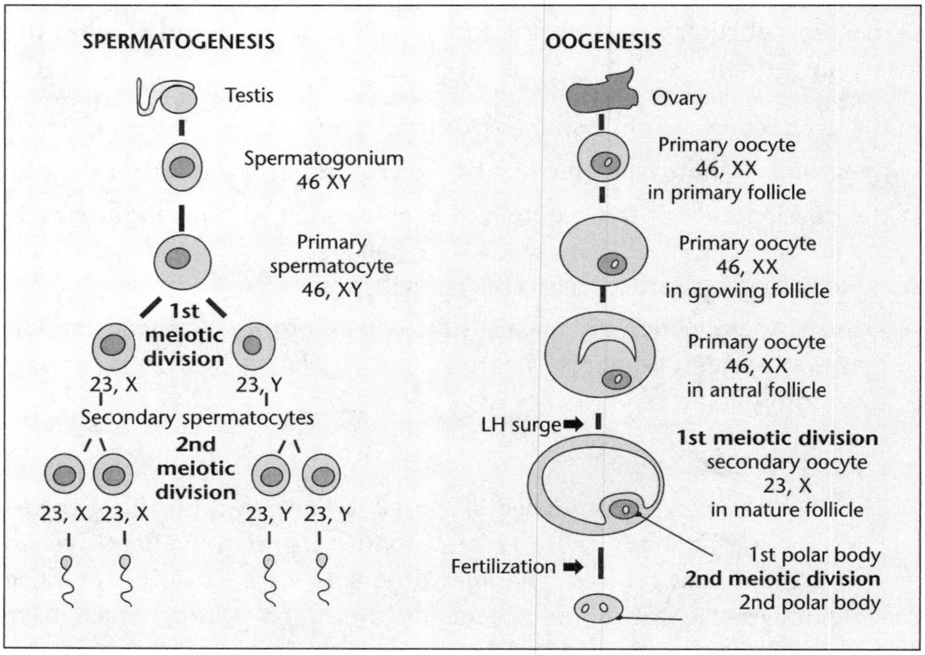

SPERMATOGENESIS

Testis

Spermatogonium
46 XY

Primary
spermatocyte
46, XY

1st
meiotic
division

23, X   23, Y

Secondary spermatocytes

2nd
meiotic
division

23, X 23, X   23, Y 23, Y

OOGENESIS

Ovary

Primary oocyte
46, XX
in primary follicle

Primary oocyte
46, XX
in growing follicle

Primary oocyte
46, XX
in antral follicle

LH surge ➡

1st meiotic division
secondary oocyte
23, X
in mature follicle

Fertilization ➡

1st polar body
2nd meiotic division
2nd polar body

Figure 2.6. Normal Gametogenesis

4. FERTILIZATION

Fertilization is the union of the egg and sperm to form a zygote with a diploid number of chromosomes.

a. External Fertilization

External fertilization occurs in vertebrates that reproduce in water (fish and amphibians). The female lays eggs in the water, and the male deposits sperm in the vicinity. The lack of direct passage of sperm from male to female reduces the chances of fertilization considerably. Many eggs must be laid to ensure some fertilization success. The sperm have flagella, enabling them to swim through the water to the eggs.

b. Internal Fertilization

Internal fertilization is practiced by terrestrial vertebrates and provides a direct route for sperm to reach the egg cell. This increases the chance for fertilization success, and females produce fewer eggs. The number of eggs produced is affected by other factors as well. If the early development of the offspring occurs outside of the mother's body, more eggs will be laid to increase the chances of offspring survival. The amount of parental care after birth is also related to the number of eggs produced. Species that care for their young produce fewer eggs.

B. Human Reproduction

1. MALE REPRODUCTIVE PHYSIOLOGY

The **testes** are located in an external pouch called the scrotum, which maintains testes temperature 2–4°C lower than body temperature, a condition essential for sperm survival. Sperm pass from the testes through the **vas deferens** to the ejaculatory duct and then to the **urethra**. The urethra passes through the penis and opens to the outside at its tip. In males, the urethra is a common passageway for both the reproductive and excretory systems. The testes are also the site of production of **testosterone**. Testosterone regulates secondary male sex characteristics, including facial and pubic hair and voice changes.

> **REMEMBER**
>
> To remember the pathway of sperm, think **Seven Up**:
> Seminiferous tubules
> Epididymis
> Vas Deferens
> Ejaculatory Duct
> (Nothing)
> Urethra
> Penis

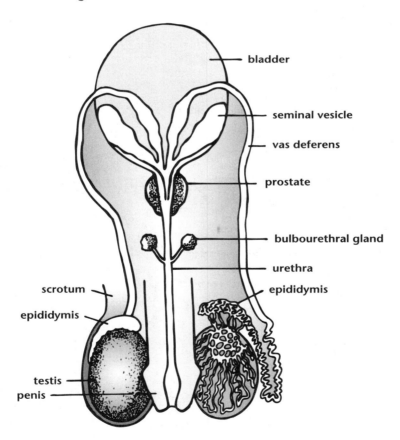

Figure 2.7. Male Reproductive Tract

2. FEMALE REPRODUCTIVE ANATOMY

The **ovaries** are found in the abdominal cavity, below the digestive system. The ovaries consist of thousands of follicles; a **follicle** is a multilayered sac of cells that contains, nourishes, and protects an immature ovum. It is actually the follicle cells that produce estrogen. Once a month, an immature ovum is released from the ovary into the abdominal cavity and drawn into the nearby **oviduct** or **fallopian tube**. Each fallopian tube opens into the upper end of a muscular chamber called the **uterus**, which is the site of fetal development. The lower, narrow end of the uterus is called the **cervix**. The cervix connects with the vaginal canal, which is the site of sperm deposition during intercourse and is also the passageway through which a baby is expelled during childbirth. Remember that at birth, all the eggs that a female will have during her lifetime are already present in the ovaries.

3. FEMALE SEX HORMONES

The ovaries synthesize and secrete the female sex hormones, including estrogens and progesterone. The secretion of both estrogens and progesterone is regulated by LH and FSH, which, in turn, are regulated by GnRH.

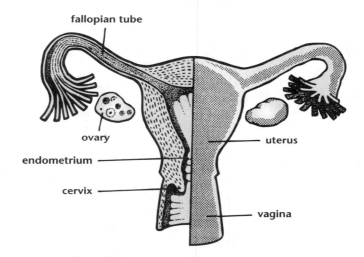

Figure 2.8. Female Reproductive Tract

a. Estrogens

Estrogens are steroid hormones necessary for normal female maturation. They stimulate the development of the female reproductive tract and contribute to the development of secondary sexual characteristics and sex drive. Estrogens are also responsible for the thickening of the **endometrium** (uterine wall). Estrogens are secreted by the ovarian follicles and the corpus luteum.

b. **Progesterone**

Progesterone is a steroid hormone secreted by the corpus luteum during the luteal phase of the menstrual cycle. Progesterone stimulates the development and maintenance of the endometrial walls in preparation for implantation of the zygote.

4. THE MENSTRUAL CYCLE

The hormonal secretions of the ovaries, the hypothalamus, and the anterior pituitary play important roles in the female reproductive cycle. From puberty through menopause, interactions among these hormones result in a monthly cyclical pattern known as the menstrual cycle. The menstrual cycle may be divided into the follicular phase, ovulation, the luteal phase, and menstruation.

a. **Follicular phase**

The follicular phase begins with the cessation of the menstrual flow from the previous cycle. It is at this point that the reproductive hormone levels are their lowest, thereby shutting off negative feedback signaling to the hypothalamus. With the removal of negative feedback, the hypothalamus can release the tropic hormone GnRH (gonadotropin-releasing hormone), which will stimulate the release of FSH from the anterior pituitary. **FSH** (follicle stimulating hormone) promotes the development of the follicle within the ovary, which grows and begins secreting estrogen.

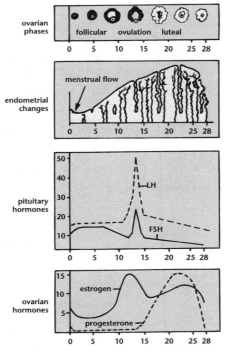

Figure 2.9. Menstrual Cycle

b. Ovulation

Midway through the cycle, **ovulation** occurs—a mature ovarian follicle bursts and releases an ovum that will be captured by the oviduct. Ovulation is caused by a surge in LH levels, which is preceded and caused in part by a peak in estrogen levels created by the mature follicle.

c. Luteal phase

Following ovulation, **LH** (luteinizing hormone) induces the ruptured follicle to develop into the **corpus luteum**, which secretes estrogen and progesterone. **Progesterone** causes the glands of the endometrium to mature and produce secretions that prepare the uterus for the implantation of an embryo. Together progesterone and estrogen are essential for the maintenance of the endometrium.

d. Menstruation

If the ovum is *not* fertilized, the corpus luteum atrophies. The resulting drop in progesterone and estrogen levels causes the endometrium (with its superficial blood vessels) to slough off, giving rise to the menstrual flow **(menses)**.

If fertilization occurs, the developing placenta produces **hCG** (human chorionic gonadotrophin). hCG maintains the corpus luteum and, thus, the supply of estrogen and progesterone that sustains the uterus, until the placenta takes over production of these hormones.

B. Sexual Reproduction in Plants

The life cycles of plants are characterized by an alternation of the diploid **sporophyte** generation and the haploid **gametophyte** generation. The relative lengths of the two stages vary with the plant type. In general, the evolutionary trend has been towards increased dominance of the sporophyte generation.

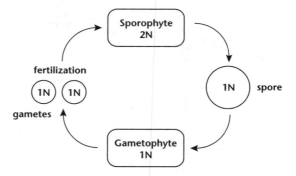

Figure 2.10. Life Cycles of Plants

1. **GAMETOPHYTE GENERATION**

   The haploid gametophyte generation produces **gametes** by mitosis. Union of the male and female gametes at fertilization restores the diploid sporophyte generation. Thus, the gametophytes reproduce sexually while the sporophyte generation reproduces asexually. An example of when the **gametophyte** is the dominant generation is in mosses. In this case, the sporophyte is a smaller short-lived organism that depends on the gametophyte for energy and nutrients.

2. **SPOROPHYTE GENERATION**

   The diploid sporophyte generation produces a haploid (monoploid) **spore** by meiosis. The spores divide by mitosis to produce the haploid or gametophyte generation. For example, in ferns, the **sporophyte** generation is the dominant, familiar form. The sporophyte releases spores from the undersides of its leaves that develop into small heart shaped gametophytes.

3. **SEXUAL REPRODUCTION IN ANGIOSPERMS**

   Flowering plants or **angiosperms** have gametophytes consisting of a few cells that exist for a very short time. The woody plant that is seen (maple, rose, etc.) is the sporophyte stage. The **flower** is the reproductive structure of angiosperms. Some species of plants have flowers that contain only **stamens** ("male plants") and other flowers that contain only **pistils** ("female plants"). Flowers have the following distinct parts:

   a. **Stamen**

      The stamen is the male organ of the flower and consists of a thin stalk-like **filament** with a terminal sac called the **anther**. The anther produces haploid spores that develop into pollen grains.

   b. **Pistil**

      The pistil is the female organ of the flower. It consists of three parts:

      - **Stigma** – the sticky top part of the pistil that catches pollen.
      - **Style** – a tube-like structure connecting the stigma to the ovary at the base of the pistil.
      - **Ovary** – the enlarged base of the pistil. It contains one or more ovules. Each ovule contains a monoploid egg nucleus.

   c. **Petals**

      Petals are specialized leaves surrounding and protecting the pistil. Their characteristic colors and odors attract insects, which transfer pollen between plants and allow for fertilization.

d. Sepals

These are green leaves that cover and product the flower bud during early development. After the flower blooms the sepals may remain, surrounding the petals.

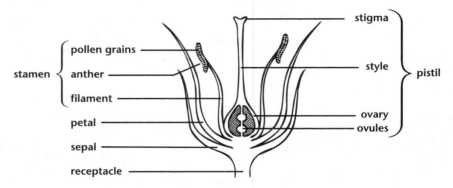

Figure 2.11. Flowering Plants

e. Fertilization

The pollen grain is the **male gametophyte**. The pollen grain contains a tube nucleus and a generative nucleus formed by mitosis of a microspore. The pollen grains are transferred from the anther to the stigma and the generative nucleus divides to form sperm nuclei which are the **male gametes**.

The **female gametophyte** develops in the ovule from one of four spores. This gametophyte is the **embryo sac** and contains nuclei including the two polar nuclei (endosperms) and an egg nucleus.

Fertilization occurs when the sperm nuclei enter the embryo sac. One sperm nucleus fuses with the egg nucleus to form the diploid zygote, which develops into the embryo. The other sperm nucleus fuses with the two polar bodies to form the endosperm (triploid or 3N). The **endosperm** provides food for the embryonic plant. In dicotyledonous plants, the endosperm is absorbed by the **seed leaves** (cotyledons).

1 sperm nucleus + 1 egg nucleus → zygote → embryo

1 sperm nucleus + 2 polar nuclei → 3N endosperm

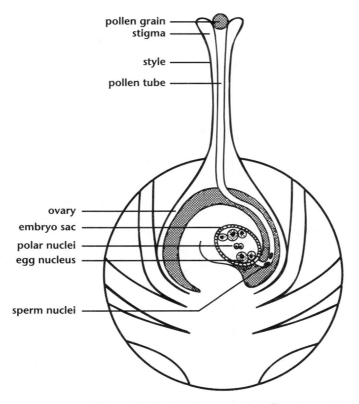

Figure 2.12. Angiosperm Fertilization

ASEXUAL REPRODUCTIVE MECHANISMS

Asexual reproduction is the production of offspring **without fertilization**. New organisms are formed by division of a single parent cell. Thus, except for random mutations, the offspring are genetically identical to the parent cells. The different types of asexual reproduction are fission, budding, regeneration, and parthenogenesis. Prokaryotes reproduce asexually. Among animals, asexual reproduction is more prevalent in invertebrates than vertebrates. All **plants**, simple and complex, use asexual reproduction in some form.

A. Fission

Binary fission is a simple form of asexual reproduction seen in prokaryotic organisms. The DNA replicates, and a new plasma membrane and cell wall grow inward along the midline of the cell, dividing it into two equally sized cells with equal amounts of cytoplasm, each containing a duplicate of the parent chromosome. A very similar process occurs in some primitive eukaryotic cells. Fission occurs in one-celled organisms, such as amoebae, paramecia, algae, and bacteria.

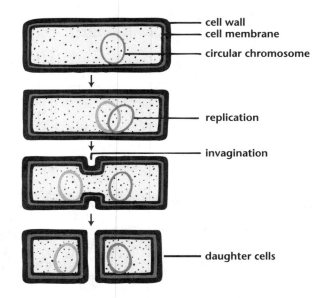

Figure 2.13. Binary Fission

B. Budding

Budding is the replication of the nucleus followed by unequal cytokinesis. The cell membrane pinches inward to form a new cell, which is smaller in size but genetically identical to the parent cell and which subsequently grows to adult size. The new cell may separate immediately from the parent, or it may remain attached to it, develop as an outgrowth, and separate at a later stage. Budding occurs in hydra and yeast.

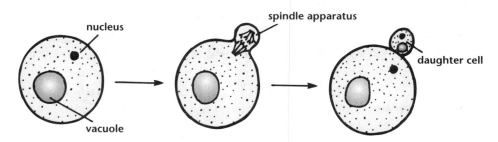

Figure 2.14. Budding

C. Regeneration

Regeneration is the regrowth of a lost or injured body part. Replacement of cells occurs by mitosis. Some lower animals, such as hydra and starfish, have extensive regenerative capabilities. If a starfish loses an arm, it can regenerate a new one; the severed arm may even be able to regenerate an entire body, as long as the arm contains a piece of an area called the **central disk.** Salamanders and tadpoles can also generate new limbs. Most often the extent of regeneration depends on the nerve damage to the severed body part.

D. Parthenogenesis

Parthenogenesis is the development of an unfertilized egg into an adult organism. This process occurs naturally in certain lower organisms. For example, in most species of bees and ants, the males develop from unfertilized eggs, while the worker bees and queen bees develop from fertilized eggs. Artificial parthenogenesis can be performed in some animals. For example, the eggs of rabbits and frogs can be stimulated to develop without fertilization by electric shock or pinprick.

E. Asexual Reproduction in Plants

1. SPORE FORMATION

All plants exhibit **alternation of generations** in which a diploid generation is succeeded by a haploid generation. The diploid **sporophyte** generation produces haploid spores that develop into the haploid **gametophyte** generation. Spores are specialized cells with hard coverings that prevent loss of water.

2. VEGETATIVE PROPAGATION

Undifferentiated tissues in plants, called **meristems,** provide a source of cells that can develop into an adult plant. Vegetative propagation can occur naturally, or through human intervention. Propagation is advantageous because it introduces no genetic variation and is a rapid form of reproduction.

a. Natural Vegetative Propagation

Vegetative propagation can occur as a natural means of plant reproduction:

- **Bulbs** split to form several bulbs as in tulips and daffodils.
- **Tubers** are underground stems with buds, like the eyes of potatoes, that can develop into adult plants.
- **Runners** are stems running above and along the ground, extending from the main stem. Runners can produce new roots and upright stems as they do in strawberry plants and lawn grasses.
- **Rhizomes** (stolons) are woody, underground stems. They can develop new upright stems as they do in ferns and iris plants.

b. **Artificial Vegetative Propagation**

Humans may use vegetative propagation in agriculture.

- A **cut** piece of stem can develop new roots in water or moist ground. Synthetic plant hormones called **auxins** can be used to accelerate root formation.

- Stems of certain plants, like blackberry and raspberry, will take root when bent to the ground and covered with soil. This process is called **layering**.

3

Genetics

Genetics is the study of how traits are inherited from one generation to the next. The basic unit of heredity is the **gene**. Genes are composed of **DNA** and are located on **chromosomes**. When a gene exists in more than one form, the alternative forms are called **alleles**. An individual's genetic makeup is known as that individual's **genotype**. The physical manifestation of the genetic makeup is the individual's **phenotype**. Some phenotypes correspond to a single genotype, while other phenotypes correspond to several different genotypes.

MENDELIAN GENETICS

In the 1860s, Gregor Mendel developed the basic principles of genetics through his experiments with the garden pea. Mendel studied the inheritance of individual traits by performing genetic **crosses**: He took **true-breeding** individuals (which, if self-crossed, produce progeny only with the parental phenotype) with different traits, mated them, and statistically analyzed the inheritance of the traits in the progeny.

A. Mendel's First Law: Law of Segregation

Mendel postulated **four principles of inheritance**:

1. Genes exist in alternative forms (**alleles**).

2. An organism has **two alleles** for each inherited trait, one inherited from each parent.

3. The two alleles **segregate** during meiosis, resulting in gametes that carry only one allele for any given inherited trait.

4. If two alleles in an individual organism are different, only one will be fully expressed, and the other will be silent. The expressed allele is said to be **dominant**; the silent allele, **recessive**. In genetics problems, dominant alleles are typically assigned capital letters, and recessive alleles are assigned lower case letters. Organisms that contain two copies of the *same* allele are **homozygous** for that trait; organisms that carry two *different* alleles are **heterozygous**.

The dominant allele appears in the phenotype. This is known as **Mendel's Law of Dominance**. For example:

Genes	Genotype	Phenotype
YY	Homozygous	Yellow
Yy	Heterozygous	Yellow
yy	Homozygous	Green

1. MONOHYBRID CROSS

The principles of Mendelian inheritance can be illustrated in a cross between two true-breeding pea plants, one with purple flowers and the other with white flowers. Since only one trait is being studied in this particular mating, it is referred to as a **monohybrid cross**. The individuals being crossed, or mated, are the **parental** or **P generation**; the progeny generations are the **filial** or **F generations**, with each generation numbered sequentially (e.g., F_1, F_2, etc.).

The purple flower parent has the genotype PP (i.e., it has two P alleles) and is homozygous dominant. The white flower parent has the genotype pp and is homozygous recessive. When these individuals are crossed, they produce F_1 plants that are 100 percent heterozygous (genotype = Pp). Since purple is dominant to white, all the F_1 progeny have the purple flower phenotype.

2. PUNNETT SQUARE

One way of predicting the possible genotypes expected from a cross is by drawing a **Punnett square diagram**. The parental genotypes are arranged around a grid. In addition, since the genotype of each progeny will be the sum of the alleles donated by the parental gametes, their genotypes can be determined by looking at the intersections on the grid (see Figure 3.1). A Punnett square indicates *all* the potential progeny genotypes, and the relative frequencies of the different genotypes. Also, expected phenotypes can be easily calculated (see Figure 3.2).

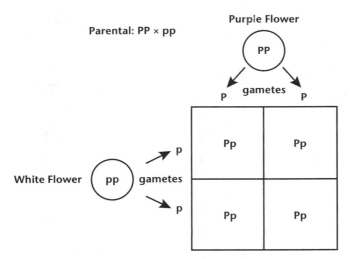

F₁ genotypes: 100% Pp (heterozygous)
F₁ phenotypes: 100% purple flowers

Figure 3.1. Monohybrid Cross

When the F₁ generation from our monohybrid cross is self-crossed (i.e., Pp × Pp) the F₂ progeny are more genotypically and phenotypically diverse than their parents. Since the F₁ plants are heterozygous, they will donate a P allele to half of their descendants and a p allele to the other half. One-fourth of the F₂ plants will have the genotype PP, 50 percent will have the genotype Pp, and 25 percent will have the genotype pp. Since the homozygous dominant and heterozygous genotypes both produce the dominant phenotype, purple flowers, 75 percent of the F₂ plants will have purple flowers, and 25 percent will have white flowers (see Figure 3.2).

This is a standard pattern of Mendelian inheritance. Its hallmarks are the disappearance of the silent (recessive) phenotype in the F₁ generation and its subsequent reappearance in 25 percent of the individuals in the F₂ generation.

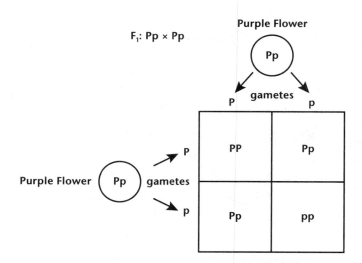

F$_1$: Pp × Pp

Purple Flower

Pp

gametes

P   p

Purple Flower   Pp   gametes

P

p

	PP	Pp
	Pp	pp

F$_2$ genotypes: 1:2:1; 1PP: 2Pp:1pp)
F$_2$ phenotypes: 3:1; 3 purple:1 white

Figure 3.2. Self-Cross of F1 Generation

3. TESTCROSS

Only with a recessive phenotype can genotype be predicted with 100 percent accuracy. If the dominant phenotype is expressed, the genotype can be either homozygous dominant or heterozygous. Thus, homozygous recessive organisms always breed true. This fact can be used to determine the unknown genotype of an organism with a dominant phenotype. In a procedure known as a **testcross** or **backcross**, an organism with a dominant phenotype of unknown genotype (A x) is crossed with a phenotypically recessive organism (genotype aa). Since the recessive parent is homozygous, it can donate only the recessive allele, a, to the progeny. If the dominant parent's genotype is AA, all of its gametes will carry an A, and thus *all* of the progeny will have genotype Aa. If the dominant parent's genotype is Aa, half of the progeny will be Aa and express the dominant phenotype, and half will be aa and express the recessive phenotype. In a testcross, the appearance of the recessive phenotype in the progeny indicates that the phenotypically dominant parent is genotypically heterozygous.

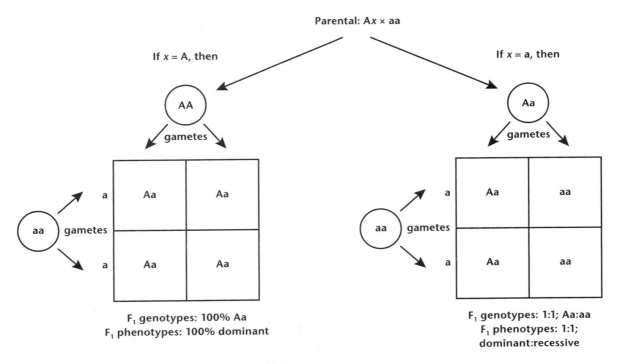

Figure 3.3. Testcross

B. Mendel's Second Law: Law of Independent Assortment

1. DIHYBRID CROSS

The principles of the monohybrid cross can be extended to a **dihybrid cross** in which the parents differ in **two traits**, as long as the genes are on separate chromosomes and assort independently during meiosis. Genes on the same chromosome will stay together, unless **crossing over** occurs. Crossing over occurs during meiosis and exchanges information between chromosomes that may break the linkage of certain patterns. For example, red hair is usually linked with freckles, but some blondes and brunettes have freckles as well.

This pattern of traits being transmitted to offspring independently is known as Mendel's law of independent assortment.

In the following example, a purple-flowered tall pea plant is crossed with a white-flowered dwarf pea plant; both plants are doubly homozygous (tall is dominant to dwarf, T = tall allele, t = dwarf allele; purple is dominant to white, P = purple allele, p = white allele). The purple parent's genotype is TTPP, so it produces only TP gametes; the white parent's genotype is ttpp and produces only tp gametes. The F$_1$ progeny, therefore, will all have the genotype TtPp and will be phenotypically dominant for both traits.

When the F_1, generation is self-crossed (TtPp × TtPp), it produces four different phenotypes: tall purple, tall white, dwarf purple, and dwarf white, in the ratio **9:3:3:1**, respectively. This is the typical pattern for Mendelian inheritance in a dihybrid cross between heterozygotes with independently assorting traits.

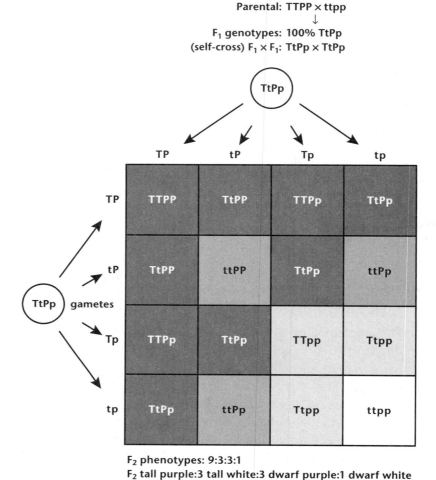

Parental: TTPP × ttpp
↓
F_1 genotypes: 100% TtPp
(self-cross) F_1 × F_1: TtPp × TtPp

F_2 phenotypes: 9:3:3:1
F_2 tall purple:3 tall white:3 dwarf purple:1 dwarf white

Figure 3.4. Dihybrid Cross

C. Non-Mendelian Inheritance Patterns

In real life, inheritance patterns are often more complicated than Mendel might have hoped. One major source of complications is in the relationship between **phenotype** and **genotype**. In theory, 100 percent of individuals with the recessive phenotype have a homozygous recessive genotype, and 100 percent of individuals with the dominant phenotype have either homozygous dominant or heterozygous genotypes. However, such clean concordance between genotype and phenotype is not always the case.

1. INCOMPLETE DOMINANCE

Some progeny phenotypes are apparently **blends** of the parental phenotypes. The classic example is flower color in snapdragons: Homozygous dominant red snapdragons, when crossed with homozygous recessive white snapdragons, produce 100 percent *pink* progeny in the F_1 generation. When F_1 progeny are self-crossed, they produce red, pink, and white progeny in the ratio of 1:2:1, respectively. The pink color is the result of the combined effects of the red and white genes in heterozygotes. An allele is **incompletely dominant** if the phenotype of the heterozygote is an intermediate of the phenotypes of the homozygotes.

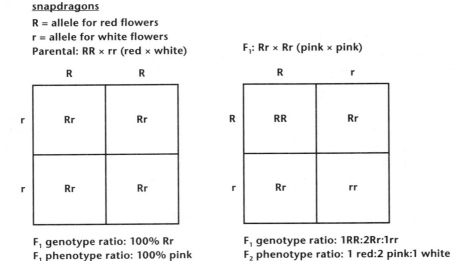

<u>snapdragons</u>
R = allele for red flowers
r = allele for white flowers
Parental: RR × rr (red × white)

F_1: Rr × Rr (pink × pink)

F_1 genotype ratio: 100% Rr
F_1 phenotype ratio: 100% pink

F_1 genotype ratio: 1RR:2Rr:1rr
F_2 phenotype ratio: 1 red:2 pink:1 white

Figure 3.5. Incomplete Dominance

2. CODOMINANCE

Codominance occurs when **multiple alleles** exist for a given gene and more than one of them is **dominant**. Each dominant allele is fully dominant when combined with a recessive allele, but when two dominant alleles are present, the phenotype is the result of the expression of both dominant alleles simultaneously.

The classic example of codominance and multiple alleles is the inheritance of **ABO blood groups** in humans. Blood type is determined by three different alleles, I^A, I^B, and i. Only two alleles are present in any single individual, but the population contains all three alleles. I^A and I^B are both dominant to i. Individuals who are homozygous I^A or heterozygous I^Ai have blood type A, individuals who are homozygous I^B or heterozygous I^Bi have blood type B, while individuals who are homozygous ii have blood type O. However, I^A and I^B are codominant; individuals who are heterozygous $I^A I^B$ have a distinct blood type, AB, which combines characteristics of both the A and B blood groups.

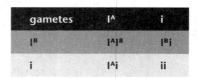

gametes	I^A	i
I^B	$I^A I^B$	$I^B i$
i	$I^A i$	ii

Figure 3.6. Blood Type Alleles

D. Sex Determination

Different species vary in their systems of sex determination. In sexually differentiated species, most chromosomes exist as pairs of homologues called **autosomes**, but sex is determined by a pair of **sex chromosomes**. For example, all humans have 22 pairs of autosomes; females also have a pair of homologous X chromosomes, while males have a pair of heterologous chromosomes, an X and a Y chromosome. The sex chromosomes pair during meiosis and segregate during the first meiotic division. Since females can produce only gametes containing the X chromosome, the gender of a **zygote** is determined by the genetic contribution of the **male gamete**. If the sperm carries a Y chromosome, the zygote will be male; if it carries an X chromosome, the zygote will be female. For *every* mating, there is a 50 percent chance that the zygote will be male and a 50 percent chance that it will be female. This is because fertilization is an independent event.

Genes that are located on the X or Y chromosome are called **sex-linked**. In humans, most sex-linked genes are located on the X chromosome, though some Y-linked traits have been found (e.g., hair on the outer ears).

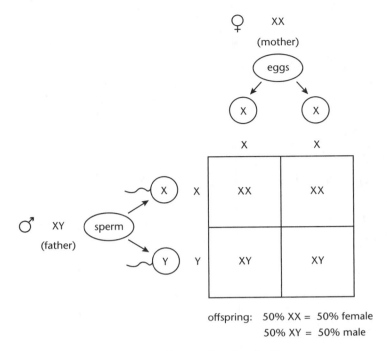

offspring: 50% XX = 50% female
            50% XY = 50% male

Figure 3.7. Sex Determination in Humans

E. Sex-Linkage

In humans, females have two X chromosomes, and males have only one. As a result, recessive genes that are carried on the X chromosome will produce the recessive phenotypes whenever they occur in males, since no dominant allele is present to mask them. The recessive phenotype will thus be much more frequently found in males. Examples of sex-linked recessives in humans are the genes for **hemophilia** and for **color-blindness**.

The pattern of inheritance for a sex-linked recessive gene is somewhat complicated (see Figure 3.8). Since the gene is carried on the X chromosome, and males pass the X chromosome only to their daughters, affected males cannot pass the trait to their male offspring. Affected males will, however, pass the gene to all of their daughters. Unless the daughter also receives the affected gene from her mother as well, she will be a phenotypically normal carrier of the trait. Since all of the daughter's male children will receive their only X chromosome from her, potentially half of her sons will receive the recessive sex-linked allele (X^n). Thus, sex-linked recessives generally affect only males; they cannot be passed from father to son, but they can be passed from father to grandson via a daughter who is a **carrier**, thereby skipping a generation.

GAMETES	Mother (carrier)	
Father (normal)	X^N	X^n
X^N	$X^N X^N$	$X^N X^n$
Y	$X^N Y$	$X^n Y$

Figure 3.8. Inheritance of Sex-Linked Genes

F. *Drosophila Melanogaster*

Modern work with the fruit fly (*Drosophila melanogaster*) helped to provide explanations and insights into the genetic patterns Mendel observed. The fruit fly provides several advantages for genetic research:

- It reproduces often (short life cycle).
- It reproduces in large numbers (large sample size).
- Its chromosomes (especially in the salivary gland) are large and easily recognizable in size and shape.
- Its chromosomes are few (4 pairs, 2N = 8).
- Mutations occur relatively frequently.

Through genetic and mutational analyses of *D. melanogaster*, scientists have elucidated the patterns of embryological development, thereby uncovering how genes expressed early in development can affect the adult organism.

G. Environmental Factors

The environment can often affect the expression of a gene. Interaction between the environment and the genotype produces the phenotype. For example, *Drosophila* with a given set of genes have crooked wings at low temperature but straight wings at higher temperature.

Temperature also influences the hair color of the Himalayan hare. The same genes for color result in white hair on the warmer parts of the body and black hair on colder parts. If the naturally warm portions are cooled (e.g., by the application of ice), the hair will grow in black.

GENETIC PROBLEMS

Although genetic replication is accurate, chromosome number and structure can be altered by abnormal cell division during meiosis or by mutagenic agents.

A. Nondisjunction

Nondisjunction is either the failure of homologous chromosomes to separate properly during meiosis I or the failure of sister chromatids to separate properly during meiosis II. The resulting **zygote** might have either three copies of that chromosome, called **trisomy** (somatic cells will have 2N + 1 chromosomes), or a single copy of that chromosome, called **monosomy** (somatic cells will have 2N − 1 chromosomes). A classic case of trisomy is the birth defect **Down syndrome**, which is caused by trisomy of **chromosome 21**. Most monosomies and trisomies are lethal, causing the embryo to abort spontaneously early in the pregnancy.

Nondisjunction of the sex chromosomes may also occur, resulting in individuals with extra or missing copies of the X and/or Y chromosomes.

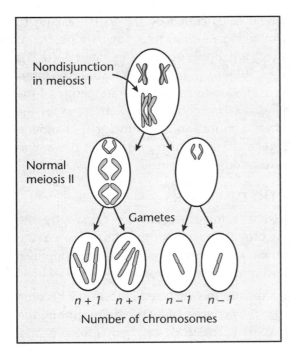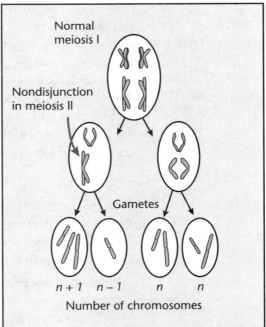

Figure 3.9. Nondisjunction

B. Chromosomal Breakage

Chromosomal breakage may occur spontaneously or be induced by environmental factors, such as mutagenic agents and X-rays. The chromosome that loses a fragment is said to have a deficiency.

C. Mutations

Mutations are changes in the genetic information of a cell, coded in the DNA. Mutations that occur in **somatic** cells can lead to tumors in the individual. Mutations that occur in the sex cells (**gametes**) will be transmitted to the offspring. Most mutations occur in regions of DNA that do not code for proteins and are **silent** (not expressed in the phenotype). Mutations that *do* change the sequence of amino acids in proteins are most often recessive and deleterious.

1. MUTAGENIC AGENTS

Mutagenic agents induce mutations. These include cosmic rays, X-rays, ultraviolet rays, and radioactivity, as well as chemical compounds such as **colchicine** (which inhibits spindle formation, thereby causing polyploidy) or **mustard gas**. Mutagenic agents are generally also **carcinogenic**.

2. MUTATION TYPES

In a gene mutation, nitrogen bases can be **added, deleted,** or **substituted**. These changes can potentially create different genes because they may change the amino acids coded by the gene, leading to inappropriate amino acids being inserted into polypeptide chains when the gene is translated. When this occurs, a mutated protein is produced. However, not every gene mutation will lead to the insertion of a different amino acid. Due to the degenerate nature of the genetic code, a change in the DNA sequence may still code for the same amino acid. Therefore, a **mutation** is a permanent change in the DNA sequence of a gene that may or may not alter the amino acid sequence of the corresponding protein.

3. EXAMPLES OF GENETIC DISORDERS

- **Phenylketonuria** (PKU) is a molecular disease caused by the inability to produce the proper enzyme for the metabolism of the amino acid **phenylalanine**. A degradation product (phenylpyruvic acid) accumulates, causing physiologic problems.

- **Sickle-cell anemia** is a disease in which red blood cells become crescent shaped because they contain defective **hemoglobin**, the molecule that carries oxygen. The sickle-cell hemoglobin is misshapen and therefore carries less oxygen. This disease is caused by a substitution of valine (GUA or GUG) for glutamic acid (GAA or GAG) because of a single base pair substitution in the gene coding for hemoglobin.

MOLECULAR GENETICS

Genes are composed of **DNA** (deoxyribonucleic acid), which contains genetic information **coded** in the sequence of its base pairs, providing the cell with a blueprint for protein synthesis. These proteins regulate all life functions. Furthermore, DNA has the ability to **self-replicate**, which is crucial for cell division and, hence, for organismal reproduction. DNA is the basis of **heredity**; self-replication ensures that its coded sequence will be passed on to successive generations.

In addition, DNA is **mutable** and can be altered under certain conditions, altering the corresponding characteristics in the organism. Changes in DNA are stable and can be passed from generation to generation, providing the basis for evolution.

A. Structure of DNA

The basic unit of DNA is the **nucleotide**, which is composed of **deoxyribose** (a sugar) bonded to both a phosphate group and a nitrogenous base. There are two types of bases: **purines** and **pyrimidines**. The purines in DNA are **adenine** (A) and **guanine** (G), and the pyrimidines are **cytosine** (C) and **thymine** (T).

REMEMBER

To remember the different categories of base, just think: **CUT** the **PY** (Cytosine, Uracil, Thymine are **PY**rimidines) and **PUR** As Gold (**PUR**ines are Adenine and Guanine).

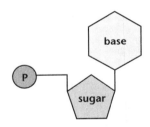

Figure 3.10. Nuczleotide

The phosphate and sugar form a chain, with the bases arranged as side groups off the chain.

A DNA molecule is a **double-stranded helix** with the sugar-phosphate chains on the outside of the helix and the bases on the inside. T always forms two hydrogen bonds with A; G always forms three hydrogen bonds with C. This base-pairing forms "rungs" on the interior of the double helix that link the two polynucleotide chains together. This is known as the **Watson-Crick DNA Model**.

Because of complementary base pairing in DNA, the amount of A will equal the amount of T, and G will equal C. Also, because G is triple bonded to C, the higher the G/C content of DNA, the more tightly bound the two strands will be.

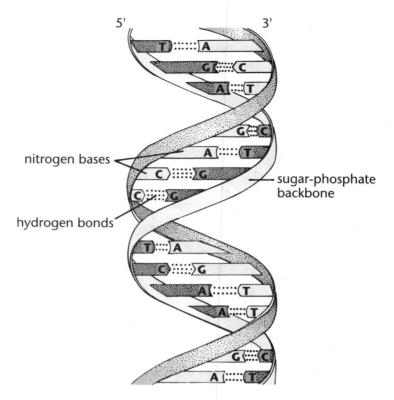

5'   3'

nitrogen bases

sugar-phosphate
backbone

hydrogen bonds

Figure 3.11. DNA Molecule

B. Function of DNA

1. DNA REPLICATION

In order for the process of DNA replication to begin, the double stranded DNA helix is unwound by **helicase** and **gyrase** enzymes. Replication of DNA actually starts with the addition of an **RNA primer** onto the 5' end of the new strand. This primer gives **DNA polymerase** a place to start adding nucleotides. DNA polymerase works on both the template strands simultaneously. Since replication occurs in the 5' to 3' direction of the new strand, this results in two strand types: the **leading strand** (adds nucleotides continuously) and the **lagging strand** (adds nucleotides in pieces called **Okazaki fragments** that are later joined together by **DNA ligase**).

DNA replication is a **semiconservative process**. This is because each strand of double stranded DNA acts as a template in the synthesis of two new daughter strands. Each new daughter strand contains complementary base pairs to one of the original parent strands, creating two DNA double helices that are identical to each other and the parent DNA.

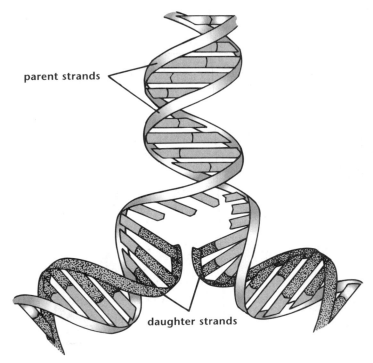

parent strands

daughter strands

Figure 3.12. Semiconservative Replication

2. THE GENETIC CODE

The language of DNA consists of four "letters": A, T, C, and G. The language of **proteins** consists of 20 "words": the **20 amino acids**. Therefore, the DNA nucleotide code within the genes needs to be interpreted in such a way as to produce the 20 amino acids that form proteins. This interpretation occurs through the process of transcription, in which the DNA code is read to produce an mRNA nucleotide transcript. There are a series of triplet codes on mRNA transcripts, known as **codons**, which can be read and translated into their corresponding amino acids. A sequence of three consecutive bases codes for a particular amino acid (e.g., the codon GGC specifies glycine, and the codon GUG specifies valine). The genetic code is **universal** for almost all organisms.

Given that 64 different codons are possible based on the triplet code and only 20 amino acids need to be coded for, the code must contain synonyms. In other words, most amino acids have more than one codon specifying them. This property is referred to as the **degeneracy** or **redundancy** of the genetic code.

Second Base

		U	C	A	G	
First Base (5′)	U	UUU UUC } Phe UUA UUG } Leu	UCU UCC UCA UCG } Ser	UAU UAC } Tyr UAA UAG } Stop	UGU UGC } Cys UGA } Stop UGG } Trp	U C A G
	C	CUU CUC CUA CUG } Leu	CCU CCC CCA CCG } Pro	CAU CAC } His CAA CAG } Gln	CGU CGC CGA CGG } Arg	U C A G
	A	AUU AUC AUA } Ile AUG } Start or Met	ACU ACC ACA ACG } Thr	AAU AAC } Asn AAA AAG } Lys	AGU AGC } Ser AGA AGG } Arg	U C A G
	G	GUU GUC GUA GUG } Val	GCU GCC GCA GCG } Ala	GAU GAC } Asp GAA GAG } Glu	GGU GGC GGA GGG } Gly	U C A G

Third Base (3′)

Figure 3.13. The Genetic Code

C. RNA

1. THE STRUCTURE OF RNA

RNA, ribonucleic acid, is a polynucleotide structurally similar to DNA except that its sugar is **ribose** instead of deoxyribose, it contains **uracil** (U) instead of thymine, and it is usually **single stranded** instead of double-stranded. RNA can be found in both the nucleus and the cytoplasm. There are several types of RNA, all of which are involved in some aspect of protein synthesis: mRNA, tRNA, and rRNA.

a. Messenger RNA (mRNA)

mRNA carries the complement of a DNA sequence and transports it from the **nucleus** to the **ribosomes**, where protein synthesis occurs. During transcription, mRNA is assembled from ribonucleotides that are complementary to the "sense" strand of the DNA. The mRNA has the "inverted" **complementary** codes of the original DNA. For example, since the DNA code for the amino acid valine is AAC, then the mRNA is the complementary GUU. mRNA is **monocistronic** (one mRNA strand codes for one polypeptide) in most eukaryotes, but **polycistronic** (one mRNA strand codes for more than one polypeptide) in prokaryotes.

b. **Transfer RNA (tRNA)**

tRNA is a small RNA found in the cytoplasm that aids in the translation of mRNA's nucleotide code into a sequence of amino acids. tRNA brings amino acids to the ribosomes during protein synthesis. There is at least one type of tRNA for each amino acid; there are approximately 40 known types of tRNA.

c. **Ribosomal RNA (rRNA)**

rRNA, a structural component of ribosome, is the most abundant of all RNA types. rRNA is synthesized in the **nucleolus** (a structure within the nucleus).

D. Protein Synthesis

1. TRANSCRIPTION

Transcription is the process in which information coded in the base sequence of DNA is turned into a strand of mRNA. mRNA (unlike DNA) can move through the nuclear pores into the cytoplasm, where it is translated to protein.

There are three main parts to transcription: **initiation, elongation**, and **termination**. In the **initiation** phase, **RNA polymerase** (the enzyme that adds RNA nucleotides) must first recognize a sequence of DNA called the **promoter** (most commonly the **TATA box** sequence), which indicates the location where transcription should begin. Just as in DNA replication, the DNA helix also needs to unwind before transcription can begin.

In the **elongation** phase of transcription, **RNA polymerase** adds nucleotides to the growing RNA transcript in the 5' to 3' direction using a *single* strand of the DNA double helix as a template. The RNA polymerase enzyme needs the assistance of other molecules known as **transcription factors** to help with the elongation process. Transcription **terminates** when the RNA polymerase recognizes a particular sequence on the new transcript and releases from the transcribing complex (e.g. the GC-rich **hairpin loop** in prokaryotes).

The termination of transcription in prokaryotes produces a complete mRNA transcript that is ready for translation into protein, but in eukaryotes, termination of transcription produces only an intermediate RNA molecule (**hnRNA**) that must undergo **post-translational processing**. This processing includes removing **introns** (sequences that do not code for genes), splicing together **exons** (sequences of genes), and protecting the transcript against the harsh cytoplasmic environment with a **5' cap** and a **poly A tail**. Once these modifications are complete, the mRNA is then ready to move into the cytoplasm and complete the process of translation.

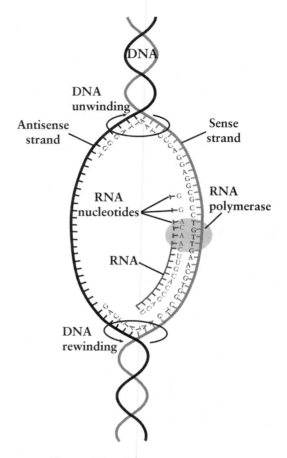

Figure 3.14. Transcription

2. TRANSLATION

Translation is the process whereby mRNA codons are translated into a sequence of amino acids. Translation occurs in the cytoplasm and involves tRNA, ribosomes, mRNA, amino acids, enzymes, and other proteins.

a. tRNA

tRNA brings amino acids to the **ribosomes** in the correct sequence for polypeptide synthesis because tRNA "recognizes" both the amino acid and the mRNA codon. This dual function is reflected in its three-dimensional structure: One end contains a three-nucleotide sequence, the **anticodon**, which is complementary to one of the mRNA codons; the other end is the site of amino acid attachment. Each amino acid has its own **aminoacyl-tRNA synthetase**, which is an enzyme that has an active site that binds to both the amino acid and its corresponding tRNA, catalyzing their attachment to form an aminoacyl-tRNA complex.

b. Ribosomes

Ribosomes are composed of two subunits (consisting of proteins and rRNA), one large and one small, that bind together only during the initiation of protein synthesis. Ribosomes have three binding sites: one for mRNA and two for tRNA. The latter are the **P site** (peptidyl-tRNA binding site) and the **A site** (aminoacyl-tRNA complex binding site). The P site binds to the tRNA attached to the growing polypeptide chain, while the A site binds to the incoming aminoacyl-tRNA complex.

c. Polypeptide synthesis

Polypeptide synthesis can be divided into **three distinct stages**: initiation, elongation, and termination. Initiation of synthesis occurs when the ribosome binds to the mRNA near its 5' end. The ribosome scans the mRNA until it binds to a **start codon** (AUG). The initiator aminoacyl-tRNA complex, methionine-tRNA (with the anticodon 3'-UAC-5'), base-pairs with the start codon.

In **elongation**, hydrogen bonds form between the mRNA codon in the A site and its complementary anticodon on the incoming aminoacyl-tRNA complex. A peptide bond is formed between the amino acid attached to the tRNA in the A site and the methionine attached to the tRNA in the P site. Following peptide bond formation, a ribosome carries uncharged tRNA (one in which the amino acid is no longer attached) in the P site and peptidyl-tRNA in the A site. The cycle of adding one amino acid is completed by **translocation**, in which the ribosome advances three nucleotides along the mRNA in the 5' to 3' direction. In a concurrent action, the uncharged tRNA from the P site is expelled, and the peptidyl-tRNA from the A site moves into the P site. The ribosome then has an empty A site ready for entry of the aminoacyl-tRNA corresponding to the next codon.

Polypeptide synthesis **terminates** when one of three special mRNA **termination codons** (UAA, UAG, or UGA) arrives in the A site. These codons signal the ribosome to terminate translation; they do not code for amino acids. Frequently, many ribosomes simultaneously translate a single mRNA molecule, forming a structure known as a **polyribosome**.

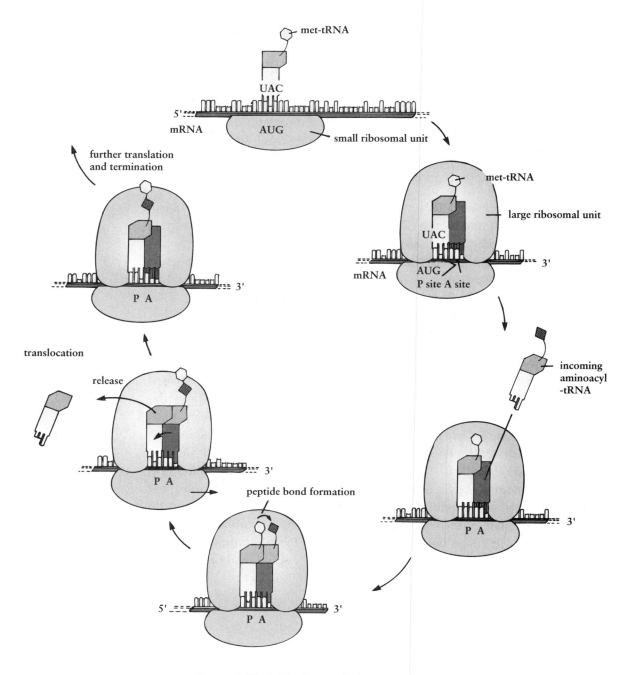

Figure 3.15. Initiation and Elongation

Following the release of the newly formed protein from the ribosome, it immediately assumes its characteristic native conformation. This conformation is determined by the **primary** sequence of amino acids. Furthermore, the polypeptide chains can form intramolecular and intermolecular cross-bridges with **disulfide bonds**. The resulting secondary structure is a complex, intertwined functional protein.

E. Cytoplasmic Inheritance

Heredity systems exist outside the nucleus. For example, **DNA** is found in **chloroplasts**, **mitochondria**, and other cytoplasmic bodies. These cytoplasmic genes may interact with nuclear genes and are important in determining the characteristics of their organelles. Drug resistance in many microorganisms is regulated by cytoplasmic rings of DNA known as **plasmids**, which contain one or more genes.

F. Bacterial Genetics

1. BACTERIAL GENOME

The bacterial genome consists of a single circular chromosome located in the **nucleoid** region of the cell (since there is no membrane bound nucleus in bacteria). Many bacteria also contain smaller circular rings of DNA called **plasmids**, which contain accessory genes. **Episomes** are plasmids that are capable of integration into the bacterial genome.

2. REPLICATION

Replication of the bacterial chromosome begins at a unique origin of replication (ORI) and proceeds in both directions simultaneously. DNA is synthesized in the 5' to 3' direction (as in eukaryotes).

3. GENETIC VARIANCE

Bacterial cells reproduce by **binary fission** and proliferate very rapidly under favorable conditions. Although binary fission is an **asexual** process, bacteria have three mechanisms for increasing the genetic variance of a population: **transformation**, **conjugation**, and **transduction**.

a. Transformation

Transformation is the process by which a foreign chromosome fragment **(plasmid)** is incorporated into the bacterial chromosome via recombination, creating new, inheritable genetic combinations.

b. Conjugation

Conjugation can be described as **sexual mating** in bacteria; it is the transfer of genetic material between two bacteria that are temporarily joined. A cytoplasmic **conjugation bridge** is formed between the two cells, and genetic material is transferred from the donor male (+) type to the recipient female (–) type. Only bacteria containing plasmids called **sex factors** are capable of conjugating. The best studied sex factor is the **F factor** in *E. coli*. Bacteria possessing this plasmid are termed F+ cells; those without it are called F− cells. During conjugation between an F+ and an F− cell, the F+ cell replicates its F factor and donates the copy to the recipient, converting it to an F+ cell. Genes that code for other characteristics, such as antibody resistance, may be found on the plasmids and transferred into recipient cells along with these factors.

Sometimes the sex factor becomes integrated into the bacterial genome. During conjugation, the entire bacterial chromosome replicates and begins to move from the donor cell into the recipient cell. The conjugation bridge usually breaks before the entire chromosome is transferred, but the bacterial genes that enter the recipient cell can easily recombine with the bacterial genes already present to form novel genetic combinations. Recombination occurs by breakage and rearrangement of adjacent regions of DNA. Bacteria with the sex factor integrated into the genome are called **Hfr** cells, meaning that they have a **high frequency of recombination**.

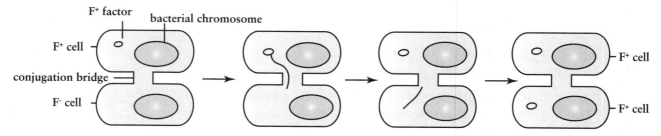

Figure 3.16. Conjugation

c. Transduction

Transduction occurs when fragments of the bacterial chromosome become packaged into viral progeny made during a viral infection. These virions may infect other bacteria and introduce new genetic arrangements through recombination with the new host cell's DNA. The closer two genes are to one another on a chromosome, the more likely they will be to transduce together.

This fact allows geneticists to map genes to a high degree of precision.

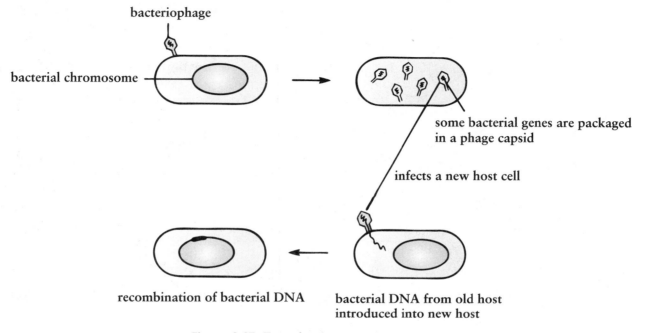

bacteriophage

bacterial chromosome

some bacterial genes are packaged in a phage capsid

infects a new host cell

recombination of bacterial DNA

bacterial DNA from old host introduced into new host

Figure 3.17. Transduction

4. GENE REGULATION

The regulation of gene expression (**transcription**) in bacteria enables them to control their metabolism. Regulation of transcription is based on the accessibility of **RNA polymerase** to the genes being transcribed. Therefore, regulation is directed by an **operon**, which consists of structural genes, an operator gene, and a promoter gene. **Structural genes** contain sequences of DNA that code for **proteins**. The **operator** gene is the sequence of nontranscribable DNA that is the repressor binding site. The **promoter gene** is the noncoding sequence of DNA that serves as the initial binding site for RNA polymerase. There is also a **regulator** gene, which codes for the synthesis of a **repressor** molecule. The repressor binds to the operator and blocks RNA polymerase from transcribing the structural genes.

Regulatory systems function by preventing or permitting the RNA polymerase to pass on to the structural genes. Regulation may be via **inducible systems** or **repressible systems**. Inducible systems are those that require the presence of a substance, called an **inducer**, for transcription to occur. Repressible systems are in a constant state of transcription unless a **corepressor** is present to inhibit transcription.

KEY CONCEPT

- RNA polymerase binds to promoter → structural genes transcribed.
- Repressor binds to operator → structural genes NOT transcribed.
- Inducer binds to repressor → no binding to operator → structural genes transcribed.

a. Inducible Systems

In an **inducible system**, the repressor binds to the operator, thereby preventing RNA polymerase from transcribing the structural genes. For transcription to occur, an inducer must bind to the repressor, forming an **inducer-repressor complex**. This complex cannot bind to the operator, thus releasing the block and permitting transcription. The proteins synthesized are then said to be inducible. In most cases, the structural genes typically code for an enzyme, and the inducer is usually the substrate, or a derivative of the substrate, upon which the enzyme normally acts. When the substrate (inducer) is present, enzymes are synthesized; when it is absent, enzyme synthesis is negligible. In this manner, enzymes are transcribed only when they are actually needed.

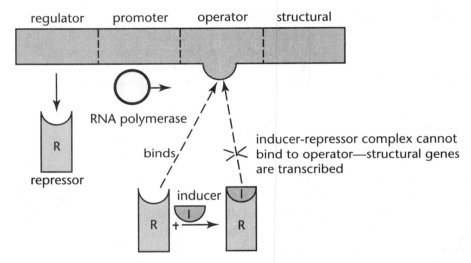

Figure 3.18. Inducible System

b. Repressible Systems

In a **repressible system**, the repressor is inactive until it combines with the corepressor. The repressor can bind to the operator and prevent transcription only when it has formed a **repressor- corepressor complex**. Corepressors are often the **end products** of the biosynthetic pathways they control. The proteins produced (usually enzymes) are said to be repressible since they are normally being synthesized; transcription and translation occur until the corepressor is synthesized. Operons containing mutations, such as deletions or whose regulator genes code for defective repressors, are incapable of being turned off and have enzymes that are always being synthesized. These operons are referred to as **constitutive**.

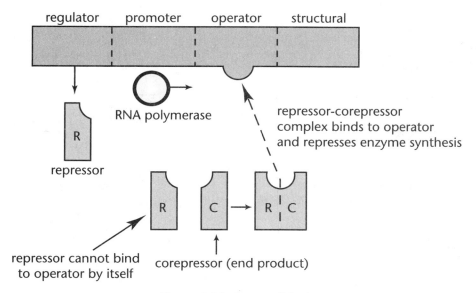

regulator   promoter   operator   structural

RNA polymerase

R

repressor

repressor-corepressor complex binds to operator and represses enzyme synthesis

R   C → R | C

repressor cannot bind to operator by itself

corepressor (end product)

Figure 3.19. Repressible System

G. Bacteriophage

A **bacteriophage** is a virus that infects its host bacterium by attaching to it, boring a hole through the bacterial cell wall, and injecting its DNA while its protein coat remains attached to the cell wall. Once inside its host, the bacteriophage enters either a **lytic cycle** or a **lysogenic cycle**.

1. LYTIC CYCLE

The phage DNA takes control of the bacterium's genetic machinery and manufactures numerous progeny. The bacterial cell then bursts **(lyses)**, releasing new virions, each capable of infecting other bacteria. Bacteriophages that replicate by the lytic cycle, killing their host cells, are called **virulent**. If the initial infection takes place on a bacterial **lawn** (a plated culture), then very shortly a **plaque** or clearing in the lawn occurs corresponding to the area of lysed bacteria. The physical characteristics of a plaque are useful in identifying mutant phage strains that may arise.

2. LYSOGENIC CYCLE

If the bacteriophage does not lyse its host cell, it becomes **integrated** into the bacterial genome in a harmless form (**prophage**), lying dormant for one or more generations. The virus may stay integrated indefinitely, replicating along with the bacterial genome. However, either spontaneously or as a result of environmental circumstances (e.g., radiation, ultraviolet light, or chemicals), the prophage can re-emerge and enter a lytic cycle. Bacteria containing prophages are resistant to further infection ("superinfection") by similar phages.

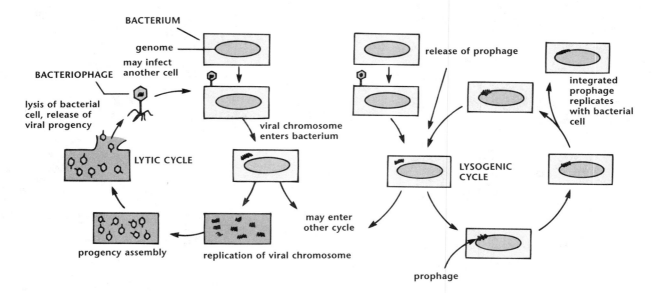

Figure 3.20. Bacteriophage Lifecycle

GENETIC TECHNOLOGY

Several techniques have proven very useful in the study of molecular genetics. **Gel electrophoresis** is used to separate molecules of different sizes using a charge gradient. When trying to separate DNA molecules of different sequence lengths, an **agarose** gel is used. In contrast, synthetic polymer gels like **polyacrylamide** are used to separate proteins of various amino acid lengths.

Blotting is a procedure used to detect molecules and preserve the sample for future use. **Southern blotting** allows for the detection of a specific DNA sequence in a sample of DNA. In this process, DNA is cleaved into fragments by specific restriction endonucleases. The fragments are then separated using electrophoresis and transferred to an inert membrane using blotting techniques. Finally, the desired sequence is detected by exposing the blot to a radioactively labeled probe. Utilizing similar procedures, **Northern blotting** is used for the detection of RNA, while **Western blotting** is used for the detection of specific proteins.

DNA amplification can be accomplished by performing **PCR (Polymerase Chain Reaction)**. There are three steps critical for PCR: denaturation, primer annealing, and primer extension. First, heat is used to **denature** the DNA so that the strands separate and the desired sequence for amplification can be used as a template. In the **annealing** step, complimentary nucleotides called primers attach to the single stranded templates at the start of the desired sequence. Then, DNA polymerase **extends the primer** by attaching bases that are complementary to the template.

Another way to amplify genes is through **DNA cloning**. Usually the DNA sequence of interest is joined to **vectors** (self-replicating phages or plasmids) via **DNA ligase.** Once this recombinant molecule is formed, it can be inserted into a bacterial strain through **transformation**. The bacteria will then produce identical copies of the DNA using its natural DNA replication processes.

Analysis of DNA includes but is not limited to **DNA sequencing**. The most popular method for sequencing DNA is the **chain termination method. The method** uses dideoxynucleotides (ddNTPs or nucleotides modified to prevent addition of more nucleotides) in replication reactions and then separates the resulting single-stranded DNA molecules (which can differ in length by a single nucleotide) by electrophoresis.

DNA is also analyzed for the presence of disease genes using **restriction fragment length polymorphisms (RFLPs). Restriction enzymes** bind to and cut the double stranded DNA at specific sequences. A variation in the fragment length will result when there is a difference in that specific sequence within an individual. Knowledge of the DNA sequence and its expected length, as well as the specific restriction enzymes necessary to cut the DNA, enables researchers to identify genetically the unique fragment patterns for disease and maybe even the specific genes involved.

4

Embryology

Embryology is the study of the development of a unicellular zygote into a complete multicellular organism. For example, in the course of nine months, a unicellular human zygote undergoes cell division, cellular differentiation, and morphogenesis in preparation for life outside the uterus.

EARLY DEVELOPMENTAL STAGES IN VERTEBRATES

A. Fertilization

An egg can be fertilized within 12–24 hours following ovulation. Fertilization occurs in the lateral, widest portion of the oviduct (fallopian tube) when sperm traveling from the vagina encounter an egg. If more than one egg is fertilized, **fraternal twins** may be conceived.

B. Cleavage

Early embryonic development is characterized by a series of rapid mitotic divisions known as **cleavage**. These divisions lead to an increase in cell number without a corresponding growth in cell **protoplasm** (i.e., the total volume of cytoplasm remains constant). Thus, cleavage results in progressively smaller cells, with an increasing ratio of nuclear to cytoplasmic material. Cleavage also increases the surface-to-volume ratio of each cell, thereby improving gas and nutrient exchange. An **indeterminate cleavage** is one that results in cells that maintain the ability to develop into a complete organism. **Identical twins** are the result of an indeterminate cleavage. A **determinate cleavage** results in cells whose future differentiation pathways are determined at an early developmental stage. **Differentiation** is the specialization of cells that occurs during development.

The first complete cleavage of the zygote occurs approximately 32 hours after fertilization. The second cleavage occurs after 60 hours, and the third cleavage after approximately 72 hours, at which point the eight-celled embryo reaches the uterus. As cell division continues, a solid ball of embryonic cells, known as the **morula,** is formed. **Blastulation** begins when the morula develops a fluid-filled cavity called the **blastocoel**, which by the fourth day becomes a hollow sphere of cells called the **blastula**. It is at this stage that the embryo adheres or implants on the uterine wall.

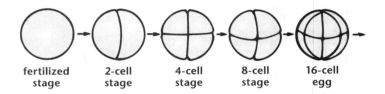

fertilized stage   2-cell stage   4-cell stage   8-cell stage   16-cell egg

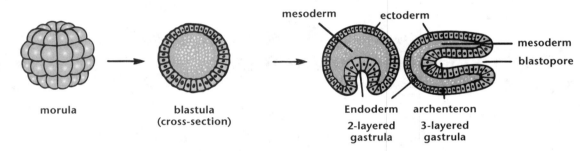

Figure 4.1. Zygote Cleavage and Gastrulation

C. Gastrulation

Once implanted in the uterus, cell migrations transform the single-cell layer of the blastula into a three-layered structure called a **gastrula**. These three primary germ layers are responsible for the differential development of the tissues, organs, and systems of the body at later stages of growth.

- **Ectoderm:** Integument (including the epidermis; hair; nails; and epithelium of the nose, mouth, and anal canal), the lens of the eye, the retina, and the nervous system

- **Endoderm:** Epithelial linings of the digestive and respiratory tracts (including the lungs) and parts of the liver, pancreas, thyroid, and bladder lining

- **Mesoderm:** Musculoskeletal system, circulatory system, excretory system, gonads, connective tissue throughout the body, and portions of digestive and respiratory organs

D. Types of Development

1. EXTERNAL DEVELOPMENT

The early development of many animals occurs outside of the mother's body, on land or in the water. **Fish** and **amphibians** lay eggs that are fertilized externally in the water. The embryo develops within the egg, feeding on nutrients stored in the yolk. **Reptiles**, **birds**, and some **mammals** (like the duck-billed platypus) develop externally on land. Fertilization occurs internally, and the fertilized egg is then laid. Egg shells provide protection for the developing embryo. The eggs also include the following embryonic membranes that facilitate development:

- **Chorion**: The chorion lines the inside of the shell. It is a moist membrane that permits gas exchange.

- **Allantois**: This saclike structure is involved in respiration and excretion, and it contains numerous blood vessels to transport O_2, CO_2, water, salt, and nitrogenous wastes.

- **Amnion**: This membrane encloses the amniotic fluid. **Amniotic fluid** provides an aqueous environment that protects the developing embryo from shock.

- **Yolk sac**: The yolk sac encloses the yolk. Blood vessels in the yolk sac transfer food to the developing embryo.

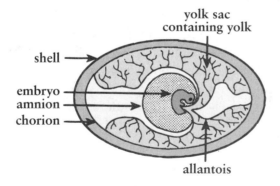

Figure 4.2. Amniote Egg

2. NONPLACENTAL INTERNAL DEVELOPMENT

Early development within the body of the mother protects the young. Certain animals, including **marsupials** and some tropical fish, develop in the mother **without** a placenta. Without a placenta, exchange of food and oxygen between the young and the mother is limited. The offspring may be born very young.

3. PLACENTAL INTERNAL DEVELOPMENT

The growing fetus (see Figure 4.3) receives oxygen directly from its mother through a specialized circulatory system. This system not only supplies oxygen and nutrients to the fetus but removes carbon dioxide and metabolic wastes as well. The two key components of this system are the **placenta** and the **umbilical cord**, which both develop in the first few weeks following fertilization. Remember, gas exchange in the fetus occurs across the placenta. Fetal lungs do not become functional until birth.

The placenta and the umbilical cord are outgrowths of the four extra-embryonic membranes formed during development: the **amnion, chorion, allantois,** and **yolk sac.** The **amnion** is a thin, tough membrane containing a watery fluid called amniotic fluid. Amniotic fluid acts as a shock absorber of external pressure and localized pressure from uterine contractions during labor. Placenta formation begins with the **chorion,** a membrane that completely surrounds the amnion. A third membrane, the **allantois,** develops as an outpocketing of the gut. The blood vessels of the allantoic wall enlarge and become the umbilical vessels, which will connect the fetus to the developing placenta. The **yolk sac,** the site of early development of blood vessels, becomes associated with the umbilical vessels.

E. Birth and Maturation in Vertebrates

Childbirth is accomplished by **labor,** a series of strong uterine contractions. Labor can be divided into three distinct stages. In the first stage, the **cervix** thins and dilates and the amniotic sac ruptures, releasing its fluids. During this time, contractions are relatively mild. The second stage is characterized by rapid contractions, resulting in the birth of the baby (and usually followed by the cutting of the umbilical cord). During the final stage, the uterus contracts, expelling the placenta and the umbilical cord.

The embryo develops into the adult through the process of maturation, which involves cell division, growth, and differentiation. In some animals, maturation is suspended in a temporary state; for example, arthropods have a pupal stage. Mammals develop uninterrupted. Differentiation of cells is complete when all organs reach adult form.

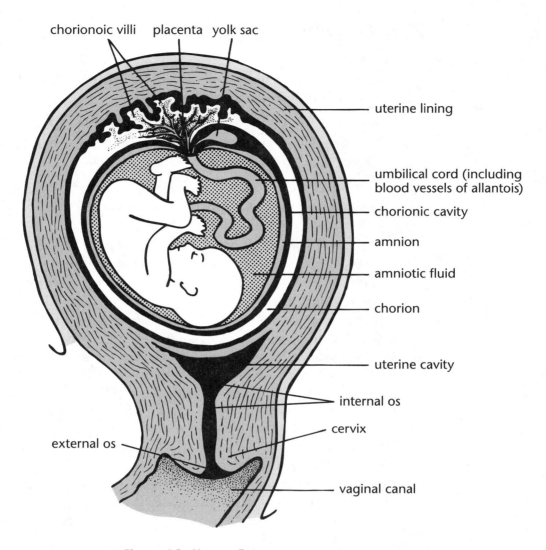

chorionoic villi placenta yolk sac

uterine lining

umbilical cord (including blood vessels of allantois)

chorionic cavity

amnion

amniotic fluid

chorion

uterine cavity

internal os

cervix

external os

vaginal canal

Figure 4.3. Human Fetus

PLANT EMBRYOLOGY

A. Seed Formation

The zygote divides mitotically to form the mass of cells called the embryo. The embryo consists of the following parts:

- **Epicotyl** – this is the precursor of the upper stem and leaves.
- **Cotyledons** – these are the seed leaves. Dicots have two seed leaves while monocots have only one.
- **Hypocotyl** – this develops into the lower stem and root.
- **Endosperm** – the endosperm grows and feeds the embryo. In dicots, the cotyledon absorbs the endosperm.
- **Seed coat** – develops from the outer covering of the ovule. The embryo and its seed coat together comprise the seed.

B. Seed Dispersal

The fruit, in which most seeds develop, is formed from the ovary walls, the base of the flower, and other consolidated flower pistil components. The fruit may be fleshy like a tomato or dry like a nut. It serves as a means of seed dispersal. The fruit enables the seed to be carried more frequently or effectively by air, water, or animals (ingestion and subsequent elimination). The seed is released from the ovary, and will germinate under proper conditions of temperature, moisture, and oxygen.

C. Plant Development

Growth in higher plants is restricted to the embryonic (undifferentiated) cells called **meristem** cells. These tissues undergo active cell reproduction. Gradually, the cells elongate and differentiate into cell types characteristic of the species.

1. APICAL MERISTEM

The apical meristem is found in the tips of roots and stems. Growth in length occurs only at these points.

2. LATERAL MERISTEM

The lateral meristem or **cambium** is located between the xylem and phloem. This tissue permits growth in diameter and can differentiate into new xylem and phloem cells. It is not an active tissue in monocots (grasses) or herbaceous dicots (alfalfa) but is predominant in woody dicots like oaks.

5

Circulatory Systems and Immunology

TRANSPORT SYSTEMS IN PLANTS

Transport in plants must supply plant cells with nutrients and remove waste products. In plants, circulation is called **translocation**. The plant **stem** is the primary organ of transport in the plant. **Vascular bundles** run up and down the stem. The **fibrovascular bundle** at the center of the stem contains xylem, phloem and cambium cells.

A. Xylem

Xylem cells are **thick-walled**, often hollow cells located on the **inside** of the vascular bundle (towards the center of the stem). They carry water and minerals **up** the plant and their thick walls give the plant its rigid support. The outer layer of xylem is alive and is called the **sapwood**. Two types of xylem cells have been differentiated: **vessel cells** and **tracheids**. The rise of water in the xylem is explained by the following:

- **Transpiration pull**—As water evaporates from the leaves of plants, a vacuum is created that pulls water up the stem
- **Capillary action**—Any liquid in a thin tube will rise due to the surface tension of the liquid and interactions between the liquid and the tube.
- **Root pressure**—Water entering the root hairs exerts a pressure that pushes water up the stem.

B. Phloem

Phloem cells are **thin-walled** cells on the **outside** of the vascular bundle. They usually transport nutrients (especially carbohydrates produced in the leaves) **down** the stem. The phloem cells are living and include **sieve tube cells,** and **companion cells**.

C. Cambium

Cambium cells (two layers thick) are the actively dividing, undifferentiated cells that give rise to xylem and phloem. They are between the xylem and phloem cell layers; as they divide, the cells near the phloem differentiate into phloem cells and the cells near the xylem differentiate into xylem cells.

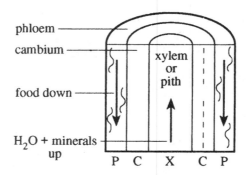

Figure 5.1a. Fibrovascular Bundle

Therefore, proceeding from the outside inwards, the following layers occur: epidermis (outer-bark), cortex, phloem, cambium, xylem, and pith (tissue involved in storage of nutrients and plant support).

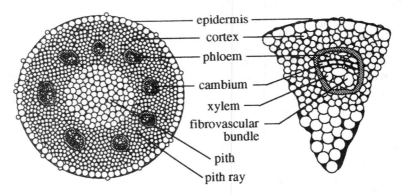

Figure 5.1b. Root Structure

D. Root

The root functions to **absorb** materials through the root hairs and **anchor** the plant. Some roots provide storage for energy reserves (such as turnips and carrots). **Root hairs** are specialized cells of the root epidermis with thin-walled projections. They increase the surface area for absorption of water and minerals from the soil. Like the stem, the root has the following layers: epidermis, cortex, phloem, xylem and cambium. The epidermis contains the root hair cells.

CIRCULATION IN INVERTEBRATES

A. Protozoans

In protozoans, movement of gases and nutrients is accomplished by simple diffusion within the cell.

B. Cnidarians

Hydra and other cnidarians have body walls that are two cells thick. All cells are in direct contact with either the internal or external environments, so there is no need for a specialized circulatory system.

C. Arthropods

Arthropods have **open circulatory systems** in which blood (interstitial fluid) is in direct contact with the body tissues. The blood is circulated primarily by body movements. Blood flows through a **dorsal vessel** and into spaces called **sinuses**, where exchange occurs.

D. Annelids

The earthworm (annelida) uses a **closed circulatory system** (Figure 5.2) to deliver materials to cells that are not in direct contact with the external environment. In a closed circulatory system, blood is confined to blood vessels. Blood moves towards the head in the dorsal vessel, which functions as the main heart by coordinated contractions. Five pairs of vessels called **aortic loops** connect the dorsal vessel to the ventral vessel and function as additional pumps. Earthworm blood lacks any red blood cells, but has instead a hemoglobin-like pigment dissolved in aqueous solution.

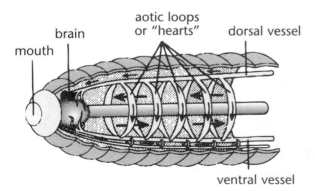

Figure 5.2. Earthworm

FUNCTIONS OF THE CIRCULATORY SYSTEM IN HUMANS

Blood transports nutrients and O_2 to tissues and removes wastes and CO_2 from tissues. Platelets are involved in injury repair. Leukocytes are the main component of the immune system.

A. Transport Of Gases

Erythrocytes transport O_2 throughout the circulatory system and, therefore, the body. Actually, it is the hemoglobin molecules in erythrocytes that bind to O_2. Hemoglobin also binds to CO_2 once O_2 has dissociated.

One of the most important functions of CO_2 gas in the body, including the blood, is to provide an important reactant for the **bicarbonate buffering system**. In this system, CO_2 combines with H_2O to make H_2CO_3 (carbonic acid). The critical part of the system is that H_2CO_3 easily dissociates into **HCO_3^-** (bicarbonate, a weak base) and **H^+** (acidic hydrogen ions). Therefore, simple shifts in the chemical equilibrium of this system (shown below) via respiration in the lungs or the cells, can accommodate many pH imbalances that may occur in the body. Blood plays an important buffering role, as it is a carrier for the crucial gases and ions used in the system.

$$CO_2 + H_2O \leftrightarrow H_2CO_3 \leftrightarrow H^+ + HCO_3^-$$

B. Transport of Nutrients and Wastes

Amino acids and **simple sugars** are absorbed into the bloodstream at the intestinal capillaries. After processing, they are transported throughout the body, where metabolic **waste products** (e.g., water, urea, and carbon dioxide) diffuse into capillaries from surrounding cells. These wastes are then delivered to the appropriate excretory organs.

CIRCULATION IN HUMANS

A. Adult Circulation

The human **cardiovascular system** is composed of a muscular, four-chambered heart, a network of blood vessels, and the blood itself. Oxygenated blood is pumped from the left ventricle of the heart to the **aorta**, which branches into a series of arteries. The **arteries** branch into **arterioles** and then into microscopic **capillaries**. Exchange of gases, nutrients, and cellular waste products occurs via diffusion across the capillary walls.

Eventually, the capillaries converge into **venules** and eventually into **veins**, channeling deoxygenated blood through the **inferior and superior vena**

cava back towards the heart. This blood enters the right atrium and then the right ventricle, which pumps the blood through the **pulmonary arteries** to the lungs so that it can pick up oxygen. Oxygenated blood returns to the heart via the **pulmonary vein** to enter the left atrium, which sends the blood to the left ventricle.

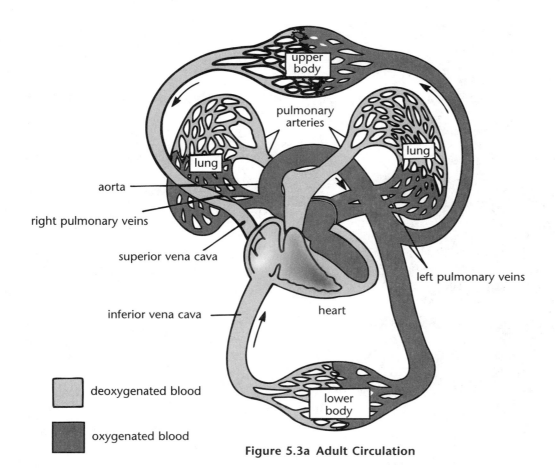

Figure 5.3a Adult Circulation

B. Fetal Circulation

There are notable differences between adult and fetal circulation because the fetal circulation aims to distribute gases and nutrients throughout the developing fetus while bypassing the lungs (it is one of the last organs to mature). One such difference is the **foramen ovale,** which is a hole between the right and left atrium of the fetal heart that shunts blood away from the right ventricle (which leads into the pulmonary circulation). Another is the **ductus arteriosus**, a connection between the aorta and the pulmonary artery that also prevents any blood in the right ventricle from entering the circulation of the developing lungs. A different kind of shunt, the **ductus venosus,** moves oxygenated blood from the umbilical vein to the inferior vena cava of the fetus, allowing oxygenated blood to bypass the liver and travel more directly to the developing fetal brain. These three structures are the hallmarks of fetal circulation in humans.

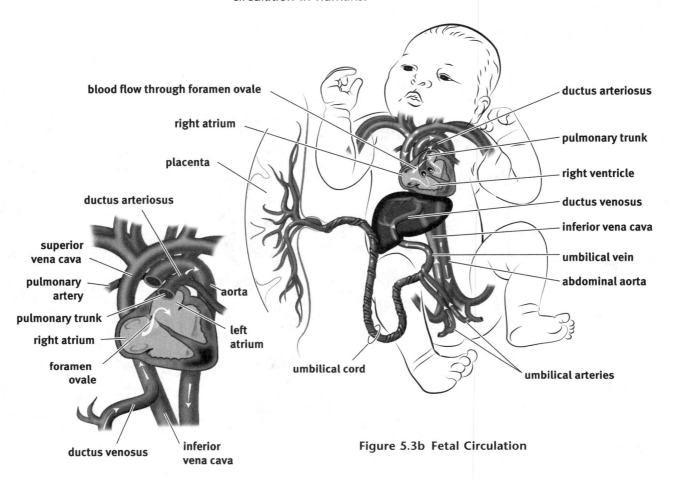

Figure 5.3b Fetal Circulation

A. The Heart

The heart is the driving force of the circulatory system. The right and left halves can be viewed as two pumps: The right side of the heart pumps **deoxygenated** blood into **pulmonary** circulation (towards the lungs), while the left side pumps **oxygenated** blood into **systemic** circulation (throughout the body). The two upper chambers are called atria, and the two lower chambers are called ventricles. The atria are thin walled, while the ventricles are extremely muscular since they "push" the blood to its appropriate destination.

B. Blood Vessels

The three main types of blood vessels are **arteries, veins,** and **capillaries. Arteries** are thick-walled, muscular, elastic vessels that transport oxygenated blood away from the heart—*except* for the pulmonary arteries, which transport deoxygenated blood from the heart to the lungs (in either case, blood is carried *away* from the heart by *ar*teries). **Veins** are relatively thinly walled, inelastic vessels that conduct deoxygenated blood towards the heart—*except* for the pulmonary veins, which carry oxygenated blood from the lungs to the heart (either way, ve*ins* carry blood *in*to the heart). Much of the blood flow in veins depends on their compression by skeletal muscles during movement rather than on the pumping of the heart. Venous circulation is often at odds with gravity; thus, larger veins, especially those in the legs, have valves that prevent backflow. **Capillaries** have very thin walls composed of a single layer of endothelial cells across which respiratory gases, nutrients, and wastes can readily diffuse. Capillaries have the smallest diameter of all three types of vessels; red blood cells must often travel through them single file.

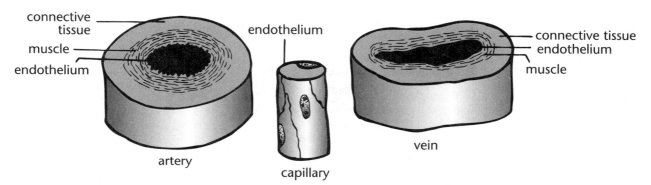

Figure 5.4. Types of Blood Vessels

C. Lymph Vessels

The **lymphatic system** is a secondary circulatory system distinct from the cardiovascular circulation. Its vessels transport excess **interstitial fluid**, called **lymph,** to the cardiovascular system, thereby keeping fluid levels in the body constant. **Lymph nodes** are swellings along lymph vessels containing phagocytic cells **(leukocytes)** that filter the lymph, removing and destroying foreign particles and pathogens.

D. Blood

On the average, the human body contains four to six liters of blood. Blood has both liquid (55%) and cellular components (45%). **Plasma** is the liquid portion of the blood. It is an aqueous mixture of nutrients, salts, respiratory gases, wastes, hormones, and blood proteins (e.g., immunoglobulins, albumin, and fibrinogen). The **cellular components** of the blood are erythrocytes, leukocytes, and platelets.

1. ERYTHROCYTES (RED BLOOD CELLS)

Erythrocytes are the oxygen-carrying components of blood. An erythrocyte contains approximately 250 million molecules of hemoglobin, each of which can bind up to four molecules of oxygen. When hemoglobin binds oxygen, it is called **oxyhemoglobin**. This is the primary form of oxygen transport in the blood. Erythrocytes have a distinct biconcave, disklike shape, which gives them both increased surface area for gas exchange and greater flexibility for movement through the tiny capillaries. Erythrocytes are formed from stem cells in the **bone marrow**, where they lose their nuclei, mitochondria, and membranous organelles (to make more room for oxygen-carrying capacity). Once mature, red blood cells (RBCs) circulate in the blood for about 120 days, after which they are phagocytized by special cells in the spleen and liver.

2. LEUKOCYTES (WHITE BLOOD CELLS)

Leukocytes are larger than erythrocytes and serve protective functions. Some white blood cells (WBCs) selectively and exclusively phagocytize foreign matter and organisms such as bacteria. Others migrate from the blood to tissue, where they mature into stationary cells called **macrophages** , which can either phagocytize pathogens or activate an immune response. Other WBCs, called **lymphocytes,** are involved in immune response and the production of antibodies (**B cells**) or cytolysis (cell death) of infected cells (**T cells**).

3. PLATELETS

Platelets are **cell fragments** that lack nuclei and are involved in clot formation as a response to tissue injury.

Clotting occurs when platelets come into contact with the exposed collagen of a damaged vessel. They release a chemical that causes neighboring platelets to adhere to one another, forming a **platelet plug**. Subsequently, both the platelets and the damaged tissue release the clotting factor **thromboplastin**. Thromboplastin, with the aid of its cofactors calcium and vitamin K, converts the inactive plasma protein **prothrombin** to its active form, **thrombin**. Thrombin then converts **fibrinogen** (another plasma protein) into fibrin. Threads of **fibrin** coat the damaged area and trap blood cells to form a clot. Clots prevent extensive blood loss while the damaged vessel heals itself. The fluid left after blood clotting is called serum.

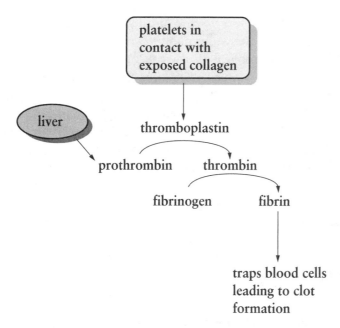

Figure 5.5. Clotting Process

IMMUNOLOGICAL REACTIONS

The body has the ability to distinguish between "self" and "nonself" and to "remember" nonself entities **(antigens)** that it has previously encountered. These defense mechanisms are an integral part of the **immune system**. The immune system is composed of two *specific* defense mechanisms: **humoral** immunity, which involves the production of antibodies, and cell-mediated immunity, which involves cells that combat fungal and viral infection. **Lymphocytes** are responsible for both of these immune mechanisms. The body also has a number of *nonspecific* defense mechanisms.

A. Humoral Immunity

One of the body's specific defense mechanisms is the production of **antibodies**. These responses are specialilzed to the antigen involved. Humoral immunity is responsible for the proliferation of antibodies following exposure to antigens. Antibodies, also called **immunoglobulins (Igs)**, originate from **B cells** and are complex proteins that recognize and bind to specific antigens and trigger the immune system to remove them. Antibodies either attract other cells (such as leukocytes) to phagocytize the antigen directly or cause the antigens to clump together **(agglutinate)** and form large, insoluble complexes, facilitating their removal by phagocytic cells.

Active immunity refers to the production of antibodies during an immune response. Active immunity can be conferred by **vaccination**; an individual is injected with a weakened, inactive, or related form of a particular antigen, which stimulates the immune system to produce specific antibodies against it. Active immunity may require weeks to build up. **Passive immunity** involves the transfer of antibodies produced by another individual or organism. Passive immunity is acquired either passively or by injection. For example, during pregnancy, some maternal antibodies cross the placenta and enter fetal circulation, conferring passive immunity upon the fetus. Although passive immunity is acquired immediately, it is very short-lived, lasting only as long as the antibodies circulate in the blood system. Passive immunity is usually not very specific. **Gamma globulin**, the fraction of the blood containing a wide variety of antibodies, can be used to confer temporary protection against hepatitis and other diseases by passive immunity.

Cell-mediated immunity is another method of specific immune defense. It uses antigen-specific cytotoxic **T lymphocytes** to mediate attacks against foreign material, using activated **macrophages, natural killer cells**, and **cytokines** instead of antibodies. This type of immunity is primarily directed against microbes such as viruses, fungi, and other pathogens. However, it also plays a major role in transplant rejection. The recipient's body recognizes the transplant as foreign and could potentially activate this cell-mediated immune response against the transplant. Immunosuppressing drugs can be used to lower the immune response and decrease the likelihood of rejection.

B. Nonspecific Defense Mechanisms

The body employs a number of nonspecific defenses against foreign material:

- **Skin** is a physical barrier against bacterial invasion. In addition, pores on the skin's surface secrete sweat, which contains an enzyme that attacks bacterial cell walls.
- Passages (e.g., the respiratory tract) are lined with ciliated, **mucous-coated epithelia**, which filter and trap foreign particles.
- **Macrophages** engulf and destroy foreign particles.
- An **inflammatory** response is initiated by the body in response to physical damage. Injured cells release **histamine**, which causes blood vessels to dilate, thereby increasing blood flow to the damaged region. **Granulocytes** attracted to the injury site phagocytize antigenic **material**. An inflammatory response is often accompanied by a **fever**.

- Proteins called **interferons** are produced by cells under viral attack. Interferons diffuse to other cells, where they help prevent the spread of the virus.

Inappropriate response to certain foods and pollen can cause the body to form antibodies and release histamine. These responses are called **allergic** reactions.

BLOOD TYPING

Erythrocytes have characteristic cell-surface proteins **(antigens)**. Remember, antigens are macromolecules that are foreign to the host organism and trigger an immune response. The two major groups of red blood cell antigens are the **ABO group** and the **Rh factor**.

A. ABO Blood Types

Blood Type	Antigen on Red Blood Cell	Antibodies Produced
A	A	anti-B
B	B	anti-A
AB (universal recipient)	A and B	none
O (universal donor)	none	anti-A and anti-B

Type A blood has the A antigen present. Therefore, type A individuals will recognize type A antigen as self and will not respond to it. It is extremely important during blood transfusions that **donor** and **recipient** blood types be appropriately matched. The aim is to avoid transfusion of red blood cells that will be clumped ("rejected") by antibodies present in the recipient's plasma. The rule of blood matching is as follows: If the donor's antigens are already in the recipient's blood, no clumping occurs. **Type AB** blood is termed the "**universal recipient**," as it has neither anti-A nor anti-B antibodies; it can accept blood from any type. **Type O** blood is considered to be the "**universal donor**" as it will not elicit a response from the recipient's immune system since it does not possess any surface antigens.

B. Rh Factor

The Rh factor is another antigen that may be present on the surface of red blood cells. Individuals may be Rh+, possessing the Rh antigen, or Rh–, lacking the Rh antigen. Consideration of the Rh factor is particularly important during **pregnancy**. An Rh– woman can be sensitized by an **Rh+ fetus** if fetal red blood cells (which will have the Rh factor) enter maternal circulation during birth. If this woman subsequently carries another Rh+ fetus, the anti-Rh antibodies she produced when sensitized by the first birth may cross the placenta and destroy fetal red blood cells. This results in a severe anemia for the fetus, known as **erythroblastosis fetalis**. Erythroblastosis is not caused by ABO blood type mismatches between mother and fetus, since anti-A and anti-B antibodies cannot cross the placenta.

6

Endocrinology

CHEMICAL REGULATION IN ANIMALS

The **endocrine system** acts as a means of internal communication, coordinating the activities of the organ systems. Endocrine glands synthesize and secrete chemical substances called **hormones** directly into the circulatory system. (In contrast, **exocrine glands**, such as the salivary glands, secrete substances that are transported by ducts.)

MECHANISM OF HORMONE ACTION

Hormones are classified on the basis of their chemical structure into two major groups: peptide hormones and steroid hormones.

A. Peptides

Peptide hormones range from simple short peptides (amino acid chains) (such as ADH), to complex polypeptides (such as insulin). Peptide hormones act as first messengers. By binding to **specific extracellular receptors** on the surface of their target cells, they trigger a series of enzymatic reactions within each cell. The first is usually the conversion of ATP to cyclic adenosine monophosphate (cAMP), a reaction catalyzed by the membrane-bound enzyme adenylate cyclase. **Cyclic AMP** acts as a **second messenger**, relaying messages from the extracellular peptide hormone to cytoplasmic enzymes, thereby initiating a series of successive reactions in the cell. This is an example of a **cascade effect**; with each step, the hormone's effects are amplified. Cyclic AMP activity is inactivated by the cytoplasmic enzyme phosphodiesterase. Peptide hormone function is usually fast acting and short lived.

B. Steroids

Steroid hormones, such as estrogen and aldosterone, belong to a class of lipid-derived molecules with a characteristic ring structure. Because they are lipid soluble, steroid hormones enter their target cells directly and bind to **specific intracellular receptor** proteins in the cytoplasm. This

---

KEY CONCEPT

Peptide hormones:
- surface receptors
- generally act via secondary messengers

Steroid hormones:
- intracellular receptors
- hormone/receptor binding to DNA promotes transcription of specific genes

---

receptor-hormone complex enters the nucleus and directly activates the expression of specific genes by binding to receptors on the chromatin. This induces a change in mRNA transcription and protein synthesis.

ENDOCRINE GLANDS

Glands that synthesize and/or secrete hormones include the pituitary, hypothalamus, thyroid, parathyroids, adrenals, pancreas, testes, ovaries, pineal, kidneys, gastrointestinal glands, heart, and thymus (see Figure 6.1). Some hormones regulate a single type of cell or organ, while others have more widespread actions. The **specificity** of hormonal action is usually determined by the presence of specific receptors on or in the target cells.

A. Adrenal Glands

The adrenal glands are situated on top of the **kidneys** and consist of the **adrenal cortex** and the **adrenal medulla**.

1. ADRENAL CORTEX

In response to stress, **ACTH** (produced by the anterior pituitary) stimulates the adrenal cortex to synthesize and secrete the steroid hormones, which are collectively known as **corticosteroids.** The corticosteroids, derived from cholesterol, include glucocorticoids, mineralocorticoids, and cortical sex hormones.

a. Glucocorticoids

Glucocorticoids, such as **cortisol** and **cortisone,** are involved in glucose regulation and protein metabolism. Glucocorticoids raise blood glucose levels by promoting protein breakdown and using the products in **gluconeogenesis** (a metabolic pathway that generates glucose from non-carbohydrates), as well as decreasing protein synthesis. Glucocorticoids raise the plasma glucose levels and are antagonistic to the effects of insulin.

b. Mineralocorticoids

Mineralocorticoids, particularly **aldosterone**, regulate plasma levels of sodium and potassium and, consequently, the total extracellular water volume. Aldosterone causes active reabsorption of sodium and passive reabsorption of water in the **nephron**, the functional unit of the kidney. This results in a rise in both blood volume and blood pressure. Excess production of aldosterone results in excess retention of water with resulting **hypertension** (high blood pressure).

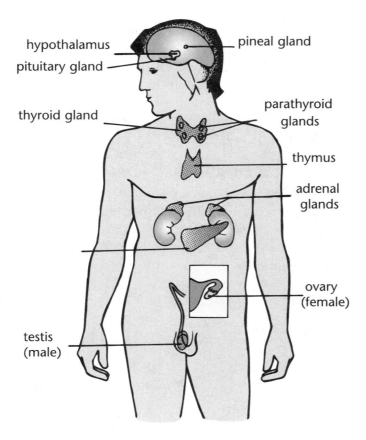

hypothalamus

pituitary gland

pineal gland

thyroid gland

parathyroid glands

thymus

adrenal glands

ovary (female)

testis (male)

Figure 6.1. Human Endocrine System

c. Cortical Sex Hormones

The adrenal cortex secretes small quantities of **androgens** (male sex hormones) like androstenedione and dehydroepiandrosterone in both males and females. Since, in males, most of the androgens are produced by the **testes,** the physiologic effect of the adrenal androgens is quite small. In females, however, overproduction of the adrenal androgens may have masculinizing effects, such as excessive facial hair.

2. ADRENAL MEDULLA

The adrenal medulla produces **epinephrine** (adrenaline) and **norepinephrine** (noradrenaline), both of which belong to a class of amino acid-derived compounds called **catecholamines.**

Epinephrine increases the conversion of glycogen to glucose in liver and muscle tissue, causing a rise in blood glucose levels and an increase in the basal metabolic rate. Both epinephrine and norepinephrine increase the rate and strength of the heartbeat, and they dilate and constrict blood vessels in such a way as to increase the blood supply to skeletal muscle, the heart, and the brain, while decreasing the blood supply to the kidneys, skin, and digestive tract. These effects are known as the **"fight or flight response"** and are elicited by sympathetic nervous stimulation in response to stress. Epinephrine will inhibit certain "vegetative" functions, like digestion, which are not immediately important for survival. Both of these hormones are also **neurotransmitters** (chemicals important for signaling in the nervous system).

3. CONTROL OF ADRENAL HORMONES

Release of adrenal cortical hormones is under the control of adrenocorticotrophic hormone (ACTH), a hormone secreted by the **anterior pituitary gland**. ACTH stimulates the production of glucocorticoids and sex steroids; aldosterone production is controlled by the renin-angiotensin mechanism.

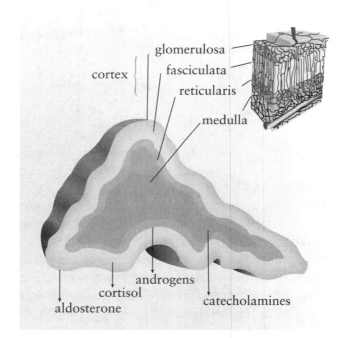

Figure 6.2. Adrenal Gland

B. Pituitary Gland

The pituitary (**hypophysis**) is a small, trilobed gland lying at the base of the brain. The two main lobes, anterior and posterior, are functionally distinct. (In humans, the third lobe, the intermediate lobe, is rudimentary.)

1. ANTERIOR PITUITARY

The anterior pituitary synthesizes both **direct hormones**, which directly stimulate their target organs, and **tropic hormones**, which stimulate other endocrine glands to release hormones. The hormonal secretions of the anterior pituitary are regulated by hypothalamic secretions called releasing/inhibiting hormones or factors.

a. Direct Hormones

i. Growth hormone (GH, somatotropin)

GH promotes bone and muscle growth. In children, a GH deficiency can lead to stunted growth (**dwarfism**), while overproduction of GH results in **gigantism.** Overproduction of GH in adults causes **acromegaly,** a disorder characterized by a disproportionate overgrowth of bone, localized especially in the skull, jaw, feet, and hands.

ii. Prolactin

Prolactin stimulates milk production and secretion in female mammary glands.

iii. Endorphins

Endorphins are neurotransmitters that behave like opioids, providing an internal mechanism for pain relief and producing pleasurable sensations.

b. Tropic Hormones

i. Adrenocorticotropic hormone (ACTH)

ACTH stimulates the adrenal cortex to synthesize and secrete glucocorticoids and is regulated by the releasing hormone corticotrophin-releasing factor (CRF).

ii. Thyroid-stimulating hormone (TSH)

TSH stimulates the thyroid gland to synthesize and release thyroid hormones, including thyroxine.

iii. Luteinizing hormone (LH)

In females, LH stimulates ovulation and formation of the **corpus luteum**, which secretes progesterone and estrogen. In males, LH stimulates the interstitial cells of the testes to synthesize testosterone.

iv. Follicle-stimulating hormone (FSH)

In females, FSH causes maturation of ovarian follicles, which then secrete estrogen; in males, FSH stimulates maturation of the seminiferous tubules and sperm production.

REMEMBER

To help remember the hormones of the anterior pituitary, think FLAT PEG:

FSH	Prolactin
LH	Endorphins
ACTH	GH
TSH	

2. POSTERIOR PITUITARY

The posterior pituitary (**neurohypophysis**) does not synthesize hormones; it stores and releases the peptide hormones **oxytocin** and **ADH**, both of which are produced by the neurosecretory cells of the hypothalamus. Hormone secretion occurs when action potentials descend from the hypothalamus in response to the body's signaling.

a. Oxytocin

Oxytocin, which is secreted during childbirth, increases the strength and frequency of uterine muscle contractions. Oxytocin release during childbirth represents a positive feedback control mechanism; oxytocin release causes uterine contractions, and uterine contractions stimulate the release of more oxytocin. The process repeats until the baby is born. Oxytocin secretion is also induced by suckling, as it also stimulates milk secretion in the mammary glands.

b. Antidiuretic hormone (ADH or vasopressin)

ADH increases the permeability of the **collecting duct** in the nephron (functional unit of the kidney) to water, thereby promoting water reabsorption and decreasing blood osmolarity by increasing blood volume. ADH is secreted when plasma osmolarity increases, as sensed by osmoreceptors in the hypothalamus, or when blood volume decreases, as sensed by baroreceptors in the circulatory system.

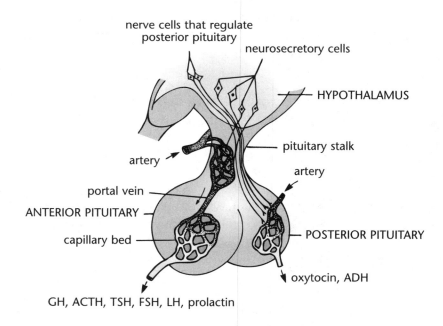

Figure 6.3. Hypothalamus and Pituitary Gland

C. Hypothalamus

The hypothalamus is part of the forebrain and is located directly above the pituitary gland. The hypothalamus receives neural transmissions from other parts of the brain and peripheral nerves, which trigger specific responses from its neurosecretory cells. The neurosecretory cells regulate pituitary gland secretions via negative feedback mechanisms and through the actions of inhibiting and releasing hormones.

1. INTERACTIONS WITH ANTERIOR PITUITARY

Hypothalamic-releasing hormones stimulate or inhibit the secretions of the anterior pituitary. For example, **GnRH** stimulates the anterior pituitary to secrete **FSH** and **LH.** Releasing hormones are secreted into the **hypothalamic-hypophyseal portal system**. In this circulatory pathway, blood from the capillary bed in the hypothalamus flows through a portal vein into the anterior pituitary, where it diverges into a second capillary network. In this way, releasing hormones can immediately reach the anterior pituitary.

A complicated feedback system regulates the secretions of the endocrine system. For example, when the plasma levels of adrenal cortical hormones drop, hypothalamic cells release ACTH-releasing factor (ACTH-RF) into the portal system. When the plasma concentration of corticosteroids exceeds the normal plasma level, the steroids themselves exert an inhibitory effect on the hypothalamus (via a negative feedback mechanism).

2. INTERACTIONS WITH POSTERIOR PITUITARY

Neurosecretory cells in the hypothalamus synthesize both **oxytocin** and **ADH** and transport them via their axons into the posterior pituitary for storage and secretion.

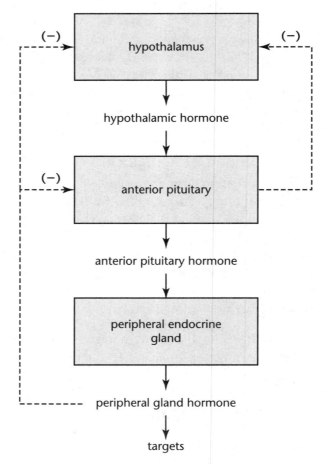

Figure 6.4. Feedback Mechanisms for Hypothalamus and Pituitary

D. Thyroid

The thyroid gland is a bi-lobed structure located on the ventral surface of the trachea. It produces and secretes thyroxine and triiodothyronine (the thyroid hormones) and calcitonin.

1. THYROID HORMONES (THYROXINE AND TRIIODOTHYRONINE)

Thyroxine (T_4) and triiodothyronine (T_3) are derived from the iodination of the amino acid **tyrosine.** Thyroid hormones are necessary for growth and neurological development in children. They also increase the rate of metabolism throughout the body.

In **hypothyroidism**, thyroid hormones are undersecreted or not secreted at all. Common symptoms of hypothyroidism include a slowed heart rate and respiratory rate, fatigue, cold intolerance, and weight gain. Hypothyroidism in newborn infants, called **cretinism,** is characterized by mental retardation and short stature. In

hyperthyroidism, the thyroid is overstimulated, resulting in the over-secretion of thyroid hormones. Symptoms often include increased metabolic rate, feelings of excessive warmth, profuse sweating, palpitations, weight loss, and protruding eyes. In both disorders, the thyroid often enlarges, forming a bulge in the neck called a **goiter.**

2. CALCITONIN

Calcitonin decreases plasma Ca^{2+} concentration by inhibiting the release of Ca^{2+} from bone. Calcitonin secretion is regulated by plasma Ca^{2+} levels. Calcitonin is antagonistic to parathyroid hormone.

E. Pancreas

The pancreas is both an **exocrine** organ and an **endocrine** organ. The exocrine function is performed by the cells that secrete digestive enzymes into the small intestine via a series of ducts. The endocrine function is performed by small glandular structures called the **islets of Langerhans,** which are composed of alpha and beta cells. Alpha cells produce and secrete glucagon; beta cells produce and secrete insulin.

1. GLUCAGON

Glucagon stimulates protein and fat degradation, the conversion of glycogen to glucose, and gluconeogenesis, all of which serve to increase blood glucose levels. Glucagon's actions are largely antagonistic to those of insulin.

KEY CONCEPTS

- Insulin decreases plasma glucose.
- Glucagon increases plasma glucose.

2. INSULIN

Insulin is a protein hormone secreted in response to a high blood glucose concentration. It stimulates the uptake of glucose by muscle and adipose cells and the storage of glucose as glycogen in muscle and liver cells, thus lowering blood glucose levels. It also stimulates the synthesis of fats from glucose and the uptake of amino acids. Insulin's actions are antagonistic to those of **glucagon** and the **glucocorticoids. (**Don't forget that growth hormone, the glucocorticoids, and epinephrine are also capable of increasing plasma glucose.) Underproduction of insulin, or an insensitivity to insulin, leads to **diabetes mellitus,** which is characterized by hyperglycemia (high blood glucose levels).

F. Parathyroid Glands

The parathyroid glands are four small, pea-shaped structures embedded in the posterior surface of the thyroid. These glands synthesize and secrete **parathyroid hormone (PTH),** which regulates plasma Ca^{2+} concentration. PTH raises the Ca^{2+} concentration in the blood by increasing bone resorption and decreasing Ca^{2+} excretion in the kidneys. Calcium

KEY CONCEPTS

- PTH increases Ca^{2+}.
- CalciTONIN decreases Ca^{2+}. (or TONES down Ca^{2+}.)

in bone is bonded to phosphate, and breakdown of the bone releases phosphate as well as calcium. Parathyroid hormone compensates for this by stimulating excretion of phosphate by the kidneys.

G. Kidneys

When blood volume falls, the kidneys produce **renin**—an enzyme that converts the plasma protein angiotensinogen to **angiotensin I**. Angiotensin I is converted to **angiotensin II**, which stimulates the adrenal cortex to secrete **aldosterone**. Aldosterone helps to restore blood volume by increasing sodium reabsorption at the kidney, leading to an increase in water. This removes the initial stimulus for renin production and helps maintain homeostasis.

H. Gastrointestinal Hormones

Ingested food stimulates the stomach to release the hormone gastrin. **Gastrin** is carried to the gastric glands and stimulates the glands to secrete HCl in response to food in the stomach. Secretion of pancreatic juice, the exocrine secretion of the pancreas, is also under hormone control: The hormone **secretin** is released by the small intestine when acidic food material enters from the stomach. Secretin stimulates the secretion of an alkaline bicarbonate solution from the pancreas, which neutralizes the acidity of the **chyme** (partially digested food coming from the stomach). The hormone **cholecystokinin** is released from the small intestine in response to the presence of fats and causes the contraction of the gallbladder and release of bile into the small intestine. **Bile** is involved in the digestion of fats. Cholecystokinin is a special hormone because it also travels to the brain's satiation center to indicate the sensation of being "full."

I. Pineal Gland

The pineal gland is a tiny structure at the base of the brain that secretes the hormone **melatonin**. The role of melatonin in humans is unclear, but it is believed to play a role in the regulation of **circadian rhythms**—physiological cycles lasting 24 hours. Melatonin secretion is regulated by light and dark cycles in the environment. In primitive vertebrates, melatonin lightens the skin by concentrating pigment granules in melanophores.

REGULATION IN PLANTS

Plant hormones are primarily involved in the regulation of growth. They are produced by actively growing parts of the plant, such as the **meristematic tissues** in the apical region (apical meristem) of shoots and roots. They are also produced in young, growing leaves and developing seeds.

A. Auxins

Auxins are an important class of plant hormones associated with several types of growth patterns.

1. PHOTOTROPISM

Auxins are responsible for **phototropism**, the tendency of the shoots of plants to bend towards light sources (particularly the sun). When light strikes the tip of a plant from one side, the auxin supply on that side is **reduced**. Thus, the illuminated side of the plant grows more slowly than the shaded side. This asymmetrical growth in the cells of the stem causes the plant to bend towards the light side. **Indoleacetic acid** is one of the auxins associated with phototropism.

2. GEOTROPISM

Geotropism is the growth of portions of plants towards or away from gravity.

- **Negative geotropism** causes shoots to grow upward, away from the acceleration of gravity. If a plant is turned on its side (horizontally), the shoot will eventually turn upward again. Gravity increases the concentration of auxin on the lower side of the horizontally placed plant, while the concentration on the upper side decreases. This unequal distribution of auxins stimulates cells on the lower side to elongate faster than cells on the upper side, causing the plant to grow vertically.

- **Positive geotropism** causes roots to grow towards the pull of gravity. Horizontally placed roots have the same auxin distribution as horizontally placed stems, but the effect on the root cells is opposite. Cells exposed to a higher concentration of auxin are inhibited from growing, while the cells with lower concentration continue to grow. This causes the root to turn downwards.

3. INHIBITION OF LATERAL BUDS

Auxins produced in the terminal bud of a plant's growing tip move downward in the shoot and inhibit development of lateral buds. Conversely, auxins also initiate the formation of lateral roots, while they inhibit root elongation.

B. Gibberellins

Gibberellins stimulate rapid stem elongation, particularly in plants that normally do not grow tall (e.g., dwarf plants). They **inhibit** the formation of new roots and stimulate the production of **new phloem** cells by the **cambium** (whereas auxins stimulate the production of new **xylem** cells). Gibberellins also terminate the dormancy of seeds and buds. They induce some biennial plants to flower during their first year of growth.

C. Kinins

Kinins also promote cell division. **Kinetin** is an important type of cytokinin. The ratio of kinetin to auxin is of particular importance in the determination of the timing of the differentiation of new cells. The action of kinetin is enhanced when auxin is present.

D. Ethylene

Ethylene stimulates fruit ripening. Ethylene also induces **senescence** or aging.

E. Inhibitors

Inhibitors block cell division and serve an important role in growth regulation. They are particularly important to the maintenance of dormancy in the lateral buds and seeds of plants during autumn and winter. Inhibitors break down gradually with time (and in some cases are destroyed by cold), so that buds and seeds can become active in the next growing season. **Abscisic acid** is one of the most important inhibitors.

F. Anti-Auxins

Anti-auxins regulate the activity of auxins. For example, **indoleacetic acid oxidase** regulates the concentration of **indoleacetic acid**. An increase in the concentration of indoleacetic acid increases the amount of indoleacetic acid oxidase produced.

7

Nervous System

The **nervous system** enables organisms to receive and respond to **stimuli** from their external and internal environments. **Neurons** are the functional units of the nervous system. A neuron converts stimuli into **electrochemical signals,** which are conducted through the nervous system. The nervous system responds to stimuli more rapidly than the endocrine system.

INVERTEBRATE NERVOUS SYSTEMS

A. Protozoa

Unicellular organisms possess no organized nervous system. These single-celled organisms may respond to stimuli such as touch, heat, light, and chemicals.

B. Cnidaria

Cnidarians have a simple nervous system called a **nerve net**. This network of nerve cells may have limited centralization. Some jellyfish have clusters of cells and pathways that coordinate the relatively complex movements required for swimming.

C. Annelida

Earthworms possesses a primitive **central nervous system**, consisting of a defined ventral nerve cord and an anterior "brain" of fused ganglia (i.e., clusters of nerve cell bodies). Definite nerve pathways lead from receptors to effectors.

D. Arthropoda

Arthropod brains are similar to those of annelids, but more specialized sense organs are present (e.g., **compound** or **simple eyes, tympanum** for detecting sound).

VERTEBRATE NERVOUS SYSTEMS

NEURON

A. Structure

A neuron is the basic building block of the nervous system. It is an elongated cell consisting of several dendrites, a cell body, and a single axon. **Dendrites** are cytoplasmic extensions of the cell body that receive information and transmit it towards the cell. The **cell body (soma)** contains the nucleus and controls the metabolic activity of the neuron. The **axon** is a long cellular process that transmits impulses away from the cell body. Most mammalian axons are sheathed by an insulating substance known as **myelin**, which allows axons to conduct impulses faster. Myelin is produced by cells known as glial cells. (**Oligodendrocytes** produce myelin in the central nervous system, and **Schwann cells** produce myelin in the peripheral nervous system.) The gaps between segments of myelin are called **nodes of Ranvier**. The axons end as swellings known as **synaptic terminals** (sometimes also called synaptic boutons or knobs). **Neurotransmitters** are released from these terminals into the **synapse** (or synaptic cleft), which is the gap between the axon terminals of one cell and the dendrites of the next cell.

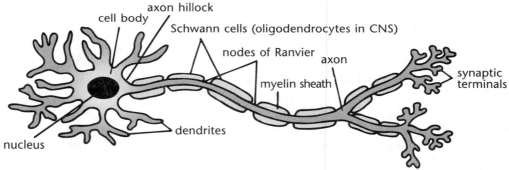

Figure 7.1. Peripheral Nerve

B. Function

Neurons are specialized to receive signals from sensory receptors or from other neurons in the body and transfer this information along the length of the axon. Impulses, known as **action potentials**, travel the length of the axon and invade the nerve terminal, thereby causing the release of neurotransmitter into the synapse. When a neuron is at rest, the potential difference between the extracellular space and the intracellular space is called the **resting potential**.

1. RESTING POTENTIAL

Even at rest, a neuron is **polarized**. This potential difference is the result of an unequal distribution of ions between the inside and outside of the cell. A typical resting membrane potential is **−70 millivolts** (mV), which means that the inside of the neuron is more negative than the outside. This difference is due to selective ionic permeability of the neuronal cell membrane and is maintained by the **active transport** by the **Na⁺/K⁺ pump** (also called the Na⁺/K⁺ ATPase). Because the transmission of action potentials lead to the disruption of the ionic gradients, the gradients must be restored by the Na⁺/K⁺ pump. This pump, using ATP energy, transports 3 Na⁺ out for every 2 K⁺ it transports into the cell.

So, at rest the pump ensures that the concentration of K⁺ is higher inside the neuron than outside and that the concentration of Na⁺ is higher outside than inside. The resting potential is created because the neuron is **selectively permeable** to K⁺, so K⁺ diffuses down its concentration gradient, leaving a net negative charge inside. (Neurons at rest are relatively **impermeable** to Na⁺, so the cell remains polarized.) Additionally, negatively charged proteins are trapped inside the cell.

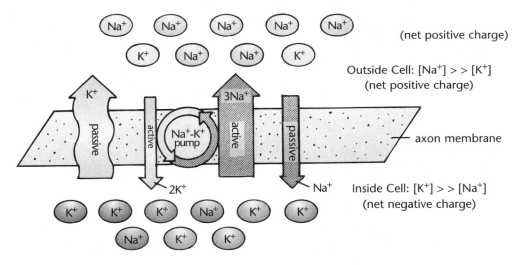

Figure 7.2. Resting Potential of a Neuron

2. ACTION POTENTIAL

The nerve cell body receives both excitatory and inhibitory impulses from other cells. If the cell becomes sufficiently excited or **depolarized** (i.e., the inside of the cell becomes less negative), an **action potential** is generated. The minimum **threshold** membrane potential (usually around −50 mV) is the level at which an action potential is initiated.

Ion channels located in the nerve cell membrane open in response to these changes in voltage and are, therefore, called voltage-gated ion channels. An action potential begins when **voltage-gated Na⁺ channels** open in response to small fluctuations in membrane potential leading to some depolarization, allowing Na⁺ to rush down its electrochemical gradient into the cell, causing a rapid further depolarization of that segment of the cell. The voltage-gated Na⁺ channels close just as quickly as they opened, and **voltage-gated K⁺ channels** open, allowing K⁺ to rush out down its electrochemical gradient. This returns the cell to a more negative potential, a process known as **repolarization**. In fact, the neuron may shoot past the resting potential and become even more negative inside than normal; this is called **hyperpolarization**. Immediately following an action potential, it may be very difficult or impossible to initiate another action potential. This period of time is called the **refractory period** and it represents the time the Na⁺ channels need to recover from inactivation.

The action potential is often described as an **all-or-none response**. This means that the nerve fires either maximally or not at all. Whenever the threshold membrane potential is reached, an action potential with a consistent size and duration is produced. Stimulus intensity is coded by the **frequency** of action potentials.

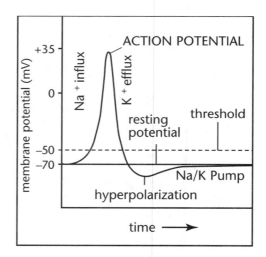

Figure 7.3. Action Potential

3. IMPULSE PROPAGATION

Although axons can theoretically propagate action potentials bidirectionally, information transfer will occur only in one direction: from dendrite to synaptic terminal. Synapses operate only in one direction because refractory periods make the backward travel of action potentials impossible. Different axons can propagate action potentials at **different speeds**. The greater the **diameter** of the axon and the more heavily it is **myelinated**, the faster the impulses will travel. Myelin increases the conduction velocity by insulating segments of the axon, so the membrane is permeable to ions only in the nodes of Ranvier. In this way, the action potential "jumps" from node to node.

SYNAPSE

The synapse is the gap between the **axon terminal** of one neuron (called the **presynaptic neuron** because it is before the synapse) and the **dendrites** of another neuron **(postsynaptic neuron)**. Neurons may also communicate with postsynaptic cells other than neurons, such as cells in muscles or glands; these are called **effector cells**. The nerve terminal contains thousands of membrane-bound vesicles full of chemical messengers known as **neurotransmitters**. When the action potential arrives at the nerve terminal and depolarizes it, the synaptic vesicles fuse with the presynaptic membrane and release neurotransmitter into the synapse. The neurotransmitter **diffuses** across the synapse and acts on receptor proteins embedded in the postsynaptic membrane. The neurotransmitter can lead to depolarization of the postsynaptic cell and consequent firing of an action potential. Neurotransmitter is removed from the synapse in a variety of ways: It may be taken back up into the nerve terminal (via a protein known as an uptake carrier), where it may be reused or degraded; it may be degraded by enzymes located in the synapse (e.g., **acetylcholinesterase** inactivates the neurotransmitter **acetylcholine**); or it may simply diffuse out of the synapse.

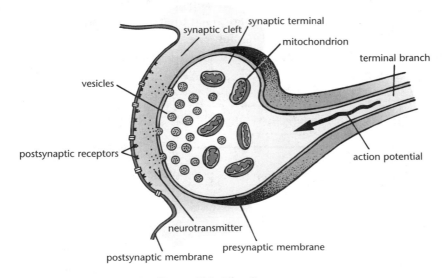

Figure 7.4. The Synapse

A. Drug Effects on Synapses

- **Curare** blocks the postsynaptic acetylcholine receptors so that acetylcholine is unable to interact with the receptor. This leads to paralysis by blocking nerve impulses to muscles.

- **Botulism toxin** prevents the release of acetylcholine from the presynaptic membrane and also results in paralysis.

- **Anticholinesterases** are used as nerve gases and in the insecticide parathion. As the name implies, these substances inhibit the activity of the **acetylcholinesterase** enzyme. As a result, the acetylcholine is not degraded in the synapse and continues to affect the postsynaptic membrane. Therefore, no coordinated muscular contractions can take place.

VERTEBRATE NERVOUS SYSTEM ORGANIZATION

There are many different kinds of neurons in the vertebrate nervous system. Neurons that carry **sensory** information about the external or internal environment to the brain or spinal cord are called **afferent neurons**. Neurons that carry **motor** commands from the brain or spinal cord to various parts of the body (e.g., muscles or glands) are called **efferent neurons**. Some neurons **(interneurons)** participate only in local circuits. They link sensory and motor neurons in the brain and spinal cord, plus their cell bodies and nerve terminals are in the same location.

Nerves are essentially **bundles of axons** covered with connective tissue. A network of nerve fibers is called a **plexus**. Neuronal cell bodies often cluster together. Such clusters are called **ganglia** in the periphery, and in the central nervous system, they are called **nuclei**. The nervous system itself is divided into two major systems, the **central** nervous system and the **peripheral** nervous system.

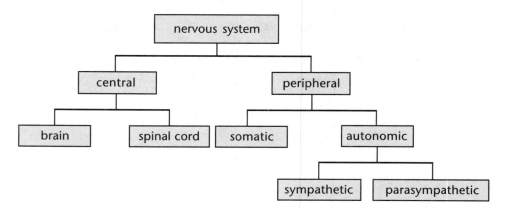

Figure 7.5. Organization of Vertebrate Nervous

A. Central Nervous System

The central nervous system (CNS) consists of the brain and spinal cord.

1. BRAIN

The brain is a mass of neurons that resides in the skull. Its functions include interpreting sensory information, forming motor plans, and cognitive function (thinking). The brain consists of an outer portion called the gray matter (cell bodies) and an inner white matter (myelinated axons). The brain can be divided into the forebrain, midbrain, and hindbrain.

a. Forebrain

The forebrain consists of the **telencephalon** and the **diencephalon**. A major component of the telencephalon is the **cerebral cortex**, which is the highly convoluted gray matter that can be seen on the surface of the brain. The cortex processes and integrates sensory input and motor responses and is important for memory and creative thought. On the inferior portion of the forebrain is the **olfactory bulb**, the center for reception and integration of olfactory or odor input.

The **diencephalon** contains the thalamus and hypothalamus. The **thalamus** is a relay and integration center for the spinal cord and cerebral cortex. The **hypothalamus** controls visceral functions, such as hunger, thirst, sex drive, water balance, blood pressure, and temperature regulation. It also plays an important role in the control of the endocrine system via feedback mechanisms.

b. Midbrain (Mesencephalon)

The midbrain is a relay center for visual and auditory impulses. It also plays an important role in motor control.

c. Hindbrain

The hindbrain is the **posterior** part of the brain and consists of the cerebellum, the pons, and the medulla. The **cerebellum** helps to modulate motor impulses initiated by the cerebral cortex and is important in the maintenance of balance, hand-eye coordination, and the timing of rapid movements. One function of the **pons** is to act as a relay center to allow the cortex to communicate with the cerebellum. The **medulla** (also called the medulla oblongata) controls many vital functions, such as breathing, heart rate, and gastrointestinal activity. Together, the midbrain, pons, and medulla constitute the **brainstem**.

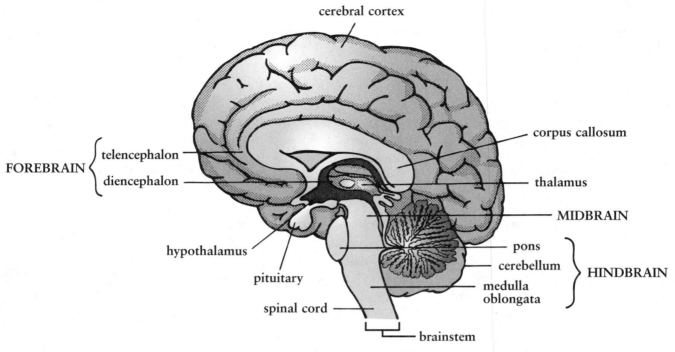

FOREBRAIN { telencephalon — diencephalon —

cerebral cortex

corpus callosum

thalamus

MIDBRAIN

pons
cerebellum } HINDBRAIN
medulla
oblongata

hypothalamus

pituitary

spinal cord —

brainstem

Figure 7.6. Human Brain

2. SPINAL CORD

The spinal cord is an elongated extension of the brain that acts as the conduit for sensory information to the brain and motor information from the brain. The spinal cord can also integrate simple motor responses (e.g., **reflexes**) by itself. A cross section of the spinal cord reveals an outer white matter area containing motor and sensory axons and an inner gray matter area containing nerve cell bodies. Sensory information enters the spinal cord through the **dorsal horn**; the cell bodies of these sensory neurons are located in the dorsal root ganglia. All motor information exits the spinal cord through the **ventral horn**. For simple reflexes, like the knee-jerk reflex, sensory fibers (entering through the dorsal root ganglion) synapse directly on ventral horn motor fibers. Other reflexes include interneurons between the sensory and motor fibers, which allow for some processing in the spinal cord.

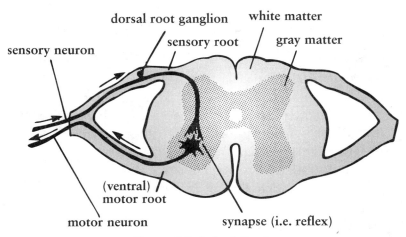

Figure 7.7. Spinal Cord

B. Peripheral Nervous System

The peripheral nervous system (PNS) consists of nerves and ganglia. The sensory nerves, which enter the CNS, and the motor nerves, which leave the CNS, are part of the peripheral nervous system. The PNS has two primary divisions, the **somatic** and the **autonomic** nervous systems, each of which has both motor and sensory components.

1. SOMATIC NERVOUS SYSTEM

The somatic nervous system (SNS) innervates **skeletal muscles** and is responsible for voluntary movement.

2. AUTONOMIC NERVOUS SYSTEM

The autonomic nervous system (ANS) is sometimes also called the **involuntary nervous system** because it regulates the body's internal environment without the aid of conscious control. The autonomic innervation of the body includes both sensory and motor fibers. The ANS innervates **cardiac** and **smooth muscle**. Smooth muscle is located in areas such as the blood vessels, digestive tract, bladder, and bronchi, so it isn't surprising that the ANS is important in blood pressure control, gastrointestinal motility, excretory processes, respiration, and reproductive processes. The ANS is comprised of two subdivisions, the **sympathetic** and the **parasympathetic** nervous systems, which generally act in opposition to one another.

a. Sympathetic Nervous System

The sympathetic division is responsible for the **"flight or fight"** responses that ready the body for action in an emergency situation. For example, it increases blood pressure and heart rate, increases blood flow to skeletal muscles, and decreases gut motility. It also dilates the bronchioles to increase gas exchange. The sympathetic nervous system uses **norepinephrine** as its primary neurotransmitter.

b. **Parasympathetic Nervous System**

The parasympathetic division acts to conserve energy and restore the body to resting activity levels following exertion (**"rest and digest"**). It acts to lower heart rate and to increase gut motility. One very important parasympathetic nerve that innervates many of the thoracic and abdominal viscera is called the **vagus nerve.** It uses **acetylcholine** as its primary neurotransmitter.

SPECIAL SENSES

The body has a number of organs that are specialized receptors, designed to detect stimuli.

A. The Eye

The eye detects light energy (as **photons**) and transmits information about intensity, color, and shape to the brain. The eyeball is covered by a thick, opaque layer known as the **sclera**, which is also known as the white of the eye. Beneath the sclera is the **choroid** layer, which helps to supply the retina with blood. The choroid is a dark, pigmented area that reduces reflection in the eye. The innermost layer of the eye is the **retina**, which contains the **photoreceptors** that sense light.

The transparent **cornea** at the front of the eye bends and focuses light rays. The rays then travel through an opening called the **pupil**, whose diameter is controlled by the pigmented, muscular **iris**. The iris responds to the intensity of light in the surroundings (light makes the pupil constrict). The light continues through the lens, which is suspended behind the pupil. The **lens**, the shape and **focal length** of which is controlled by the **ciliary muscles**, focuses the image onto the retina.

In the retina are **photoreceptors**, which transduce light into action potentials. There are two main types of photoreceptors: cones and rods. **Cones** respond to high-intensity illumination and are sensitive to color, while **rods** detect low-intensity illumination and are important in night vision. The cones and rods contain various pigments that absorb specific wavelengths of light. The cones contain three different pigments that absorb red, green, and blue wavelengths; the rod pigment, **rhodopsin**, absorbs a single wavelength. The photoreceptor cells synapse onto **bipolar cells**, which in turn synapse onto **ganglion cells**. Axons of the ganglion cells bundle to form the optic nerves, which conduct visual information to the brain. The point at which the optic nerve exits the eye is called the **blind spot** because photoreceptors are not present there. A small area of the retina, called the **fovea**, is densely packed with cones and is important for high-acuity vision.

The eye contains a **jellylike material,** called **vitreous humor,** which helps maintain its shape and optical properties. **Aqueous humor** is formed by the eye and exits through ducts to join the venous blood.

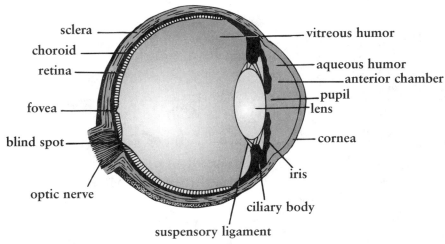

sclera
choroid
retina
fovea
blind spot
optic nerve
vitreous humor
aqueous humor
anterior chamber
pupil
lens
cornea
iris
ciliary body
suspensory ligament

Figure 7.8. Human Eye

1. DISORDERS OF THE EYE

- **Myopia (nearsightedness)** occurs when the image is focused in front of the retina.

- **Hyperopia (farsightedness)** occurs when the image is focused behind the retina.

- **Astigmatism** is caused by an irregularly shaped cornea.

- **Cataracts** cause the lens to become opaque; light cannot enter the eye, and blindness results.

- **Glaucoma** is an increase of **pressure** in the eye due to the blocking of the outflow of the aqueous humor.

B. The Ear

The ear transduces **sound** energy **(pressure waves)** into impulses perceived by the brain as sound. Sound waves pass through three regions as they enter the ear. First, they enter the **outer ear**, which consists of the auricle (external ear) and the **auditory canal**. At the end of the auditory canal is the **tympanic membrane** (eardrum) of the middle ear, which vibrates at the same frequency as the incoming sound. Next, the three ear bones, or **ossicles** (malleus, incus, and stapes), amplify the stimulus and transmit it through the oval window, which leads to the fluid-filled **inner ear**. The inner ear consists of the **cochlea** and the **vestibular**

apparatus, which is involved in maintaining equilibrium. Vibration of the ossicles exerts pressure on the fluid in the cochlea, stimulating **hair cells** in the **basilar membrane** to transduce the pressure into action potentials, which travel via the auditory (cochlear) nerve to the brain for processing.

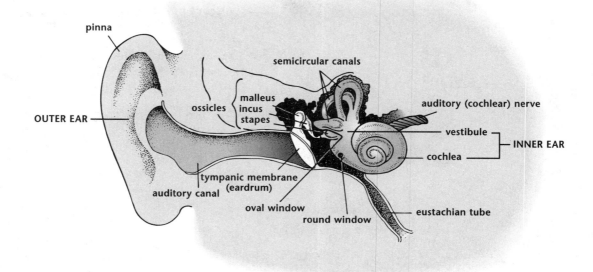

Figure 7.9. Human Ear

8

Respiration

Respiration refers to the utilization of **oxygen** by an organism. This process includes the intake of oxygen from the environment, the transport of oxygen in the blood, and the ultimate oxidation of fuel molecules in the cell. **External respiration** refers to the entrance of air into the lungs and the gas exchange between the alveoli and the blood. **Internal respiration** includes the exchange of gas between the blood and the cells and the intracellular processes of respiration.

OVERVIEW OF CELLULAR RESPIRATION

Photosynthesis converts the energy of the sun into chemical energy held within the bonds of compounds such as glucose. **Respiration** involves the conversion of the chemical energy in these bonds into a form of energy needed to drive the processes of living cells.

Carbohydrates and fats are the favored **fuel** molecules in living cells. The C–H bond is energy-rich; in fact, compared with other bonds, it is capable of releasing the largest amount of energy per mole. As hydrogen is removed, this bond energy is made available. In contrast, carbon dioxide contains little usable energy. It is the stable, "energy-exhausted" end product of respiration.

During respiration, high-energy hydrogen atoms are removed from organic molecules. This is called **dehydrogenation** and is an oxidation reaction. The subsequent acceptance of hydrogen by a hydrogen acceptor (oxygen in the final step) is the reduction component of the redox reaction. Energy released by this reduction is used to form a high-energy phosphate bond in ATP. Although the initial oxidation step requires an energy input, the net result of the redox reaction is energy production. If all of this energy were released in a single step, little could be harnessed. Instead, the reductions occur in a series of steps called the **electron transport chain**.

GLUCOSE CATABOLISM

The degradative oxidation of glucose occurs in two stages, **glycolysis** and **cellular respiration**.

A. Glycolysis

The first stage of glucose catabolism is glycolysis (see Figure 8.1). Glycolysis is a series of reactions that lead to the oxidative breakdown of glucose into two molecules of **pyruvate** (the ionized form of pyruvic acid), the production of ATP, and the reduction of NAD^+ into NADH. All of these reactions occur in the **cytoplasm** and are mediated by specific enzymes.

1. GLYCOLYTIC PATHWAY

Note that at step 4, fructose 1,6-diphosphate is split into 2 three-carbon molecules: dihydroxyacetone phosphate and **glyceraldehyde 3-phosphate (PGAL)**. **Dihydroxyacetone phosphate** is isomerized into PGAL so that it can be used in subsequent reactions. Thus, 2 molecules of PGAL are formed per molecule of glucose, and all of the subsequent steps occur twice for each glucose molecule.

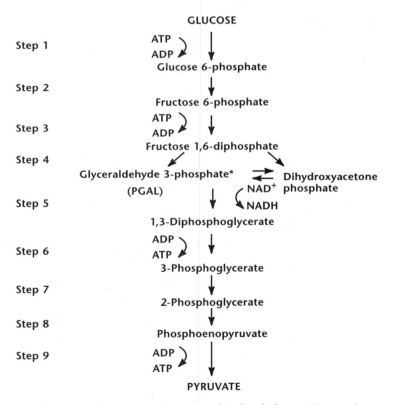

*NOTE: Steps 5–9 occur twice per molecule of glucose (see text).

Figure 8.1. Glycolysis

From 1 molecule of glucose (a six-carbon molecule), 2 molecules of pyruvate (a three-carbon molecule) are obtained. During this sequence of reactions, 2 ATP are used (in steps 1 and 3), and 4 ATP are generated (2 in step 6 and 2 in step 9). Thus, there is a net production of 2 ATP per glucose molecule. This type of phosphorylation is called **substrate-level phosphorylation**, since ATP synthesis is directly coupled with the degradation of glucose without the participation of an intermediate molecule such as NAD^+. One NADH is produced per PGAL, for a total of 2 NADH per glucose.

The net reaction for glycolysis is as follows:

Glucose + 2ADP + $2P_i$ + $2NAD^+$ →

2Pyruvate + 2ATP + 2NADH + $2H^+$ + $2H_2O$

At this stage, much of the initial energy stored in the glucose molecule has not been released and is still present in the chemical bonds of pyruvate. Depending on the capabilities of the organism, pyruvate degradation can proceed in one of two directions. Under **anaerobic** conditions (in the absence of oxygen), pyruvate is reduced during the process of fermentation. Under **aerobic** conditions (in the presence of oxygen), pyruvate is further oxidized during cell respiration in the mitochondria.

2. FERMENTATION

NAD^+ must be regenerated for glycolysis to continue in the absence of O_2. This is accomplished by reducing pyruvate into ethanol or lactic acid. **Fermentation** refers to all of the reactions involved in this anaerobic process—glycolysis and the additional steps leading to the formation of ethanol or lactic acid. Fermentation produces only 2 ATP per glucose molecule.

Alcohol fermentation commonly occurs only in yeast and some bacteria. The pyruvate produced in glycolysis is converted to ethanol. In this way, NAD^+ is regenerated, and glycolysis can continue.

Lactic acid fermentation occurs in certain fungi and bacteria and in human muscle cells during strenuous activity. When the oxygen supply to muscle cells lags behind the rate of glucose catabolism, the pyruvate generated is reduced to lactic acid. As in alcohol fermentation, the NAD^+ used in step 5 of glycolysis is regenerated when pyruvate is reduced.

B. Cellular Respiration

Cellular respiration (aerobic respiration) is the most efficient catabolic pathway used by organisms to harvest the energy stored in **glucose** because of its utilization of oxygen. Whereas glycolysis (anaerobic respiration) yields only **2 ATP** per molecule of glucose, cellular respiration can yield **36–38 ATP**. In this **aerobic** process, **oxygen** acts as the final acceptor of the electrons that are passed from carrier to carrier during the final stage of glucose oxidation. The metabolic reactions of cell respiration occur in the eukaryotic mitochondrion and are catalyzed by reaction-specific enzymes.

Cellular respiration can be divided into three stages: pyruvate decarboxylation, the citric acid cycle, and the electron transport chain.

1. PYRUVATE DECARBOXYLATION

The pyruvate formed during glycolysis is transported from the cytoplasm into the mitochondrial matrix where it is decarboxylated (i.e., it loses a CO_2), and the acetyl group that remains is transferred to coenzyme A to form acetyl CoA. In the process, NAD^+ is reduced to NADH.

2. CITRIC ACID CYCLE

The citric acid cycle is also known as the **Krebs cycle**. The cycle begins when the two-carbon acetyl group from acetyl CoA combines with oxaloacetate, a four-carbon molecule, to form the six-carbon citrate. Through a complicated series of reactions, 2 CO_2 molecules are released, and oxaloacetate is regenerated for use in another turn of the cycle.

For each turn of the citric acid cycle, 1 ATP is produced by substrate-level phosphorylation via a GTP intermediate. In addition, electrons are transferred to NAD^+ and FAD, generating NADH and $FADH_2$, respectively. These coenzymes then transport the electrons to the electron transport chain, where more ATP is produced via oxidative phosphorylation (see below). When studying the cycle, keep in mind that for each molecule of glucose, 2 pyruvates are decarboxylated and channeled into the citric acid cycle. Overall:

$$2 \times 3 \text{ NADH} \rightarrow 6 \text{ NADH}$$
$$2 \times 1 \text{ FADH}_2 \rightarrow 2 \text{ FADH}_2$$
$$2 \times 1 \text{ GTP (ATP)} \rightarrow 2 \text{ ATP}$$

The net reaction of the citric acid cycle per glucose molecule is as follows:

$$2\text{Acetyl CoA} + 6NAD^+ + 2FAD + 2GDP + 2P_i + 4H_2O \rightarrow$$
$$4CO_2 + 6NADH + 2FADH_2 + 2GTP(ATP) + 4H^+ + 2CoA$$

3. ELECTRON TRANSPORT CHAIN

The Electron Transport Chain (ETC) is a complex carrier mechanism located on the inside of the **inner mitochondrial membrane**. During oxidative phosphorylation, ATP is produced when high-energy potential electrons are transferred from NADH and $FADH_2$ to oxygen by a series of carrier molecules located in the inner mitochondrial membrane. As the electrons are transferred from carrier to carrier, free energy is released, which is then used to form ATP. Most of the molecules of the ETC are **cytochromes**, electron carriers that resemble hemoglobin in the structure of their active site. The functional unit contains a central iron atom, which is capable of undergoing a reversible redox reaction; that is, it can be alternatively reduced and oxidized. Sequential redox reactions continue to occur as the electrons are transferred from one carrier to the next; each carrier is reduced as it accepts an electron and is then oxidized when it passes it on to the next carrier. The last carrier of the ETC passes its electron to the final electron acceptor, O_2. In addition to the electrons, O_2 picks up a pair of hydrogen ions from the surrounding medium, forming water.

$$2H^+ + 2e^- + O_2 \rightarrow H_2O$$

C. Total Energy Production

To calculate the net amount of ATP produced per molecule of glucose, we need to tally the number of ATP produced by substrate-level phosphorylation and the number of ATP produced by oxidative phosphorylation.

1. SUBSTRATE-LEVEL PHOSPHORYLATION

Degradation of 1 glucose molecule yields a net of 2 ATP from glycolysis and 1 ATP for each turn of the citric acid cycle. Thus, a total of 4 ATP are produced by substrate-level phosphorylation.

2. OXIDATIVE PHOSPHORYLATION

Two pyruvate decarboxylations yield 1 NADH each for a total of 2 NADH. Each turn of the citric acid cycle yields 3 NADH and 1 $FADH_2$, for a total of 6 NADH and 2 $FADH_2$ per glucose molecule. Each $FADH_2$ generates 2 ATP, as previously discussed. Each NADH generates 3 ATP except for the 2 NADH that were reduced during glycolysis; these NADH cannot cross the inner mitochondrial membrane and must transfer their electrons to an intermediate carrier molecule, which delivers the electrons to the second carrier protein complex, Q. Therefore, these NADH generate only 2 ATP per glucose. So the 2 NADH of glycolysis yield 4 ATP, the other 8 NADH yield 24 ATP, and the 2 $FADH_2$ produce 4 ATP for a total of 32 ATP by oxidative phosphorylation.

The total amount of ATP produced per glucose molecule during eukaryotic glucose catabolism is, therefore, 4 via substrate level phosphorylation plus 32 via oxidative phosphorylation for a total of 36 ATP. (For prokaryotes, the yield is 38 ATP, because the 2 NADH of glycolysis don't have any mitochondrial membranes to cross and therefore don't lose energy.)

Eukaryotic ATP Production per Glucose Molecule

Glycolysis

2 ATP invested (steps 1 and 3)	–	2	ATP
4 ATP generated (steps 6 and 9)	+	4	ATP (substrate)
2 NADH × 2 ATP/NADH (step 5)	+	4	ATP (oxidative)

Pyruvate Decarboxylation

2 NADH × 3 ATP/NADH	+	6	ATP (oxidative)

Citric Acid Cycle

6 NADH × 3 ATP/NADH	+	18	ATP (oxidative)
2 $FADH_2$ × 2 ATP/$FADH_2$	+	4	ATP (oxidative)
2 GTP × 1 ATP/GTP	+	2	ATP (substrate)
Total	+	**36**	**ATP**

ALTERNATE ENERGY SOURCES

When glucose supplies run low, the body utilizes other energy sources. These sources are used by the body in the following preferential order: other carbohydrates, fats, and proteins. These substances are first converted to either glucose or glucose intermediates, which can then be degraded in the glycolytic pathway and the citric acid cycle.

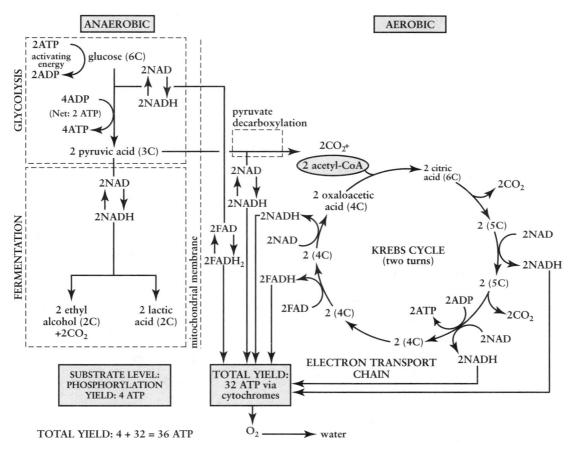

Figure 8.2. Glucose Catabolism

A. Carbohydrates

Disaccharides are hydrolyzed into monosaccharides, most of which can be converted into glucose or glycolytic intermediates. Glycogen stored in the liver can be converted, when needed, into a glycolytic intermediate.

B. Fats

Fat molecules are stored in adipose tissue in the form of triglycerides. When needed, they are hydrolyzed by **lipases** to **fatty acids** and **glycerol** and are carried by the blood to other tissues for oxidation. Glycerol can be converted into PGAL, a glycolytic intermediate. A fatty acid must first be "activated" in the cytoplasm; this process requires 2 ATP. Once activated, the fatty acid is transported into the mitochondrion and taken through a series of beta-oxidation cycles that convert it into two-carbon fragments, which are then converted into acetyl CoA. Acetyl CoA then enters the TCA cycle. With each round of β oxidation of a saturated fatty acid, 1 NADH and 1 FADH$_2$ are generated.

Of all the high-energy compounds used in cellular respiration, fats yield the greatest number of ATP per gram. This makes them extremely efficient energy-storage molecules. Thus, while the amount of glycogen stored in humans is enough to meet the short-term energy needs of about a day, the stored fat reserves can meet the long-term energy needs of about a month.

C. Proteins

The body degrades proteins only when not enough carbohydrate or fat is available. Most amino acids undergo a **transamination reaction** in which they exchange an amino group for the ketone group of another acid to form an α-keto acid. The carbon atoms of most amino acids are converted into acetyl CoA, pyruvate, or one of the intermediates of the citric acid cycle. These intermediates enter their respective metabolic pathways, allowing cells to produce fatty acids, glucose, or energy in the form of ATP.

Another way for amino acids to convert to keto acids is by **oxidative deamination**, which removes an ammonia molecule directly from the amino acid. **Ammonia** is a toxic substance in vertebrates. Fish can excrete ammonia, insects and birds convert it to uric acid, and mammals convert it into urea for excretion.

PHOTOSYNTHESIS

All green plants use photosynthesis to convert carbon dioxide and water into **glucose** and oxygen. Glucose can be stored as starch or used as an energy source. In plants, photosynthesis takes place in a specialized organelle called a **chloroplast**. Photosynthetic bacteria lack chloroplasts but have membranes that function in a similar manner.

A. Overview of Photosynthesis

Photosynthesis involves the reduction of CO_2 to carbohydrate accompanied by release of oxygen from water. The net reaction is the reverse of respiration—reduction occurs instead of oxidation. This net reaction is shown below:

$$6CO_2 + 12\ H_2O + \text{light energy} \rightarrow C_6H_{12}O_6 + 6O_2 + 6\ H_2O$$

Photosynthesis can be divided into two distinct reactions, the light reactions and the dark reactions. The **light reactions** convert solar energy into chemical energy in the form of **ATP** (by photophosphorylation) and **NADPH**. These reactions must take place in the light. The **dark reactions** are coupled to the light reactions. They incorporate CO_2 into organic molecules in a process called **carbon fixation**. The dark reactions are also called **reduction synthesis** because carbohydrates are produced by reducing CO_2. Both reactions take place in the chloroplasts, a highly organized organelle containing the complex **chlorophyll** molecule within **thylakoid membranes**. Chlorophyll absorbs photons of light to drive the reactions of photosynthesis.

B. The Light Reactions

The light reactions, also called **photolysis** reactions, begin with the absorption of a photon of light by a chlorophyll molecule. When light strikes the special chlorophyll a P700 molecule, it excites electrons to a higher energy level. These high energy electrons can flow along two pathways, giving cyclic electron flow or noncyclic electron flow.

1. CYCLIC ELECTRON FLOW

In cyclic electron flow, the excited electrons of P700 move along a chain of electron carriers. A series of redox reactions ultimately returns the electrons to P700. The reactions are harnessed to produce **ATP** from ADP and P_i in a process called **cyclic photophosphorylation**.

2. NONCYCLIC ELECTRON FLOW

This is the key pathway of the light reactions. Again, photons of light excite electrons in P700. However, instead of returning to P700 along the carrier chain, the high-energy electrons are transferred to the electron acceptor **$NADP^+$**. $NADP^+$ is very similar to NAD^+ which functions in cellular respiration. $NADP^+$ accepts the high energy electrons and forms **NADPH**. P700 is left with electron "holes" and thus is a powerful oxidizing agent.

When light strikes P680, another special chlorophyll absorbing at a wavelength of 680, electrons are excited. These electrons travel down the same electron carrier chain used by cyclic electron flow until they reach P700 and fill the electron "holes". This cascade produces ATP by **noncyclic photophosphorylation**.

P680 is a strong enough oxidizing agent to oxidize water and fill its holes. Water is split into two hydrogen ions and an oxygen atom and the electrons produced reduce P680. Oxygen atoms combine to form O_2. The net result of noncyclic electron flow is the production of NADPH and ATP, as well as and the photolysis (breakdown) of water (not carbon dioxide).

C. The Dark Reactions

The dark reactions use the ATP and NADPH produced by the light reactions to reduce CO_2 to carbohydrates. Although these reactions do not directly require light, they will only occur during the day, when the light reactions are replenishing the supply of ATP and NADPH. The dark reactions are also called **carbon-fixation** or **reduction synthesis** reactions.

CO_2 is the source of carbon for carbohydrate production in the **Calvin cycle**. The product of the cycle is the **three carbon** sugar **phospho-glyceraldehyde (PGAL)**. In order to produce a three carbon sugar from CO_2, the cycle must take place three times.

The Calvin cycle is similar to the **Krebs cycle** in reverse: (1) carbon dioxide is fed into the cycle; in the Krebs cycle it was produced and released; (2) reducing power is utilized during the cycle (NADPH); in the Krebs cycle NADH was used; (3) energy is used in the cycle (conversion of ATP to ADP); in the Krebs cycle, energy was produced when ATP was formed from ADP and inorganic phosphate.

SUMMARY OF THE CALVIN CYCLE

Carbon dioxide is fixed to RBP (ribulose bisphosphate), a five-carbon sugar. The resulting unstable six-carbon molecule splits to form 2 molecules of PGA (phosphoglyceric acid). PGA is then phosphorylated and reduced (by ATP and NADPH) to form PGAL. Most of the PGAL is recycled to RBP by a complex series of reactions. In six turns of the Calvin cycle, 12 PGAL are formed from 6 carbon dioxide and 6 RBP. The 12 PGAL recombine to form 6 RBP and 1 molecule of glucose, the net product.

PGAL is generally considered the prime end product of photosynthesis, and it can be used as an immediate food nutrient; combined and rearranged to form monosaccharide sugars (e.g., glucose), which can be transported to other cells; or packaged for storage as insoluble polysaccharides, such as starch.

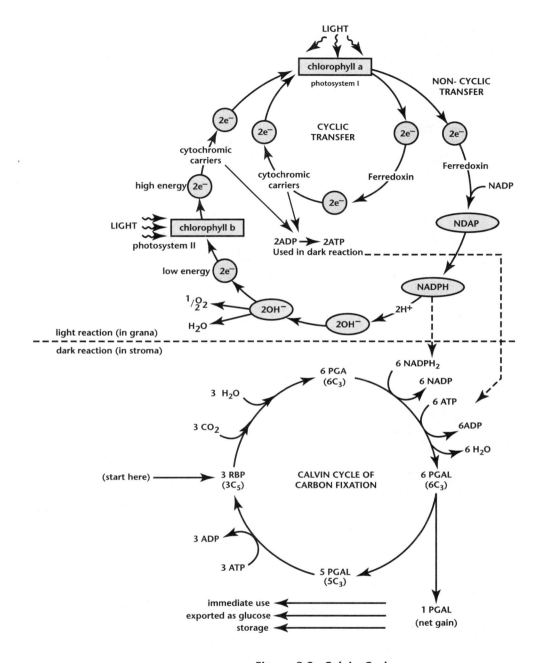

Figure 8.3. Calvin Cycle

RESPIRATION IN INVERTEBRATES

A. Unicellular and Simple Multicellular Organisms

1. PROTOZOA AND HYDRA (PHYLUM: CNIDARIA)

In these organisms, every cell is in contact with the external environment (water), and respiratory gases can be exchanged between the cell and the environment by simple diffusion through the cell membrane.

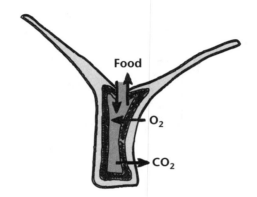

Figure 8.4. Hydra

B. Annelids

Mucus secreted by cells on the external surface of the earthworm's body provides a moist surface for gaseous exchange by diffusion. The circulatory system brings O_2 to the cells and waste products, such as CO_2, back to the skin for excretion. The vascularity under the skin makes cutaneous respiration highly efficient. Meanwhile, aquatic annelids use branchial repiration, via gills or parapodia, for gas exchange.

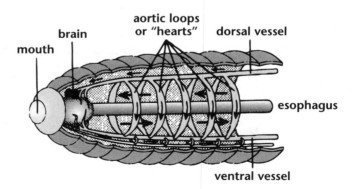

Figure 8.5. Earthworm

C. Arthropod Phylum

The respiratory system of a grasshopper consists of a series of respiratory tubules, called **tracheae**, whose branches reach to almost every cell. These tubes access the surface in openings called **spiracles.** This system thus permits the intake, distribution, and removal of respiratory gases directly between the air and the body cells by diffusion. No carrier of oxygen is needed in this respiratory system, and the efficiency of this system allows insects to have a relatively effortless open circulatory system.

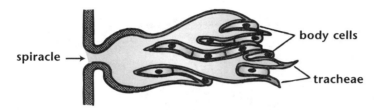

spiracle

body cells

tracheae

Figure 8.6. Grasshopper

RESPIRATION IN HUMANS

In the human respiratory system, air enters the **lungs** after traveling through a series of respiratory **airways**. The air passages consist of the nose, pharynx (throat), larynx, trachea, bronchi, bronchioles, and the alveoli. Gas exchange between the air in the lungs and the blood in the circulatory system occurs across the very thin walls of the **alveoli,** or air-filled sacs at the terminals of the airway branches. Three hundred million alveoli provide approximately 100 m^2 of moist respiratory surface for gas exchange. Following gas exchange, air rushes back through the respiratory pathway and is exhaled.

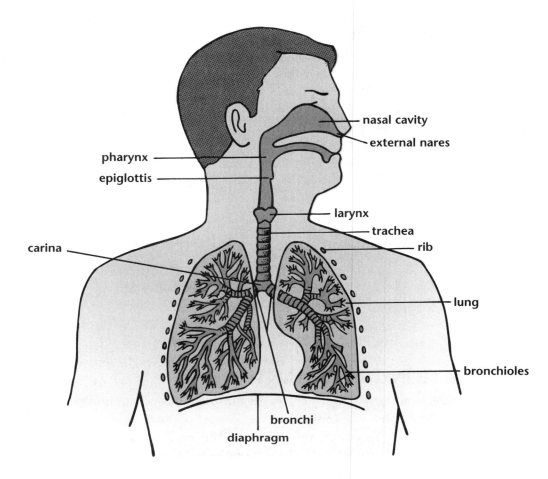

Figure 8.7. Human Respiratory System

A. Ventilation

Ventilation of the lungs (breathing) is the process by which air is **inhaled** and **exhaled**. The purpose of ventilation is to take in oxygen from the atmosphere and eliminate carbon dioxide from the body.

During **inhalation**, the muscular diaphragm contracts and flattens, and the external intercostal muscles contract, pushing the rib cage and chest wall up and out. This causes the thoracic cavity to increase in **volume**. This volume increase, in turn, reduces the pressure in the lungs, causing them to expand and fill with air.

Exhalation is generally a passive process. The lungs and chest wall are highly elastic and tend to recoil to their original positions following inhalation. The diaphragm and external intercostal muscles relax, and the chest wall moves inward. The consequent decrease in thoracic cavity volume causes the air pressure to increase. This causes the lungs to deflate, forcing air out of the alveoli.

B. Control of Ventilation

Ventilation is regulated by collections of neurons (referred to as **respiratory centers**) located in the **medulla oblongata**, whose rhythmic discharges stimulate the intercostal muscles and/or the diaphragm to contract. When the partial pressure of CO_2 rises, the medulla oblongata stimulates an increase in the rate of ventilation.

C. Gas Exchange

Ventilation, or breathing, produces the pressure gradient that permits simple diffusion of gases between the alveoli and the pulmonary capillaries (a dense network of minute blood vessels surrounding the alveoli). Gases, like oxygen and carbon dioxide, generally move from regions of higher partial pressure to regions of lower partial pressure. Specifically, oxygen will diffuse from the alveolar air into the blood, while carbon dioxide will move from the blood into the alveoli to be exhaled by the lungs. The walls of the alveoli, however, are coated with a thin layer of water that may hinder gas exchange. The water molecules tend to be more attracted to each other than the gases in the lungs, and this creates a force called surface tension that could lead to alveolar collapse. Fortunately, the alveolar cells secrete a detergent-like substance called **pulmonary surfactant** that coats the alveolar walls and reduces surface tension, thereby allowing for easier gas exchange and better **pulmonary compliance** (lung elasticity).

RESPIRATION IN PLANTS

In all plants and animals, respiration is continuous, occurring both day and night. In contrast, photosynthesis only takes place during the day. Note also that photosynthesis produces glucose and gives off oxygen while respiration requires oxygen to degrade glucose.

Plants undergo aerobic respiration similar to animals. The bonds of glucose are broken in glycolysis to produce 2 ATP and pyruvic acids. The gases diffuse into the air space entering (or leaving) through the stomata of the leaf or the lenticels (openings) of woody stems. 36 ATP molecules are produced per molcule of glucose. Anaerobic respiration takes place in simple plants when molecular oxygen is lacking, in a manner similar to animals.

9

Muscles and Locomotion

The **musculoskeletal system** forms the basic internal framework of the vertebrate body. Muscles and bones work in close coordination to produce voluntary movement in addition to a number of other independent functions. Physical support and locomotion are the functions of animal skeletal systems, while the muscular system generates force. Invertebrates have developed a number of systems for locomotion. Unicellular organisms, for example, may rely on specialized organelles for locomotion.

UNICELLULAR LOCOMOTION

Protozoans and primitive algae may move by beating **cilia** or **flagella**. The cilia and flagella of all eukaryotic cells possess the same basic structure. Each contains a cylindrical stalk of 11 microtubules—9 paired microtubules arranged in a circle with 2 single microtubules in the center. Flagella achieve movement by means of the **power stroke**, a thrusting movement generated by the sliding action of microtubules. Return of the cilium or flagellum to its original position is termed the **recovery stroke**. Amoeba extend **pseudopodia** for locomotion; the advancing cell membrane extends forward, allowing the cell to move.

INVERTEBRATE LOCOMOTION

A. Hydrostatic Skeletons

1. FLATWORMS

The muscles within the body wall of advanced **flatworms**, such as **planaria**, are arranged in two antagonistic layers, **longitudinal** and **circular.** The muscles contract against the resistance of the **incompressible fluid** within the animal's tissues (this fluid is termed the **hydrostatic skeleton**). Contraction of the circular layer of muscles causes the incompressible interstitial fluid to flow longitudinally, lengthening the animal. Conversely, contraction of the longitudinal layer of muscles shortens the animal.

2. **SEGMENTED WORMS (ANNELIDS)**

The same type of hydrostatic skeleton seen in flatworms assists in the locomotion of **annelids**, in which each segment of the animal can expand or contract independently. For example, bristles in the lower part of each segment, called **setae**, anchor an earthworm temporarily in the earth while muscles push it ahead.

B. Exoskeleton

An exoskeleton is a **hard skeleton** that covers all muscles and organs of some invertebrates. Exoskeletons are found principally in **arthropods** (e.g., insects). Insect exoskeletons are composed of **chitin**. All exoskeletons are composed of noncellular material secreted by the epidermis. While offering the animal some protection, exoskeletons impose limitations on growth. Thus, periodic **molting** and deposition of a new skeleton are necessary to permit body growth.

VERTEBRATE SKELETON

An **endoskeleton** serves as the framework within all vertebrate organisms. For example, muscles are attached to the bones, permitting movement. The endoskeleton also provides protection by surrounding delicate vital organs in bone. The rib cage protects the thoracic organs (heart and lungs), while the skull and vertebral column protect the brain and spinal cord respectively. The two major components of the skeleton are cartilage and bone.

A. Structure of the Skeleton

1. CARTILAGE

Cartilage is a type of **connective tissue** that is softer and more flexible than bone. Cartilage is retained in adults in places where firmness and flexibility are needed—for example, in humans, the external ear, the nose, the walls of the larynx and trachea, and the skeletal joints all contain cartilage.

2. BONE

Bone is a specialized type of mineralized **connective tissue** that has the ability to withstand physical stress. Ideally designed for body support, bone tissue is hard and strong while, at the same time, somewhat elastic and lightweight. There are two basic types of bone: **compact bone** and **spongy bone**.

- **Compact bone** is dense bone that does not appear to have any cavities when observed with the naked eye. The bony matrix is deposited in structural units called **osteons (Haversian systems)**. Each osteon consists of a central microscopic channel, called a

Haversian canal, surrounded by a number of concentric circles of bony matrix (calcium phosphate) called **lamellae**.

- **Spongy bone** is much less dense and consists of an interconnecting lattice of bony spicules (**trabeculae**); the cavities between the spicules are filled with yellow and/or red bone marrow. Yellow marrow is inactive and infiltrated by adipose tissue; red marrow is involved in blood cell formation.

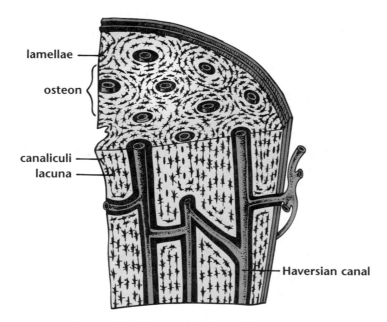

lamellae

osteon

canaliculi
lacuna

Haversian canal

Figure 9.1. Microscopic Bone Structure

3. OSTEOCYTES

Two other types of cells found in bone tissue are osteoblasts and osteoclasts. **Osteoblasts** synthesize and secrete the organic constituents of the bone matrix; once they have become surrounded by their matrix, they mature into osteocytes. **Osteoclasts** are large, multinucleated cells involved in bone resorption or breakdown.

4. BONE FORMATION

Bone formation occurs by either **endochondral ossification** or by **intramembranous ossification**. In endochondral ossification, existing **cartilage** is replaced by bone. Long bones arise primarily through endochondral ossification. In intramembranous ossification, mesenchymal (embryonic, undifferentiated) connective tissue is transformed into, and replaced by, bone.

KEY CONCEPTS

- OsteoBLASTS: Build bone.
- OsteoCLASTS: Destroy bone (also called bone resorption).

B. Organization of Vertebrate Skeleton

The **axial skeleton** is the basic framework of the body, consisting of the skull, vertebral column, and the rib cage. It is the point of attachment of the **appendicular** skeleton, which includes the bones of the appendages and the pectoral and pelvic girdles.

Bones are held together in a number of ways. **Sutures** or immovable joints hold the bones of the skull together. Bones that do move relative to one another are held together by **movable joints** and are additionally supported and strengthened by **ligaments**. Ligaments serve as bone-to-bone connectors. **Tendons** attach skeletal muscle to bones and bend the skeleton at the movable joints.

The point of attachment of a muscle to a stationary bone (the proximal end in limb muscles) is called the **origin**. The point of attachment of a muscle to the bone that moves (distal end in limb muscles) is called the **insertion**. **Extension** indicates a straightening of a joint, while **flexion** refers to a bending of a joint.

MUSCULAR SYSTEM

Muscle tissue consists of bundles of specialized **contractile fibers** held together by connective tissue. There are three morphologically and functionally distinct types of muscle in mammals: **skeletal muscle**, **smooth muscle**, and **cardiac muscle**.

A. Skeletal Muscle

Skeletal muscle is responsible for **voluntary** movements and is innervated by the somatic nervous system. Each fiber is a **multinucleated** cell created by the fusion of several mononucleated embryonic cells. Embedded in the fibers are filaments called **myofibrils**, which are further divided into contractile units called **sarcomeres**. The myofibrils are enveloped by a modified endoplasmic reticulum that stores calcium ions and is called the **sarcoplasmic reticulum**. The cytoplasm of a muscle fiber is called sarcoplasm, and the cell membrane is called the sarcolemma. The sarcolemma is capable of propagating an action potential and is connected to a system of **transverse tubules** (T system) oriented perpendicularly to the myofibrils. The T system provides channels for ion flow throughout the muscle fibers and can also propagate an action potential. Because of the high energy requirements of contraction, **mitochondria** are very abundant in muscle cells, distributed along the myofibrils. The repeating unit of the sarcomere gives skeletal muscle its **striations** of light-and dark bands; it is, therefore, also referred to as **striated muscle**.

1. THE SARCOMERE

a. Structure

The sarcomere is composed of **thin** and **thick** filaments. The thin filaments are chains of **actin** molecules. The thick filaments are composed of organized bundles of **myosin** molecules.

Electron microscopy reveals that the sarcomere is organized as follows: **Z lines** define the boundaries of a single sarcomere and anchor the thin filaments. The **M line** runs down the center of the sarcomere. The **I band** is the region containing thin filaments only. The **H zone** is the region containing thick filaments only. The **A band** spans the entire length of the thick filaments and any overlapping portions of the thin filaments. Note that during contraction, the A band is not reduced in size, while the H zone and I band are.

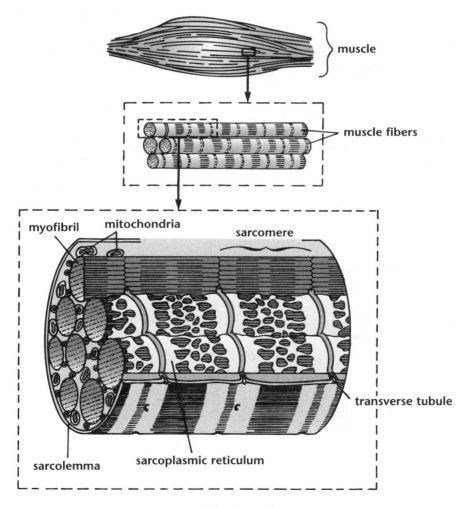

Figure 9.2. Skeletal Muscle

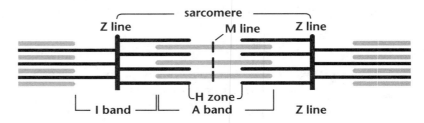

Figure 9.3. Sarcomere

b. Contraction

Muscle contraction is stimulated by a message from the somatic nervous system sent via a motor neuron. The link between the nerve terminal (synaptic bouton) and the sarcolemma of the muscle fiber is called the **neuromuscular junction**. The space between the two is known as the synapse, or synaptic cleft. Depolarization of the motor neuron results in the release of neurotransmitters (e.g., **acetylcholine**) from the nerve terminal. The neurotransmitter diffuses across the synaptic cleft and binds to special receptor sites on the sarcolemma. If enough of these receptors are stimulated, the permeability of the sarcolemma is altered, and an action potential is generated.

Once an action potential is generated, it is conducted along the sarcolemma and the T system and into the interior of the muscle fiber. This causes the sarcoplasmic reticulum to release **calcium ions** into the sarcoplasm. Calcium ions initiate the contraction of the sarcomere by binding to **tropomyosin**, thereby allowing actin and myosin to slide past each other, and the sarcomere to contract.

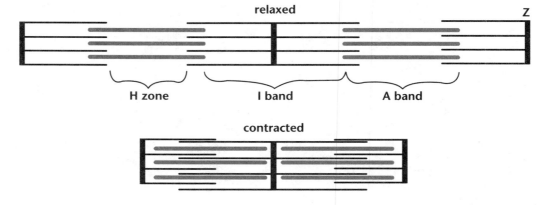

Figure 9.4. Contraction

2. STIMULUS AND MUSCLE RESPONSE

Individual muscle fibers generally exhibit an **all-or-none response**; only a stimulus above a minimal value, called the **threshold value**, can elicit contraction. The strength of the contraction of a single muscle fiber cannot be increased, regardless of the strength of the stimulus. However, the strength of contraction of the entire muscle can be increased by **recruiting** more muscle fibers.

a. Simple twitch

A simple twitch is the response of a single muscle fiber to a brief stimulus at or above the **threshold** stimulus. It consists of a latent period, a contraction period, and a relaxation period. The **latent period** is the time between stimulation and the onset of contraction. During this time lag, the action potential spreads along the sarcolemma, and Ca^{2+} ions are released into the sarcoplasm. Following the **contraction period**, there is a brief **relaxation period** in which the muscle is unresponsive to a stimulus; this is known as the **absolute refractory period**.

b. Summation and tetanus

When the fibers of a muscle are exposed to very frequent stimuli, the muscle cannot fully relax. The contractions begin to combine, becoming stronger and more prolonged. This is known as temporal **summation**. Since the contractions become continuous when the stimuli are so frequent, the muscle cannot relax at all. This type of contraction is known as **tetanus** and is stronger than a simple twitch of a single fiber. If tetanus is maintained, the muscle will eventually fatigue, and the contraction will weaken.

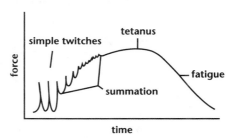

Figure 9.5. Simple Twitch and Summation / Tetanus

c. Tonus

Tonus is a state of partial contraction. Muscles are never completely relaxed and maintain a partially contracted state at all times.

B. Smooth Muscle

Smooth muscle is responsible for involuntary actions and is innervated by the **autonomic nervous system**. Smooth muscle is found in the digestive tract, bladder, uterus, and blood vessel walls, among other places. Smooth muscle cells possess **one** centrally located nucleus. In addition, smooth muscles lack the striations of skeletal muscle.

C. Cardiac Muscle

The muscle tissue of the heart is composed of cardiac muscle fibers. These fibers possess characteristics of both skeletal and smooth muscle fibers. As in skeletal muscle, actin and myosin filaments are arranged in sarcomeres, giving cardiac muscle a striated appearance. However, cardiac muscle cells generally have only one or two centrally located nuclei and are controlled primarily by the autonomic nervous system.

ENERGY RESERVES

ATP is the primary source of energy for muscle contraction. Very little ATP is actually stored in the muscles, and other forms of energy must be stored and rapidly converted to ATP to facilitate contraction.

A. Creatine Phosphate and Arginine Phosphate

In vertebrates and some invertebrates, particularly echinoderms, energy can be temporarily stored in a high-energy compound called **creatine phosphate**. Many invertebrates utilize a similar compound called arginine phosphate.

B. Myoglobin

Myoglobin is a hemoglobin-like protein found in muscle tissue. Myoglobin has a high oxygen affinity and maintains the oxygen supply in muscles by binding oxygen tightly. This oxygen can then be used to generate ATP for contraction via cellular respiration.

10

Digestion

Some organisms are **heterotrophic** and thus unable to synthesize their own nutrients. Food provides the raw material for energy, repair, and growth of tissues. In these cases, food must first be **ingested**. **Digestion** consists of the degradation of large molecules into smaller molecules, which can be **absorbed** into the bloodstream and used directly by cells. **Intracellular** digestion occurs within the cell, usually in membrane-bound vesicles. **Extra-cellular** digestion refers to a digestive process that occurs outside of the cell, within a lumen or tract.

DIGESTION IN UNICELLULAR ORGANISMS

In unicellular organisms, food capture is primarily done by **phagocytosis**. Food vacuoles form immediately following ingestion. For example, in the **amoeba** pseudopods surround and engulf food (phagocytosis) and enclose it in food vacuoles. **Lysosomes** (containing digestive enzymes) fuse with the food vacuole and release their digestive enzymes, which act upon the nutrients. The resulting simpler molecules diffuse into the cytoplasm. The unusable end products are subsequently eliminated from the vacuole.

In the paramecium (see Figure 10.1), cilia sweep food into the oral groove and **cytopharynx**. A food vacuole forms around food at the lower end of the cytopharynx. Eventually, the vacuole breaks off into the cytoplasm and progresses towards the anterior end of the cell. Enzymes are secreted into the vacuole, and the products diffuse into the cytoplasm. Solid wastes are expelled at the anal pore.

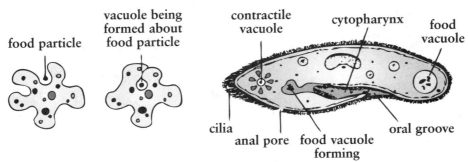

Figure 10.1. Paramecium

DIGESTION IN INVERTEBRATES

Multicellular organisms have developed numerous adaptations for food capture and ingestion, digestion, and absorption. In many animals, the **physical breakdown** of large particles of food into small particles begins by cutting and grinding in the mouth and churning in the digestive tract. The molecular composition is unchanged, but the surface area of the substrates on which the enzymes act is increased. **Chemical breakdown** of molecules is accomplished by enzymatic hydrolysis. The smaller digested nutrients (glucose, amino acids, fatty acids, and glycerol) pass through the semipermeable plasma membrane of the gut cells to be further metabolized or transported.

A. Cnidarians

The hydra uses intracellular and extracellular digestion. **Tentacles** bring food to the mouth (ingestion) and release the particles into a cup-like sac. The endodermal cells lining this gastrovascular cavity secrete enzymes into the cavity. Thus, digestion principally occurs outside the cells (extracellular). However, once the food is reduced to small fragments, the gastrodermal cells engulf the nutrients, and digestion is completed intracellularly. Every cell is exposed to the external environment, thereby facilitating intracellular digestion. Undigested food is expelled through the **mouth**.

B. Annelids

Like higher animals, **earthworms** (see Figure 10.2) have a one-way digestive tract with both a mouth and an anus. This is because of **specialization** of different parts of the digestive tract for different functions. These parts include the mouth, pharynx, esophagus, **crop** (to store the food), **gizzard** (to grind the food), **intestine** (which contains a large dorsal fold [**typholosole**] to provide increased surface area for digestion and absorption), and **anus**. Soluble nutrients pass, by diffusion, through the walls of the small intestine into the blood.

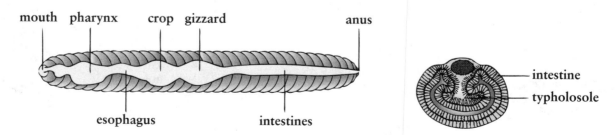

Figure 10.2. Earthworm

C. Arthropods

Insects (see Figure 10.3) have a digestive system similar to that of the earthworm. They also have jaws for chewing and **salivary glands**, which improve food digestion.

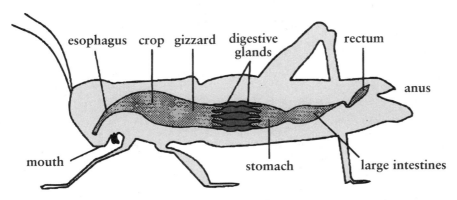

Figure 10.3. Insect

DIGESTION IN HUMANS

The human digestive tract (see Figure 10.4) begins with the **oral cavity** and continues with the **pharynx**, the **esophagus**, the **stomach**, the **small intestine**, the **large intestine**, and the anus. Accessory organs, such as the salivary glands, the pancreas, the liver, and the gall bladder, also play essential roles in digestion.

A. The Oral Cavity

The oral cavity (the mouth) is where the **mechanical** and **chemical** digestion of food begins. Mechanical digestion is the breakdown of large food particles into smaller particles through the biting and chewing action of teeth (**mastication**). Chemical digestion refers to the enzymatic breakdown of macromolecules into smaller molecules. It begins in the mouth when the salivary glands secrete **saliva**. Saliva **lubricates** food to facilitate swallowing and provides a solvent for food particles. Saliva is secreted in response to a nervous reflex triggered by the presence of food in the oral cavity. Saliva contains the enzyme **salivary amylase (ptyalin)**, which hydrolyzes starch to maltose (a disaccharide).

B. The Esophagus

The esophagus is the muscular tube leading from the mouth to the stomach. Food is moved down the esophagus by rhythmic waves of involuntary smooth muscle contractions called **peristalsis**.

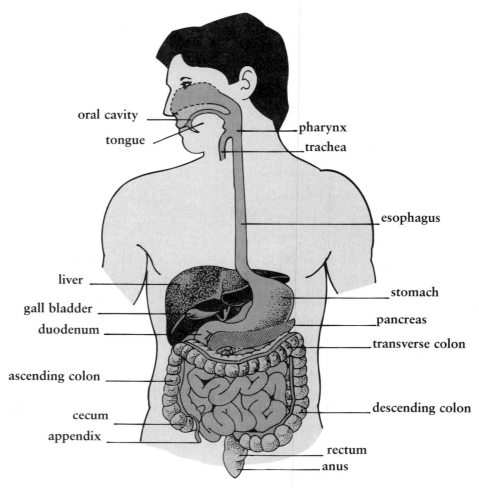

Figure 10.4. Human Digestive Tract

C. The Stomach

The stomach, a large, muscular organ located in the upper abdomen, stores and partially digests food. The walls of the stomach are lined by the thick gastric mucosa, which contains the glands. These glands secrete **mucus**, which protects the stomach lining from the harshly acidic juices (pH = 2) present in the stomach. They also secrete **pepsin**, which is a protein-hydrolyzing enzyme, and hydrochloric acid (**HCl**), which kills bacteria, dissolves the intercellular "glue" holding food tissues together, and activates certain enzymes (like pepsin). The churning of the stomach produces an acidic, semi-fluid mixture of partially digested food known as **chyme**. The chyme passes into the first segment of the small intestine, the **duodenum**, through the **pyloric sphincter**.

D. The Small Intestine

Chemical digestion is completed in the small intestine. The small intestine is divided into three sections: the duodenum, the jejunum, and the ileum. The small intestine is also highly adapted to **absorption**. To maximize the surface area available for digestion and absorption, the intestine is extremely long (greater than six meters in length) and highly coiled. In addition, numerous fingerlike projections, called **villi**, extend out of the intestinal wall (see Figure 10.5). Villi contain capillaries and **lacteals** (vessels of the lymphatic system). Amino acids and monosaccharides pass through the villi walls into the capillary system. Large fatty acids and glycerol pass into the lacteals and are then reconverted into fats (fatty acid + glycerol). Note that some nutrients are actively absorbed (i.e., requiring energy to be absorbed), such as glucose and amino acids, while others are passively absorbed.

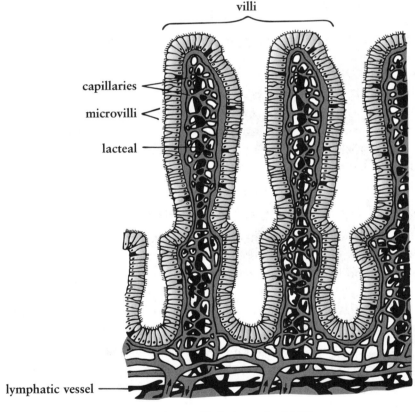

Figure 10.5. Intestinal Villi

Most digestion in the small intestine occurs in the duodenum, where the secretions of the intestinal glands, pancreas, liver, and gall bladder mix with the acidic chyme entering from the stomach. The intestinal mucosa secretes **lipases** (for fat digestion), **aminopeptidases** (for polypeptide digestion) and **disaccharidases** (for the digestion of maltose, lactose, and sucrose). The disaccharidase **lactase** breaks down lactose (milk sugar). This enzyme is present in infants, but many adults lack the enzyme and are **lactose-intolerant**. Lactose in the small intestine that cannot be digested is metabolized by bacteria, producing intestinal discomfort.

E. The Liver

The liver produces **bile**, which is stored in the **gall bladder** prior to release into the small intestine. Bile contains no enzymes; it **emulsifies** fats, breaking down large globules into small droplets. Emulsification of fats exposes a greater surface area of the fat to the action of pancreatic lipase. In the absence of bile, fats cannot be digested.

F. The Pancreas

The pancreas has an exocrine function that produces enzymes such as **amylase** for carbohydrate digestion, **trypsin** for protein digestion, and **lipase** for fat digestion. The pancreas secretes a bicarbonate-rich juice that neutralizes the acidic chyme arriving from the stomach. The pancreatic enzymes operate optimally at this higher pH.

G. The Large Intestine

The large intestine is approximately 1.5 meters long and functions in the absorption of salts and the absorption of any water not already absorbed by the small intestine. The **rectum** provides for transient storage of feces prior to elimination through the anus.

DIGESTION IN PLANTS AND FUNGI

Plants have no digestive system, but intracellular digestive processes similar to those of animals do occur, coordinating the utilization of nutrients along with their production.

A. Intracellular digestion

Plants store insoluble polymers, starches, lipids, and proteins in the cells. The principle storage food is starch (a glucose polysaccharide), found in large quantities in seeds, stems, and roots. When nutrients are required, the storage polymers are broken down to simpler molecules (glucose, fatty acids, glycerol, and amino acids) by enzyme **hydrolysis**. The simple products can be used in the storage cell itself or transported by diffusion to other cells.

B. Extracellular Digestion

Some heterotrophic organisms, such as fungi, must obtain preformed organic molecules (nutrients) from the environment. Enzymes are secreted, hydrolyzing complex nutrients into simpler molecules, which are then absorbed. Once inside the organism, the simpler molecules can be used for energy or to synthesize larger molecules.

For example, the **rhizoids** of bread mold, a typical saprophyte that lives on dead organic material, secrete enzymes into the external environment (the bread). Digestion produces simple soluble end products (glucose, amino acids, fatty acids, and glycerol), which are absorbed by diffusion into the rhizoid and transported throughout the mold.

In the plant kingdom, the **Venus flytrap** comes the closest to actual ingestion. When a fly arrives, certain sensitive tissues entrap the insect. **Enzymes** are secreted to digest the fly and absorb the soluble end products. This is, of course, extracellular digestion. Note that the Venus flytrap is still an autotroph—it photosynthesizes to produce glucose. It uses the insect as a **nitrate** source, because the flytrap grows in nitrogen-poor soils.

11

Excretion

Excretion refers to the removal of **metabolic wastes** produced in the body. It is distinguished from **elimination**, the removal of indigestible material. Most of the body's activities produce metabolic wastes that must be removed. **Aerobic respiration** leads to the production of **carbon dioxide** and water. **Deamination** of amino acids in the liver leads to the production of **nitrogenous wastes** like urea and ammonia. All metabolic processes lead to the production of mineral salts, which must be excreted by the kidneys.

EXCRETION IN INVERTEBRATES

A. Excretion in Protozoans and Cnidarians

In these phyla, all cells are in contact with the external, aqueous environment. Water soluble wastes, such as **ammonia** and **carbon dioxide**, can exit the cells by simple diffusion through the cell membrane. This type of excretion is **passive**. Some freshwater **protozoa**, such as the paramecium, possess a contractile **vacuole**—an organelle specialized for water excretion by active transport. Excess water, which continually diffuses into the cell from the hypotonic environment (freshwater), is collected and periodically pumped out of the cell. This homeostatic mechanism permits the cell to maintain its volume and pressure.

B. Excretion in Annelids

In earthworms, carbon dioxide excretion occurs directly through the moist skin. In addition, two pairs of **nephridia** in each body segment excrete water, mineral salts, and nitrogenous wastes in the form of urea (see Figure 11.1).

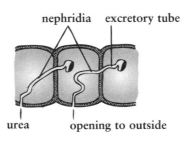

Figure 11.1. Earthworm

C. Excretion in Arthropods

In insects, carbon dioxide is released from the tissues into adjacent tube-like **tracheae**, which are continuous with the external air through openings called **spiracles**. Nitrogenous wastes are excreted in the form of solid **uric acid** crystals. The use of solid nitrogenous wastes is an adaptation for the conservation of water. Mineral salts and uric acid accumulate in the **Malphigian tubules** and are then transported to the intestine to be expelled with the solid wastes of digestion.

EXCRETION IN HUMANS

The principal organs of excretion in humans are the lungs, liver, skin, and kidneys. In the **lungs**, carbon dioxide and water vapor diffuse from the blood into the alveoli and are continually exhaled. Sweat glands in the **skin** excrete water and dissolved salts (and a small quantity of urea). Perspiration also serves to regulate body temperature, since the evaporation of sweat produces cooling. The **liver** processes nitrogenous wastes, blood pigment wastes, and other chemicals for excretion. Urea is produced by the deamination of amino acids in the liver and diffuses into the blood for ultimate excretion in the **kidneys**. Bile salts and red blood pigments are excreted as bile and pass out with the feces. In addition to excreting numerous waste products and toxic chemicals, the kidneys also function to maintain the osmolarity of the blood and conserve glucose, salt, and water.

A. The Kidneys

The kidneys regulate the concentration of salt and water in the blood through the formation and **excretion** of urine. The kidneys are bean shaped and are located behind the stomach and liver. Each kidney is composed of approximately 1 million functional units called **nephrons**.

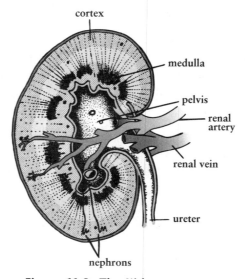

Figure 11.2. The Kidney

1. **STRUCTURE**

   The kidney is divided into three regions: the outer **cortex**, the inner **medulla**, and the renal **pelvis**. A **nephron** consists of a bulb called **Bowman's capsule**, which embraces a special capillary bed called a **glomerulus**. Bowman's capsule leads into a long, coiled tubule, which is divided into functionally distinct units: the **proximal convoluted tubule**, the **loop of Henle**, the **distal convoluted tubule**, and the **collecting duct**. The nephron is positioned such that the loop of Henle runs through the medulla, while the convoluted tubules and Bowman's capsule are in the cortex. Concentrated urine in the collecting tubules flows into the pelvis of the kidney, a funnel-like region that opens directly into the **ureter**. The ureters from each kidney empty into the **urinary bladder**, where urine collects until expelled via the **urethra**. Most of the nephron is surrounded by a complex **peritubular capillary** network to facilitate reabsorption of amino acids, glucose, salts, and water.

2. **URINE FORMATION**

   Filtration, secretion, and reabsorption are the three processes that lead to urine formation.

   a. **Filtration**

   Blood pressure forces 20 percent of the blood plasma entering the **glomerulus** through the capillary walls and into the surrounding **Bowman's capsule**. The fluid and small solutes entering the nephron are called the **filtrate**. The filtrate is isotonic with blood plasma. Particles too large to filter through the glomerulus, such as blood cells and albumin, remain in the circulatory system. Filtration is a passive process driven by the hydrostatic pressure of the blood.

   b. **Secretion**

   The nephron secretes potentially harmful substances such as acids, bases, and ions like potassium and phosphate from the interstitial fluid into the filtrate by both **passive** and **active** transport. Materials are secreted from the peritubular capillaries into the nephron tubule.

   c. **Reabsorption**

   Essential substances (**glucose**, salts, and amino acids) and water are **reabsorbed** from the filtrate and returned to the blood. Reabsorption occurs primarily in the proximal convoluted tubule (whose convolutions create increased surface area) and is an active process. Movement of these molecules is accompanied by the passive movement of water. This results in the formation of concentrated urine, which is **hypertonic** to the blood.

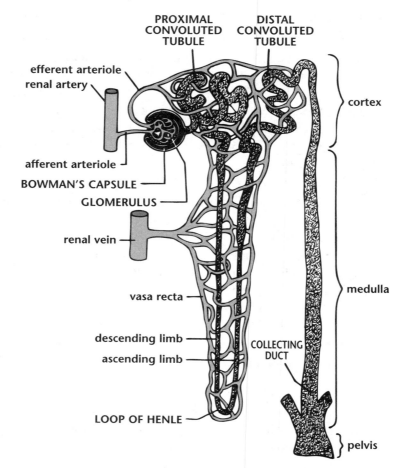

Figure 11.3. The Nephron

3. NEPHRON FUNCTION

Through the selective permeability of its walls and the maintenance of an osmolarity gradient, the nephron reabsorbs nutrients, salts, and water from the filtrate and returns them to the body, thus maintaining the bloodstream's solute concentration.

a. Osmolarity Gradient

The selective permeability of the tubules establishes an osmolarity gradient in the surrounding interstitial fluid. By exiting and then re-entering at different segments of the nephron, solutes create an osmolarity gradient, with tissue osmolarity increasing from **cortex** to **inner medulla**. The solutes that contribute to the maintenance of the gradient are urea and salt (Na^+ and Cl^-). The osmolarity of urine (determined by the concentration of dissolved particles) is established in the collecting tubule by means of this **countercurrent-multiplier system**: The anatomic arrangement of the loop of Henle within the kidney permits the establishment of a concentration gradient that permits the reabsorption of 99 percent of the filtrate in the collecting tubules. This allows for the production of as concentrated urine as possible and the conservation of as much water and salts as possible.

b. **Concentration of Urine**

The countercurrent system causes the medulla of the kidney to be **hyperosmolar** with respect to the dilute filtrate flowing in the collecting tubule. As the filtrate flowing in the collecting tubules passes through this region of the kidney on its way to the pelvis and ureter, water flows out of the collecting tubules by **osmosis**. This water is removed by capillaries flowing in the medulla. The reabsorption of water in this zone of the kidney, which permits the concentration of urine, depends on the permeability of the collecting tubules to water. Regulation of the permeability of the collecting tubule to water is accomplished by the hormone **ADH (vasopressin)**. ADH increases the permeability of the collecting duct to water, allowing more water to be absorbed and more concentrated urine to be formed in response to increased blood osmolarity.

Therefore, the primary function of the human kidney is to conserve water and solutes while simultaneously excreting dangerous waste products.

EXCRETION IN PLANTS

There is no specific excretory system in plants. While animals excrete the unusable products of metabolism as wastes, plants are able to use many of these "waste" products. These products are utilized as simple precursors in the synthesis of complex molecules; for example, **carbon dioxide** is utilized in **photosynthesis**, and nitrogen wastes can be re-utilized in the synthesis of proteins.

Any excess carbon dioxide, as well as waste oxygen and water vapor, leaves the plant by diffusion through **stomates** (pores in leaves) and **lenticels** (pores in stems). Exit of water vapor through leaf stomates is known as **transpiration**.

12

Animal Behavior

PATTERNS OF ANIMAL BEHAVIOR

A. Simple Reflexes

Reflexes are automatic responses to simple stimuli and are recognized as reliable behavioral responses following a given environmental stimulus. A **simple reflex** is controlled at the **spinal cord**, connecting a two-neuron pathway from the **receptor** (afferent neuron) to the **motor** (efferent neuron). The efferent nerve innervates the effector (e.g., a muscle or gland). Reflex behavior is important in the behavioral response of lower animals. It is less important in the behavior of higher forms of life, such as vertebrates.

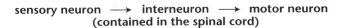

sensory neuron → interneuron → motor neuron
(contained in the spinal cord)

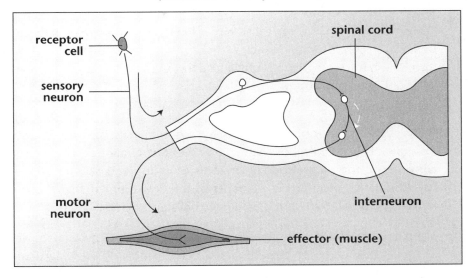

Figure 12.1. Simple Reflex

B. Complex Reflexes

More complex reflex patterns involve neural integration at a higher level—the **brainstem** or even the **cerebrum**. For example, the "**startle response**" alerts an animal to a significant stimulus. It can occur in response to potential danger or to hearing one's name called. The startle response involves the interaction of many neurons in a system termed the **reticular activating system**, which is responsible for sleep-wake transitions and behavioral motivation.

C. Fixed-Action Patterns

Fixed-action patterns are complex, coordinated, **innate** behavioral responses to specific patterns of stimulation in the environment. The stimulus that elicits the behavior is referred to as the **releaser**. Because fixed-action patterns are innate, they are relatively unlikely to be modified by learning. An animal has a repertoire of fixed-action patterns and only a limited ability to develop new ones. The particular stimuli that trigger a fixed-action pattern are more readily modified, provided certain cues or elements of the stimuli are maintained.

An example of a fixed-action pattern is the retrieval and maintenance response of many female birds to an egg of their species. Certain kinds of stimuli are more effective than others in triggering a fixed-action pattern. For example, an egg with the characteristics of that species will be more effective than one that only crudely resembles the natural egg. Another type of fixed-action pattern is the characteristic movements made by animals that herd or flock together, such as the swimming actions of fish and the flying actions of locusts.

D. Behavior Cycles

Daily cycles of behavior are called **circadian rhythms**. Animals with such behavior cycles lose their exact 24-hour periodicity if they are isolated from the natural phases of light and dark. Cyclical behavior, however, will continue with approximate day-to-day phasing. The cycle is thus initiated intrinsically but modified by external factors.

Daily cycles of eating, maintained by most animals, provide a good example of cycles with both **internal** and **external** control. The internal controls are the natural bodily rhythms of eating and satiation. External modulators include the elements of the environment that occur in familiar cyclic patterns, such as dinner bells and clocks.

Sleep and wakefulness are the most obvious example of cyclic behavior. In fact, these behavior patterns have been associated with particular patterns of brain waves.

E. Environmental Rhythms

In many situations, patterns of behavior are established and maintained mainly by periodic **environmental stimuli**. (A human example of this is the response to traffic light signals.) Also, just as environmental stimuli influence many naturally occurring biological rhythms, biological factors influence behavior governed by periodic environmental stimuli.

LEARNING

Learned behavior involves **adaptive responses** to the environment. Learning is a complex phenomenon that occurs to some extent in all animals. In lower animals, instinctual or innate behaviors are the predominant determinants of behavior patterns, and learning plays a relatively minor role in the modification of these predetermined behaviors. In higher animals, the major share of the response to the environment is learned. The capacity for learning adaptive responses is closely correlated with the degree of **neurologic development** (i.e., the capacity of the nervous system, particularly the cerebral cortex, for flexibility).

A. Habituation

Habituation is one of the simplest learning patterns, involving the suppression of the normal startle responses to stimuli. In habituation, repeated stimulation results in decreased responsiveness to that stimulus. The normal autonomic response to that stimulus would serve no useful purpose since the stimulus becomes a part of the background environment; thus, the response to the stimulus is suppressed. If the stimulus is no longer regularly applied, the response tends to recover over time. This is referred to as **spontaneous recovery**. Recovery of the response can also occur with modification of the stimulus.

B. Classical Conditioning

Classical or **Pavlovian** conditioning involves the association of a normally **autonomic** or visceral response with an environmental stimulus. For this reason, the response learned through Pavlovian conditioning is sometimes called a **conditioned reflex**. In Pavlovian conditioning, the normal, innate stimulus for a reflex is replaced by one chosen by the experimenter.

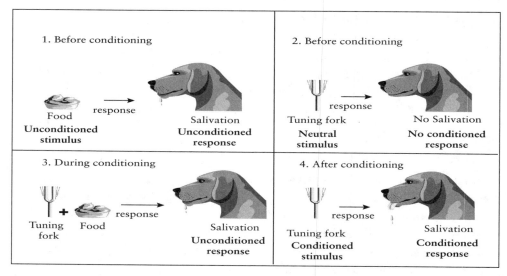

Figure 12.2. Classical (Pavlovian) Conditioning

1. PAVLOV'S EXPERIMENTS

Pavlov, who won a Nobel prize for his work on digestive physiology, studied the **salivation reflex** in dogs. In 1927, he discovered that if a dog was presented with an **arbitrary stimulus** (e.g., a bell) and then presented with food, it would eventually salivate on hearing the bell alone. The food elicited the unconditioned response of salivation. After repeated association of the bell with the food, the bell alone could elicit the salivation reflex. Thus, the innate or unconditioned response would occur with the selected stimulus. Pavlov's terminology, still used today, is described below:

- An established (innate) reflex consists of an **unconditioned stimulus** (e.g., food), and the response that is naturally elicited, termed the **unconditioned response** (e.g., salivation).

- A neutral stimulus is a stimulus that will not by itself elicit the response (prior to conditioning). During conditioning, the neutral stimulus (the bell) and the unconditioned stimulus (the food) are presented together. Eventually, the neutral stimulus is able to elicit the response in the absence of the unconditioned stimulus, and it is then called the conditioned stimulus. Pavlov's example of a conditioned stimulus is the sound of a bell for salivation.

- The product of the conditioning experience is termed the **conditioned reflex**. The conditioned reflex in Pavlov's experiment was salivation (the conditioned response) following a previously neutral stimulus (now the conditioned stimulus) such as the sound of a bell.

- Pavlov defined **conditioning** as the establishment of a new reflex (association of stimulus with response) by the addition of a new, previously neutral stimulus to the set of stimuli that are already capable of triggering the response.

2. PSEUDOCONDITIONING

Pseudoconditioning is a phenomenon that can be confused with true classical conditioning. A critical test of conditioning is the determination of whether the conditioning process is actually necessary for the production of a response by a previously "neutral stimulus." In many cases, the so-called "neutral" stimulus is able to elicit the response even before conditioning and, hence, is not really a neutral stimulus. Pseudoconditioning can be avoided by carefully evaluating all prospective stimuli before conditioning begins.

C. Operant or Instrumental Conditioning

Operant or instrumental conditioning involves conditioning responses to stimuli with the use of **reward** or **reinforcement**. When the organism exhibits a specific behavioral pattern that the experimenter would like to see repeated, the animal is rewarded. The reinforcement or reward increases the likelihood that the behavior will appear—it has been "reinforced." Although this instrumental conditioning was originally applied to conditioning responses under the voluntary control of the organism, it has been successfully applied more recently to the conditioning of visceral responses, such as changes in heartbeat.

1. EXPERIMENTS OF B. F. SKINNER

B. F. Skinner first demonstrated the principles of operant conditioning and reinforcement. In the original operant conditioning experiments, he used the well-known "Skinner box," consisting of a cage with a lever or key and a food dispenser. A food pellet was delivered whenever the animal pressed the lever. Thus, depression of the lever was the **operant response** under study. In later experiments, Skinner varied the type of reinforcement. Reinforcers fell into two categories:

a. Positive reinforcement

Positive reinforcement or **reward** includes providing food, light, or electrical stimulation of the animal's brain's "pleasure centers." Following positive reinforcement, the animal was much **more likely** to repeat the desired behavioral response (i.e., to press the bar). In a sense, the animal has developed a positive connection between the action (response) and the reward (stimulus that followed). This type of conditioning is likely to be involved in normal habit formation.

b. Negative reinforcement

Negative reinforcement also involves stimulating the brain's pleasure centers. However, in contrast to positive reinforcement, negative reinforcement links the **lack** of certain behavior with a reward (i.e., a bird may learn that it will receive a food pellet if it does *not* peck on a yellow circle in its cage).

In this case, the animal has developed a negative connection between action (response) and reward (stimulus that followed). Thus, the animal has developed a *positive* connection between the *lack* of the action and the reward, and the animal is **less likely** to repeat the behavioral response.

c. Punishment

Punishment involves conditioning an organism so that it will **stop** exhibiting a given behavior pattern. Punishment may involve painfully shocking the organism each time the chosen behavior appears. After punishment, the organism is **less likely** to repeat the behavioral response. The animal develops a negative connection between the stimulus and the response.

d. Habit family hierarchy

A stimulus is usually associated with several possible responses, each response having a different probability of occurrence. These stimulus-behavioral associations are believed to be ordered in a **habit family hierarchy**. For example, a chicken may respond to a light in many ways, but if one particular response is rewarded, it will occur with higher probability in the future. Reward strengthens a specific behavioral response and raises its order in the hierarchy. Punishment weakens a specific behavioral response and lowers its order in the hierarchy.

D. Modifications of Conditioned Behavior

1. EXTINCTION

Extinction is the gradual **elimination** of conditioned responses in the absence of reinforcement (i.e., the "unlearning" of the response pattern). In **instrumental and operant conditioning**, the response is diminished and finally eliminated in the absence of reinforcement. The response is not completely unlearned—rather, it is inhibited in the absence of reinforcement. It will rapidly reappear if the reinforcement is returned. In **classical conditioning**, extinction occurs when the unconditioned stimulus is removed or was never sufficiently paired with the conditioned stimulus. The conditioned stimulus must be paired with the unconditioned stimulus, at least part of the time, for the maintenance of the conditioned response. After sufficient time elapses following extinction, the conditioned response may again be elicited by the conditioned stimulus. The recovery of the conditioned response after extinction is called **spontaneous recovery**.

2. GENERALIZATION AND DISCRIMINATION

Stimulus generalization is the ability of a conditioned organism to respond to stimuli that are similar, but not identical, to the original conditioned stimulus. The less similar the stimulus is to the original conditioned stimulus, the less the response will be. For example, an organism may be conditioned to respond to a stimulus of a 1,000 Hz tone, but it may respond to stimuli somewhat higher or lower in pitch as well. **Stimulus discrimination** involves the ability of the learning organism to respond differentially to slightly different stimuli. For example, if rewards are given to only a very narrow range of sound (such as a tone of 990 to 1,010 Hz) but not to stimuli outside this range, the organism will also learn not to respond to stimuli that are very different in tone. A **stimulus generalization gradient** is established after the organism has been conditioned, whereby stimuli further and further away from the original conditioned stimulus elicit responses with decreasing magnitude.

LIMITS OF BEHAVIORAL CHANGE

A. Imprinting

Imprinting is a process in which environmental patterns or objects presented to a developing organism during a brief **"critical period"** in early life become accepted permanently as an element of its behavioral environment (i.e., "stamped in" and included in an animal's behavioral response). A duckling passes through a critical period in which it learns that the first large moving object it sees is its mother. In the natural environment, this is usually the case. However, other objects can be substituted during this period, and the duckling will follow anything that is substituted for its mother. This phenomenon was first identified by the ethologist **Konrad Lorenz**, who swam in a pond amongst newly hatched ducklings separated from their mother and found that they eventually followed him as if he were their mother.

B. Critical Period

Critical periods are specific time periods during an animal's early development when it is physiologically able to develop specific behavioral patterns. If the proper environmental pattern is not present during the critical period, the behavioral pattern will not develop properly. In addition to the critical period described above, some animals have a **visual critical period**. If light is not present during this period, visual effectors will not develop properly either.

INTRASPECIFIC INTERACTIONS

Intraspecific interactions occur as a means of communication between members of a species.

A. Behavioral Displays

A display may be defined as an **innate behavior** that has evolved as a signal for **communication** between members of the same species. According to this definition, a song, call, or an intentional change in an animal's physical characteristics are considered displays. Categories of displays include the following:

- **Reproductive displays** are specific behaviors found in all animals, including humans. Many animals have evolved a variety of complex actions that function as signals in preparation for mating.

- **Agonistic displays** are such things as a dog's display of appeasement when it wags its tail or the dog's **antagonistic** behavior when it directs its face straight and raises its body.

- Other displays include various **dancing** procedures exhibited by **honeybees**, especially the scout honeybee, to convey information concerning the quality and location of food sources. Displays utilizing auditory, visual, chemical, and tactile elements are often used as means of communication.

B. Pecking Order

The relationships among members of the same species living as a contained social group frequently become stable for a period of time. When food, mates, or territory are disputed, a **dominant** member of the species will prevail over a **subordinate** one. The social hierarchy is frequently referred to as the **pecking order**. It minimizes violent intraspecific aggressions by defining stable relationships among members of the group.

C. Territoriality

Members of most land-dwelling species **defend** a limited area or territory from intrusion by other members of the species. These territories are typically occupied by a male or a male-female pair and are frequently used for mating, nesting, and feeding. Territoriality serves the adaptive function of **distributing** members of the species so that the environmental resources are not depleted in a small region, in addition to reducing intraspecific competition. Although there is frequently a minimum size for any species' territory, the territory size varies with the population size and density. The larger the population, the smaller the territories are likely to be.

D. Response to Chemicals

The **olfactory sense** is immensely important as a means of communication in many animals. Many animals secrete substances, called **pheromones**, that influence the behavior of other members of the same species. Pheromones can be classified as one of two types:

1. **RELEASER PHEROMONES** trigger a reversible behavioral change in the recipient. For example, female silkworms secrete a very powerful attracting pheromone, so powerful that a male responds to 1 ten-millionth of a gram from a distance of two miles or more. **Sex-attractant** pheromones are secreted by many animals, including cockroaches, queen honeybees, and gypsy moths. In addition to sex-attracting purposes, releaser pheromones are secreted as **alarm** and **toxic defensive** substances.

2. **PRIMER PHEROMONES** produce long-term behavioral and physiological alterations in recipient animals. For example, pheromones from male mice may affect the estrous cycles of females. Pheromones have also been shown to limit sexual reproduction in areas of high animal density. Primer pheromones are important in social insects such as ants, bees, and termites, where they regulate role determination and reproductive capacities.

13

Ecology

Ecology is the study of the **interactions** between organisms and their environment. The **environment** encompasses all that is external to the organism and is necessary for its existence. An organism's environment contains two components—the physical or non-living **(abiotic)** environment and the living **(biotic)** environment. The physical environment includes climate, temperature, availability of light and water, and the local topology. The biotic environment includes all living things that directly or indirectly influence the life of the organism, including the relationships that exist between organisms.

LEVELS OF BIOLOGICAL ORGANIZATION

A. Organism

The organism is the individual unit of an ecological system, but the organism itself is composed of smaller units. The organism contains many organ systems, which are made up of **organs**. Organs are formed from **tissues**, tissues from **cells**, cells from many different **molecules**, molecules from **atoms**, and atoms from subatomic particles.

B. Population

A **species** is any group of similar organisms that are capable of reproducing fertile offspring. A **population** is a group of organisms of the same species **living together** *in a given location.* Examples of populations include dandelions on a lawn, flies in a barn, minnows of a certain species in a pond, and lions in a grassland. Environmental factors, such as nutrients, water, and sunlight limitations, aid in maintaining populations at relatively constant levels.

C. Communities

A community consists of populations of different plants and animal species interacting with each other in a given environment. The term **biotic community** is used to include only the populations and not their physical environment. An **ecosystem** includes the community and the environment. Generally, a community contains populations from all five kingdoms, monerans, protists, plants, fungi, and animals, all depending upon each other for survival. The following are examples of communities:

- A **lawn** contains dandelions, grasses, mushrooms, earthworms, nematodes, and bacteria.
- A **pond** contains dragonflies, algae, minnows, insect larvae, etc.
- A **forest** contains moss, pine, bacteria, lichens, ferns, deer, chipmunks, spiders, foxes, etc.
- The **sea** contains fish, whales, plankton, etc.

D. Ecosystem

An ecosystem or ecological community encompasses the interaction between living **biotic communities** and the **nonliving environment.** In studying the ecosystem, the biologist emphasizes the effects of the biotic community on the environment and the environment on the community. The examples listed above for communities are also examples of ecosystems.

E. Biosphere

The biosphere includes all portions of the planet that support life—the **atmosphere**, the **lithosphere** (rock and soil surface), and the **hydrosphere** (the oceans). It is a relatively thin zone extending a few feet beneath the earth's surface, several miles into the deepest sea, and several miles into the atmosphere.

THE ENVIRONMENT

A. Physical Environment

1. WATER

Water is the major component of the internal environment of all living things. Water may be readily available, or the organism may possess adaptations for storage and conservation of water.

2. TEMPERATURE

Temperature must be maintained at an optimal level. Protoplasm is destroyed at temperatures below 0°C and at high temperatures. Organisms have adaptations necessary for protection against these extremes. The temperature of a geographic location depends upon its latitude and altitude. In fact, the same changes in habitat that occur as one approaches colder polar regions (changes in latitude) occur as one ascends towards the colder regions of a mountain top (changes in altitude).

3. SUNLIGHT

Sunlight is the ultimate source of energy for all organisms. Green plants must compete for sunlight in forests. They have adapted to capture as much sunlight as possible by growing broad leaves, branching, growing to greater height, or producing vine growths. The **photic zone** in water, the top layer through which light can penetrate, is where all aquatic photosynthetic activity takes place. In the **aphotic zone**, only animal life and other heterotrophic life exist.

4. OXYGEN SUPPLY

This poses no problem for **terrestrial** life since the air contains approximately 20 percent oxygen. Aquatic plants and animals utilize the small amount of oxygen **dissolved** in water. Pollution can significantly lower oxygen content in water and threaten aquatic life.

5. SUBSTRATUM (SOIL OR ROCK)

The substratum determines the nature of plant and animal life in the soil. Soil is affected by a number of factors:

- **Acidity (pH):** Rhododendrons and pines are more suited for growth in acid soil. Acid rain may make soil pH too low for most plant growth.
- The **texture** of soil and its clay content determine the water-holding capacity of the soil. Willows require moist soil. Most plants grow well in **loams,** which contain high percentages of each type of soil.
- **Minerals,** including **nitrates** and **phosphates,** affect the type of vegetation that can be supported. Beach sand has been leached of all minerals and is generally unable to support plant life.
- **Humus** quantity is determined by the amount of decaying plant and animal life in the soil.

B. Biotic Factors in the Environment

Organisms belonging to the same or different species influence each other's development. Living things interact with other living organisms and with their physical environment.

INTERACTIONS WITHIN THE ECOSYSTEM

Complex interactions exist among the constituents of an ecosystem. These interactions involve a cyclic flow of energy and materials.

A. The Niche

The niche defines the functional role of an organism in its ecosystem. The niche is distinct from the **habitat**—the latter is the physical place where an organism lives. The characteristics of the habitat aid in defining the niche, but additional factors must also be considered. The niche describes what the organism eats, where and how it obtains its food, what climactic factors it can tolerate and which are optimal, the nature of its parasites and predators, where and how it reproduces, etc. The concept of niche embodies every aspect of an organism's existence.

It is implicit in the definition of *niche* that no two species can ever occupy the same niche in the same location. Organisms occupying the same niche compete for the same limited resources: food, water, light, oxygen, space, minerals, and reproductive sites. There may be many organisms in this niche, but they are all of the same species and thus have the same requirements. The niche is so specific that a species can be identified by the niche it occupies.

Species occupying similar niches utilize at least one resource in common. Therefore, they will compete for that resource. This competition can have a number of outcomes:

- One species may be competitively superior to the other and drive the second to **extinction**.

- One species may be competitively superior in some regions, and the other may be superior in other regions under different environmental conditions. This would result in the elimination of one species in some places and the other in other places.

- The two species may rapidly evolve in **divergent** directions under the strong selection pressure resulting from intense competition. Thus, the two species would rapidly evolve greater differences in their niches.

B. Nutritional Interactions Within the Ecosystem

1. AUTOTROPHS

Autotrophs are organisms that manufacture their own food. The green plants utilize the energy of the sun to manufacture food. Chemosynthetic bacteria obtain energy from the oxidation of inorganic sulfur, iron, and nitrogen compounds.

2. HETEROTROPHS

Heterotrophs cannot synthesize their own food and must depend upon autotrophs or other heterotrophs in the ecosystem to obtain food and energy.

a. Herbivores

These animals consume only **plants** or plant foods. The toughness of **cellulose-containing** plant tissues has led to the development of structures for crushing and grinding that can extract plant fluids. Herbivores have long digestive tracts that provide greater surface area and time for digestion. However, they cannot digest much of the food they consume. **Symbiotic bacteria** capable of digesting cellulose inhabit the digestive tracts of herbivores and allow the breakdown and utilization of cellulose.

Herbivores are more adept in **defense** than carnivores because they are often prey. Many herbivores, such as cows and horses, have hoofs instead of toes for faster movement on the grasslands. They have incisors adapted for cutting and molars adapted for grinding their food. Insects or other invertebrates can also be herbivores.

b. Carnivores

Carnivores are animals that eat only other **animals**. In general, carnivores, such as hyenas, possess pointed teeth and fanglike canine teeth for tearing flesh. They have shorter digestive tracts due to the easier digestibility of animal food.

c. Omnivores

Omnivores, such as humans, are animals that eat both **plants** and **animals**.

C. Interspecific Interactions

A community is not simply a collection of different species living within the same area. It is an **integrated system** of species that are dependent upon one another for survival. The major types of interspecific interactions are symbiosis, predation, saprophytism, and scavenging.

1. SYMBIOSIS

Symbionts live together in an intimate, often permanent association, which may or may not be beneficial to both participants. Some symbiotic relationships are **obligatory**; that is, one or both organisms cannot survive without the other. Symbiotic relationships are classified according to the benefits the symbionts receive. The types of symbiotic relationships include commensalism, mutualism, and parasitism.

a. Commensalism (+/0)

One organism is benefited (+) by the association, and the other is not affected (0). The host neither discourages nor fosters the relationship. Some examples include the following:

- **Remora and shark:** The remora (sharksucker) attaches itself by a holdfast device to the underside of a shark. Through this association, the remora obtains the food the shark discards, wide geographic dispersal, and protection from enemies. The shark is totally indifferent to the association.

- **Barnacle and whale:** The barnacle is a sessile crustacean that attaches to the whale and obtains wider feeding opportunities through the migrations of the whale.

b. Mutualism (+/+)

A symbiotic relationship from which both organisms derive some benefit (+). Some examples are the following:

- **Tick bird and rhinoceros:** The bird receives food in the form of ticks on the skin of the rhinoceros. The rhinoceros has its ticks removed and is warned of danger by the rapid departure of the bird.

- **Fungi and algae:** In a lichen, the green algae produces food for itself and the fungus by **photosynthesis**. The meshes of fungal threads support the algae and conserve rainwater. The fungus also provides carbon dioxide and nitrogenous wastes for the algae, all of which are needed for photosynthesis and protein synthesis.

- **Nitrogen-fixing bacteria and legumes:** Nitrogen-fixing bacteria invade the roots of legumes, and infected cells grow to form root nodules. In the nodule, the legume provides nutrients for the bacteria, and the bacteria fixes nitrogen (by changing it to a soluble nitrate, a mineral essential for protein synthesis by the plant). These bacteria are a major source of usable nitrogen, which is needed by all plants and animals.

- **Protozoa and termites:** Termites chew and ingest wood but are unable to digest the **cellulose**. Protozoa in the digestive tract of the termite secrete an enzyme that digests the cellulose. Both organisms share the carbohydrates. Thus, the protozoan is guaranteed protection and a steady food supply, while the termite is able to obtain nourishment from the ingested wood.

- **Intestinal bacteria and humans:** Bacteria utilize some of the food material not fully digested by humans and manufacture vitamin K.

c. **Parasitism (+/–)**

A parasite benefits (+) at the expense (–) of the host. Parasitism exists when competition for food is most intense. Few autotrophs (green plants) exist as parasites (mistletoe is an exception). Parasitism flourishes among organisms such as bacteria, fungi, and animals. Some parasites cling to the exterior surface of the host (**ectoparasites**) using suckers or clamps. They may bore through the skin and suck out blood and nutrients. Leeches, ticks, and sea lampreys employ these techniques. Other parasites (**endoparasites**) live within the host. To gain entry, they must pass through defenses such as skin, digestive juices, antibodies, and white blood cells. Parasites possess special adaptations to overcome these defenses.

Parasitism is advantageous and efficient. The parasite lives with a minimum expenditure of energy. Parasites may even have parasites of their own. Thus, a mammal may have parasitic worms, which in turn are parasitized by bacteria, which in turn are victims of bacteriophages. It is interesting to note that successful parasites do not kill their hosts; this would lead to the death of the parasite. The more dangerous the parasite, the less the chance it will survive.. Some examples are the following:

- **Virus and host cell:** All viruses are parasites. They contain nucleic acids surrounded by a protein coat and are nonfunctional outside the host. Upon entry of the viral nucleic acid into the host, the virus takes over the host cell functions and redirects them into replication of itself. The life functions of the bacterial cell slow down or cease in favor of viral replication.

- **Disease bacteria and animals:** Most bacteria are either chemosynthetic (energy-producing)or **saprophytic** (bacteria of decay). For example, diphtheria is parasitic upon humans, anthrax on sheep, and tuberculosis on cows or on humans.

- **Disease fungi and animals:** Most fungi are saprophytic. **Ringworm** is parasitic on humans.

- **Worms and animals:** An example is the parasitic relationship that exists between the tapeworm and humans.

2. PREDATION

Predators are free-living organisms that feed on other living organisms. This definition of predation includes both **carnivores** and **herbivores**. The effects of predators on their prey vary. The predator may severely limit the numbers or distribution of the prey, and the prey may become extinct. On the other hand, the predator may only slightly affect the prey, because the predator is scarce or commonly utilizes another food source. In many cases, the predator aids in controlling the numbers of the prey but not so much as to endanger the existence of the prey population. Predator-prey relationships evolve toward a balance in which the predator is a regulatory influence on the prey but not a threat to its survival. Examples of predators include the hawk, lion, human, and Venus flytrap.

3. SAPROPHYTISM

Saprophytes include those protists and fungi that **decompose** (digest) dead organic matter externally and absorb the nutrients; they constitute a vital link in the cycling of material within the ecosystem. Examples of saprophytes include mold, mushrooms, bacteria of decay, and slime molds.

4. SCAVENGERS

Scavengers are animals that consume dead animals. They therefore require no adaptations for hunting and killing their prey. Decomposers, such as the bacteria of decay, may be considered scavengers. Examples of scavengers include the vulture and hyena. The snapping turtle is an organism that may be considered both a scavenger and a predator.

D. Intraspecific Interactions

Competition is not restricted to **interspecific** interactions (relations between species). Individuals belonging to the same species utilize the same resources; if a particular resource is limited, then these organisms must compete with one another. Members of the same species compete, but they must also **cooperate**. Intraspecific cooperation may be extensive (as with the formation of societies in animal species) or may be nearly nonexistent. Relationships between individuals within a species are influenced by both disruptive and cohesive forces. Competition is the chief disruptive force. Cohesive forces include reproduction and protection from predators and destructive weather.

E. Interactions Between Organisms and Their Environment

1. OSMOREGULATION

Animals have developed many adaptations for maintaining their internal osmolarity and conserving water.

- **Saltwater fish** live in a **hyperosmotic** environment, which causes them to lose water and take in salt. They are constantly in danger of dehydration and must compensate by constant drinking and active excretion of salt across their gills.

- **Freshwater fish** live in a **hypo-osmotic** environment, which causes intake of excess water and excessive salt loss. These fish correct this condition by seldom drinking, absorbing salts through the gills, and excreting dilute urine.

- **Insects** excrete solid uric acid crystals to conserve water.

- Desert animals possess adaptations for avoiding desiccation (drying up). The **camel** can tolerate a wide range of body temperatures and possesses fat layers in regions that are exposed to solar radiation. The **horned toad** has thick, scaly skin, which prevents water loss. Other desert animals burrow in the sand during the day and search for food at night, thereby avoiding the intense heat that causes water loss.

- Plants possess adaptations for conservation of water. Nondesert plants possess waxy **cuticles** on leaf surfaces and stomata on the lower leaf surfaces only. They shed leaves in winter to avoid water loss. Desert plants have extensive root systems, **fleshy stems** to store water, **spiny leaves** to limit water loss, extra thick cuticles, and few stomata.

2. THERMOREGULATION

Cellular respiration only transfers a fraction of the energy derived from the oxidation of carbohydrates into the high-energy bonds of ATP. Roughly **60 percent** of the total energy is given off as heat. The vast majority of animals and plants are cold-blooded or **poikilothermic**, and most of their heat energy escapes to the environment. The body temperature of poikilotherms is very close to that of their surroundings. Since an organism's metabolism is closely tied to its body temperature, the activity of poikilothermic animals is radically affected by environmental temperature changes. As the temperature rises, these organisms become more active. As temperatures fall, they become sluggish and lethargic.

Some animals, notably **mammals** and **birds**, are warm-blooded or **homeothermic**. They have evolved physical mechanisms that allow them to make use of the heat produced as a consequence of respiration. Physical adaptations like fat, hair, and feathers retard heat loss. Homeotherms maintain constant body temperatures that are higher than the temperature of environment. They are less dependent upon environmental temperature than poikilothermic animals and are able to inhabit a comparatively wider range of environments.

RELATIONSHIPS WITHIN THE ECOSYSTEM

A. Energy Flow

All living things require energy to carry on their life functions. The complex pathways involved in the transfer of energy through the living components of the ecosystem (biotic community) may be mapped in the form of a **food chain** or **food web**.

1. FOOD CHAIN

A food chain is a single chain showing the transfer of energy. For example, energy from the sun enters living systems through the **photosynthetic** production of glucose by green plants. Within the food chain, energy is transferred from the original sources in green plants through a series of organisms with repeated stages of consumption and finally decomposition. Thus, there are producers, primary consumers, secondary consumers, and decomposers.

a. Producers

The **autotrophic** green plants and **chemosynthetic** bacteria are the producers. They utilize the energy of the sun and simple raw materials (carbon dioxide, water, minerals), respectively, to manufacture carbohydrates, proteins, and lipids. The radiant energy of the sun is captured and stored in the C–H bond. Producers always form the initial step in any food chain. The wheat plant is a typical producer.

b. Primary Consumers

Primary consumers are animals that consume green plants (**herbivores**). Examples include the cow, grasshopper, and elephant.

c. Secondary Consumers

Secondary consumers are animals that consume the primary consumers (**carnivores**). These include frogs, tigers, and dragonflies.

d. Tertiary Consumers

These are animals that feed on secondary consumers (also carnivores).

e. Decomposers

Decomposers include **saprophytic** organisms and organisms of decay, which include bacteria and fungi. The producers and consumers concentrate and organize materials of the environment into complex living substances. Living things give off wastes during their lifetimes and eventually die. Bacteria and fungi decompose the organic wastes and dead tissues to simpler compounds, such as nitrates and phosphates, which are returned to the environment to be used again by living organisms. These processes are demonstrated in **food webs** and **material cycles** (nitrogen, carbon, and water).

2. FOOD WEB

The food web is not a simple linear chain but an intricate collection of interconnected food chains. Almost every species is consumed by one or more other species, some of which are on different food chain levels. The result is a series of branches and cross-branches among all the food chains of a community to form a web. The greater the number of pathways in a community food web, the more stable the community. For example, owls eat rabbits. If rabbits died off because of disease, there would be more vegetation available to mice. Mice would thrive and provide substitute food for owls. Meanwhile, the decimated rabbit population would have a better chance of recovering while owls concentrated their predation on mice.

3. FOOD PYRAMIDS

Without a constant input of **energy** from the sun, an ecosystem would soon run down. As food is transferred from one level of the food chain to the next, a transfer of energy occurs. According to the second law of thermodynamics, every energy transfer involves a loss of energy. In addition to the energy lost in the transfer, each level of the food chain utilizes some of the energy it obtains from the food for its own metabolism (i.e., to support life functions) and loses some additional energy in the form of heat. A pyramid of energy is thus a fundamental property of all ecosystems at all levels.

a. Pyramid of Energy

Each member of a food chain utilizes some of the energy it obtains from its food for its own metabolism (life functions) and loses some additional energy in the form of heat. Since this means a loss of energy at each feeding level, the producer organism at the base of the pyramid contains the greatest amount of energy. Less energy is available for the primary consumer and still less for secondary and tertiary consumers. The smallest amount of available energy is thus at the top of the pyramid.

b. Pyramid of Mass

Since organisms at the upper levels of the food chain derive their food energy from organisms at lower levels and since energy is lost from one level to the next, each level can support a successively smaller biomass. Three hundred pounds of foliage (producer) may support 125 lb. of insects. This may support 50 lb. of insectivorous hens, who in turn will be just the right amount to sustain 25 lb. of hawks.

c. Pyramid of numbers

Consumer organisms that are higher in the food chain are usually larger and heavier than those further down. Since the lower organisms have a greater total mass, there must be a greater number of lower-level organisms. (A large bass eats tiny minnows but eats many of them.) With the greatest number of organisms at the base (producer level) and the smallest number at the top (final consumer level), we have a pyramid of numbers.

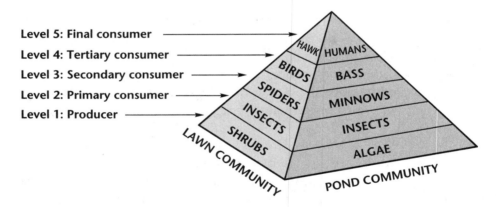

Figure 13.1. Food Pyramids

Note: Since other factors, such as the generation time and the size of the organisms must be considered, the pyramids of numbers and biomass do not apply to all levels at all times (unlike the pyramid of energy). In general, as the pyramid is ascended, there is (1) less energy content, (2) less mass, and (3) fewer organisms.

B. Material Cycles

Material is cycled and recycled between organisms and their environments, passing from inorganic forms to organic forms and then back to the inorganic forms. Many of these cycles are accomplished largely through the action of scavengers (such as hyenas and vultures) and decomposers (saprophytes such as bacteria and fungi).

1. NITROGEN CYCLE

Nitrogen is an essential component of amino acids and nucleic acids, which are the building blocks for all living things. Since there is a finite amount of nitrogen on the earth, it is important that it be recovered and reused.

- Elemental nitrogen is chemically inert and cannot be used by most organisms. Lightning and nitrogen-fixing bacteria in the roots of legumes change the nitrogen to the usable, soluble nitrates.

- The nitrates are absorbed by plants and are used to synthesize nucleic acids and plant proteins.

- Animals eat the plants and synthesize specific animal proteins from the plant proteins. Both plants and animals give off wastes and eventually die.

- The nitrogen locked up in the wastes and dead tissues is released by the action of the bacteria of decay, which convert the proteins into ammonia.

- Two fates await the ammonia (NH_3). Some is nitrified to nitrites by chemosynthetic bacteria and then to usable nitrates by nitrifying bacteria. The rest is denitrified. This means the ammonia (NH_3) is broken down to release free nitrogen, which returns to the beginning of the cycle. Note that four kinds of bacteria are involved in this cycle: **decay, nitrifying, denitrifying**, and **nitrogen fixing**. The bacteria have no use for the excretory ammonia, nitrites, nitrates, and nitrogen they produce. These materials are essential, however, for the existence of other living organisms.

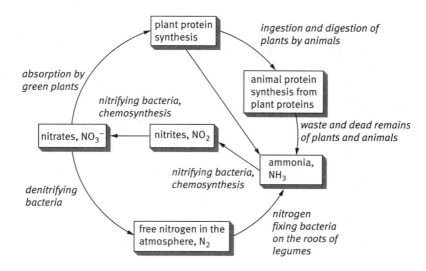

Figure 13.2. Nitrogen Cycle

2. CARBON CYCLE

- **Gaseous CO_2** enters the living world when plants use it to produce glucose via photosynthesis. The carbon atoms in CO_2 are bonded to hydrogen and other carbon atoms. The plant uses the glucose to make starch, proteins, and fat.

- Animals eat plants and use the digested nutrients to form carbohydrates, fats, and proteins characteristic of the species. A part of these organic compounds is used as fuel in respiration in both plants and animals.

- The metabolically produced CO_2 is released to the air. The rest of the organic carbon remains locked within an organism until its death (except for wastes given off), at which time decay processes by bacteria return the CO_2 to the air.

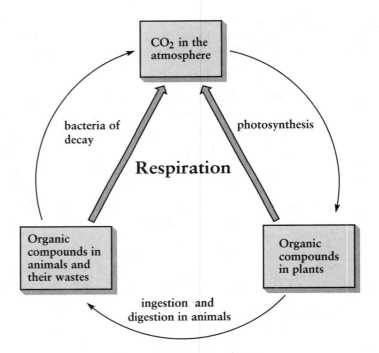

Figure 13.3. Carbon Cycle

3. OTHER CYCLES

Other cycles recycle water, oxygen, and phosphorus. These substances are used by almost all living things and must be returned by the biotic community to the environment so they can be reused.

STABILITY IN THE ECOSYSTEM

A. Conditions for Stability in an Ecosystem

An ecosystem is self-sustaining and, therefore, will be stable if three conditions are met. First, it needs a relatively stable physical environment (abiotic factors) and a relatively stable biotic community. Second, a stable ecosystem requires a constant **energy source** and a living system incorporating this energy into organic compounds. Lastly, the **cycling** of materials between the living system and its environment is critical for a stable ecosystem.

B. Ecological Succession

Ecological succession is the orderly process by which one biotic community replaces or succeeds another until a climax community is established. Each community stage, or **sere**, in an ecological succession is identified by a **dominant** species—the one that exerts control over the other species that are present. Thus, in a grassland community, grass is the dominant species.

Changes occur because each community that establishes itself changes the **environment**, making it more unfavorable for itself and more favorable for the community that is to succeed it. Successive communities are composed of populations that are able to exist under the new conditions. Finally, a stage arises in which a population alters the environment in such a way that the original conditions giving rise to that population are re-created. Replacement stops, and we have our **climax community**, the final and most stable stage of ecological succession. This climax community is permanent in the ecosystem, unless the abiotic factors are drastically altered by climactic or geologic upheavals. If this happens, a new series of successions is initiated.

- **Example 1:** Consider a barren rocky area in the northeastern United States, barren perhaps as a result of a severe forest fire. **Lichen** may be the first or **pioneer organism** to resettle this virgin area. Recall that a lichen is an association between an alga and a fungus that can live on a rocky surface. Acids produced by the lichen attack the rocks and help to form bits of soil. Since lichens thrive only on a solid surface, conditions are now worse for the lichen but better for mosses. Airborne spores of mosses land on the soil and germinate. The result is a new **sere** with the moss as the dominant species in the community. As the remains of the moss build up the soil still more, annual grasses and then perennial grasses with deeper roots become the dominant species. As time marches on, we find shrubs and then trees. The first trees are the sun-loving gray birch and poplar. As more and more trees compete for the sun, these trees are replaced by white pine and finally **maples** and **beeches**, which grow in deep shade—the climax community.

The growth of maples and beeches produces the same conditions that originally favored their appearance. And so this community remains for thousands of years. In the final maple-beech community, you would find foxes, deer, chipmunks, and plant-eating insects. These are animals that would not have been found in the original barren rock terrain. However, one forest fire can kill the entire community. Ecological succession then starts all over again, commencing with the lichen and the bare rock.

It is important to note again that the dominant species of the climax community depend on such **physical factors** as temperature, nature of the soil, rainfall, etc. Thus, the climax community in New York State at higher elevations is hemlock-beech-maple, while at lower elevations, the climax plants are more often oak-hickory. In cold Maine, the climax community is dominated by pine; in the wet areas of Wisconsin, by cypress; in sandy New Jersey, by pine; on a cold, windy mountain top, by scrub oak.

- **Example 2:** Ecological succession in a pond. A quick summary:
  - **Step 1:** Pond: Plants such as algae, pondweed. Animals such as protozoa, water insects, small fish.
  - **Step 2:** Shallow water as pond fills in: Reeds, cattails, water lilies.
  - **Step 3:** Moist land: Grass, herbs, shrubs, willow trees; frogs, snakes.
  - **Step 4:** Woodland: Climax tree—perhaps pine or oak.

C. The Climax Community

A climax community is the **stable**, living (**biotic**) part of the ecosystem described above in which populations exist in balance with each other and with the environment. The type of climax community depends upon all the abiotic factors: rainfall, soil conditions, temperature, shade, etc. A climax community persists until a major climactic or geological change disturbs the abiotic factors or a major biotic change (such as disease, mutations, etc.) affects the populations. Once the equilibrium is upset, new climax conditions are produced, and new communities will be established in the ecosystem.

WORLD BIOMES (MAJOR COMMUNITIES)

A. Terrestrial Biomes

The evolutionary **origin** of plants and animals can be traced to the seas. To survive on land, these organisms had to develop adaptations to face an environment with a (1) relative lack of water, (2) relative lack of food and supporting medium, (3) varying temperature (as compared to the oceans, which have a relatively constant temperature), and (4) varying composition of the soil as compared to the definite salt composition in the oceans. The conditions in different terrestrial and climate regions selected for plants and animals possessing suitable adaptations. Each **geographic region** is inhabited by a distinct community, called a **biome**, existing in the major climate areas.

Land biomes are characterized and named according to the **climax vegetation** of the region. The climax vegetation is the vegetation that becomes dominant and stable after years of evolutionary development. Since plants are important as food producers, they determine the nature of the inhabiting animal population, and thus the climax vegetation determines the **climax animal population**. Some types of terrestrial biomes are these:

1. DESERT BIOME

Deserts receive fewer than 10 inches of rain each year; the rain is concentrated within a few heavy cloudbursts. The growing season in the desert is restricted to those days after rainfalls. Generally, small plants and animals inhabit the desert. Most desert plants conserve water actively (cactus, sagebrush, mesquite). Desert animals live in burrows (insects and lizards). Few birds and mammals are found in the deserts except those that have developed adaptations for maintaining constant body temperatures. Examples of deserts include the Sahara in Africa and the Gobi in Asia.

2. GRASSLAND BIOME

Grasslands are characterized by a low rainfall (usually 10–30 inches per year), although considerably more than the desert biomes receive. Grasslands provide no shelter for **herbivorous mammals** (bison, antelope, cattle, zebra) from carnivorous predators. Animals that do inhabit the grasslands have developed long legs, and many are hoofed. Examples of grasslands include the prairies east of the Rockies, the steppes of the Ukraine, and the pampas of Argentina.

3. TROPICAL RAIN FOREST BIOME

Rain forests are "**jungles**" characterized by **high temperatures** and **torrential rains**. The climax community includes a dense growth of vegetation that does not shed its leaves. Vegetation such as vines and **epiphytes** (plants growing on other plants) and animals such as monkeys, lizards, snakes, and birds inhabit the tropical rain forests. Trees grow closely together; sunlight hardly reaches the forest floor. The floor is inhabited by **saprophytes**, living off dead organic matter. Tropical rain forests are found in Central Africa, Central America, the Amazon basin, and Southeast Asia.

4. TEMPERATE DECIDUOUS FOREST BIOME

Temperate deciduous forests have cold winters, warm summers, and a moderate rainfall. Trees such as **beech**, **maple**, **oaks**, and **willows** shed their leaves during the cold winter months. Animals in temperate deciduous forests include the deer, fox, woodchuck, and squirrel. These biomes are found in the northeast and central-eastern United States and in Central Europe.

5. TEMPERATE CONIFEROUS FOREST BIOME

These forests are cold, dry, and inhabited by **fir, pine,** and **spruce** trees. Much of the vegetation has evolved adaptations for water conservation, such as needle-shaped leaves. These forests are found in the extreme northern part of the United States and in southern Canada.

6. TAIGA BIOME

Taigas receive less rainfall than temperate forests. They have long, cold winters and are inhabited by a single coniferous tree: the **spruce**. The forest floors in the taiga contain moss and lichens. The chief animal inhabitant is the moose; however, the black bear, wolf, and birds are also found there. Taigas exist in the extreme northern parts of Canada and Russia.

7. TUNDRA BIOME

The tundra is a treeless, frozen plain found between the taiga lands and the northern ice sheets. There is only a very short summer and, thus, a very short growing season when the ground becomes wet and marshy. Lichens, moss, polar bears, musk oxen, and arctic hens are found in the tundra.

8. POLAR REGION

The polar region is a frozen area with no vegetation and few terrestrial animals. Animals that do inhabit polar regions generally live near the polar oceans.

B. Terrestrial Biome and Altitude

The sequence of biome between the equator and the poles is comparable to the sequence of regions on mountains. The nature of those regions are determined by the same decisive factors—temperatures and rainfall. For example, the base of the mountain would resemble the biome of a temperate deciduous area. As one ascends the mountain, one would pass a coniferous-like biome, then taiga-like, tundra-like, and polar-like biomes.

C. Aquatic Biomes

More than 70 percent of the earth's surface is covered by water. Most of the earth's plant and animal life is found in water. As much as 90 percent of the earth's food and oxygen production (**photosynthesis**) takes place in the water. Aquatic biomes are classified according to criteria quite different from the criteria used to classify terrestrial biomes. Plants have little controlling influence in communities of aquatic biomes compared to their role in terrestrial biomes. Aquatic areas are the most stable ecosystems; the conditions affecting temperature, amount of available oxygen and carbon dioxide, and amount of suspended or dissolved materials are stable over very large areas and show little tendency to change. Therefore, aquatic food webs and aquatic communities are balanced. There are two types of major aquatic biomes: **marine** and **freshwater**.

1. MARINE BIOMES

The oceans connect to form one continuous body of water, which controls the earth's temperature by absorbing solar heat. Water has the distinctive property of being able to absorb or utilize large amounts of heat without undergoing a great temperature change. Marine biomes contain a relatively constant amount of nutrient materials and dissolved salts.

Although ocean conditions are more uniform than those on land, distinct zones in the marine biomes exist.

- **Intertidal zone:** The region exposed at low tides that undergoes variations in temperature and periods of dryness. Populations in the intertidal zones include algae, sponges, clams, snails, sea urchins, starfish, and crabs.
- **Littoral zone:** The region on the continental shelf that contains ocean area with depths up to 600 feet and extends several hundred miles from the shores. Populations in littoral zone regions include algae, crabs, crustacea, and many different species of fish.

- **Pelagic zone:** Typical of the open seas, this can be divided into photic and aphotic zones (see Figure 13.4).

  - **Photic zone:** The **sunlit layer** of the open sea extending to a depth of 250–600 feet. It contains **plankton**, passively drifting masses of microscopic photosynthetic and heterotrophic organisms, and **nekton**, active swimmers such as fish, sharks, or whales that feed on plankton and smaller fish. The chief autotroph is the **diatom**, an algae.

  - **Aphotic zone:** The region beneath the photic zone that receives **no sunlight**. There is no photosynthesis in the aphotic zone, and only heterotrophs exist here. **Deep-sea organisms** in this zone have adaptations enabling them to survive in very cold water with high pressures and in complete darkness. The zone contains **nekton** and **benthos** (the crawling and sessile organisms). Some are scavengers, and some are predators. The habitat of the aphotic zone is fiercely competitive.

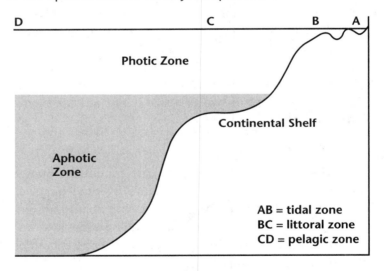

Figure 13.4. Marine Biomes

2. FRESHWATER BIOMES

Rivers, lakes, ponds, marshes—the links between the oceans and land—contain freshwater. Rivers are the routes by which ancient marine organisms reached land and evolved terrestrial adaptations. Many forms failed to adapt to land and developed adaptations for freshwater. Others developed special adaptations suitable for both land and freshwater. As in **marine biomes**, factors affecting life in freshwater include **temperature**, **transparency** (illumination due to suspended mud particles), **depth** of water, available carbon dioxide and **oxygen**, and most important, the **salt concentration**. Freshwater biomes differ from saltwater biomes in three basic ways:

1. Freshwater is **hypotonic,** creating a diffusion gradient that results in the passage of water into the cell. Freshwater organisms have homeostatic mechanisms to maintain water balance by the regular **removal** of **excess water.** These include the contractile vacuoles of protozoa and excretory systems of fish. Plant cells have rigid cell walls and thus build up cell pressure (cell **turgor**) as water flows in. This pressure counteracts the gradient pressure, stops the influx of water, and establishes a water balance.

2. In rivers and streams, strong, swift **currents** exist, and thus selection favored the survival of fish that developed strong muscles and plants with rootlike **holdfasts.**

3. Freshwater biomes, except very large lakes, are affected by variations in climate and weather. **Temperature** of freshwater bodies varies considerably; they may freeze or dry up, and mud from their floors may be stirred up by storms.

14

Classification

TAXONOMIC CLASSIFICATION

A. Taxonomy

Billions of years of evolution have led to the great diversity of living organisms we see today. Scientists have tried to categorize relationships among the vast number of different organisms. The science of classification and the nomenclature used are known as **taxonomy**. The modern classification system seeks to group organisms on the basis of **evolutionary relationships**. In this system, the bat, whale, horse, and humans are placed in the same class of animals because they have all descended from a common ancestor. Since much of early evolutionary history is not known, there is some disagreement among biologists as to the best classification system to employ, particularly with regard to groups of unicellular organisms. Taxonomy takes into account anatomical and structural characteristics; modes of excretion, movement, and digestion; genetic makeup; and biochemical capabilities. Taxonomic organization proceeds from the largest, broadest group to the smaller, more specific subgroups.

B. Classification and Subdivisions

The modern scheme of taxonomy has **five kingdoms** for all living organisms. Each kingdom is divided into several major **phyla** (in the animal kingdom) or **divisions** (in other kingdoms). A phylum or division has several **subphyla** or **subdivisions**, which are further divided into **classes**. Each class includes multiple **orders**. Orders are subdivided into **families**, and each family is made up of many **genera** (singular *genus*). The **species** is the final, smallest subdivision. Organisms of the same species can mate with one another to produce fertile offspring.

Kingdom
Phylum (Division)
Subphylum (Subdivision)
Class
Order
Family
Genus
Species

For example, the full classification of humans is **Kingdom**: Animal, **Phylum**: Chordata, **Subphylum**: Vertebrata, **Class**: Mammalia, **Order**: Primates, **Family**: Hominidae, **Genus**: *Homo,* **Species**: *sapiens.*

C. Assignment of Scientific Names

All organisms are assigned a scientific name consisting of the **genus** and **species** name of that organism. Thus, humans are *Homo sapiens,* and the common housecat is *Felis domestica*. This follows a scheme originated by the biologist Carl Linn (Carolus Linnaeus).

CLASSIFICATION INTO KINGDOMS (A MODERN APPROACH)

Biologists originally divided all living things into two categories: plants and animals. This division ignored a number of different organisms. One type of modern classification system recognizes five kingdoms: Monera, Protista, Plantae, Fungi, and Animalia. Another classification system utilizes three kingdoms: Monera, Plantae (including Fungi), and Animalia (including Protista).

A. Viruses

Viruses have not been placed in any of the five kingdoms because they do not carry out physiological or biochemical processes outside of a host. They may be considered **nonliving**, although they are highly advanced parasites. Viruses are capable of taking over their host's cellular machinery and directing the replication of the viral genome and protein coat. Viruses have **lytic** and **lysogenic** life cycles. They contain either **DNA** or **RNA** and some essential enzymes surrounded by a protein coat. Viruses that exclusively infect bacteria are called **bacteriophages**.

B. Monera

Monerans are **prokaryotes** (e.g., bacteria). They lack a nucleus or any membrane-bound organelles. All monerans are single-celled organisms that reproduce asexually.

C. Protista

The protist kingdom contains primitive **eukaryotic** organisms with both plant- and animal-like characteristics. These organisms are either single cells or colonies of similar cells with no differentiation of specialized tissues. Each protist cell possesses the capability to carry out all of the life processes. The protist kingdom contains all simple eukaryotes that cannot be classified as plants or animals. For example, the protists of the genus *Euglena* demonstrate the motility of animals and the photosynthetic capabilities of plants.

D. Fungi

Fungi may be considered nonphotosynthetic plants (i.e., they resemble plants in that they are **multicellular**, **differentiated**, and **nonmotile**). Fungi are either **saprophytic** (i.e., bread mold) or **parasitic** (i.e., athlete's foot fungus). Their modes of reproduction are varied and unique. In addition, their cell walls are composed of chitin, not cellulose (as in plants).

E. Plantae

The plant kingdom includes multicellular organisms that exhibit differentiation of tissues and are **nonmotile** and **photosynthetic**. Many plants exhibit an alternation of generations and a distinct embryonic phase.

F. Animalia

The animal kingdom contains the **multicellular**, generally **motile**, **heterotrophic** organisms that have **differentiated** tissues (and organs in higher forms).

KINGDOM MONERA

Monerans, also called **bacteria**, are prokaryotic cells. They may exist as single cells or as aggregates of cells that stick together after division.

A. Cyanobacteria

Cyanobacteria, also called blue-green algae, live primarily in fresh water but also exist in marine environments. They possess a cell wall and **photosynthetic pigments**, but they have no flagella, true nucleus, chloroplasts, or mitochondria. They can withstand extreme temperatures and are believed to be directly descended from the first organisms that developed photosynthetic capabilities.

B. Other Bacteria

Bacteria are generally single-celled prokaryotes with a single double-stranded circular loop of DNA that is not enclosed by a nuclear membrane. Almost all forms have **cell walls**. They play active roles in **biogeochemical cycles**, recycling various chemicals such as carbon, nitrogen, phosphorous, and sulfur. Bacteria may be classified by their **morphological** appearances; **cocci** (round), **bacilli** (rods), and **spirilla** (spiral). Some forms are **duplexes** (diplococci), **clusters** (staphylococci), and **chains** (streptococci). Bacteria are ubiquitous, and many possess a wide variety of complex biochemical pathways.

NOTE: Much of the information that follows concerning eukaryotic classification is presented to improve your background in the features of living things. The general trends should be understood, but the specific details need not be memorized, with the exception of the classification of higher vertebrates.

KINGDOM PROTISTA

Most protists are unicellular, but there exist some colonial forms as well as some simple multicellular organisms that are neither plants nor animals. Protists are **eukaryotes** and possess a membrane-bound nucleus and organelles. The kingdom protista includes two major categories—**protozoa** and **algae**. The kingdom is divided into many phyla, which fall primarily into these two categories.

A. Protozoa

Traditionally, protozoans are considered those single-celled organisms that are **heterotrophic**, like little animals. This category of protists includes a number of phyla. The **rhizopods**, including amoebas, move with cellular extensions called pseudopods. The **ciliophors** have cilia that are used for feeding and locomotion.

B. Algae

Algae are primarily **photosynthetic** organisms. They include the **phytoplankton**, which are important sources of food for many marine organisms. *Euglena* may be considered an algal protist because they photosynthesize. *Euglena* can also act as heterotrophs and move about with flagellum. Blue, green, and red algae can be multicellular and are sometimes placed in the animal kingdom.

C. Protists Resembling Fungi

The slime molds are often placed in kingdom fungi. However, they appear to be more directly related to the protists. They are arranged in a **coenocytic** (many nuclei) mass of **protoplasm**. The slime mold undergoes a unique life cycle containing animal-like and plantlike stages. These stages include fruiting bodies and unicellular flagellated spores. Slime molds reproduce asexually by sporulation.

KINGDOM FUNGI

Fungi are eukaryotes and primarily multicellular. All fungi are **heterotrophs**. This differentiates them from the plant kingdom. They may be **saprophytic**, decomposing dead organic material, or parasitic. In either case, fungi **absorb** their food from their environment. Fungi reproduce by asexual **sporulation** or by intricate sexual processes. Notable types are mushrooms, yeast, and lichens.

THE PLANT KINGDOM

All plants are multicellular, non-motile, photosynthetic autotrophs.

A. Differentiation of Tissues

Plants have developed complex differentiated tissues to adapt to a terrestrial life. Photosynthetic tissue layers contain **chloroplasts** for the manufacture of carbohydrates. Supportive tissues provide mechanical support facilitating the typical upright radial construction of plants. Absorptive tissues like specialized **rhizoids** or complex roots project into soil for absorption of water and minerals. **Conducting** or **vascular** tissues include specialized "tubes" that transport water, minerals and nutrients to all parts of the plant. **Waxy cuticles** on exposed surfaces minimize loss of water while permitting the transmittance of light. Cells are in direct contact with the external environment by means of **air spaces** and **stomata**; therefore elaborate respiratory and excretory systems are unnecessary.

B. Division Bryophyta

Bryophytes are simple plants with few specialized organs and tissues. They lack the water-conducting woody material (xylem) that functions as support in tracheophytes and retain flagellated sperm cells which must swim to the eggs. Bryophytes have never become successful terrestrial plants and must live in moist places.

Bryophytes undergo alternation of generations. The **gametophyte** is the dominant generation; it is the "main plant," larger and nutritionally independent. The **sporophyte** is small, short-lived, attached to the gametophyte, and grows from the **archegonium**. It resembles a heterotrophic parasite in that it obtains organic and inorganic material from the independent autotrophic gametophyte. There are two types of bryophytes: mosses and liverworts. **Mosses** are primitive bryophytes in which the sporophyte and gametophyte generations grow together. **Liverworts** are flat horizontal leaf-like plants with differentiated dorsal and ventral surfaces.

C. Division Tracheophyta

Vascular plants (**tracheophytes**) are complex plants with a great degree of cell differentiation. They contain vascular tissues: **xylem** (water-conducting) and **phloem** (food-conducting). Tracheophytes have radial symmetry about a main vertical axis and are anchored by deep roots instead of rhizoids. Their extensive **woody** or non-woody support systems allow them to grow to great heights. They have developed excellent provisions for water conservation (waxy surfaces) and gas exchange (stomata). Cellular water storage creates turgid cells.

In contrast to bryophytes, in vascular plants, the sporophyte generation is dominant. The gametophyte is short-lived, independent in primitive tracheophytes (fern); small and parasitic in more advanced tracheophytes (seed plants).

There are four divisions of vascular plants, three of which are almost extinct. Those that do remain are evidence of prior evolutionary linkage to the bryophytes.

1. DIVISION PSILOPHYTA

Psilophytes are the most primitive of the tracheophytes and contain rhizoids instead of roots and one vascular bundle (microphyll) in the leaves (e.g., *Psilotum*).

2. DIVISION LYCOPHYTA

Lycophytes belong to an ancient subdivision, have roots, are non-woody, and contain microphyll leaves (e.g., club mosses).

3. DIVISION SPHENOPHYTA

Sphenophytes possess roots, microphyll leaves, and hollow jointed stems. Whorls of leaves occur on each joint (e.g., *Equisetum* [horsetail]).

4. DIVISION PTEROPHYTA

Pterophytes are the largest division and include the familiar **fern**. They evolved from early psilopsids. Pteropsida contain large leaves (megaphylls) which possess many vascular bundles. Ferns grow lengthwise, not in diameter, and contain xylem as **tracheids**, not vessels. They do not produce seeds and their short-lived gametophyte generation possesses heart-shaped leaves. Sperm are flagellated and thus require water or moisture to facilitate fertilization. The fern's leaves are part of the sporophyte generation. They grow from an underground stem called the **rhizome**. Sporangium on the underside of the leaves produce monoploid spores which germinate to form gametophytes.

D. Division Coniferophyta

Conifers are the largest grouping of **gymnosperms**, which are naked-seeded plants. They include cycads, pines, spruce, and firs. Conifers have cones, spiral clusters of modified leaves. There are two different types of cones: large female cones whose sporangia produce **megaspores** and small male cones whose sporangia produce **microspores**.

The gametophyte stage of gymnosperms is short lived and microscopic. The male microspore produces pollen that can be carried by the wind; thus, the requirement of a water environment for flagellated sperm is eliminated and the gymnosperms are truly terrestrial. Sperm nuclei fertilize the egg with the aid of a pollen tube and the embryo develops within the exposed seed.

The presence of a specialized cambium tissue allows for secondary growth—secondary xylem (wood) and secondary phloem. Gymnosperms can grow in **diameter** as well as in length and are woody, not herbaceous (green with soft stems) plants. Most gymnosperms are evergreens (nondeciduous).

F. Division Anthophyta

This division includes the flowering plants known as **angiosperms**. They have covered seeds and are the most abundant of all plants.

Angiosperms have flowers, not cones, as their principal **reproductive structure**. The **anther** of the male **stamen** produces **microspores** (pollen grains), while the **ovary** of the female **pistil** produces **megaspores**. Successful pollination results in the germination of pollen tubes, which aid in fertilization of female eggs in the gametophyte. The embryo develops into a seed within the ovary. The ovary eventually ripens into fruit, the means by which the seeds are dispersed. Xylem conducting cells are in the form of vessels as well as tracheids, allowing for better conduction of water.

1. SUBCLASSES OF THE ANGIOSPERMS

- **Dicotyledons** (dicots)—have "net veined" leaves and vascular bundles about a ring within the central cylinder. Dicotyledons contain two cotyledons (seed leaves) within the seed. Many have cambium and can be woody. They have flower parts in multiples of four or five. Some examples of dicotyledons are the maple and apple trees, potatoes, carrots, goldenrods, and buttercups.

- Monocotyledons (monocots)—contain leaves with parallel veins, scattered vascular bundles, and seeds with single cotyledons (seed leaves). Most monocots do not possess cambium and therefore are nonwoody (herbaceous). They contain flower parts in multiples of three. Some examples are grasses such as wheat, corn, rye, and rice. Other monocots include sugar cane, pineapple, irises, bananas, orchids, and palms (woody monocots).

KINGDOM ANIMALIA

A. General Characteristics of All Animals (Metazoa)

1. DIFFERENTIATION OF TISSUES, ORGANS, AND ORGAN SYSTEMS

Simple multicellular animals, such as sponges, coelenterates, and flatworms, have minimal differentiation. Most of their cells are in direct contact with the outside environment. In these organisms, few systems (such as the digestive systems and the reproductive systems) are required to support the life processes. In more advanced animals, specialized tissues and systems facilitate digestion, locomotion, circulation, message conduction (nervous system), and support.

2. ALIMENTATION

All animals, except some parasites like the tapeworm, ingest bulk foods (are holotrophic), digest them, and then eliminate the remains.

3. LOCOMOTION

All animals employ some form of locomotion to acquire nutrients. Some are **sessile** (stationary) and create currents to trap food. Locomotion is also important for protection, mate selection, and reproduction.

4. BILATERAL SYMMETRY

Most animals have right and left sides that are mirror images. The head is directed **anteriorly**. However, some animals, such as the echinoderms and cnidarians, are radially symmetrical.

5. NERVOUS SYSTEM

Animals possess a system enabling them to receive stimuli and control their actions. They have sense organs, specialized conductors, and higher brain centers for coordination and learning.

6. CHEMICAL-COORDINATING SYSTEM

Animals secrete chemicals (**hormones**) that operate in conjunction with the nervous system to maintain a steady state or **homeostasis**.

B. Porifera (Sponges)

Sponges have two layers of cells, have pores, are sessile, and have a low degree of cellular specialization.

C. Cnidarians

Cnidarians, also called coelenterates, contain a digestive sac that is sealed at one end (gastrovascular cavity). Two layers of cells are present—the **ectoderm** and the **endoderm**. Cnidarians have many specialized features, including tentacles, stinging cells, and net nerves. Examples of cnidarians are hydra, jellyfish, sea anemone, and coral.

D. Platyhelminthes (Flatworms)

Flatworms are ribbonlike, **bilaterally symmetrical**, and possess three layers of cells, including a solid mesoderm. They do not have circulatory systems, and their nervous system consists of eyes, an anterior brain ganglion, and a pair of longitudinal nerve cords.

E. Nematoda (Round Worms)

Round worms possess long digestive tubes and an anus. A solid mesoderm is present. Nematodes lack circulatory systems. They possess nerve cords and an anterior nerve ring (examples include hookworm, trichina, and free-living soil nematodes).

F. Annelida (Segmented worms)

Segmented worms possess a **coelom** (a true body cavity) contained in the mesoderm. Annelids have well-defined systems, including nervous, circulatory, and excretory systems (e.g., earthworms, leeches).

G. Mollusca

Mollusks are soft bodied and possess mantles that often secrete calcareous (**calcium carbonate**) exoskeletons. They breathe by gills and contain chambered hearts, blood sinuses, and a pair of ventral nerve cords (e.g., clams, snails, and squid).

H. Arthropoda

Arthropods have jointed appendages, chitinous exoskeletons, and open circulatory systems (**sinuses**). The three most important classes of arthropods are insects, arachnids, and crustaceans.

- **Insects** possess three pairs of legs, spiracles, and tracheal tubes designed for breathing outside of an aquatic environment.
- **Arachnids** have four pairs of legs and "book lungs" (e.g., scorpion, spider).
- **Crustaceans** have a segmented body with a variable number of appendages and possess gills (e.g., lobster, crayfish, and shrimp).

I. Echinoderms

Echinoderms are spiny, are **radially** symmetrical, contain a water-vascular system, and possess the capacity for regeneration of parts. There is evolutionary evidence suggesting a link between echinoderms and chordates (e.g., starfish, sea urchin).

J. Chordates

Chordates are characterized by a stiff dorsal rod, called the **notochord**, present at some stage of embryologic development. They have paired gill slits and a tail extending beyond the anus at some point during development. The lancelets and tunicates (like amphioxus) are chordates but not **vertebrates**. This means they have notochords but no backbones.

Vertebrates are the most advanced subphylum of the chordates. Vertebrates include **amphibians, reptiles, birds, fish**, and **mammals**. In addition to the chordate characteristics described above, vertebrates also possess bones, called vertebrae, which form the **backbone**. Bony vertebrae replace the notochord of the embryo and protect the nerve cord; a bony case (i.e., the skull) protects the brain. Vertebrates can be divided into the following **classes**:

1. FISH

All fish possess a two-chambered heart and gills, and utilize external fertilization for reproduction.

- **Jawless fish** are eel-like; retain the notochord throughout life; and have a cartilaginous internal skeleton, no jaws, and a sucking mouth. Jawless fish include the class Agnatha. Examples include the lamprey and hagfish.
- **Cartilaginous fish** possess jaws and teeth. A reduced notochord exists as segments between cartilaginous vertebrae. An example is the shark.
- **Bony fish** are the most prevalent type of fish. They have scales and lack a notochord in the adult form. During development, cartilage is replaced by a bony skeleton. Examples include the sturgeon, trout, and tuna.

2. AMPHIBIA

The larval stage is found in water, possesses gills and a tail and has no legs. The adult amphibian lives on land; has **lungs**, two pairs of legs, no tail, a three-chambered heart, and no scales; and utilizes external fertilization. Eggs are laid in water with a jellylike secretion. Examples include the frog, salamander, toad, and newt.

3. **REPTILES**

Reptiles are **terrestrial** animals. They breathe air by means of **lungs**, lay leathery eggs, and utilize **internal fertilization**. Reptiles are cold-blooded (**poikilothermic**) and have scales and a three-chambered heart. Examples include the turtle, lizard, snake, and crocodile.

4. **BIRDS**

Birds possess a four-chambered heart. They are **warm-blooded** (homeothermic), and their eggs are surrounded by shells. Examples include the hen and eagle.

5. **MAMMALS**

Mammals are warm-blooded animals that feed their offspring with milk produced in mammary glands.

- **Monetremes** lay leathery eggs, have horny bills, and have milk (mammary) glands with numerous openings but no nipples. Examples include the duckbilled platypus and spiny anteater.

- **Marsupials** are **pouched** mammals. The embryo begins development in the uterus and completes development while attached to nipples in the abdominal pouch. Examples include the kangaroo and opossum.

- **Placental mammals** have embryos that develop fully in the uterus. The placenta attaches the embryo to the uterine wall and provides for the exchange of food, oxygen, and waste material. Examples include the bat, whale, mouse, and humans.

15

Evolution

The change in the genetic makeup of a population over time is termed **evolution**. Evolution is explained by the constant propagation of new variations in the genes of a species, some of which impart an **adaptive advantage**.

EVIDENCE OF EVOLUTION

A. Fossil Record

Fossils are the most direct evidence of evolutionary change. They represent the remains of an extinct ancestor. Fossils are generally found in sedimentary rocks.

1. TYPES OF FOSSILS

Many types of fossils can provide information. Paleontologists can find **actual remains**, including teeth, bones, etc., in rock, tar pits, ice, and amber (the fossil resin of trees). **Petrification** is the process in which minerals replace the cells of an organism. **Imprints** are impressions left by an organism (i.e., footprints). **Molds** form in hollow spaces of rocks, as the organisms within decay. **Casts** are formed by minerals deposited in molds.

B. Comparative Anatomy

1. HOMOLOGOUS STRUCTURES

Homologous structures have the same basic anatomical features and **evolutionary origins**. They demonstrate similar evolutionary patterns with late divergence of form due to differences in exposure to evolutionary forces, and may therefore have different functions. Examples of homologous structures include the wings of a bat, the flippers of a whale, the forelegs of horses, and the arms of humans.

2. ANALOGOUS STRUCTURES

Analogous structures have **similar functions** but may have different evolutionary origins and entirely different patterns of development. The wings of a fly (membranous) and the wings of a bird (bony and

> **KEY CONCEPT**
>
> Homologous =
> similar structure
> same origin
>
> Analogous =
> similar function
> different origin

covered with feathers) are analogous structures. Analogous structures demonstrate superficial resemblance that cannot be used as a basis for classification.

C. Comparative Embryology

The **stages of development** of the embryo resemble the stages in an organism's evolutionary history. The human embryo passes through the stages that demonstrate common ancestry. The **two-layer gastrula** is similar to the structure of the **hydra**, a cnidarian. The three-layer gastrula is similar in structure to the flatworm. Gill slits, which are present in the embryo, indicate a common ancestry with fish.

The similarity of stages suggests a common ancestry and development history rather than an identical early development to that of the hydra, flatworm, and fish. The earlier the stage at which the development begins to diverge, the more dissimilar the adult organisms will be. Thus, it is difficult to differentiate between the embryo of a human and that of a gorilla until relatively late in the development of each embryo.

Embryological development suggests other evidence of evolution. The avian embryo has teeth, suggesting a reptile stage. The larvae of some mollusks resemble annelids. Human embryos possess a tail.

D. Comparative Biochemistry (Physiology)

Most organisms demonstrate the same basic needs and **metabolic processes**. They require the same nutrients and contain similar cellular organelles and energy storage forms (ATP). For example, **respiratory processes** are very similar in most organisms. The similarity of the enzymes involved in these processes suggests that all organisms must contain some DNA sequences in common. The closer the organisms in the evolutionary scheme, the greater the similarity of their chemical constituents (enzymes, hormones, antibodies, blood) and **genetic information**. Thus, we can conclude that all organisms are descended from a common, primitive ancestral form. The chemical similarity of the blood of different organisms very closely parallels the evolutionary pattern. A chimpanzee's blood shows close similarity to that of a human but is quite different from that of a rabbit or fish. Thus, the more time that has elapsed since the **divergence** of two species, the more different their biochemical characteristics.

E. Vestigial Structures

Vestigial structures appear to be useless but apparently had some ancestral function. There are many examples of vestigial structures in humans, other animals, and plants.

- In humans, the **appendix** is small and useless. In herbivores, it assists in the digestion of cellulose.
- In humans, the **tail** is reduced to a few useless bones (coccyx) at the base of the spine.
- **Splints** on the legs of the horse are the vestigial remains of the two side toes of *Eohippus*.
- The **python** has legs that are reduced to useless bones embedded in the sides of the adult. The whale has similar hind-limb bones.

F. Geographic Barriers

Species multiplication is generally accompanied by **migration** to lessen **intraspecific competition**. Separation of a widely distributed population by emerging geographic barriers increases the likelihood of genetic adaptations on either side of the barrier. Each population may evolve specific adaptations to the environment in which it lives, in addition to the accumulation of **neutral** (random, nonadaptive) changes. These adaptations will remain unique to the population in which they evolve— provided that interbreeding is prevented by the barrier. In time, genetic differences will reach the point where successful interbreeding becomes impossible within the population, and **reproductive isolation** would be maintained if the barrier were removed.

- **Example: Marsupials**—A line of pouched mammals paralleling the development of placental mammals developed on the **Australian** side of a large water barrier. The geographic barrier protected the more primitive pouched mammals from competition with modern placental mammals. In addition to marsupials like the kangaroo and pouched wolf, this barrier resulted in the development of other uniquely Australian plants and animals (e.g., duckbilled platypus and eucalyptus tree).

Systematics is a field of study that constructs and studies evolutionary relationships. A **phylogeny** is the evolutionary history of a group of organisms. In phylogenetic relationships, species should be somewhat similar to their ancestors. However, keep in mind that because of genetic divergence, those similarities will fade with time since separation increases.

Cladistics is used to classify organisms based on their phylogenetic relationships. Cladograms are constructed to predict how an ancestor has evolved into its proposed descendents. Each subtree of the cladogram is called a **clade**; members of a clade possess some kind of derived characteristic that distinguishes them from other clades. In constructing these clades, scientists utilize the principal of **parsimony**; that is, the least complex explanation. So if one cladogram assumes five evolutionary events and another assumes only two, then the latter will be more accepted.

THEORIES OF EVOLUTION

A. Lamarckian Evolution

This discredited theory held that new organs or changes in existing ones arose because of the needs of the organism. The amount of change was thought to be based on the **use or disuse** of the organ. The theory of use and disuse was based upon a **fallacious** understanding of genetics. Any useful characteristic acquired in one generation was thought to be transmitted to the next. An example was that of early giraffes, who were thought to have stretched their necks to reach for leaves on higher branches of trees. The offspring were believed to have inherited the valuable trait of longer necks as a result of this excessive use.

Modern genetics has disproved theories of acquired characteristics. **Only changes in the DNA of the sex cells can be inherited.** Changes acquired during an individual's life are changes in the characteristics and organization of somatic cells. Weissman showed that these changes are not inherited in an experiment in which he cut off the tails of mice for 20 generations (somatic change) only to find that the 21st generation was born with tails.

B. Darwin's Theory of Natural Selection

In Darwin's theory, pressures in the environment select for the organism **most fit to survive and reproduce**. Darwin outlined a number of basic agents leading to evolutionary change:

1. OVERPOPULATION

More offspring are produced than can survive, so there is insufficient food, air, light, and space to support the entire population.

2. VARIATIONS

Offspring naturally show differences (variations) in their characteristics compared to their parents. Darwin did not know the source of these differences. De Vries later suggested **mutations** as the cause of variations. Some mutations are beneficial, although most are harmful.

3. COMPETITION (STRUGGLE FOR SURVIVAL)

The developing population must compete for the necessities of life. Many young must die, and the number of adults in the population generally remains constant from generation to generation.

4. NATURAL SELECTION

Some organisms in a species have variations that give them an advantage over other members of the species. For example, a giraffe with a variation of a longer neck would be able to get more food from higher branches of a tree and would be more fit for survival. This principle is encapsulated in the phrase "**survival of the fittest.**"

5. INHERITANCE OF THE VARIATIONS

The individuals that survive (those with the favorable variations) live to adulthood, reproduce their own kind, and thus **transmit** these favorable variations or adaptations to their offspring. These favored genes gradually dominate the gene pool.

6. EVOLUTION OF NEW SPECIES

Over many generations of natural selection, the favorable changes (adaptations) are perpetuated in the species. The accumulation of these favorable changes eventually results in such significant changes of the gene pool that we can say a new species has evolved. These physical changes in the gene pool were perpetuated or selected for by environmental conditions.

- **Example**—The rapid evolution of **DDT-resistant** insects illustrates the theory of natural selection. A change in the environment, such as the introduction of DDT, constitutes a favorable change for the DDT-resistant mutant flies. These mutants existed before the environmental change. Now, conditions select for survival of DDT-resistant mutants.

> **KEY CONCEPT**
>
> **Natural Selection:**
> - Chance variations occur thanks to mutation and recombination.
> - If the variation is "selected for" by the environment, that individual will be more "fit" and more likely to survive to reproductive age.
> - Survival of the fittest leads to an increase of those favorable genes in the gene pool.

FORCES OF EVOLUTION

A. Population Genetics

A **population** includes all members of a particular species inhabiting a given location. The **gene pool** of a population is the sum total of all the alleles for any given trait in the population. **Gene frequency** is the decimal fraction representing the presence of an allele for all members of a population that have this particular gene locus. The letter p is used for the frequency of the **dominant allele** of a particular gene locus. The letter q represents the frequency of the **recessive allele**. For a given gene locus, $p + q = 1$.

1. THE HARDY-WEINBERG PRINCIPLE

Evolution can be viewed as a result of changing gene frequencies within a population. Gene frequency is the relative frequency of a particular allele. When the gene frequencies of a population are not changing, the gene pool is stable, and the population is not evolving. However, this is true only in ideal situations in which the following five conditions are met:

1. The population is very large.
2. There are no mutations that affect the gene pool.
3. Mating between individuals in the population is random.
4. There is no net migration of individuals into or out of the population.
5. The genes in the population are all equally successful at reproducing.

Under these idealized conditions, a certain equilibrium will exist among all of the genes in a gene pool, which is described by the **Hardy-Weinberg equation**.

For a gene locus with only two alleles, T and t, p = the frequency of allele T and q = the frequency of allele t. By definition, for a given gene locus, $p + q = 1$, since the combined frequencies of the alleles must total 100%. Thus $(p + q)^2 = (1)^2$ and

$$p2 + 2pq + q2 = 1$$

where p^2 = frequency of TT (dominant homozygotes)

$2pq$ = frequency of Tt (heterozygotes)

q^2 = frequency of tt (recessive homozygotes)

The Hardy-Weinberg equation may be used to determine gene frequencies in a large population in the absence of microevolutionary change (defined by the five conditions given above). For example, individuals from a nonevolving population can be randomly crossed to demonstrate that the gene frequencies remain constant from generation to generation. Assume that in the original gene pool the gene frequency of the dominant gene for tallness, T, is 0.80, and the gene frequency of the recessive gene for shortness, t, is 0.20. Thus, $p = 0.80$ and $q = 0.20$. In a cross between two heterozygotes, the resulting F_1 genotype frequencies are 64% TT, 16% + 16% = 32% Tt, and 4% tt (see the Punnett square below).

	$p = 0.80$ (T)	$q = 0.20$ (t)
$p = 0.80$ (T)	$(p^2 = 0.64)$ (TT = 64%	$(pq = 0.16)$ Tt = 16%
$q = 0.20$ (t)	$(pq = 0.16)$ Tt = 16%	$(q^2 = 0.04)$ tt = 4%

The gene frequencies of the F_1 generation can be calculated as follows:

$$64\% \ TT = 64\% \ T \ allele + \ \ 0\% \ t \ allele.$$
$$32\% \ Tt = 16\% \ T \ allele + 16\% \ t \ allele.$$
$$4\% \ tt = \ \ 0\% \ T \ allele + \ \ 4\% \ t \ allele.$$

Gene frequencies $= 80\% \ T$ allele $+ 20\% \ t$ allele.

Thus, $p = 0.80$ and $q = 0.20$. These frequencies are the same as those in the parent generation, demonstrating Hardy-Weinberg equilibrium in a nonevolving population.

B. Microevolution

No population can be represented indefinitely by the Hardy-Weinberg equilibrium, because such idealized conditions do not exist in nature. Real populations have **unstable** gene pools and **migrating** populations. The agents of microevolutionary change—natural selection, mutation, assortive mating, genetic drift, and gene flow—are all deviations from the five conditions of a Hardy-Weinberg population.

1. NATURAL SELECTION

Genotypes with favorable variations are selected through natural selection, and the frequency of favorable genes increases within the gene pool. Genotypes with low adaptive values tend to disappear.

2. MUTATION

Gene mutations change allele frequencies in a population, shifting gene equilibria.

3. ASSORTIVE MATING

If mates are not randomly chosen, but rather selected according to criteria such as phenotype and proximity, the relative genotype ratios will be affected and will depart from the predictions of the Hardy-Weinberg equilibrium. On the average, the allele frequencies in the gene pool remain unchanged.

4. GENETIC DRIFT

Genetic drift refers to changes in the composition of the gene pool due to chance. Genetic drift tends to be more pronounced in small populations, where it is sometimes called the **founder effect** since a small change due to chance will have a greater relative effect.

5. GENE FLOW

Migration of individuals between populations will result in a loss or gain of genes and thus change the composition of a population's gene pool.

C. Speciation

Speciation is the evolution of new species, which are groups of individuals who can interbreed freely with each other but not with members of other species. Different selection pressures act upon the gene pools of each group, causing them to evolve independently. Changes in the environment change the survival value of certain traits, and the gene frequencies for these traits change accordingly. Eventually, the populations will become sufficiently different from each other as to become reproductively isolated. They are then considered to be distinct **species**.

1. DEMES

A deme is a **small local population** of interbreeding organisms of the same species. For example, all the beavers along a specific portion of a river form a deme. Many demes may belong to a specific species. Members of a deme resemble one another more closely than they resemble the members of other demes. They are closely related genetically, since mating between members of the same deme occurs more frequently. Also they are influenced by similar environmental factors and thus are subject to the same selection processes.

2. DEVELOPMENT OF NEW SPECIES

If the gene pools within a species become sufficiently different so that two individuals cannot mate and produce fertile offspring, two different species have developed. Gene flow is impossible between two species. Genetic **variation**, changes in the **environment, migration** to new environments, **adaptation** to new environments, **natural selection**, and **isolation** are all factors that lead to speciation.

3. ADAPTIVE RADIATION

Adaptive radiation is the emergence of a number of lineages from a **single ancestral species**. A single species may **diverge** into a number of distinct species; the differences between them are those adaptive to a distinct lifestyle, or **niche**. A classic example is Darwin's finches of the Galapagos island chain. Over a comparatively short period of time, a single species of finch underwent adaptive radiation, resulting in 13 species of finches, some of them on the same island. Such adaptations minimized the competition among the birds, enabling each emerging species to become firmly established in its own environmental niche.

4. EVOLUTIONARY HISTORY

Dissimilar species have been found to have evolved from a common ancestor. Biologists seek to understand the evolutionary relationships among the species alive today. This evolutionary history is termed **phylogeny**. Evolutionary history may be visualized as a branching tree, where the common ancestor is found at the trunk and the modern species at the tips of the branches. It is interesting to note that groups on different branches develop in similar ways when exposed to similar environments. This is known as **convergent evolution**. For example, fish and dolphins have come to resemble one another physically, although they belong to different classes of vertebrates. They evolved certain similar features in adapting to the conditions of aquatic life.

Descendants of an ancestral **pouched mammal** include the pouched wolf, anteater, mouse, and mole. They have developed **parallel** to the placental wolf, anteater, mouse, and mole. These pouched mammals and their placental counterparts faced similar though geographically separate environments; thus, they developed similar adaptations.

The concepts of **adaptive radiation** and **phylogeny** form the basis for the methods employed in developing a system for the classification of living things.

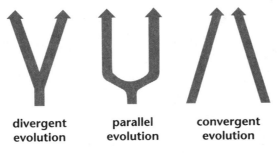

divergent
evolution

parallel
evolution

convergent
evolution

Figure 15.1. Evolutionary Patterns

5. ISOLATION

Genetic isolation often results from the **geographic isolation** of a population into two groups. When groups are isolated from each other, no gene flow occurs between them. Any difference arising from mutations or new combinations of genes will be maintained in the isolated population. This is known as **divergent evolution**. Over time, these genetic differences may become significant enough to make mating impossible. In this way, new species are formed.

GENERAL CHEMISTRY

Atomic Structure

Chemistry is the study of the nature and behavior of matter. The **atom** is the basic building block of matter, representing the smallest unit of a chemical element. An atom in turn is composed of subatomic particles called **protons, neutrons,** and **electrons.** The protons and neutrons in an atom form the **nucleus,** the core of the atom. The electrons exist outside the nucleus in characteristic regions of space called **orbitals.** All atoms of an **element** show similar chemical properties and cannot be further broken down by chemical means.

SUBATOMIC PARTICLES

A. Protons

Protons carry a single positive charge and have a mass of approximately one **atomic mass unit** or amu. The **atomic number** (Z) of an element is equal to the number of protons found in an atom of that element. All atoms of a given element have the same atomic number.

B. Neutrons

Neutrons carry no charge and have a mass only slightly larger than that of protons. Different isotopes of one element have different numbers of neutrons but the same number of protons. The **mass number** of an atom is equal to the total number of protons and neutrons added together. The convention $^A_Z X$ is used to show both the atomic number and mass number of an X atom, where Z is the atomic number and A is the mass number.

C. Electrons

Electrons carry a charge equal in magnitude but opposite in sign to that of protons. An electron has a very small mass—approximately 1/1,837th the mass of a proton or neutron—which is negligible for most purposes. The electrons farthest from the nucleus are known as **valence electrons.** The farther the valence electrons are from the nucleus, the weaker the attractive force of the positively charged nucleus, and the more likely the-valence electrons are to be influenced by other atoms. Generally, the valence electrons and their activity determine the **reactivity** of an atom. In a neutral atom, the number of electrons is equal to the number of protons. A positive or negative charge on an atom is due to a loss or gain of electrons; the result is called an **ion.**

Some basic features of the three subatomic particles are shown in Table 1.1.

Table 1.1

Subatomic Particle	Symbol	Relative Mass	Charge	Location
Proton	^1_1H	1	+1	Nucleus
Neutron	^1_0n	1	0	Nucleus
Electron	e^-	0	−1	Electron orbitals

Example: Determine the number of protons, neutrons, and electrons in a Nickel-58 atom and in a Nickel-60 2+ cation.

Solution: ^{58}Ni has an atomic number of 28 and a mass number of 58. Therefore, ^{58}Ni has 28 protons, 28 electrons, and 58 − 28, or 30, neutrons.

In the $^{60}Ni^{2+}$ species, the number of protons is the same as in the neutral ^{58}Ni atom. However, $^{60}Ni^{2+}$ has a positive charge because it has lost two electrons; thus, Ni^{2+} 26 electrons. Also, the mass number is two units higher than for the ^{58}Ni atom, and this difference in mass must be due to two extra neutrons; thus, it has a total of 32 neutrons.

ATOMIC WEIGHTS AND ISOTOPES

A. Atomic Weights

The atomic mass of an atom is the relative mass of that atom compared to the mass of a carbon-12 atom, which is used as a standard with an assigned mass of 12.000. Atomic masses are expressed in terms of atomic mass units (amu), with one amu being defined as exactly one-twelfth the mass of the carbon-12 atom, approximately 1.66×10^{-24} grams (g). A more common convention used to define the mass of an atom is **atomic weight.** The atomic weight is the weight in grams of one mole (mol) of a given element and is expressed in terms of g/mol. A mole is a unit used to count particles and is represented by **Avogadro's number,** 6.022×10^{23} particles. For example, the atomic weight of carbon is 12.0 g/mol, which means that 6.022×10^{23} carbon atoms weigh 12.0 g (see "Molecules and Moles").

B. Isotopes

For a given element, multiple species of atoms with the same number of protons (same atomic number) but different numbers of neutrons (different mass numbers) exist; these are called **isotopes** of the element. Isotopes are referred to either by the convention described above or, more commonly, by the name of the element followed by the mass number. For example, carbon-12 ($^{12}_{6}$C) is a carbon atom with 6 protons and 6 neutrons, while carbon-14 ($^{14}_{6}$C) is a carbon atom with 6 protons and 8 neutrons. Since isotopes have the same number of protons and electrons, they generally exhibit the same chemical properties.

In nature, almost all elements exist as a collection of two or more isotopes, and these isotopes are usually present in the same proportions in any sample of a naturally occurring element. The presence of these isotopes accounts for the fact that the accepted atomic weight for most elements is not a whole number. The masses listed in the periodic table are weighted averages that account for the relative abundance of various isotopes.

Example: Element Q consists of three different isotopes: A, B, and C. Isotope A has an atomic mass of 40.00 amu and accounts for 60.00% of naturally occurring Q. The atomic mass of isotope B is 44.00 amu and accounts for 25.00% of Q. Finally, isotope C has an atomic mass of 41.00 amu and a natural abundance of 15.00%. What is the atomic weight of element Q?

Solution: 0.60(40 amu) + 0.25(44 amu) + 0.15(41 amu)

   = 24.00 amu + 11.00 amu + 6.15 amu = 41.15 amu

The atomic weight of element Q is 41.15 g/mol.

BOHR'S MODEL OF THE HYDROGEN ATOM

In 1911, Ernest Rutherford provided experimental evidence that an atom has a dense, positively charged nu cleus that accounts for only a small portion of the volume of the atom. In 1900, Max Planck developed the first **quantum theory,** proposing that energy emitted as electromagnetic radiation from matter comes in discrete bundles called **quanta**. The energy value of a quantum is given by the equation $E = hf$ where h is a proportionality constant known as **Planck's constant,** equal to 6.626×10^{-34} J·s, and f (sometimes designated ν) is the **frequency** of the radiation.

A. The Bohr Model

In 1913, Niels Bohr used the work of Rutherford and Planck to develop his model of the electronic structure of the hydrogen atom. Starting from Rutherford's findings, Bohr assumed that the hydrogen atom consisted of a central proton around which an electron travelled in a circular orbit and that the centripetal force acting on the electron as it revolved around the nucleus was the electrical force between the positively charged proton and the negatively charged electron.

Bohr's model used the quantum theory of Planck in conjunction with concepts from classical physics. In classical mechanics, an object, such as an electron, revolving in a circle may assume an infinite number of values for its radius and velocity. Therefore, the **angular momentum** ($L = mvr$) and **kinetic energy** ($KE = mv^2/2$) can take on any value. However, by incorporating Planck's quantum theory into his model, Bohr placed conditions on the value of the angular momentum. Like Planck's energy, the angular momentum of an electron is quantized according to the following equation:

$$\text{angular momentum} = nh/2\pi$$

where h is Planck's constant and n is a quantum number that can be any positive integer. Since h, 2, and π are constants, the angular momentum changes only in discrete amounts with respect to the quantum number, n.

Bohr then equated the allowed values of the angular momentum to the energy of the electron. He obtained the following equation:

$$E = -R_H/n^2$$

where R_H is an experimentally determined constant (known as the Rydberg constant) equal to 2.18×10^{-18} J/electron. Therefore, like angular momentum, the energy of the electron changes in discrete amounts with respect to the quantum number.

A value of zero energy was assigned to the state in which the proton and electron were separated completely, meaning that there was no attractive force between them. Therefore, the electron in any of its quantized states in the atom would have a negative energy as a result of the attractive forces between the electron and proton. This explains the negative sign in the above equation for energy.

B. Applications of the Bohr Model

In his model of the structure of hydrogen, Bohr postulated that an electron can exist only in certain fixed energy states. In terms of quantum theory, the energy of an electron is **quantized**. Using this model, certain generalizations concerning the characteristics of electrons can be made. The energy of the electron is related to its orbital radius: The smaller the radius, the lower the energy state of the electron. The smallest orbit (radius) an electron can have corresponds to $n = 1$, which is the ground state of the hydrogen electron. At the **ground state** level, the electron is in its lowest energy state. The Bohr model is also used to explain the atomic emission spectrum and atomic absorption spectrum of hydrogen, and it is helpful in interpretation of the spectra of other atoms.

1. ATOMIC EMISSION SPECTRA

At room temperature, the majority of atoms in a sample are in the ground state. However, electrons can be excited to higher energy levels, by heat or other energy, to yield the excited state of the atom. Because the lifetime of the excited state is brief, the electrons will return rapidly to the ground state, emitting energy in the form of photons. The electromagnetic energy of these photons may be determined using the following equation:

$$E = hc/\lambda$$

where h is Planck's constant, c is the velocity of light (3.00×10^8 m/s), and λ is the wavelength of the radiation.

The different electrons in an atom will be excited to different energy levels. When these electrons return to their ground states, each will emit a photon with a wavelength characteristic of the specific transition it undergoes. The quantized energies of light emitted under these conditions do not produce a continuous spectrum (as expected from classical physics). Rather, the spectrum is composed of light at specific frequencies and is thus known as a line spectrum, where each line on the emission spectrum corresponds to a specific electronic transition. Because each element can have its electrons excited to different distinct energy levels, each possesses a unique **atomic emission spectrum**, which can be used as a fingerprint for the element. One application of atomic emissions spectroscopy is in the analysis of stars; while a physical sample can not be taken, the light from a star can be resolved into its component wavelengths, which are then matched to the known line spectra of the elements.

The Bohr model of the hydrogen atom explained the atomic emission spectrum of hydrogen, which is the simplest emission spectrum among all the elements. The group of hydrogen emission lines corresponding to transitions from upper levels $n > 2$ to $n = 2$ is known as the **Balmer series** (four wavelengths in the visible region), while the group corresponding to transitions between upper levels $n > 1$ to $n = 1$ is known as the **Lyman series** (higher energy transitions, occur in the UV region).

KEY CONCEPT

Note that all systems tend towards minimal energy. Thus, atoms of any element will generally exist in the ground state unless subjected to extremely high temperatures or irradiation.

When the energy of each frequency of light observed in the emission spectrum of hydrogen was calculated according to Planck's quantum theory, the values obtained closely matched those expected from energy level transitions in the Bohr model. That is, the energy associated with a change in the quantum number from an initial value n_i to a final value n_f is equal to the energy of Planck's emitted photon. Thus,

$$E = hc/\lambda = - R_H[1/(n_i)^2 - 1/(n_f)^2]$$

and the energy of the emitted photon corresponds to the precise difference in energy between the higher-energy initial state and the lower-energy final state.

2. ATOMIC ABSORPTION SPECTRA

When an electron is excited to a higher energy level, it must absorb energy. The energy absorbed as an electron jumps from an orbital of low energy to one of higher energy is characteristic of that transition. This means that the excitation of electrons in a particular element results in energy absorptions at specific wavelengths. Thus, in addition to an emission spectrum, every element possesses a characteristic **absorption spectrum**. Not surprisingly, the wavelengths of absorption correspond directly to the wavelengths of emission since the energy difference between levels remains unchanged. Absorption spectra can thus be used in the identification of elements present in a gas phase sample.

QUANTUM MECHANICAL MODEL OF ATOMS

While the concepts put forth by Bohr offered a reasonable explanation for the structure of the hydrogen atom and ions containing only one electron (such as He^+ and Li^{2+}), they did not explain the structures of atoms containing more than one electron. This is because Bohr's model does not take into consideration the repulsion between multiple electrons surrounding one nucleus. Modern quantum mechanics has led to a more rigorous and generalized study of the electronic structure of atoms. The most important difference between the Bohr model and modern quantum mechanical models is that Bohr's assumption that electrons follow a circular orbit at a fixed distance from the nucleus is no longer considered valid. Rather, electrons are described as being in a state of rapid motion within regions of space around the nucleus called **orbitals.** An orbital is a representation of the probability of finding an electron within a given region. In the current quantum mechanical description of electrons, pinpointing the exact location of an electron at any given point in time is impossible. This idea is best described by the **Heisenberg uncertainty principle**, which states that it is impossible to determine, with perfect accuracy, the momentum and the position of an electron simultaneously. This means that if the momentum of the electron is being measured accurately, its position will change, and vice versa.

A. Quantum Numbers

Modern atomic theory states that any electron in an atom can be completely described by four **quantum numbers:** n, ℓ, m_ℓ, and m_s. Furthermore, according to the **Pauli exclusion principle,** no two electrons in a given atom can possess the same set of four quantum numbers. The position and energy of an electron described by its quantum numbers is known as its **energy state.** The value of n limits the values of ℓ, which in turn limits the values of m_ℓ. The values of the quantum numbers qualitatively give information about the orbitals: n about the size, ℓ about the shape, and m_ℓ about the orientation of the orbital. All four quantum numbers are discussed below.

1. PRINCIPAL QUANTUM NUMBER

The first quantum number is commonly known as the **principal quantum number** and is denoted by the letter n. This is the quantum number used in Bohr's model that can theoretically take on any positive integer value. The larger the integer value of n, the higher the energy level and radius of the electron's orbit. The maximum number of electrons in energy level n (electron shell n) is $2n^2$. The difference in energy between adjacent shells decreases as the distance from the nucleus increases, since it is related to the expression $(1/n_2^2 - 1/n_1^2)$. For example, the energy difference between the third and fourth shells ($n = 3$ to $n = 4$) is less than that between the second and third shells ($n = 2$ to $n = 3$).

2. AZIMUTHAL QUANTUM NUMBER

The second quantum number is called the **azimuthal (angular momentum) quantum number** and is designated by the letter ℓ. The second quantum number refers to the **subshells** or **sublevels** that occur within each principal energy level. For any given n, the value of ℓ can be any integer in the range of 0 to $n - 1$. The four subshells corresponding to $\ell = 0, 1, 2$, and 3 are known as the s, p, d, and f subshells, respectively. The maximum number of electrons that can exist within a subshell is given by the equation $4\ell + 2$. The greater the value of ℓ, the greater the energy of the subshell. However, the energies of subshells from different principal energy levels may overlap. For example, the $4s$ subshell will have a lower energy than the $3d$ subshell because its average distance from the nucleus is smaller.

KEY CONCEPT

For any principal quantum number n, there will be n possible values for ℓ.

3. MAGNETIC QUANTUM NUMBER

The third quantum number is the **magnetic quantum number** and is designated m_ℓ. An orbital is a specific region within a subshell that may contain no more than two electrons. The magnetic quantum number specifies the particular orbital within a subshell where an electron is highly likely to be found at a given point in time. The possible values of m_ℓ are all integers from ℓ to $-\ell$, including 0. Therefore, the *s* subshell, where there is one possible value of m_ℓ (0), will contain 1 orbital; likewise, the *p* subshell will contain 3 orbitals, the *d* subshell will contain 5 orbitals, and the *f* subshell will contain 7 orbitals. The shape and energy of each orbital are dependent upon the subshell in which the orbital is found. For example, a *p* subshell has three possible m_ℓ values (–1, 0, +1). The three dumbbell-shaped orbitals are oriented in space around the nucleus along the *x*, *y*, and *z* axes and are often referred to as *px*, *py*, and *pz*.

> **REMEMBER**
>
> For any value of ℓ, there will be $2\ell+1$ possible values for m_ℓ. For any *n*, this produces n^2 possible values of m_ℓ (i.e., n^2 orbitals).

4. SPIN QUANTUM NUMBER

The fourth quantum number, also called the **spin quantum number**, is denoted by m_s. The spin of a particle is its intrinsic angular momentum and is a characteristic of a particle, like its charge. In classical mechanics, an object spinning about its axis has an angular momentum; however, this does not apply to the electron. Classical analogies often are inapplicable in the quantum world.

In any case, the two spin orientations are designated $+\frac{1}{2}$ and $-\frac{1}{2}$.

Whenever two electrons are in the same orbital, they must have opposite spins. Electrons in different orbitals with the same m_s values are said to have **parallel** spins.

The quantum numbers for the orbitals in the second principal energy level, with their maximum number of electrons noted in parentheses, are shown in Table 1.2. Electrons with opposite spins in the same orbital are often referred to as **paired**.

Table 1.2

> **REMEMBER**
>
> For any value of *n*, there will be a maximum of $2n^2$ electrons (i.e., two per orbital).

n	2(8)			
ℓ	0(2)	1(6)		
m_ℓ	0(2)	+1(2)	0(2)	–1(2)
m_s	$+\frac{1}{2}, -\frac{1}{2}$	$+\frac{1}{2}, -\frac{1}{2}$	$+\frac{1}{2}, -\frac{1}{2}$	$+\frac{1}{2}, -\frac{1}{2}$

B. Electron Configuration and Orbital Filling

For a given atom or ion, the pattern by which subshells are filled and the number of electrons within each principal level and subshell are designated by an **electron configuration**. In electron configuration notation, the first-number denotes the principal energy level, the letter designates the subshell, and the superscript gives the number of electrons in that subshell. For example, $2p^4$ indicates that there are four electrons in the second (p) subshell of the second principal energy level.

When writing the electron configuration of an atom, it is necessary to remember the order in which subshells are filled. Subshells are filled from lowest to highest energy, and each subshell will fill completely before electrons begin to enter the next one. The $(n + \ell)$ rule is used to rank subshells by increasing energy. This rule states that the lower the values of the first and second quantum numbers, the lower the energy of the subshell. If two subshells possess the same $(n + \ell)$ value, the subshell with the lower n value has a lower energy and will fill first. The order in which the subshells fill is shown in the following chart.

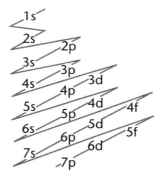

Figure 1.1

Example: Which will fill first, the 3d subshell or the 4s subshell?

Solution: For 3d, $n = 3$ and $\ell = 2$, so $(n + \ell) = 5$. For 4s, $n = 4$ and $\ell = 0$, so $(n + \ell) = 4$. Therefore, the 4s subshell has lower energy and will fill first. This can also be determined from the chart by examination.

To determine which subshells are filled, you must know the number of electrons in the atom. In the case of uncharged atoms, the number of electrons equals the atomic number. If the atom is charged, the number of electrons is equal to the atomic number plus the extra electrons if the atom is negative, or the atomic number minus the electrons if the atom is positive.

In subshells that contain more than one orbital, such as the $2p$ subshell with its three orbitals, the orbitals will fill according to **Hund's rule.** Hund's rule states that within a given subshell, orbitals are filled such that there are a maximum number of half-filled orbitals with parallel spins. Electrons "prefer" empty orbitals to half-filled ones, because a pairing energy must be overcome for two electrons carrying repulsive negative charges to exist in the same orbital.

Example: What are the written electron configurations for nitrogen (N) and iron (Fe) according to Hund's rule?

Solution: Nitrogen has an atomic number of 7. Thus, its electron configuration is $1s^2\ 2s^2\ 2p^3$. According to Hund's rule, the two s-orbitals will fill completely, while the three p-orbitals will each contain one electron, all with parallel spins.

$$\underset{1s^2}{\uparrow\downarrow} \qquad \underset{2s^2}{\uparrow\downarrow} \qquad \underset{2p^3}{\uparrow\ \uparrow\ \uparrow}$$

Iron has an atomic number of 26, and its $4s$ subshell fills before the $3d$. Using Hund's rule, the electron configuration will be

$$\underset{1s^2}{\uparrow\downarrow} \quad \underset{2s^2}{\uparrow\downarrow} \quad \underset{2p^6}{\uparrow\downarrow\,\uparrow\downarrow\,\uparrow\downarrow} \quad \underset{3s^2}{\uparrow\downarrow} \quad \underset{3p^6}{\uparrow\downarrow\,\uparrow\downarrow\,\uparrow\downarrow} \quad \underset{3d^6}{\uparrow\downarrow\,\uparrow\ \uparrow\ \uparrow} \quad \underset{4s^2}{\uparrow\downarrow}$$

Iron's electron configuration is written as $1s^2\ 2s^2\ 2p^6\ 3s^2\ 3p^6\ 3d^6\ 4s^2$. Subshells may be listed either in the order in which they fill (e.g., $4s$ before $3d$) or with subshells of the same principal quantum number grouped together, as shown here. Both methods are correct.

One notable exception to traditional orbital filling rules is that of transition metals such as chromium and copper. Chromium would be expected to have an electron configuration of $1s^2 2s^2 2p^6 3s^2 3p^6 3d^4 4s^2$, but this is not the case. Rather, an electron from the 4s subshell is "promoted" to the 3d subshell in order to form a half-filled 3d shell. Because the stability gained from the half-filled 3d shell outweighs the energy cost of promoting the electron, the actual electron configuration of chromium will be $1s^2 2s^2 2p^6 3s^2 3p^6 \mathbf{3d^5 4s^1}$. In the case of copper, we would expect a configuration of $1s^2 2s^2 2p^6 3s^2 3p^6 3d^9 4s^2$. In reality, however, we again see an electron from the 4s subshell promoted to the 3d subshell in order to completely fill 3d. Thus, the actual electron configuration of copper is $1s^2 2s^2 2p^6 3s^2 3p^6 \mathbf{3d^{10} 4s^1}$.

The presence of paired or unpaired electrons affects the chemical and magnetic properties of an atom or molecule. If the material has unpaired electrons, a magnetic field will align the spins of these electrons and weakly attract the atom. These materials are said to be **paramagnetic.** Materials that have no unpaired electrons and are slightly repelled by a magnetic field are said to be **diamagnetic.**

C. Valence Electrons

The valence electrons of an atom are those electrons that are in its outer energy shell *or* that are available for bonding. For elements in Groups IA and IIA, only the outermost *s* electrons are valence electrons. For elements in Groups IIIA through VIIIA, the outermost *s* and *p* electrons in the highest energy shell are valence electrons. For transition elements, the valence electrons are those in the outermost *s* subshell and in the *d* subshell of the next-to-outermost energy shell. For the inner transition elements, the valence electrons are those in the *s* subshell of the outermost energy shell, the *d* subshell of the next-to-outermost energy shell, and the *f* subshell of the energy shell two levels below the outermost shell.

Group IIIA–VIIA elements beyond Period II might, under some circumstances, accept electrons into their empty *d* subshell, which gives them more than eight valence electrons.

Example: Which are the valence electrons of elemental iron, elemental selenium, and the sulfur atom in a sulfate ion?

Solution: Iron has 8 valence electrons: 2 in its 4*s* subshell and 6 in its 3*d* subshell.

Selenium has 6 valence electrons: 2 in its 4*s* subshell and 4 in its 4*p* subshell. Selenium's 3*d* electrons are not part of its valence shell.

Sulfur in a sulfate ion has 12 valence electrons: its original 6 plus 6 more from the oxygens to which it is bonded. Sulfur's 3*s* and 3*p* subshells can only contain 8 of these 12 electrons; the other 4 electrons have entered the sulfur atom's 3*d* subshell, which in elemental sulfur is empty (see chapter 3, Figure 3.1).

KEY CONCEPT

Period II elements cannot expand their octets, since the energy gap between the 2*p* and the 3*s* sublevels is too large.

Periodic Table of the Elements

Group	1	2		3	4	5	6	7	8	9	10	11	12	13	14	15	16	17	18
Period																			
1	1 H																		2 He
2	3 Li	4 Be												5 B	6 C	7 N	8 O	9 F	10 Ne
3	11 Na	12 Mg												13 Al	14 Si	15 P	16 S	17 Cl	18 Ar
4	19 K	20 Ca		21 Sc	22 Ti	23 V	24 Cr	26 Mn	26 Fe	27 Co	28 Ni	29 Cu	30 Zn	31 Ga	32 Ge	33 Ss	34 Se	35 Br	36 Kr
5	37 Rb	38 Sr		39 Y	40 Zr	41 Nb	42 Mo	42 Tc	44 Ru	45 Rh	46 Pd	47 Ag	48 Cd	49 In	50 Sn	51 Sb	52 Te	53 I	54 Xe
6	55 Cs	56 Ba	*	71 Lu	72 Hf	73 Ta	74 W	75 Re	76 Os	77 Ir	78 Pt	79 Au	80 Hg	81 Ti	82 Pb	83 Bi	84 Po	85 At	86 Rn
7	87 Fr	88 Ra	**	103 Lr	104 Rf	105 Db	106 Sg	107 Bh	108 Hs	109 Mt	110 Ds	111 Rg	112 Cn	113 Uut	114 Fl	115 Uup	116 Lv	117 Uus	118 Uuo

*Lanthanoids	*	57 La	58 Ce	59 Pr	60 Nd	61 Pm	62 Sm	63 Eu	64 Gd	65 Tb	66 Dy	67 Ho	68 Er	69 Tm	70 Yb
**Actinoids	**	89 Ac	90 Th	91 Pa	92 U	93 Np	94 Pu	95 Am	96 Cm	97 Bk	98 Cf	99 Es	100 Fm	101 Md	102 No

2

The Periodic Table

In 1869, the Russian chemist Dmitri Mendeleev published the first version of his periodic table, in which he showed that ordering the elements according to atomic weight produced a pattern where similar properties periodically recurred. This table was later revised, using the work of the physicist Henry Moseley, to organize the elements on the basis of increasing atomic number. Using this revised table, the properties of certain elements that had not yet been discovered were predicted: A number of these predictions were later borne out by experimentation. The substance of this work is summarized in the **periodic law**, which states that the chemical properties of the elements are dependent, in a systematic way, upon their atomic numbers.

In the periodic table used today, the elements are arranged in **periods** (rows) and **groups** (columns). There are seven periods, representing the principal quantum numbers $n = 1$ to $n = 7$, and each period is filled sequentially. Groups represent elements that have the same electronic configuration in their **valence**, or outermost shell, and share similar chemical properties. The electrons in the outermost shell are called **valence electrons.** They are involved in chemical bonding and determine the chemical reactivity and properties of the element. The Roman numeral above each group represents the number of valence electrons. There are two sets of groups, designated A and B. The A elements are the **representative elements**, which have either s or p sublevels as their outermost orbitals. The B elements are the **non-representative elements,** including the **transition elements,** which have partly filled d sublevels, and the **lanthanide** and **actinide series,** which have partly filled f sublevels. The electron configuration for the valence electrons is given by the Roman numeral and letter designations. For example, an element in Group VA will have a valence electron configuration of s^2p^3 (2 + 3 = 5 valence electrons).

PERIODIC PROPERTIES OF THE ELEMENTS

The properties of the elements exhibit certain trends, which can be explained in terms of the position of the element in the periodic table or in terms of the electron configuration of the element. All elements seek to gain or lose valence electrons so as to achieve the stable octet formation possessed by the **inert** or **noble gases** of Group VIII. Two other important trends exist within the periodic table. First, as one goes from left to right across a period, electrons are added one at a time; the electrons of the outermost shell experience an increasing amount of nuclear attraction, becoming closer and more tightly bound to the nucleus. Second, as one goes down a given column, the outermost electrons become less tightly bound to the nucleus. This is because the number of filled principal energy levels (which shield the outermost electrons from attraction by the nucleus) increases downward within each group. These trends help explain elemental properties such as atomic radius, ionization potential, electron affinity, and electronegativity.

A. Atomic Radii

The **atomic radius** of an element is equal to one-half the distance between the centers of two atoms of that element that are just touching each other. In general, the atomic radius decreases across a period from left to right and increases down a given group; the atoms with the largest atomic radii will be located at the bottom of groups and in Group I.

As one moves from left to right across a period, electrons are added one at a time to the outer energy shell. Electrons within a shell cannot shield one another from the attractive pull of protons. Therefore, since the number of protons is also increasing, producing a greater positive charge attracting the valence electrons, the effective nuclear charge increases steadily across a period. This causes the atomic radius to decrease.

As one moves down a group of the periodic table, the number of electrons and filled electron shells will increase, but the number of valence electrons will remain the same. Thus, the outermost electrons in a given group will feel the same amount of effective nuclear charge, but electrons will be found farther from the nucleus as the number of filled energy shells increases. Thus, the atomic radii will increase.

B. Ionization Energy

The **ionization energy** (IE), or **ionization potential,** is the energy required to remove an electron completely from a gaseous atom or ion. Removing an electron from an atom always requires an input of energy (is **endothermic**). The closer and more tightly bound an electron is to the nucleus, the more difficult it will be to remove, and the higher the ionization energy will be. The **first ionization energy** is the energy required to remove one valence electron from the parent atom, the **second ionization energy** is the energy needed to remove a second valence electron from the univalent ion to form the divalent ion, and so on. Successive ionization energies grow increasingly large (i.e., the second ionization energy is always greater than the first ionization energy). For example:

$$Mg\ (g) \longrightarrow Mg^+\ (g)\ +\ e^-\qquad \text{First Ionization Energy}\quad =\ 7.646\ eV$$

$$Mg^+\ (g) \longrightarrow Mg^{2+}\ (g)\ +\ e^-\qquad \text{Second Ionization Energy}\ =\ 15.035\ eV$$

Ionization energy increases from left to right across a period as the atomic radius decreases. Moving down a group, the ionization energy decreases as the atomic radius increases. Group I elements have low ionization energies because the loss of an electron results in the formation of a stable octet.

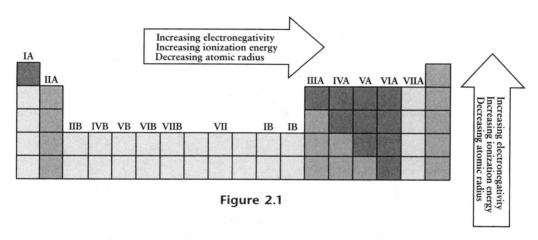

Figure 2.1

C. Electron Affinity

Electron affinity is the energy change that occurs when an electron is added to a gaseous atom, and it represents the ease with which the atom can accept an electron. The stronger the attractive pull of the nucleus for electrons (**effective nuclear charge**, or Z_{eff}), the greater the electron affinity will be. In discussing electron affinities, two sign conventions are used. The more common one states that a positive electron affinity value represents energy release when an electron is added to an atom; the other states that a negative electron affinity represents a release of energy. In this discussion, the first convention will be used.

Generalizations can be made about the electron affinities of particular groups in the periodic table. For example, the Group IIA elements, or **alkaline earths,** have low electron affinity values. These elements are relatively stable because their s subshell is filled. Group VIIA elements, or **halogens,** have high electron affinities because the addition of an electron to the atom results in a completely filled shell, which represents a stable electron configuration. Achieving the stable octet involves a release of energy, and the strong attraction of the nucleus for the electron leads to a high energy change. The Group VIII elements, or **noble gases,** have electron affinities on the order of zero, since they already possess a stable octet and cannot readily accept an electron. Elements of other groups generally have low values of electron affinity.

REMEMBER

L → R Atomic Radius ↓
       Ionization Energy ↑
       Electronegativity ↑

Top → Bottom
       Atomic Radius ↑
       Ionization Energy ↓
       Electronegativity ↓

REMEMBER

To recall the various trends, remember this: Cesium, Cs, is the largest, most metallic, and least electronegative of all naturally occurring elements. It also has the smallest ionization energy and the least exothermic electron affinity.

D. Electronegativity

Electronegativity is a measure of the attraction an atom has for electrons in a chemical bond. The greater the electronegativity of an atom, the greater its attraction for bonding electrons. Electronegativity values are not determined directly. The most common electronegativity scale is the Pauling electronegativity scale, where the values range from 0.7 for the most electropositive elements, like cesium, to 4.0 for the most electronegative element, fluorine. Electronegativities are related to ionization energies: Elements with low ionization energies have low electronegativities because their nuclei do not attract electrons strongly, while elements with high ionization energies have high electronegativities because of the strong pull the nucleus has on electrons. Therefore, electronegativity increases from left to right across periods. In any group, the electronegativity decreases as the atomic number increases as a result of the increased distance between the valence electrons and the nucleus (i.e., greater atomic radius).

TYPES OF ELEMENTS

The elements of the periodic table may be classified into three categories: **metals,** located on the left side and in the middle of the periodic table; **nonmetals,** located on the right side of the table; and **metalloids (semimetals),** found along a diagonal line between the other two.

A. Metals

Metals are shiny solids (except for mercury) at room temperature and generally have high melting points and densities. Metals have the characteristic ability to be deformed without breaking. The ability of a metal to be hammered into shapes is called **malleability,** and the ability to be drawn into wires is called **ductility.** Many of the characteristic properties of metals, such as large atomic radius, low ionization energy, and low electronegativity, are due to the fact that the few electrons in the valence shell of a metal atom can easily be removed. Because the valence electrons can move freely, metals are good conductors of heat and electricity. Groups IA and IIA represent the most reactive metals and will be discussed below. The transition elements, also discussed later, are metals that have partially filled *d*-orbitals.

B. Nonmetals

Nonmetals are generally brittle in the solid state and show little or no metallic luster. They have high ionization energies and electronegativities and are usually poor conductors of heat and electricity. Most nonmetals share the ability to gain electrons easily, but otherwise they display a wide range of chemical behaviors and reactivities. The nonmetals are located on the upper right side of the periodic table; they are separated from the metals by a line cutting diagonally through the region of the periodic table containing elements with partially filled *p*-orbitals.

C. Metalloids

The metalloids or semimetals are found along the line between the metals and nonmetals in the periodic table, and their properties vary considerably. Their densities, boiling points, and melting points fluctuate widely. The electronegativities and ionization energies of metalloids lie between those of metals and nonmetals; therefore, these elements possess characteristics of both those classes. For example, silicon has a metallic luster, yet it is brittle and is not an efficient conductor. The reactivity of metalloids is dependent upon the element with which they are reacting. For example, boron (B) behaves as a nonmetal when reacting with sodium (Na) and as a metal when reacting with fluorine (F). The elements classified as metalloids are boron, silicon, germanium, arsenic, antimony, and tellurium.

THE CHEMISTRY OF GROUPS

A. Alkali Metals

The **alkali metals** are the elements of Group IA. They possess most of the physical properties common to metals, yet their densities are lower than those of other metals. The alkali metals have only one loosely bound electron in their outermost shell, giving them the largest atomic radii of all the elements in their respective periods. Their metallic properties and high reactivity are determined by the fact that they have low ionization energies; thus, they easily lose their valence electron to form univalent cations. Alkali metals have low electronegativities and react very readily with nonmetals, especially halogens.

B. Alkaline Earths

The **alkaline earths** are the elements of Group IIA, which also possess many characteristically metallic properties. Like the alkali metals, these properties are dependent upon the ease with which they lose electrons. The alkaline earths have two electrons in their outer shell and thus have smaller atomic radii than the alkali metals. However, the two valence electrons are not held very tightly by the nucleus, so they can be removed to form divalent cations. Alkaline earths have low electronegativities and electron affinities.

C. Halogens

The **halogens**, Group VIIA, are highly reactive nonmetals with seven valence electrons (one short of the favored octet configuration). Halogens are highly variable in their physical properties. For instance, the halogens range from gaseous (F_2 and Cl_2) to liquid (Br_2) to solid (I_2) at room temperature. Their chemical properties are more uniform: The electronegativities of halogens are very high, and they are particularly reactive towards alkali metals and alkaline earths, which "want" to donate electrons to the halogens to form stable ionic crystals. Fluorine (F) has the highest electronegativity of all the elements.

D. Noble Gases

The **noble gases**, also called the **inert gases,** are found in Group VIII (also called Group O). They are fairly nonreactive because they have a complete valence shell, which is an energetically favored arrangement. This gives them little or no tendency to gain or lose electrons, high ionization energies, and no real electronegativities. They possess low boiling points and are all gases at room temperature.

E. Transition Elements

The **transition elements**, Groups IB to VIIIB, are all considered metals; hence, they are also called the **transition metals.** These elements are very hard and have high melting points and boiling points. As one moves across a period, the five d-orbitals become progressively more filled. The d electrons are held only loosely by the nucleus and are relatively mobile, contributing to the malleability and high electrical conductivity of these elements. Chemically, transition elements have low ionization energies and may exist in a variety of positively charged forms or **oxidation states.** This is because transition elements are capable of losing various numbers of electrons from the s- and d-orbitals of their valence shell. Theoretically, the transition metals in Group VIIIB could have eight different oxidation states, from +1 to +8; however, they typically do not exhibit so many. For instance, copper (Cu), in Group IB, can exist in either the +1 or the +2 oxidation state, and manganese (Mn), in Group VIIB, occurs in the +2, +3, +4, +6, or +7 state. Because of this ability to attain positive oxidation states, transition metals form many different ionic and partially ionic compounds. The dissolved ions can form **complex ions** with either molecules of water **(hydration complexes)** or with nonmetals, forming highly colored solutions and compounds (e.g., $CuSO_4 \cdot 5H_2O$), and this complexation may enhance the relatively low solubility of certain compounds (e.g., AgCl is insoluble in water but quite soluble in aqueous ammonia due to the formation of the complex ion $[Ag(NH_3)_2]^+$). The formation of complexes causes the d-orbitals to be split into two energy sublevels. This enables many of the complexes to absorb certain frequencies of light—those containing the precise amount of energy required to raise electrons from the lower to the higher d sublevel. The frequencies not absorbed—known as the **subtraction frequencies**—give the complexes their characteristic colors.

3

Bonding and Chemical Interactions

The atoms of many elements can combine to form **molecules**. The atoms in most molecules are held together by strong attractive forces called **chemical bonds**. These bonds are formed via the interaction of the valence electrons of the combining atoms. The chemical and physical properties of the resulting molecules are often very different than their constituent elements. In addition to the very strong forces within a molecule, there are weaker intermolecular forces between molecules. These **intermolecular forces,** although weaker than the intramolecular chemical bonds, are of considerable importance in understanding the physical properties of many substances.

BONDING

Many molecules contain atoms bonded according to the **octet rule,** which states that an atom tends to bond with other atoms until it has eight electrons in its outermost shell, thereby forming a stable electron configuration similar to that of the Group VIII (noble gas) elements. **Exceptions** to this rule are as follows: **hydrogen,** which can have only two valence electrons; lithium and beryllium, which bond to attain two and four valence electrons, respectively; boron, which bonds to attain six; and elements beyond the second row, such as phosphorus and sulfur, which can expand their octets to include more than eight electrons by incorporating d-orbitals.

When classifying chemical bonds, it is helpful to introduce two distinct types: ionic bonds and covalent bonds. In **ionic bonding,** an electron(s) from an atom with a smaller ionization energy is transferred to an atom with a greater electron affinity, and the resulting ions are held together by electrostatic forces. In **covalent bonding,** an electron pair is shared between two atoms. In many cases, the bond is partially covalent and partially ionic; we call such bonds **polar covalent bonds.**

IONIC BONDS

When two atoms with large differences in electronegativity react, there is a complete transfer of electrons from the less electronegative atom to the more electronegative atom. The atom that loses electrons becomes a positively charged ion, or **cation**, and the atom that gains electrons becomes a negatively charged ion, or **anion**. For this transfer to occur, the difference in electronegativity must be greater than 1.7. In general, the elements of Groups I and II (low electronegativities) bond ionically to elements of Group VII (high electronegativities). Elements of Groups I and II give up their electrons to achieve a noble gas configuration, while Group VII elements gain an electron to achieve the noble gas configuration. For example, Na + Cl → Na$^+$ Cl$^-$ (sodium chloride). The electrostatic force of attraction between the charged ions is called an **ionic** or **electrovalent bond**.

Ionic compounds have characteristic physical properties. They have high melting and boiling points due to the strong electrostatic forces between the ions. They can conduct electricity in the liquid and aqueous states, though not in the solid state. Ionic solids form crystal lattices consisting of infinite arrays of positive and negative ions in which the attractive forces between ions of opposite charge are maximized, while the repulsive forces between ions of like charge are minimized.

REMEMBER

The *t* in *cation* looks like a plus sign: ca+ion.

COVALENT BONDS

When two or more atoms with similar electronegativities interact, the energy required to form ions is greater than the energy that would be released upon the formation of an ionic bond (i.e., the process is not energetically favorable). However, since a complete transfer of electrons cannot occur, such atoms achieve a noble gas electron configuration by **sharing** electrons in a covalent bond. The binding force between the two atoms results from the attraction that each electron of the shared pair has for the two positive nuclei.

Covalent compounds contain discrete molecular units with weak intermolecular forces. Consequently, they are low-melting solids and do not conduct electricity in the liquid or aqueous states.

A. Properties of Covalent Bonds

Atoms can share more than one pair of electrons. Two atoms sharing one, two, or three electron pairs are said to be joined by a **single**, **double**, or **triple covalent bond**, respectively. The number of shared electron pairs between two atoms is called the **bond order;** hence, a single bond has a bond order of one, a double bond has a bond order of two, and a triple bond has a bond order of three.

A covalent bond can be characterized by two features: **bond length** and **bond energy**.

1. BOND LENGTH

Bond length is the average distance between the two nuclei of the atoms involved in the bond. As the number of shared electron pairs increases, the two atoms are pulled closer together, leading to a decrease in bond length. Thus, for a given pair of atoms, a triple bond is shorter than a double bond, which is shorter than a single bond.

2. BOND ENERGY

Bond energy is the energy required to separate two bonded atoms. For a given pair of atoms, the strength of a bond (and therefore the bond energy) increases as the number of shared electron pairs increases.

B. Covalent Bond Notation

The shared valence electrons of a covalent bond are called the **bonding electrons**. The valence electrons not involved in the covalent bond are called **nonbonding electrons**. The unshared electron pairs can also be called **lone electron pairs**. A convenient notation, called a **Lewis structure**, is used to represent the bonding and nonbonding electrons in a molecule, facilitating chemical "bookkeeping." The number of valence electrons attributed to a particular atom in the Lewis structure of a molecule is not necessarily the same as the number would be in the isolated atom, and the difference accounts for what is referred to as the **formal charge** of that atom. Often, more than one Lewis structure can be drawn for a molecule; this phenomenon is called **resonance**. Lewis structures, formal charge, and resonance are discussed in detail below.

1. LEWIS STRUCTURES

A Lewis structure, or **Lewis dot diagram**, is the chemical symbol of an element surrounded by dots, each representing one of the s and/or p valence electrons of the atom. The Lewis symbols of the elements found in the second period of the periodic table are shown in Table 3.1.

Table 3.1

·Li	Lithium	·N̈·	Nitrogen
·Be·	Beryllium	·Ö:	Oxygen
·Ḃ·	Boron	·F̈:	Fluorine
·Ċ·	Carbon	:N̈e:	Neon

Just as a Lewis symbol is used to represent the distribution of valence electrons in an atom, it can also be used to represent the distribution of valence electrons in a molecule. For example, the Lewis symbol of an F ion is $: \ddot{F} \; :$; the Lewis structure of an F_2 molecule is $: \ddot{F} \overline{} \ddot{F} :$.

Certain steps must be followed in assigning a Lewis structure to a molecule. These steps are outlined below, using HCN as an example.

- Write the skeletal structure of the compound (i.e., the arrangement of atoms). In general, the least electronegative atom is the central atom. Hydrogen (always) and the halogens F, Cl, Br, and I (usually) occupy the end position.

In HCN, H must occupy an end position. Of the remaining two atoms, C is the least electronegative and, therefore, occupies the central position. The skeletal structure is as follows:

$$H - C - N$$

- Count all the valence electrons of the atoms. The number of valence electrons of the molecule is the sum of the valence electrons of all atoms present:

    H has 1 valence electron;
    C has 4 valence electrons;
    N has 5 valence electrons; therefore,
    HCN has a total of 10 valence electrons.

- Draw single bonds between the central atom and the atoms surrounding it. Place an electron pair in each bond (bonding electron pair).

$$H : C : N$$

Each bond has 2 electrons, so $10 - 4 = 6$ valence electrons remain.

- Complete the octets (8 valence electrons) of all atoms bonded to the central atom, using the remaining valence electrons still to be assigned. (Recall that H is an exception to the octet rule since it can have only 2 valence electrons.) In this example, H already has 2 valence electrons in its bond with C.

$$H : C : \ddot{N} :$$

- Place any extra electrons on the central atom. If the central atom has less than an octet, try to write double or triple bonds between the central and surrounding atoms using the nonbonding, unshared lone electron pairs.

The HCN structure above does not satisfy the octet rule for C because C possesses only 4 valence electrons. Therefore, 2 lone electron pairs from the N atom must be moved to form two more bonds with C, creating a triple bond between C and N. Finally, bonds are drawn as lines rather than pairs of dots.

$$H - C \equiv N:$$

Now the octet rule is satisfied for all three atoms, since C and N have 8 valence electrons and H has 2 valence electrons.

2. FORMAL CHARGES

The number of electrons officially assigned to an atom in a Lewis structure does not always equal the number of valence electrons of the free atom. The difference between these two numbers is the **formal charge** of the atom. Formal charge can be calculated using the following formula:

$$\text{Formal charge} = V - \frac{1}{2}N_{\text{bonding}} - N_{\text{nonbonding}}$$

where V is the number of valence electrons in the free atom, N_{bonding} is the number of bonding electrons, and $N_{\text{nonbonding}}$ is the number of nonbonding electrons.

The formal charge of an ion or molecule is equal to the sum of the formal charges of the individual atoms comprising the ion or molecule.

Example: Calculate the formal charge on the central N atom of $[NH_4]^+$.

Solution: The Lewis structure of $[NH_4]^+$ is

$$\left[\begin{array}{c} H \\ | \\ H - N - H \\ | \\ H \end{array} \right]^+$$

Nitrogen is in Group VA; thus, it has 5 valence electrons.

In $[NH_4]^+$, N has 4 bonds (i.e., 8 bonding electrons and no nonbonding electrons).

So $V = 5$; $N_{\text{bonding}} = 8$; $N_{\text{nonbonding}} = 0$.

Formal charge $= 5 - \dfrac{1}{2}(8) - 0 = +1$.

Thus, the formal charge on the N atom in $[NH_4]^+$ is +1.

3. RESONANCE

For some molecules, two or more nonidentical Lewis structures can be drawn; these are called **resonance structures.** The molecule doesn't actually exist as either one of the resonance structures but is rather a composite, or hybrid, of the two. For example, SO_2 has three resonance structures, two of which are minor: O = S – O and O – S = O. The actual molecule is a hybrid of these three structures (spectral data indicate that the two S–O bonds are identically equivalent). This phenomenon is known as resonance, and the actual structure of the molecule is called the **resonance hybrid.** Resonance structures are expressed with a double-headed arrow between them; thus,

$$\ddot{O}\!=\!\ddot{S}\!=\!\ddot{O} \longleftrightarrow \ddot{O}\!=\!\ddot{S}\!-\!\ddot{O}\!: \longleftrightarrow :\!\ddot{O}\!-\!\ddot{S}\!=\!\ddot{O}$$

represents the resonance structures of SO_2.

The last two resonance structures of sulfur dioxide shown above have equivalent energy or stability. Often, nonequivalent resonance structures may be written for a molecule. In these cases, the more stable the structure, the more that structure contributes to the character of the resonance hybrid. Conversely, the less stable the resonance structure, the less that structure contributes to the resonance hybrid. The structure on the left of the diagram above is the most stable. Formal charges are often useful for qualitatively assessing the stability of a particular resonance structure. The following guidelines are used:

- A Lewis structure with small or no formal charges is preferred over a Lewis structure with large formal charges.
- A Lewis structure in which negative formal charges are placed on more electronegative atoms is more stable than one in which the formal charges are placed on less electronegative atoms.

Example: Write the resonance structures for [NCO]⁻.

Solution: 1.   C is the least electronegative of the three given atoms, N, C, and O. Therefore, the C atom occupies the central position in the skeletal structure of [NCO]⁻.

N C O

2.   N has 5 valence electrons;

C has 4 valence electrons;

O has 6 valence electrons;

and the species itself has one negative charge.

Total valence electrons = 5 + 4 + 6 + 1 = 16.

3. Draw single bonds between the central C atom and the surrounding atoms, N and O. Place a pair of electrons in each bond.

$$N : C : O$$

4. Complete the octets of N and O with the remaining $16 - 4 = 12$ electrons.

$$:\overset{..}{\underset{..}{N}}:C:\overset{..}{\underset{..}{O}}:$$

5. The C octet is incomplete. There are three ways in which double and triple bonds can be formed to complete the C octet. Two lone pairs from the O atom can be used to form a triple bond between the C and O atoms:

$$:\overset{..}{N}-C\equiv O:$$

Or 1 lone electron pair can be taken from both the O and the N atoms to form two double bonds, one between N and C and the other between O and C:

$$:\overset{..}{N}=C=\overset{..}{O}:$$

Or 2 lone electron pairs can be taken from the N atom to form a triple bond between the C and N atoms:

$$:N\equiv C-\overset{..}{\underset{..}{O}}:$$

These three are all resonance structures of [NCO]⁻.

6. Assign formal charges to each atom of each resonance structure.

The most stable structure is

$$:N\equiv C-\overset{..}{\underset{..}{O}}:$$

since the negative formal charge is on the most electronegative atom, O.

4. EXCEPTIONS TO THE OCTET RULE

Atoms found in or beyond the third period can have more than eight valence electrons, since some of the valence electrons may occupy *d*-orbitals. These atoms can be assigned more than four bonds in Lewis structures. When drawing the Lewis structure of the sulfate ion, giving the sulfur 12 valence electrons permits three of the five atoms to be assigned a formal charge of zero. The sulfate ion can

---

REMEMBER

The octet "rule" is really not much of a rule. It always applies to neutral atoms and anions of C, N, O, and F only. It often (not always!) applies to the halogens and other representative elements, but it never applies to H, He, Li, Be, or to neutral B and Al.

be drawn in six resonance forms, each with the two double bonds attached to a different combination of oxygen atoms.

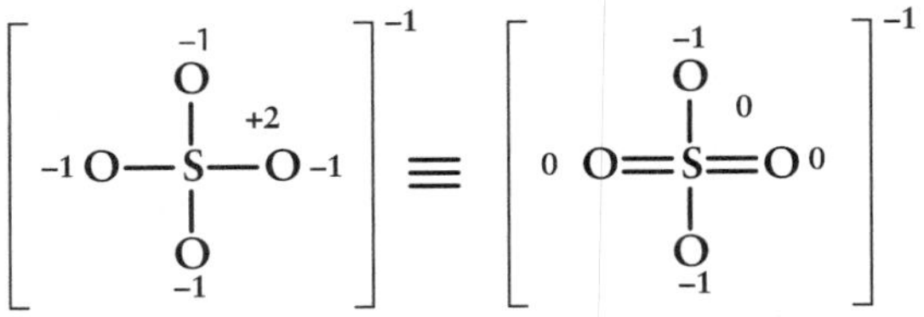

$$
\begin{bmatrix}
\overset{-1}{O} \\
\overset{\mid}{}\,{}^{+2} \\
{}^{-1}O\!-\!S\!-\!O^{-1} \\
\overset{\mid}{O} \\
{}_{-1}
\end{bmatrix}^{-1}
\equiv
\begin{bmatrix}
\overset{-1}{O} \\
\overset{\mid}{}\,{}^{0} \\
{}_{0}\,O\!=\!S\!=\!O\,{}^{0} \\
\overset{\mid}{O} \\
{}_{-1}
\end{bmatrix}^{-1}
$$

Figure 3.1

C. Types of Covalent Bonding

The nature of a covalent bond depends on the relative electronegativities of the atoms sharing the electron pairs. Covalent bonds are considered to be **polar** or **nonpolar** depending on the difference in electronegativities between the atoms.

1. POLAR COVALENT BOND

Polar covalent bonding occurs between atoms with small differences in electronegativity, generally in the range of 0.4 to 1.7 Pauling units. The bonding electron pair is not shared equally but is pulled more towards the element with the higher electronegativity. As a result, the more electronegative atom acquires a partial negative charge, δ^-, and the less electronegative atom acquires a partial positive charge, δ^+, giving the molecule partially ionic character. For instance, the covalent bond in HCl is polar because the two atoms have a small difference in electronegativity (approx. 0.9). Chlorine, the more electronegative atom, attains a partial negative charge, and hydrogen attains a partial positive charge. This difference in charge between the atoms is indicated by an arrow crossed (like a plus sign) at the positive end pointing to the negative end, as shown in Figure 3.2.

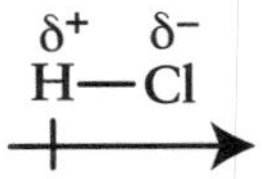

$$
\overset{\delta^+ \quad \delta^-}{H\!-\!Cl}
$$
$$
\longmapsto
$$

Figure 3.2

A molecule that has such a separation of positive and negative charges is called a polar molecule. The **dipole moment** itself is a vector quantity, μ, defined as the product of the charge magnitude (q) and the distance between the two partial charges (r):

$$\mu = qr$$

The dipole moment is denoted by an arrow pointing from the positive to the negative charge and is measured in Debye units (coulomb-meters).

2. NONPOLAR COVALENT BOND

Nonpolar covalent bonding occurs between atoms that have the same electronegativities. The bonding electron pair is shared equally, with no separation of charge across the bond. Not surprisingly, nonpolar covalent bonds occur in diatomic molecules, such as H_2, Cl_2, O_2, and N_2.

3. COORDINATE COVALENT BOND

In a coordinate covalent bond, the shared electron pair comes from the lone pair of one of the atoms in the molecule. Once such a bond forms, it is indistinguishable from any other covalent bond. Distinguishing such a bond is useful only in keeping track of the valence electrons and formal charges. Coordinate bonds are typically found in Lewis acid-base compounds. A **Lewis acid** is a compound that can accept an electron pair to form a covalent bond; a **Lewis base** is a compound that can donate an electron pair to form a covalent bond. For example, Figure 3.3 shows the reaction between borontrifluoride (BF_3) and ammonia (NH_3).

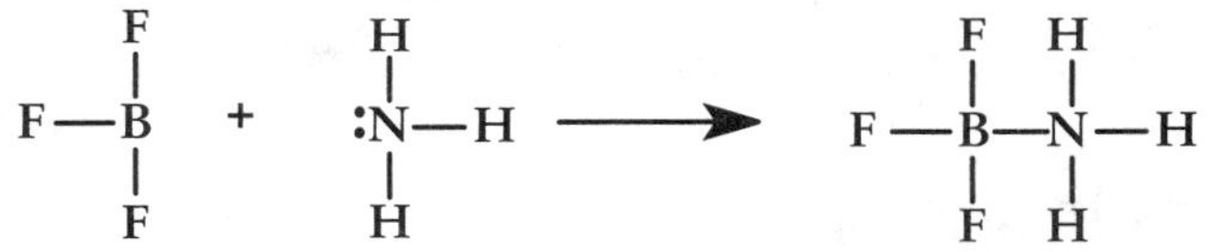

Lewis acid   Lewis base   Lewis acid–base compound

Figure 3.3

NH_3 donates a pair of electrons to form a coordinate covalent bond; thus, it acts as a Lewis base. BF_3 accepts this pair of electrons to form the coordinate covalent bond; thus, it acts as a Lewis acid.

D. Geometry and Polarity of Covalent Molecules

1. THE VALENCE SHELL ELECTRON-PAIR REPULSION THEORY

The valence shell electron-pair repulsion (VSEPR) theory uses Lewis structures to predict the molecular geometry of covalently bonded molecules. It states that the three-dimensional arrangement of atoms surrounding a central atom is determined by the repulsions between the bonding and the nonbonding electron pairs in the valence shell of the central atom. These electron pairs arrange themselves as far apart as possible, thereby minimizing repulsion.

The following steps are used to predict the geometrical structure of a molecule using the VSEPR theory.

1. Draw the Lewis structure of the molecule.

2. Count the total number of bonding and nonbonding electron pairs in the valence shell of the central atom.

3. Arrange the electron pairs around the central atom so that they are as far apart from each other as possible. For example, the compound AX_2 has the Lewis structure X : A : X. A has two bonding electron pairs in its valence shell. To make these electron pairs as far apart as possible, their geometric structure should be linear:

$$X - A - X$$

Valence electron arrangements are summarized in Table 3.2.

Table 3.2

Regions of Electron Density	Example	Geometric Arrangement of Electron Pairs Around the Central Atom	Shape	Angle between Electron Pairs
2	$BeCl_2$	X—A—X	linear	180.0°
3	BH_3	120°	trigonal planar	120.0°
4	CH_4	109.5°	tetrahedral	109.5°
5	PCl_5	axial 90° 120° equatorial axial	trigonal bipyramidal	90.0°, 120°, 180°
6	SF_6	90°	octahedral	90.0°, 180.0°

Example: Predict the geometry of NH_3.

Solution: 1. The Lewis structure of NH_3 is

$$\begin{array}{c} H \\ | \\ H-N-H \\ \cdot\cdot \end{array}$$

2. The central atom, N, has 3 bonding electron pairs and 1 nonbonding electron pair for a total of 4 electron pairs.

3. The 4 electron pairs will be farthest apart when they occupy the corners of a tetrahedron. Since 1 of the 4 electron pairs is a lone pair, the observed geometry is trigonal pyramidal (see Figure 3.4).

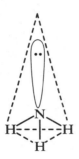

Figure 3.4

In describing the shape of a molecule, only the arrangement of atoms (not electrons) is considered. Even though the electron pairs are arranged tetrahedrally, the shape of NH_3 is pyramidal. It is not trigonal planar because the lone pair repels the 3 bonding electron pairs, causing them to move as far away as possible.

Example: Predict the geometry of CO_2.

Solution: The Lewis structure of CO_2 is $\overset{\cdot\cdot}{\underset{\cdot\cdot}{O}} :: C :: \overset{\cdot\cdot}{\underset{\cdot\cdot}{O}}$.

The double bond behaves just like a single bond for purposes of predicting molecular shape. This compound has two groups of electrons around the carbon. According to the VSEPR theory, the two sets of electrons will orient themselves 180° apart, on opposite sides of the carbon atom, minimizing electron repulsion. Therefore, the molecular structure of CO_2 is linear: $\overset{\cdot\cdot}{O}=C=\overset{\cdot\cdot}{\underset{\cdot\cdot}{O}}$.

2. POLARITY OF MOLECULES

A molecule with a net dipole moment is called **polar**, as previously mentioned, because it has positive and negative poles. The polarity of a molecule depends on the polarity of the constituent bonds and on the shape of the molecule. A molecule with nonpolar bonds is always nonpolar; a molecule with polar bonds may be polar or nonpolar depending on the orientation of the bond dipoles.

A molecule of two atoms bound by a polar bond must have a net dipole moment and, therefore, be polar. The two equal and opposite partial charges are localized at the ends of the molecule on the two atoms. A molecule consisting of more than two atoms bound with polar bonds may be either polar or nonpolar, since the overall dipole moment of a molecule is the vector sum of the individual bond dipole moments. If the molecule has a particular shape such that the bond dipole moments cancel each other (i.e., if the vector sum is zero), then the result is a nonpolar molecule. For instance, CCl_4 has four polar C–Cl bonds. According to the VSEPR theory, the shape of CCl_4 is tetrahedral. The four bond dipoles point to the vertices of the tetrahedron and cancel each other, resulting in a nonpolar molecule (see Figure 3.5).

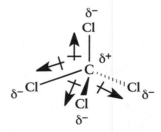

Figure 3.5. No Net Dipole Moment

However, if the orientation of the bond dipoles are such that they do not cancel out, the molecules will have a net dipole moment and, therefore, be polar. For instance, H_2O has two polar O–H bonds. According to the VSEPR model, its shape is angular. The two dipoles add together to give a net dipole moment to the molecule, making the H_2O molecule polar (see Figure 3.6).

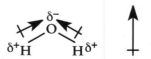

Figure 3.6. Net Dipole Moment

E. Atomic and Molecular Orbitals

An understanding of quantum numbers is necessary for an accurate description of orbitals. The azimuthal quantum number ℓ describes the orbitals of each n shell. The shapes of these orbitals represent the probability of finding an electron at any given instant. When $\ell = 0$, the orbital is an s-orbital. s-orbitals are spherically symmetric. The 1s-orbital ($n = 1$, $\ell = 0$) is plotted in Figure 3.7.

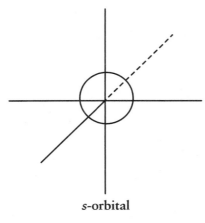

s-orbital

Figure 3.7

When $\ell = 1$, there are three possible orbitals (since the magnetic quantum number, m_ℓ, may equal –1, 0, or 1). These are called p-orbitals and have a dumbbell shape. The three p-orbitals, designated px, py, and pz, are oriented at right angles to each other; the px-orbital is plotted in Figure 3.8.

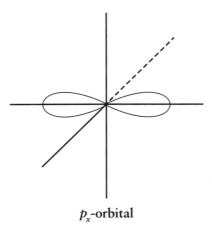

p_x-orbital

Figure 3.8

Plus and minus signs, determined from the mathematics of the wave function, are assigned to each lobe of the p-orbitals. The shapes of the five d-orbitals ($\ell = 2$, $m_\ell = -2, -1, 0, 1, 2$) and the seven f-orbitals

($\ell = 3$, $m_\ell = -3, -2, -1, 0, 1, 2, 3$) are more complex and need not be memorized. When two atoms bond to form a molecule, the atomic orbitals interact to form a **molecular orbital,** which describes the probability of finding the bonding electrons. Molecular orbitals are obtained by adding the wave functions of the atomic orbitals. Qualitatively, this is described by the **overlap** of two atomic orbitals. If the signs of the two atomic orbitals are the same, a **bonding orbital** is formed. If the signs are different, an **antibonding orbital** is formed. In addition, two different types of overlap are possible. When orbitals overlap head-to-head, the resulting bond is called a **sigma** (σ) bond. When the orbitals are parallel, a **pi** (π) bond is formed.

FLASHBACK

Quantum numbers revisited:
- For any value of n, there are n values of ℓ ($0 \rightarrow n - 1$).
- $\ell = 0 \rightarrow s$
  $\ell = 1 \rightarrow p$
  $\ell = 2 \rightarrow d$
- For any value of ℓ, there are $2\ell + 1$ values of m_ℓ (number of orbitals); values themselves will range from $-\ell$ to ℓ.

THE INTERMOLECULAR FORCES

The attractive forces that exist between molecules are collectively known as **intermolecular forces.** These include **dipole-dipole interactions, hydrogen bonding,** and **dispersion forces.** Dipole-dipole interactions and dispersion forces are often referred to as **van der Waals forces.**

A. Dipole-Dipole Interactions

Polar molecules tend to orient themselves such that the positive region of one molecule is close to the negative region of another molecule. This arrangement is energetically favorable because an attractive dipole force is formed between the two molecules.

Dipole-dipole interactions are present in the solid and liquid phases but become negligible in the gas phase because the molecules are generally much farther apart. Polar species tend to have higher boiling points than nonpolar species of comparable molecular weight.

B. Hydrogen Bonding

REMEMBER

The elements that result in hydrogen bonds can be remembered by the phrase "Chemistry is FON!" referring to Fluorine, Oxygen, and Nitrogen.

Hydrogen bonding is a specific, unusually strong form of dipole-dipole interaction, which may be either intra- or intermolecular. When hydrogen is bound to a highly electronegative atom, such as fluorine, oxygen, or nitrogen, the hydrogen atom carries little of the electron density of the covalent bond. This positively charged hydrogen atom interacts with the partial negative charge located on the electronegative atoms of nearby molecules. Substances that display hydrogen bonding tend to have unusually high boiling points compared with compounds of similar molecular weight that do not hydrogen bond. The difference derives from the energy required to break the hydrogen bonds. Hydrogen bonding is particularly important in the behavior of water, alcohols, amines, and carboxylic acids (see the Organic Chemistry section for further discussion).

C. Dispersion Forces

The bonding electrons in covalent bonds may appear to be equally shared between two atoms, but at any particular point in time, they will be located randomly throughout the orbital. This permits unequal sharing of electrons, causing rapid polarization and counterpolarization of the electron cloud and formation of short-lived dipoles. These dipoles interact with the electron clouds of neighboring molecules, inducing the formation of more dipoles. The attractive interactions of these short-lived dipoles are called dispersion or **London forces.**

Dispersion forces are generally weaker than other intermolecular forces. They do not extend over long distances and are, therefore, most important when molecules are close together. The strength of these interactions within a given substance depends directly on how easily the electrons in the molecules can move (i.e., be polarized). Large molecules in which the electrons are far from the nucleus are relatively easy to polarize and, therefore, possess greater dispersion forces. If not for dispersion forces, the noble gases would not liquefy at any temperature, since no other intermolecular forces exist between the noble gas atoms. The low temperature at which the noble gases liquefy is to some extent indicative of the magnitude of dispersion forces between the atoms.

KEY CONCEPT

These intermolecular forces are the binding forces that keep a substance together in its solid or liquid state. These same forces determine whether two substances are miscible or immiscible in the solution phase.

4

Compounds and Stoichiometry

A **compound** is a pure substance that is composed of two or more elements in a fixed proportion. Compounds can be broken down chemically to produce their constituent elements or other compounds. All elementa, except for some of the noble gases, can react with other elements or compounds to form new compounds. These new compounds can react further to form yet different compounds.

MOLECULES AND MOLES

A **molecule** is a combination of two or more atoms held together by covalent bonds. It is the smallest unit of a compound displaying the properties of that compound. Molecules may contain two atoms of the same element, as in N_2 and O_2, or may be comprised of two or more different atoms, as in CO_2 and $SOCl_2$. Molecules are usually discussed in terms of molecular weights and moles.

Ionic compounds do not form true molecules. In the solid state, they can be considered to be a nearly infinite, three-dimensional array of the charged particles of which the compound is composed. Since no actual molecule exists, molecular weight becomes meaningless, and the term **formula weight** is used in its place.

A. Molecular Weight

Like atoms, molecules can be characterized by their weight. The molecular weight is the sum of the atomic weights (in amu) of the atoms in the molecule. Similarly, the formula weight of an ionic compound is found by adding up the atomic weights according to the empirical formula of the substance.

FLASHBACK

Ionic compounds form from combinations of elements that are likely to form ions, such as sodium or potassium with chlorine or bromine. Molecular compounds form from the combination of elements of similar electronegativity, such as carbon or hyd

Example: What is the molecular weight of $SOCl_2$?

Solution: To find the molecular weight of SOCl2, add together the atomic weights of each of the atoms.

$$1\ S = 1 \times 32\ amu\quad = 32\ amu$$
$$1\ O = 1 \times 16\ amu\quad = 16\ amu$$
$$2\ Cl = 2 \times 35.5\ amu = 71\ amu$$
$$molecular\ weight = 119\ amu$$

B. Mole

A mole is defined as the amount of a substance that contains the same number of particles that are found in a 12.000 g sample of carbon-12. This quantity, **Avogadro's number,** is equal to 6.022×10^{23}. One mole of a compound has a mass in grams equal to the molecular weight of that compound in amu and contains 6.022×10^{23} molecules of the compound. For example, 62 g of H_2CO_3 represents one mole of carbonic acid and contains 6.022×10^{23} H_2CO_3 molecules. The mass of 1 mole of a compound is called its **molar weight** or **molar mass** and is usually expressed as g/mol. Therefore, the molar mass of H_2CO_3 is 62 g/mol.

The following formula is used to determine the number of moles present:

$$mol =$$

Example: How many moles are in 9.52 g of $MgCl_2$?

Solution: First, find the molar mass of $MgCl_2$.

$$1(24.31\ g/mol) + 2(35.45\ g/mol) = 95.21\ g/mol$$

Now, solve for the number of moles.

$$\frac{9.52\ g}{95.21\ g/mol} = 0.10\ mol\ of\ MgCl_2$$

C. Equivalent Weight

For some substances, it is useful to define a measure of reactive capacity. This expresses the fact that some molecules are more potent than others in performing certain reactions. An example of this is the ability of different acids to donate protons (H^+ ions) in solution (see Acids and Bases). For instance, 1 mole of HCl can donate 1 mole of hydrogen ions, while 1 mole of H_2SO_4 can donate 2 moles of hydrogen ions. This difference is expressed using the term **equivalent:** 1 mole of HCl contains 1 equivalent of hydrogen ions, while 1 mole of H_2SO_4 contains 2 equivalents of hydrogen ions. To determine the number of equivalents a compound contains, a new measure of weight called **gram-equivalent weight (GEW)** was developed.

$$\text{Equivalents} = \frac{\text{Weight of Compound}}{\text{Gram Equivalent Weight}}$$

and

$$\text{Gram Equivalent Weight} = \frac{\text{Molar Mass}}{n}$$

where n is usually either the number of hydrogens used per molecule of acid in a reaction or the number of hydroxyl groups used per molecule of base in a reaction. This value is strictly dependent on reaction conditions. By using equivalents, it is possible to say that one equivalent of acid will neutralize one equivalent of base, a statement that may not necessarily be true when dealing with moles.

REPRESENTATION OF COMPOUNDS

A. Law of Constant Composition

The **law of constant composition** states that any sample of a given compound will contain the same elements in the identical mass ratio. For instance, every sample of H_2O will contain two atoms of hydrogen for every atom of oxygen, or, in other words, one gram of hydrogen for every eight grams of oxygen.

B. Empirical and Molecular Formulas

There are two ways to express a formula for a compound. The **empirical formula** gives the simplest whole number ratio of the elements in the compound. The **molecular formula** gives the exact number of atoms of each element in the compound and is usually a multiple of the empirical formula. For example, the empirical formula for benzene is CH, while the molecular formula is C_6H_6. For some compounds, the empirical and molecular formulas are the same, as in the case of H_2O. An ionic compound, such as NaCl or $CaCO_3$, will have only an empirical formula.

C. Percent Composition

The percent composition by mass of an element is the weight percent of the element in a specific compound. To determine the percent composition of an element X in a compound, the following formula is used:

$$\text{\% Composition} = \frac{\text{Mass of X in Formula}}{\text{Formula Weight of Compound}} \times 100\%$$

The percent composition of an element may be determined using either the empirical or molecular formula. If the percent compositions are known, the empirical formula can be derived. It is possible to determine the molecular formula if both the percent compositions and molecular weight of the compound are known.

Example: What is the percent composition of chromium in $K_2Cr_2O_7$?

Solution: The formula weight of $K_2Cr_2O_7$ is calculated as follows:

2(39 g/mol) + 2(52 g/mol) + 7(16 g/mol) = 294 g/mol

$$\% \text{ composition of Cr} = \frac{2(52 g/mol)}{294 g/mol} = \times 100\%$$

$$= 0.354 \times 100\%$$

$$= 35.4\%$$

Example: What are the empirical and molecular formulas of a compound that contains 40.9% carbon, 4.58% hydrogen, and 54.52% oxygen and has a molecular weight of 264 g/mol?

Method One: First, determine the number of moles of each element in the compound by assuming a 100 gram sample; this converts the percentage of each element present directly into grams of that element. Then convert grams to moles:

$$\text{\#mol of C} = \frac{40.9 \text{ g}}{12 \text{ g/mol}} = 3.41 \text{ mol}$$

$$\text{\#mol of H} = \frac{4.58 \text{ g}}{1 \text{ g/mol}} = 4.58 \text{ mol}$$

$$\text{\#mol of O} = \frac{54.52 \text{ g}}{16 \text{ g/mol}} = 3.41 \text{ mol}$$

Next, find the simplest whole number ratio of the elements by dividing the number of moles by the smallest number obtained in the previous step.

C: $\frac{3.41}{3.41} = 1.00$ H: $\frac{4.58}{3.41} = 1.33$ O: $= \frac{3.41}{3.41} = 1.00$

Finally, the empirical formula is obtained by converting the numbers obtained into whole numbers (multiplying them by an integer value).

$$C_1H_{1.33}O_1 \times 3 = C_3H_4O_3$$

$C_3H_4O_3$ is the empirical formula. To determine the molecular formula, divide the molecular weight by the weight represented by the empirical formula. The resultant value is the number of empirical formula units in the molecular formula.

The empirical formula weight of $C_3H_4O_3$ is calculated as follows:

$$3(12 \text{ g/mol}) + 4(1 \text{ g/mol}) + 3(16 \text{ g/mol}) = 88 \text{ g/mol}$$

$$\frac{264 \text{ g/mol}}{88 \text{ g/mol}} = 3$$

$C_3H_4O_3 \times 3 = C_9H_{12}O_9$ is the molecular formula.

Method Two: When the molecular weight is given, it is generally easier to find the molecular formula first. This is accomplished by multiplying the molecular weight by the given percentages to find the grams of each element present in one mole of compound, then dividing by the respective atomic weights to find the mole ratio of the elements:

$$\#\text{mol of C} = \frac{(0.409)(264) \text{ g}}{12 \text{ g/mol}} = 9 \text{ mol}$$

$$\#\text{mol of H} = \frac{(0.0458)(264) \text{ g}}{1 \text{ g/mol}} = 12 \text{ mol}$$

$$\#\text{mol of O} = \frac{(0.5452)(264) \text{ g}}{16 \text{ g/mol}} = 9 \text{ mol}$$

Thus, the molecular formula, $C_9H_{12}O_9$, is the direct result.

The empirical formula can now be found by reducing the subscript ratio to the simplest integer values.

TYPES OF CHEMICAL REACTIONS

There are many ways in which elements and compounds can react to form other species; memorizing every reaction would be impossible, as well as unnecessary. However, nearly every inorganic reaction can be classified into at least one of four general categories.

A. Combination Reactions

Combination reactions are reactions in which two or more **reactants** form one **product**. The formation of sulfur dioxide by burning sulfur in air is an example of a combination reaction.

$$S \ (s) + O_2 \ (g) \rightarrow SO_2 \ (g)$$

B. Decomposition Reactions

A **decomposition reaction** is defined as one in which a compound breaks down into two or more substances, usually as a result of heating or electrolysis. An example of a decomposition reaction is the breakdown of mercury (II) oxide (the sign Δ represents the addition of heat).

$$2 \text{ HgO } (s) \rightarrow 2 \text{ Hg } (\ell) + \text{O}_2 \text{ } (g)$$

C. Single-Displacement Reactions

Single-displacement reactions occur when an atom (or ion) of one compound is replaced by an atom of another element. For example, zinc metal will displace copper ions in a copper sulfate solution to form zinc sulfate.

$$\text{Zn } (s) + \text{CuSO}_4 \text{ } (aq) \rightarrow \text{Cu } (s) + \text{ZnSO}_4 \text{ } (aq)$$

Single-displacement reactions are often further classified as **redox** reactions.

D. Double-Displacement Reactions

In **double-displacement reactions**, also called **metathesis reactions**, elements from two different compounds displace each other to form two new compounds. This type of reaction occurs when one of the products is removed from the solution as a precipitate or gas or when two of the original species combine to form a weak electrolyte that remains undissociated in solution. For example, when solutions of calcium chloride and silver nitrate are combined, insoluble silver chloride forms in a solution of calcium nitrate.

$$\text{CaCl}_2 \text{ } (aq) + 2 \text{ AgNO}_3 \text{ } (aq) \rightarrow \text{Ca(NO}_3)_2 \text{ } (aq) + 2 \text{ AgCl } (s)$$

NET IONIC EQUATIONS

Because reactions such as displacements often involve ions in solution, they can be written in ionic form. In the example where zinc is reacted with copper sulfate, the **ionic equation** would be

$$\text{Zn } (s) + \text{Cu}^{2+} \text{ } (aq) + \text{SO}_4^{2-} \text{ } (aq) \rightarrow \text{Cu } (s) + \text{Zn}^{2+} \text{ } (aq) + \text{SO}_4^{2-} \text{ } (aq)$$

When displacement reactions occur, there are usually **spectator ions** that do not take part in the overall reaction but simply remain in solution throughout. The spectator ion in the equation above is sulfate, which does not undergo any transformation during the reaction. A **net ionic reaction** can be written showing only the species that actually participate in the reaction:

$$\text{Zn } (s) + \text{Cu}^{2+} \text{ } (aq) \rightarrow \text{Cu } (s) + \text{Zn}^{2+} \text{ } (aq)$$

Net ionic equations are important for demonstrating the actual reaction that occurs during a displacement reaction.

NEUTRALIZATION REACTIONS

Neutralization reactions are a specific type of double displacements that occur when an acid reacts with a base to produce a solution of a salt and water. For example, hydrochloric acid and sodium hydroxide will react to form sodium chloride and water:

$$HCl \ (aq) + NaOH \ (aq) \rightarrow NaCl \ (aq) + H_2O \ (\ell)$$

A. Balancing Equations

Chemical equations express how much and what type of reactants must be used to obtain a given quantity of product. From the **law of conservation of mass**, the mass of the reactants in a reaction must be equal to the mass of the products. More specifically, chemical equations must be balanced so that there are the same number of atoms of each element in the products as there are in the reactants. **Stoichiometric coefficients** are used to indicate the number of moles of a given species involved in the reaction. For example, the reaction for the formation of water is:

$$2 \ H_2 \ (g) + O_2 \ (g) \rightarrow 2 \ H_2O \ (g)$$

The coefficients indicate that two moles of H_2 gas must be reacted with one mole of O_2 gas to produce two moles of water. In general, stoichiometric coefficients are given as whole numbers.

Example: Balance the following reaction.

$$C_4H_{10} \ (\ell) + O_2 \ (g) \rightarrow CO_2 \ (g) + H_2O \ (\ell)$$

Solution: First, balance the carbons in the reactants and products.

$$C_4H_{10} + O_2 \rightarrow 4 \ CO_2 + H_2O$$

Second, balance the hydrogens in the reactant and the products.

$$C_4H_{10} + O_2 \rightarrow 4 \ CO_2 + 5 \ H_2O$$

Third, balance the oxygens in the reactants and products.

$$2 \ C_4H_{10} + 13 \ O_2 \rightarrow 8 \ CO_2 + 10 \ H_2O$$

Finally, check that all of the elements and the total charges, are balanced correctly. If there is a difference in total charge between the reactants and products, then the charge will also have to be balanced.

KEY CONCEPT

When balancing equations, focus on the least represented elements first and work your way to the most represented element of the reaction (usually oxygen or hydrogen).

B. Applications of Stoichiometry

Once an equation has been balanced, the ratio of moles of reactant to moles of products is known, and that information can be used to solve many types of stoichiometry problems. It is important to use proper units when solving such problems. If and when you are faced with doing the calculations, the units should cancel out so that the units obtained in the answer represent those asked for in the problem.

Example: How many grams of calcium chloride are needed to prepare 72 g of silver chloride according to the following equation?

$$CaCl_2 \ (aq) + 2AgNO_3 \ (aq) \rightarrow Ca(NO_3)_2 \ (aq) + 2AgCl \ (s)$$

Solution: Noting first that the equation is balanced, 1 mole of $CaCl_2$ yields 2 moles of AgCl when it is reacted with 2 moles of $AgNO_3$. The molar mass of $CaCl_2$ is 110 g, and the molar mass of AgCl is 144 g.

$$72g \ AgCl \times \frac{1 \ mol \ AgCl}{144 \ g \ AgCl} \times \frac{1 \ mol \ CaCl_2}{2 \ mol \ AgCl} \times \frac{110 \ g \ CaCl_2}{1 \ mol \ CaCl_2} =$$

$$27.5 \ g \ CaCl_2$$

Thus, 27.5 g of $CaCl_2$ are needed to produce 72 g of AgCl.

1. LIMITING REACTANT

When reactants are mixed, they are seldom added in the exact stoichiometric proportions as shown in the balanced equation. Therefore, in most reactions, one of the reactants will be consumed first. This reactant is known as the **limiting reactant** because it limits the amount of product that can be formed in the reaction. The reactant that remains after all of the limiting reactant is used up is called the **excess reactant.**

Example: If 28 g of Fe react with 24 g of S to produce FeS, what would be the limiting reactant? How many grams of excess reactant would be present in the vessel at the end of the reaction?

The balanced equation is Fe + S $\xrightarrow{\Delta}$ FeS.

Solution: First, the number of moles for each reactant must be determined.

$$28 \ g \ Fe \times \frac{1 \ mol \ Fe}{56 \ g} = 0.5 \ mol \ Fe$$

$$24 \ g \ S \times \frac{1 \ mol \ S}{32 \ g} = 0.75 \ mol \ S$$

Since 1 mole of Fe is needed to react with 1 mole of S, and there are 0.5 moles Fe for every 0.75 moles S, the limiting reagent is Fe. Thus, 0.5 moles of Fe will react with 0.5 moles of S, leaving an excess of 0.25 moles of S in the vessel. The mass of the excess reactant will be

$$\text{mass of S} = 0.25 \text{ mol S} \times \frac{32 \text{ g}}{1 \text{ mol S}}$$
$$= 8 \text{ g of S}$$

2. YIELDS

The **yield** of a reaction, which is the amount of product predicted or obtained when the reaction is carried out, can be determined or predicted from the balanced equation. There are three distinct ways of reporting yields. The **theoretical yield** is the amount of product that can be predicted from a balanced equation, assuming that all of the limiting reagent has been used, that no competing side reactions have occurred, and all of the product has been collected. The theoretical yield is seldom obtained; therefore, chemists speak of the **actual yield**, which is the amount of product that is isolated from the reaction experimentally.

The term **percent yield** is used **to** express the relationship between the actual yield and the theoretical yield and is given by the following equation:

$$\textbf{Percent Yield} = \frac{\text{Actual Yield}}{\text{Theoretical Yield}} \times 100\%$$

Example: What is the percent yield for a reaction in which 27 g of Cu is produced by reacting 32.5 g of Zn in excess $CuSO_4$ solution?

Solution: The balanced equation is as follows:

$$\text{Zn } (s) + CuSO_4 \ (aq) \rightarrow \text{Cu } (s) + ZnSO_4 \ (aq)$$

Calculate the theoretical yield for Cu.

$$32.5 \text{ g Zn} \times \frac{1 \text{ mol Zn}}{65 \text{ g}} = 0.5 \text{ mol Zn}$$

$$0.5 \text{ mol Zn} \times \frac{1 \text{ mol Cu}}{1 \text{ mol Zn}} = 0.5 \text{ mol Cu}$$

$$0.5 \text{ mol Cu} \times \frac{64 \text{ g}}{1 \text{ mol Cu}} = 32 \text{g Cu} = \text{theoretical yield}$$

Finally, determine the percent yield.

$$\frac{27 \text{ g}}{32 \text{ g}} \times 100\% = 84\%$$

5

Chemical Kinetics and Equilibrium

When studying a chemical reaction, it is important to consider not only the chemical properties of the reactants but also the **conditions** under which the reaction occurs, the **mechanism** by which it takes place, the rate at which it occurs, and the **equilibrium** (or steady state) towards which it proceeds.

CHEMICAL KINETICS

Chemical kinetics is the study of the rates of reactions, the effect of reaction conditions on these rates, and the mechanisms implied by such observations.

A. Reaction Mechanisms

The **mechanism** of a reaction is the actual series of steps through which a chemical reaction occurs. Knowing the accepted mechanism of a reaction often helps to explain the reaction's rate, position of equilibrium, and thermodynamic characteristics. Consider the reaction below:

$$\text{Overall reaction: } A_2 + 2\,B \rightarrow 2\,AB$$

This equation seems to imply a mechanism in which two molecules of B collide with one molecule of A_2 to form two molecules of AB. But suppose instead that the reaction actually takes place in two steps.

$$\text{Step 1:} \quad A_2 + B \rightarrow A_2B \quad \text{(Slow)}$$
$$\text{Step 2:} \quad A_2B + B \rightarrow 2\,AB \quad \text{(Fast)}$$

Note that these two steps add up to the overall (net) reaction. A_2B, which does not appear in the overall reaction because it is neither a reactant nor a product, is called an **intermediate**. Reaction intermediates are often difficult to detect, but a proposed mechanism can be supported through kinetic experiments.

The slowest step in a proposed mechanism is called the **rate-determining step,** because the overall reaction cannot proceed faster than that step.

B. Reaction Rates

1. DEFINITION OF RATE

Consider a reaction $2A + B \rightarrow C$ in which 1 mole of C is produced from every 2 moles of A and 1 mole of B. The rate of this reaction may be described in terms of either the disappearance of reactants over time or the appearance of products over time.

$$\text{rate} = \frac{\text{decrease in concentration of reactants}}{\text{time}}$$

$$= \frac{\text{increase in concentration of products}}{\text{time}}$$

Because the concentration of a reactant decreases during the reaction, a minus sign is placed before a rate that is expressed in terms of reactants. For the reaction above, the rate of reaction with respect to A is $-\Delta[A]/\Delta t$, with respect to B is $-\Delta[B]/\Delta t$, and with respect to C is $\Delta[C]/\Delta t$. In this particular reaction, the three rates are not equal. According to the stoichiometry of the reaction, A is used up twice as fast as B ($-\frac{1}{2}\Delta[A]/\Delta t = -\Delta[B]/\Delta t$), and A is consumed twice as fast as C is produced ($-\frac{1}{2}\Delta[A]/\Delta t = \Delta[C]/\Delta t$). To show a standard rate of reaction in which the rates with respect to all substances are equal, the rate for each substance should be divided by its stoichiometric coefficient.

$$\text{rate} = -\frac{1}{2}\frac{\Delta[A]}{\Delta t} = -\frac{\Delta[B]}{\Delta t} = \frac{\Delta[C]}{\Delta t}$$

In general, for the reaction

$$a A + b B \rightarrow c C + d D,$$

$$\text{rate} = -\frac{1}{a}\frac{\Delta[A]}{\Delta t} = -\frac{1}{b}\frac{\Delta[B]}{\Delta t} = \frac{1}{c}\frac{\Delta[C]}{\Delta t} = \frac{1}{d}\frac{\Delta[D]}{\Delta t}$$

Rate is expressed in the units of moles per liter per second (mol/L·s) or molarity per second (M/s).

2. RATE LAW

For nearly all forward, irreversible reactions, the rate is proportional to the product of the concentrations of the reactants, each raised to some power. For the general reaction

$$a \, A + b \, B \rightarrow c \, C + d \, D$$

the rate is proportional to $[A]^x \, [B]^y$; that is,

$$\text{rate} = k \, [A]^x \, [B]^y$$

This expression is the **rate law** for the general reaction above, where k is the **rate constant**. Multiplying the units of k by the concentration factors raised to the appropriate powers gives the rate in units of concentration/time. The exponents x and y are called the **orders of reaction**; x is the order with respect to A, and y is the order with respect to B. These exponents may be integers, fractions, or zero and must be determined experimentally.

It is important to note that the exponents of the rate law are *not* necessarily equal to the stoichiometric coefficients in the overall reaction equation. (The exponents *are* equal to the stoichiometric coefficients of the rate-determining step. If one of the reactants or products in this step is an intermediate not included in the overall reaction, then calculating the rate law in terms of the original reactants is more complex.)

The **overall order of a reaction** (or the **reaction order**) is defined as the sum of the exponents, here equal to $x + y$.

a. Experimental determination of rate law

The values of k, x, and y in the rate law equation (rate = k $[A]^x$ $[B]^y$) must be determined experimentally for a given reaction at a given temperature. The rate is usually measured as a function of the **initial** concentrations of the reactants, A and B.

Example: Given the data in Table 5.1, find the rate law for the following reaction at 300 K.

$$A + B \rightarrow C + D$$

Table 5.1

Trial	$[A]_{initial}(M)$	$[B]_{initial}(M)$	$r_{initial}(M/s)$
1	1.00	1.00	2.0
2	1.00	2.00	8.1
3	2.00	2.00	15.9

Solution: First, look for two trials in which the concentrations of all but one of the substances are held constant.

a) In trials 1 and 2, the concentration of A is kept constant, while the concentration of B is doubled. The rate increases by a factor of 8.1/2.0, approximately 4. Write down the rate expression of the two trials.

Trial 1: $r_1 = k[A]x [B]y = k(1.00)x (1.00)y$

Trial 2: $r_2 = k[A]x [B]y = k(1.00)x (2.00)y$

Divide the second equation by the first:

$$\frac{r_2}{r_1} = \frac{8.1}{2.0} = \frac{k(1.00)^x (2.00)^y}{k(1.00)^x (1.00)^y} = (2.00)^y$$

$$4 = (2.00)^y$$

$$y = 2$$

b) In trials 2 and 3, the concentration of B is kept constant, while the concentration of A is doubled; the rate is increased by a factor of 15.9/8.1, approximately 2. The rate expression of the two trials are as follows:

Trial 2: $r_2 = k(1.00)x (2.00)y$

Trial 3: $r_3 = k(2.00)x (2.00)y$

Divide the second equation by the first:

$$\frac{r_3}{r_2} = \frac{15.9}{8.1} = \frac{k(2.00)^x (2.00)^y}{k(1.00)^x (2.00)^y} = (2.00)^x$$

$$2 = (2.00)^x$$

$$x = 1$$

So $r = k[A] [B]^2$

The order of the reaction with respect to A is 1 and with respect to B is 2; the overall reaction order is $1 + 2 = 3$.

To calculate k, substitute the values from any one of the above trials into the rate law, for Example,

$$2.0 \text{ M/s} = k \times 1.00 \text{ M} \times (1.00 \text{ M})^2$$

$$k = 2.0 \text{ M}^{-2} \text{ s}^{-1}$$

Therefore, the rate law is $r = 2.0 \text{ M}^{-2} \text{ s}^{-1} [A][B]^2$

KEY CONCEPT

The temperature, 300 K, doesn't enter into the calculation of the rate law; it is reported in the initial data just to make the results meaningful, since the rates of most reactions are temperature dependent.

3. REACTION ORDERS

Chemical reactions are often classified on the basis of kinetics as zero-order, first-order, second-order, mixed-order, or higher-order reactions. The general reaction $a \text{ A} + b \text{ B} \rightarrow c \text{ C} + d \text{ D}$ will be used in the discussion below.

a. Zero-order reactions

A zero-order reaction has a constant rate, which is independent of the reactants' concentrations. Thus, the rate law is rate = k, where k has units of Ms^{-1}.

b. First-order reactions

A first-order reaction (order = 1) has a rate proportional to the concentration of one reactant.

$$\text{rate} = k[A] \text{ or rate} = k[B]$$

First-order rate constants have units of s^{-1}.

The classic example of a first-order reaction is the process of radioactive decay. The concentration of radioactive substance A at any time t can be expressed mathematically as

$$[A_t] = [A_o] \, e^{-kt}$$

where $[A_o]$ = initial concentration of A

$[A_t]$ = concentration of A at time t

k = rate constant

t = elapsed time

The half-life ($t_{1/2}$) of a reaction is the time needed for the concentration of the radioactive substance to decrease to one-half of its original value. Half-lives can be calculated from the rate law as follows:

$$t_{1/2} = \ln(2)/k = 0.693/k$$

where k is the first-order rate constant.

c. **Second-order reactions**

A second-order reaction (order = 2) has a rate proportional to the product of the concentration of two reactants or to the square of the concentration of a single reactant; for example, rate = $k[A]^2$, rate = $k[B]^2$ or rate = $k[A][B]$. The units of second-order rate constants are $M^{-1}\ s^{-1}$.

d. **Higher-order reactions**

A higher-order reaction has an order greater than 2.

e. **Mixed-order reactions**

A mixed-order reaction has a fractional order (e.g., rate = $k[A]^{1/3}$).

4. **EFFICIENCY OF REACTIONS**

a. **Collision theory of chemical kinetics**

For a reaction to occur, molecules must collide with each other. The **collision theory of chemical kinetics** states that the rate of a reaction is proportional to the number of collisions per second between the reacting molecules.

Not all collisions, however, result in a chemical reaction. An **effective collision** (one that leads to the formation of products) occurs only if the molecules collide with correct orientation and sufficient force to break the existing bonds and form new ones. The minimum energy of collision necessary for a reaction to take place is called the **activation energy, E_a,** or the **energy barrier.** Only a fraction of colliding particles have enough kinetic energy to exceed the activation energy. This means that only a fraction of all collisions are effective. The rate of a reaction can therefore be expressed as follows:

$$\text{rate} = fZ$$

where Z is the total number of collisions occurring per second and f is the fraction of collisions that are effective.

b. Transition state theory

When molecules collide with sufficient energy, they form a **transition state** in which the old bonds are weakened and the new bonds are beginning to form. The transition state then dissociates into products, and the new bonds are fully formed. For a reaction $A_2 + B_2 \rightarrow 2AB$, the change along the reaction coordinate (a measure of the extent to which the reaction has progressed from reactants to products) can be represented as shown in Figure 5.1.

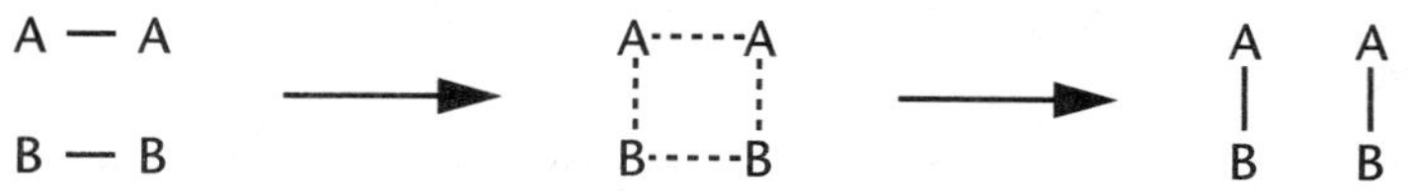

Figure 5.1

The **transition state**, also called the **activated complex**, has greater energy than either the reactants or the products and is denoted by the symbol ‡. The activation energy is required to bring the reactants to this energy level. Once an activated complex is formed, it can either dissociate into the products or revert to reactants without any additional energy input. Transition states are distinguished from intermediates in that, existing as they do at energy maxima, transition states have an extremely short, finite lifetime.

A **potential energy diagram** illustrates the relationship among the activation energy, the heats of reaction, and the potential energy of the system. The most important factors in such diagrams are the **relative** energies of the products and reactants. The **enthalpy change** of the reaction (ΔH) is the difference between the potential energy of the products and the potential energy of the reactants. A negative enthalpy change indicates an exothermic reaction (where heat is given off), and a positive enthalpy change indicates an endothermic reaction (where heat is absorbed). The activated complex exists at the top of the energy barrier. The difference in potential energies between the activated complex and the reactants is the activation energy of the forward reaction; the difference in potential energies between the activated complex and the products is the activation energy of the reverse reaction.

For example, consider the formation of HCl from H_2 and Cl_2. Figure 5.2, which gives the energy profile of the reaction

$$H_2 + Cl_2 \rightleftharpoons 2\,HCl$$

> **REMEMBER**
>
> $-\Delta H$ = exothermic = heat given off.
>
> $+\Delta H$ = endothermic = heat absorbed.

shows that the reaction is exothermic. The potential energy of the products is less than the potential energy of the reactants; heat is evolved, and the heat of reaction is negative.

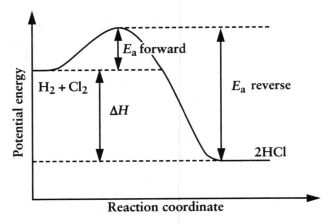

Figure 5.2

5. FACTORS AFFECTING REACTION RATE

The rate of a chemical reaction depends upon the individual species undergoing reaction and upon the reaction environment. The rate of reaction will increase if either of the following occurs: an increase in the number of effective collisions or a stabilization of the activated complex compared to the reactants.

a. Reactant concentrations

The greater the concentrations of the reactants (the more particles per unit volume), the greater will be the number of effective collisions per unit time. Therefore, the reaction rate will increase for all but zero-order reactions. For reactions occurring in the gaseous state, the partial pressures of the reactants can serve as a measure of concentration (see "Dalton's Law of Partial Pressures").

b. Temperature

For nearly all reactions, the reaction rate will increase as the temperature of the system increases. Since the temperature of a substance is a measure of the particles' average kinetic energy, increasing the temperature increases the average kinetic energy of the molecules. Consequently, the proportion of molecules having energies greater than E_a (thus capable of undergoing reaction) increases with higher temperature.

c. Medium

The rate of a reaction may also be affected by the medium in which it takes place. Certain reactions proceed more rapidly in

d. Catalysts

Catalysts are substances that increase reaction rate without themselves being consumed; they do this by lowering the activation energy. Catalysts are important in biological systems and in industrial chemistry; enzymes are biological catalysts. Catalysts may increase the frequency of collision between the reactants; change the relative orientation of the reactants, making a higher percentage of collisions effective; donate electron density to the reactants; or reduce intramolecular bonding within reactant molecules. Figure 5.3 compares the energy profiles of catalyzed and uncatalyzed reactions.

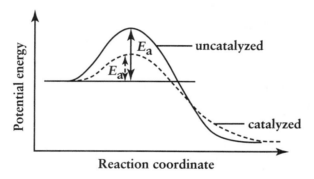

Figure 5.3

The energy barrier for the catalyzed reaction is much lower than the energy barrier for the uncatalyzed reaction. Note that the rates of both the forward and the reverse reactions are increased by catalysis, since E_a of the forward and reverse reactions is lowered by the same amount. Therefore, the presence of a catalyst causes the reaction to proceed more quickly toward equilibrium.

EQUILIBRIUM

A. The Dynamic Concept of Equilibrium

So far, reaction rates have been discussed under the assumption that the reactions were **irreversible** (i.e., only proceeded in one direction) and that the reactions proceeded to completion. However, a **reversible** reaction often does not proceed to completion, because (by definition) the products can react to reform the reactants. This is particularly true of reactions occurring in closed systems, where products are not allowed to escape. When there is no **net** change in the concentrations of the products and reactants during a reversible chemical reaction, **equilibrium** exists. This is not to say that a reaction in equilibrium is static; change continues to occur in both the forward and reverse directions. Equilibrium can be thought of as a balance between the two reaction directions.

Consider the following reaction:

$$A \rightleftharpoons B$$

At equilibrium, the concentrations of A and B are constant, yet the reactions A → B and B → A continue to occur at equal rates.

B. Law of Mass Action

Consider the following **one-step** reaction:

$$2A \rightleftharpoons B + C$$

Since the reaction occurs in one step, the rates of the forward and reverse reaction are given by

$$rate_f = k_f[A]^2 \text{ and } rate_r = k_r[B][C]$$

When $rate_f = rate_r$, equilibrium is achieved. Since the rates are equal, it can be stated that

$$k_f[A]^2 = k_r[B][C] \text{ or } \frac{k_f}{k_r} = \frac{[B][C]}{[A]^2}$$

Since k_f and k_r are both constants, this equation may be rewritten:

$$K_c = \frac{[B][C]}{[A]^2} \qquad \text{(see below for the general equation)}$$

where K_c is called the **equilibrium constant**, and the subscript c indicates that it is in terms of concentration (when dealing with gases, the equilibrium constant is referred to as K_p, and the subscript p indicates that it is in terms of pressure). For dilute solutions, K_c and K_{eq} are used interchangeably; the symbol K is also often used, though it is not completely correct to do so.

While the forward and reverse reaction rates are equal at equilibrium, the molar concentrations of the reactants and products usually are not equal. This means that the forward and reverse rate constants, k_f and k_r, are also usually unequal. For the **one-step** reaction described above,

$$k_f [A]^2 = k_r[B][C]$$

$$k_f = k_r \left(\frac{[B][C]}{[A]^2} \right)$$

In a reaction of more than one step, the equilibrium constant for the overall reaction is found by multiplying together the equilibrium constants for each step of the reaction. When this is done, the equilibrium constant for the overall reaction is equal to the concentrations of products divided by reactants in the overall reaction, each raised to its stoichiometric coefficient. The forward and reverse rate constants for any step n are designated k_n and k_{-n} respectively. For example, if the reaction

$$a \text{ A} + b \text{ B} \rightleftharpoons c \text{ C} + d \text{ D}$$

occurs in three steps, then

$$k_c = \frac{k_1 k_2 k_3}{k_{-1} k_{-2} k_{-3}} \text{ will equal } \frac{[C]^c [D]^d}{[A]^a [B]^b}.$$

This expression is known as the **Law of Mass Action.**

Example: What is the expression for the equilibrium constant for the following reaction?

$$3 \text{ H}_2 \, (g) + \text{N}_2 \, (g) \rightleftharpoons 2 \text{ NH}_3 \, (g)$$

Solution: $K_c = \dfrac{[NH_3]^2}{[H_2]^3 [N_2]}$

The **reaction quotient**, Q, is a measure of the degree to which a reaction has gone to completion. Q_c is equal to

$$\frac{[C]^c [D]^d}{[A]^a [B]^b}$$

Q_c is a constant only at equilibrium, when it is equal to K_c.

KEY CONCEPT

Remember that the exponents of the concentrations of the reactants and products are equal to their stoichiometric coefficients in the equilibrium expression but not in the kinetic rate law. Equilibrium expressions thus depend on the form in which the balanced equation is written, while rate laws do not.

C. Properties of the Equilibrium Constant

The equilibrium constant, K_{eq}, has the following characteristics:

- Pure solids and liquids do not appear in the equilibrium constant expression.
- K_{eq} is characteristic of a given system at a given temperature.
- If the value of K_{eq} is very large compared to 1, an equilibrium mixture of reactants and products will contain very little of the reactants compared to the products.

- If the value of K_{eq} is very small compared to 1 (i.e., less than 0.1), an equilibrium mixture of reactants and products will contain very little of the products compared to the reactants.
- If the value of K_{eq} is close to 1, an equilibrium mixture of products and reactants will contain approximately equal amounts of reactants and products.

D. Le Châtelier's Principle

The French chemist Henry Louis Le Châtelier stated that a system to which a stress is applied tends to change so as to relieve the applied stress. This rule, known as **Le Châtelier's principle**, is used to determine the direction in which a reaction at equilibrium will proceed when subjected to a stress, such as a change in concentration, pressure, temperature, or volume.

1. CHANGES IN CONCENTRATION

Increasing the concentration of a species will tend to shift the equilibrium away from the species that is added to re-establish its equilibrium concentration, and vice versa. For example, in the reaction

$$A + B \rightleftharpoons C + D$$

if the concentration of A and/or B is increased, the equilibrium will shift towards (or favor production of) C and D. Conversely, if the concentration of C and/or D is increased, the equilibrium will shift away from the production of C and D, favoring production of A and B. Similarly, decreasing the concentration of a species will tend to shift the equilibrium towards the production of that species. For example, if A and/or B is removed from the above reaction, the equilibrium will shift so as to favor increasing concentration of A and B.

This effect is often used in industry to increase the yield of a useful product or drive a reaction to completion. If D were constantly removed from the above reaction, the net reaction would produce more D and concurrently more C. Likewise, using an excess of the least expensive reactant helps to drive the reaction forward.

2. CHANGES IN PRESSURE OR VOLUME

In a system at constant temperature, a change in pressure causes a change in volume, and vice versa. Since liquids and solids are practically incompressible, a change in the pressure or volume of systems involving only these phases has little or no effect on their equilibrium. Reactions involving gases, however, may be greatly affected by changes in pressure or volume, since gases are highly compressible.

Pressure and volume are inversely related. An increase in the pressure of a system will shift the equilibrium so as to decrease the number of moles of gas present. This reduces the volume of the system and relieves the stress of the increased pressure. Consider the following reaction:

$$N_2\ (g) + 3\ H_2\ (g) \rightleftharpoons 2\ NH_3\ (g)$$

The left side of the reaction has 4 moles of gaseous molecules, whereas the right side has only 2 moles. When the pressure of this system is increased, the equilibrium will shift so that the side of the reaction producing fewer moles is favored. Since there are fewer moles on the right, the equilibrium will shift towards the right. Conversely, if the volume of the same system is increased, its pressure immediately decre- ases, which, according to Le Châtelier's principle, leads to a shift in the equilibrium to the left.

3. CHANGES IN TEMPERATURE

Changes in temperature also affect equilibrium. To predict this effect, heat may be considered as a product in an exothermic reaction and as a reactant in an endothermic reaction. Consider the following exothermic reaction:

$$A \rightleftharpoons B + heat$$

If this system were placed in an ice bath, its temperature would decrease, driving the reaction to the right to replace the heat lost. Conversely, if the system were placed in a boiling-water bath, the reaction equilibrium would shift to the left due to the increased "concentration" of heat.

Not only does a temperature change alter the position of the equilibrium, it also alters the numerical value of the equilibrium constant. In contrast, changes in the concentration of a species in the reaction, in the pressure, or in the volume will alter the position of the equilibrium without changing the numerical value of the equilibrium constant.

KEY CONCEPT

$$A + B \rightleftharpoons C + heat$$

will shift to

1. If more A or B added
2. If C taken away
3. If pressure applied or volume reduced (assuming A, B, and C are gases)
4. If temp. reduced

will shift to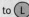

1. If more C added
2. If A or B taken away
3. If pressure reduced or volume increased (assuming A, B, and C are gases)
4. If temp. increaced

6

Thermochemistry

All chemical reactions are accompanied by energy changes. Thermal, chemical, potential, and kinetic energies are all interconvertible, as they must obey the **Law of Conservation of Energy.** Energy changes determine whether reactions can occur and how easily they will do so. Thus, an understanding of **thermodynamics** is essential to an understanding of chemistry. In chemistry, thermodynamics helps determine whether a chemical reaction is **spontaneous** (i.e., if under a given set of conditions it can occur by itself without outside assistance). A spontaneous reaction may or may not proceed to completion, depending upon the rate of the reaction, which is determined by chemical kinetics.

The application of thermodynamics to chemical reactions is called **thermochemistry.** Several thermodynamic definitions are very useful in thermochemistry. A **system** is the particular part of the universe being studied; everything outside the system is considered the **surroundings** or **environment.** A system may be:

- **isolated:** It cannot exchange energy or matter with the surroundings, as with an insulated bomb reactor.
- **closed:** It can exchange energy but not matter with the surroundings, as with a steam radiator.
- **open:** It can exchange both matter and energy with the surroundings, as with a pot of boiling water.

A system undergoes a **process** when one or more of its properties changes. A process is associated with a change of state. An **isothermal** process occurs when the temperature of the system remains constant, an **adiabatic** process occurs when no heat exchange occurs, and an **isobaric** process occurs when the pressure of the system remains constant. Isothermal and isobaric processes are common, since it is usually easy to control temperature and pressure.

HEAT

A. Definition

Heat is a form of energy that can easily transfer to or from a system, the result of a temperature difference between the system and its surroundings; this transfer will occur spontaneously from a warmer system to a cooler system. According to convention, heat absorbed by a system (from its surroundings) is considered positive, while heat lost by a system (to its surroundings) is considered negative.

Heat change is the most common energy change in chemical processes. Reactions that absorb heat energy are said to be **endothermic**, while those that release heat energy are said to be **exothermic**. Heat is commonly measured in **calories (cal)** or **joules (J)** and, more commonly, in kcal or kJ (1 cal = 4.184 J).

B. Calorimetry

Calorimetry measures heat changes. The terms **constant-volume calorimetry** and **constant-pressure calorimetry** are used to indicate the conditions under which the heat changes are measured. The heat (q) absorbed or released in a given process is calculated from this equation:

$$q = mc\Delta T$$

where m is the mass, c is the **specific heat**, and ΔT is the change in temperature.

1. CONSTANT-VOLUME CALORIMETRY

In constant-volume calorimetry, the volume of the container holding the reacting mixture does not change during the course of the reaction. The heat of reaction is measured using a device called a bomb calorimeter. This apparatus consists of a steel bomb into which the reactants are placed. The bomb is immersed in an insulated container containing a known amount of water. The reactants are electrically ignited, and heat is absorbed or evolved as the reaction proceeds. The heat of the reaction, q_{rxn}, can be determined as follows.

Since no heat enters or leaves the system, the net heat change for the system is zero; therefore, the heat change for the reaction is compensated for by the heat change for the water (q_{water}) and the bomb (q_{steel}), which is easy to measure.

$$q_{system} = q_{rxn} + q_{water} + q_{steel} = 0$$

Thus: $q_{rxn} = -(q_{water} + q_{steel})$

$$= -(m_{water}\, c_{water}\, \Delta T + m_{steel}\, c_{steel}\, \Delta T)$$

Note that the overall system, as defined, is adiabatic, since no net heat gain or loss occurs. However, the heat exchange between the various components makes it possible to determine the heat of reaction.

STATES AND STATE FUNCTIONS

The state of a system is described by the macroscopic properties of the system. Examples of macroscopic properties include temperature (T), pressure (P), and volume (V). When the state of a system changes, the values of the properties also change. Properties whose magnitude depends only on the initial and final states of the system, and not on the path of the change (how the change was accomplished), are known as **state functions**. Pressure, temperature, and volume are important state functions. Other examples are **enthalpy (H)**, **entropy (S)**, **free energy (G)** (all discussed below) and **internal energy (E or U)**. Although independent of path, state functions are not necessarily independent of one another.

A set of **standard conditions** (25°C and 1 atm) is normally used for measuring the enthalpy, entropy, and free energy of a reaction. A substance in its most stable form under standard conditions is said to be in its **standard state**. Examples of substances in their standard states include hydrogen as $H_2(g)$, water as $H_2O(<)$, and salt as $NaCl(s)$. The changes in enthalpy, entropy, and free energy that occur when a reaction takes place under standard conditions are called the **standard enthalpy**, **standard entropy**, and **standard free energy** changes respectively and are symbolized by $\Delta H°$, $\Delta S°$, and $\Delta G°$.

KEY CONCEPT

Standard conditions in thermodynamics must not be confused with standard temperature and pressure (STP) in gas law calculations.

A. Enthalpy

Most reactions in the lab occur under constant pressure (at 1 atm, in open containers). To express heat changes at constant pressure, chemists use the term **enthalpy (H)**. The change in enthalpy (ΔH) of a process is equal to the heat absorbed or evolved by the system at constant pressure. The enthalpy of a process depends only on the enthalpies of the initial and final states, *not* on the path. Thus, to find the enthalpy change of a reaction, ΔH_{rxn}, one must subtract the enthalpy of the reactants from the enthalpy of the products:

$$\Delta H_{rxn} = H_{products} - H_{reactants}$$

A positive ΔH corresponds to an endothermic process, and a negative ΔH corresponds to an exothermic process.

Unfortunately, it is not possible to measure H directly; only ΔH can be measured and, even then, only for certain fast and spontaneous processes. Thus, several standard methods have been developed to calculate ΔH for any process.

1. STANDARD HEAT OF FORMATION

The enthalpy of formation of a compound, $\Delta H°_f$, is the enthalpy change that would occur if one mole of a compound were formed directly from its elements in their standard states. Note that $\Delta H°_f$ of an element in its standard state is zero. The $\Delta H°_f$ of most known substances have been calculated.

2. STANDARD HEAT OF REACTION

The standard heat of a reaction, $\Delta H°_{rxn}$, is the hypothetical enthalpy change that would occur if the reaction were carried out under standard conditions (i.e., when reactants in their standard states are converted to products in their standard states at 298 K). It can be expressed as follows:

$$\Delta H°_{rxn} = \text{(sum of } \Delta H°_f \text{ of products)} - \text{(sum of } \Delta H°_f \text{ of reactants)}$$

3. HESS'S LAW

Hess's Law states that enthalpies of reactions are additive. When *thermochemical equations* (chemical equations for which energy changes are known) are added to give the net equation for a reaction, the corresponding heats of reaction are also added to give the net heat of reaction. Because enthalpy is a state function, the enthalpy of a reaction does not depend on the path taken but only on the initial and final states. For example, consider this reaction:

$$Br_2 (\ell) \rightarrow Br_2 (g) \quad \Delta H = (31 \text{ kJ/mol})(1 \text{ mol}) = 31 \text{ kJ}$$

The enthalpy change of the above reaction, called the **heat of vaporization**, $\Delta H°_{vap}$, will always be 31 kJ/mol, provided that the same initial and final states, $Br_2(\ell)$ and $Br_2(g)$ respectively, exist at standard conditions. $Br_2(\ell)$ could instead be decomposed to Br atoms and then recombined to form $Br_2(g)$, but since the net reaction is the same, the change in enthalpy will always be the same.

$$\begin{array}{lll} Br_2 (\ell) & \rightarrow 2\ Br\ (g) & \Delta H_1 \\ 2\ Br\ (g) & \rightarrow Br_2\ (g) & \Delta H_2 \\ \hline Br_2\ (\ell) & \rightarrow Br_2\ (g) & \Delta H = \Delta H_1 + \Delta H_2 = 31\ \text{kJ} \end{array}$$

Example: Given the following thermochemical equations,

a) $C_3H_8 (g) + 5 O_2 (g) \rightarrow 3 CO_2 (g) + 4 H_2O (\ell)$ $\Delta H_a = -2220.1$ kJ

b) $C (graphite) + O_2 (g) \rightarrow CO_2 (g)$ $\Delta H_b = -393.5$ kJ

c) $H_2 (g) + 1/2\ O_2 (g) \rightarrow H_2O (\ell)$ $\Delta H_c = -285.8$ kJ

calculate ΔH for this reaction:

d) $3 C (graphite) + 4 H_2 (g) \rightarrow C_3H_8 (g)$

Solution: Equations a, b, and c must be combined to obtain equation d. Since equation d contains only C, H_2, and C_3H_8, we must eliminate O_2, CO_2, and H_2O from the first three equations. Equation a is reversed to get C_3H_8 on the product side (this gives equation e).

e) $3 CO_2 + (g) + 4 H_2O + (\ell) \rightarrow C_3H_8 (g) + 5 O_2 (g)$ $\Delta H_e = 2220.1$ kJ

Next, equation b is multiplied by 3 (this gives equation f) and c by 4 (this gives equation g). The following addition is done to obtain the required equation d: 3b + 4c + e.

f) $3 CO_2 (g) + 4 H_2O (\ell) \rightarrow C_3H_8 (g) + 5 O_2$ $\Delta H_e = 2220.1$ kJ

g) $3 \times [C (graphite) + O_2 (g) \rightarrow CO_2 (g)]$ $\Delta H_f = 3 \times -393.5$ kJ

h) $4 \times [H_2 (g) + \dfrac{1}{2}O_2 (g) \rightarrow H_2O (\ell)]$ $\Delta H_g = 4 \times -285.8$ kJ

$3 C (graphite) + 4 H_2 (g) \rightarrow C_3H_8 (g)$ $\Delta H_d = -103.6$ kJ

where $\Delta H_d = \Delta H_e + \Delta H_f + \Delta H_g$.

It is important to note that the reverse of any reaction has an enthalpy of the same magnitude as that of the forward reaction, but its sign is opposite.

4. BOND DISSOCIATION ENERGY

Heats of reaction are related to changes in energy associated with the breakdown and formation of chemical bonds. **Bond energy,** or **bond dissociation energy,** is an average of the energy required to break a particular type of bond in one mole of gaseous molecules. It is calculated as the positive value of the energy absorbed as the bonds are broken. For example:

$$H_2 (g) \rightarrow 2H (g) \quad \Delta H = 436 \text{ kJ}$$

A molecule of H_2 gas is cleaved to produce two gaseous, unassociated hydrogen atoms. For each mole of H_2 gas cleaved, roughly 436 kJ of energy is absorbed by the system. The reaction is therefore endothermic. For bonds found in other than diatomic molecules,

KEY CONCEPT

Since it takes energy to pull two atoms apart, bond breakage is always endothermic. Bond formation is the reverse process and, thus, must always be exothermic.

many compounds have been measured and the energy requirements averaged. For example, the C–H bond dissociation energy one would find in a table (415 kJ/mol) was compiled from measurements on thousands of different organic compounds. (See the Organic Chemistry section.)

Bond energies can be used to estimate enthalpies of reactions. The enthalpy change of a reaction is given by

$$\Delta H_{rxn} = (\Delta H \text{ of bonds broken}) + (\Delta H \text{ of bonds formed})$$

$$= \text{total energy input} - \text{total energy released}$$

Example: Calculate the enthalpy change for the following reaction:

$$C\ (s) + 2\ H_2\ (g) \rightarrow CH_4\ (g)\quad \Delta H = ?$$

Bond dissociation energies of H–H and C–H bonds are 436 kJ/mol and 415 kJ/mol, respectively. ΔH_f of C (g) = 715 kJ/mol.

Solution: CH_4 is formed from free elements in their standard states (C in solid and H_2 in gaseous state).

Thus here, $\Delta H_{rxn} = \Delta H_f$.

The reaction can be written as three steps:

a) $C\ (s) \rightarrow C\ (g)$ $\qquad\qquad\qquad \Delta H_1$

b) $2\ [H_2\ (g) \rightarrow 2\ H\ (g)]$ $\qquad\quad 2\Delta H_2$

c) $C\ (g) + 4\ H\ (g) \rightarrow CH_4\ (g)$ $\quad \Delta H_3$

and $\Delta H_f = [\Delta H_1 + 2\Delta H_2] + [\Delta H_3]$.

$\qquad \Delta H_1 = \Delta H_f\ C(g) = 715$ kJ/mol

ΔH_2 is the energy required to break the H–H bond of one mole of H_2,

so

$$\Delta H_2 = \text{bond energy of } H_2$$

$$= 436 \text{ kJ/mol}$$

ΔH_3 is the energy released when 4 C–H bonds are formed,

so

$$\Delta H_3 = -(4 \times \text{bond energy of C–H})$$

$$= -(4 \times 415 \text{ kJ/mol})$$

$$= -1,660 \text{ kJ/mol}$$

[Note: Since energy is released when bonds are formed, ΔH_3 is negative.]

Therefore:

$$\Delta H_{rxn} = \Delta H_f = [715 + 2(436)] - 1{,}660 \text{ kJ/mol} = -73 \text{ kJ/mol}$$

5. HEATS OF COMBUSTION

One more type of standard enthalpy change that is often used is the standard heat of combustion, $\Delta H°_{comb}$. As stated earlier, a requirement for relatively easy measurement of ΔH is that the reaction be fast and spontaneous; combustion generally fits this description. The reactions used in the C_3H_8 (g) example above were combustion reactions, and the corresponding values ΔH_a, ΔH_b, and ΔH_c were thus heats of combustion.

B. Entropy

Entropy (S) is a measure of the disorder, or randomness, of a system. The units of entropy are energy/temperature, commonly J/K or cal/K. The greater the order in a system, the lower the entropy; the greater the disorder or randomness, the higher the entropy. At any given temperature, a solid will have lower entropy than a gas, because individual molecules in the gaseous state are moving randomly, while individual molecules in a solid are constrained in place. Entropy is a state function, so a change in entropy depends only on the initial and final states:

$$\Delta S = S_{final} - S_{initial}$$

A change in entropy is also given by

$$\Delta S = \frac{q_{rev}}{T}$$

where q_{rev} is the heat added to the system undergoing a reversible process (a process that proceeds with infinitesimal changes in the system's conditions) and T is the absolute temperature.

A standard entropy change for a reaction, $\Delta S°$, is calculated using the standard entropies of reactants and products:

$$\Delta S°_{rxn} = (\text{sum of } S°_{products}) - (\text{sum of } S°_{reactants})$$

The second law of thermodynamics states that all spontaneous processes proceed such that the entropy of the system plus its surroundings (i.e., the entropy of the universe) increases:

$$\Delta S_{universe} = \Delta S_{system} + \Delta S_{surroundings} > 0$$

KEY CONCEPT

Entropy changes accompanying phase changes can be easily estimated, at least qualitatively. For example, freezing is accompanied by a decrease in entropy, as the relatively disordered liquid becomes a well-ordered solid. Meanwhile, boiling is accompanied by a large increase in entropy, as the liquid becomes a much more highly disordered gas. For any substance, sublimation will be the phase transition with the greatest entropy change.

A system reaches its maximum entropy at **equilibrium,** a state in which no observable change takes place as time goes on. For a reversible process, $\Delta S_{universe}$ is zero:

$$\Delta S_{universe} = \Delta S_{system} + \Delta S_{surroundings} = 0$$

A system will spontaneously tend towards an equilibrium state if left alone.

C. Gibbs Free Energy

1. SPONTANEITY OF REACTION

The thermodynamic state function, **G** (known as the **Gibbs free energy**), combines the two factors that affect the spontaneity of a reaction—changes in enthalpy, ΔH, and changes in entropy, ΔS. The change in the free energy of a system, ΔG, represents the maximum amount of energy released by a process, occurring at constant temperature and pressure, that is available to perform useful work. ΔG is defined by this equation:

$$\Delta G = \Delta H - T\Delta S$$

where T is the absolute temperature and $T\Delta S$ represents the total amount of heat absorbed by a system when its entropy increases reversibly.

In the equilibrium state, free energy is at a minimum. A process can occur spontaneously if the Gibbs function decreases (i.e., $\Delta G < 0$).

1. If ΔG is negative, the reaction is spontaneous.

2. If ΔG is positive, the reaction is not spontaneous.

3. If ΔG is zero, the system is in a state of equilibrium;

   thus, $\Delta G = 0$ and $\Delta H = T\Delta S$.

Because the temperature is always positive (i.e., in Kelvins), the effects of the signs of ΔH and ΔS and the effect of temperature on spontaneity can be summarized as follows:

ΔH	ΔS	Outcome
–	+	spontaneous at all temperatures
+	–	nonspontaneous at all temperatures
+	+	spontaneous only at high temperatures
–	–	spontaneous only at low temperatures

It is very important to note that the **rate** of a reaction depends on the **activation energy,** not the ΔG.

2. STANDARD FREE ENERGY

Standard free energy, $\Delta G°$, is defined as the ΔG of a process occurring at 25°C and 1 atm pressure, and for which the concentrations of any solutions involved are 1 M. The standard free energy of formation of a compound, $\Delta G°_f$, is the free-energy change that occurs when 1 mol of a compound in its standard state is formed from its elements in their standard states under standard conditions. The standard free energy of formation of any element in its most stable form (and, therefore, its standard state) is zero. The standard free energy of a reaction, $\Delta G°_{rxn}$, is the free energy change that occurs when that reaction is carried out under standard state conditions (i.e., when the reactants in their standard states are converted to the products in their standard states, at standard conditions of T and P). For example: Conversion of C(*diamond*) to C(*graphite*) is spontaneous under standard conditions. However, its rate is so slow that the reaction is never observed.

$$\Delta G°_{rxn} = \text{(sum of } \Delta G°_f \text{ of products)} - \text{(sum of } \Delta G°_f \text{ of reactants)}$$

REMEMBER

Recall that thermodynamics and kinetics are separate topic areas. In thermodynamics, *spontaneous* does not necessarily mean *instantaneous*.

3. REACTION QUOTIENT

$\Delta G°_{rxn}$ can also be derived from the equilibrium constant for the equation:

$$\Delta G° = -RT \ln K_{eq}$$

where K_{eq} is the equilibrium constant, R is the gas constant, and T is the temperature in K.

BRIDGE

Note the similarity of this equation to Hess's Law. Almost any state function could be substituted for ΔG here.

Once a reaction commences, however, the standard state conditions no longer hold. K_{eq} must be replaced by another parameter, the **reaction quotient (Q)**. For the reaction $a\, A + b\, B \rightleftharpoons c\, C + d\, D$,

$$Q = \frac{[C]^c\, [D]^d}{[A]^a\, [B]^b}$$

Likewise, ΔG must be used in place of $\Delta G°$. The relationship between the two is as follows:

$$\Delta G = \Delta G° + RT \ln Q$$

where R is the gas constant and T is the temperature in K.

4. EXAMPLES

a. Vaporization of water at one atmosphere pressure

$$H_2O\, (\ell) + \text{heat} \rightarrow H_2O\, (g)$$

When water boils, hydrogen bonds (H-bonds) are broken. Energy is absorbed (the reaction is endothermic), and thus ΔH is positive. Entropy increases as the closely packed molecules of the liquid become the more randomly moving molecules of a gas; thus, $T\Delta S$ is also positive. Since ΔH and $T\Delta S$ are each positive, the reaction will proceed spontaneously only if $T\Delta S > \Delta H$. This is true only at temperatures above 100°C. Below 100°C, ΔG is positive, and the water remains a liquid. At 100°C, $\Delta H = T\Delta S$ and $\Delta G = 0$: An equilibrium is established between water and water vapor. The opposite is true when water vapor condenses. H-bonds are formed, and energy is released; the reaction is exothermic (ΔH is negative) and entropy decreases, since a liquid is forming from a gas ($T\Delta S$ is negative). Condensation will be spontaneous only if $\Delta H < T\Delta S$. This is the case at temperatures below 100°C. Above 100°C, $T\Delta S$ is more negative than H, ΔG is positive, and condensation is not spontaneous. Again, at 100°C, an equilibrium is established.

b. **The combustion of C_6H_6 (benzene)**

$$2\ C_6H_6\ (\ell) + 15\ O_2\ (g) \rightarrow 12\ CO_2\ (g) + 6\ H_2O\ (g) + heat$$

In this case, heat is released (ΔH is negative) as the benzene burns and the entropy is increased ($T\Delta S$ is positive), because two gases (18 moles total) have greater entropy than a gas and a liquid (15 moles gas and 2 liquid). ΔG is negative, and the reaction is spontaneous.

7

The Gas Phase

Matter can exist in three different physical forms, called **phases** or **states: gas, liquid,** and **solid.**

The gaseous phase, the subject of this chapter, is the simplest to understand, since all gases display similar behavior and follow similar laws regardless of their identity. The atoms or molecules in a gaseous sample move rapidly and are far apart from each other. In addition, only very weak intermolecular forces exist between gas particles; this results in certain characteristic physical properties, such as the ability to expand to fill any volume and to take on the shape of a container. Furthermore, gases are easily, though not infinitely, compressible.

The state of a gaseous sample is generally defined by four variables: pressure (P), volume (V), temperature (T), and number of moles (n). Gas pressures are usually expressed in units of atmospheres (atm) or millimeters of mercury (mm Hg or torr), which are related as follows:

$$1 \text{ atm} = 760 \text{ mm Hg} = 760 \text{ torr}$$

Volume is generally expressed in liters (L) or milliliters (mL). The temperature of a gas is usually given in Kelvin (K, *not* °K). Gases are often discussed in terms of **standard temperature and pressure (STP),** which refers to conditions of 273.15 K (0°C) and 1 atm.

Note: It is important not to confuse **STP** with **standard conditions**—the two standards involve different temperatures and are used for different purposes. STP (0°C or 273 K) is generally used for gas law calculations; standard conditions (25°C or 298 K) is used when measuring standard enthalpy, entropy, Gibbs free energy, and voltage.

IDEAL GASES

When examining the behavior of gases under varying conditions of temperature and pressure, scientists speak of ideal gases. An ideal gas represents a hypothetical gas whose molecules have no intermolecular forces and occupy no volume. Although gases actually deviate from this idealized behavior, at relatively low pressures (atmospheric pressure) and high temperatures, many gases behave in a nearly ideal fashion. Therefore, the assumptions used for ideal gases can be applied to real gases with reasonable accuracy.

A. Boyle's Law

Experimental studies performed by Robert Boyle in 1660 led to the formulation of Boyle's Law. His work showed that for a given gaseous sample held at constant temperature (isothermal conditions), the volume of the gas is inversely proportional to its pressure:

$$PV = k \text{ or } P_1V_1 = P_2V_2$$

where k is a proportionality constant and the subscripts 1 and 2 represent two different sets of conditions. A plot of pressure versus volume for a gas is shown in Figure 7.1.

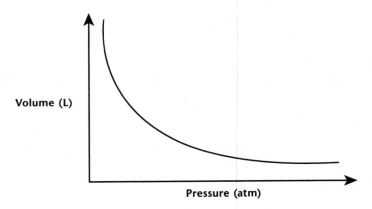

Figure 7.1

Example: Under isothermal conditions, what would be the volume of a 1 L sample of helium after its pressure is changed from 12 atm to 4 atm?

Solution:

$P_1 = 12$ atm $P_2 = 4$ atm

$V_1 = 1$ L $V_2 = x$

$P_1V_1 = P_2V_2$

12 atm (1 L) = 4 atm (x)

$$\frac{12 \text{ atm (1L)}}{4 \text{ atm}} = x$$

$x = 3$ L

B. Law of Charles and Gay-Lussac

The Law of Charles and Gay-Lussac, or simply Charles' Law, was developed during the early 19th century. The law states that at constant pressure, the volume of a gas is directly proportional to its absolute temperature. The absolute temperature is the temperature expressed in Kelvin, which can be calculated from the expression $T_K = T_{^\circ C} + 273.15$.

$$\frac{V}{T} = k \quad \text{or} \quad \frac{V_1}{T_1} = \frac{V_2}{T_2}$$

where k is a constant and the subscripts 1 and 2 represent two different sets of conditions. A plot of temperature versus volume is shown in Figure 7.2.

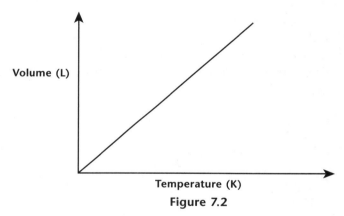

Figure 7.2

Example: If the absolute temperature of 2 L of gas at constant pressure is changed from 283.15 K to 566.30 K, what would be the final volume?

Solution:

$$T_1 = 283.15 \text{ K} \qquad V_1 = 2 \text{ L}$$
$$T_2 = 566.30 \text{ K} \qquad V_2 = x$$

$$\frac{V_1}{T_1} = \frac{V_2}{T_2}$$

$$\frac{2 \text{ L}}{283.15 \text{ K}} = \frac{x}{566.30 \text{ K}}$$

$$x = \frac{2 \text{ L}(566.30 \text{ K})}{283.15 \text{ K}}$$

$$x = 4 \text{ L}$$

C. Avogadro's Principle

In 1811, Amedeo Avogadro proposed that for all gases at a constant temperature and pressure, the volume of the gas will be directly proportional to the number of moles of gas present; therefore, all gases have the same number of moles in the same volume.

$$\frac{n}{V} = k \text{ or } \frac{n_1}{V_1} = \frac{n_2}{V_2}$$

The subscripts 1 and 2 once again apply to two different sets of conditions with the same temperature and pressure.

D. Ideal Gas Law

The ideal gas law combines the relationships outlined in Boyle's Law, Charles' Law, and Avogadro's Principle to yield an expression that can be used to predict the behavior of a gas. The ideal gas law shows the relationship among four variables that define a sample of gas—pressure (P), volume (V), temperature (T), and number of moles (n)—and is represented by the equation

$$PV = nRT$$

The constant R is known as the **gas constant.** Under STP conditions (273.15 K and 1 atmosphere), 1 mole of gas was shown to have a volume of 22.4 L. Substituting these values into the ideal gas equation gave R = 8.21×10^{-2} L · atm/(mol · K).

The gas constant may be expressed in many other units: Another common value is 8.314 J/(K · mol), which is derived when SI units of pascals (for pressure) and cubic meters (for volume) are substituted into the ideal gas law. **When carrying out calculations based on the ideal gas law, it is important to choose a value of R that matches the units of the variables.**

Example: What volume would 12 g of helium occupy at 20°C and a pressure of 380 mm Hg?

Solution: The ideal gas law can be used, but first, all of the variables must be converted to yield units that will correspond to the expression of the gas constant as 0.0821 L · atm/(mol · K).

$$P = 380 \text{ mm Hg} \times \frac{1 \text{ atm}}{760 \text{ mm Hg}} = 0.5 \text{ atm}$$

$$T = 20°C + 273.15 = 293.15 \text{ K}$$

$$n = 12 \text{ g He} \times \frac{1 \text{mol He}}{4.0 \text{ Hg}} = 3 \text{ mol He}$$

Substitute to the ideal gas equation:

$$PV = nRT$$

$$(0.5 \text{ atm})(V) = (3 \text{ mol})(0.0821 \text{ L} \cdot \text{atm}/(\text{mol} \cdot \text{K})(293.15 \text{ K})$$

$$V = 144.4 \text{ L}$$

In addition to standard calculations to determine the pressure, volume, or temperature of a gas, the ideal gas law may be used to determine the **density** and molar mass of the gas.

1. DENSITY

Density is defined as the mass per unit volume of a substance and, for gases, is usually expressed in units of g/L. By rearrangement, the ideal gas equation can be used to calculate the density of a gas.

$$PV = nRT$$

$$\text{where} \quad n = \frac{m}{MM} = \frac{(\text{mass in g})}{(\text{molar mass})}$$

$$\text{therefore} \quad PV = \frac{m}{MM} RT$$

$$\text{and} \quad d = \frac{m}{V} = \frac{P(MM)}{RT}$$

Another way to find the density of a gas is to start with the volume of a mole of gas at STP, 22.4 L; calculate the effect of pressure and temperature on the volume; and finally calculate the density by dividing the mass by the new volume. The following equation, derived from Boyle's and Charles' Laws, is used to relate changes in the temperature, volume, and pressure of a gas:

$$\frac{P_1 V_1}{T_1} = \frac{P_2 V_2}{T_2}$$

where the subscripts 1 and 2 refer to the two states of the gas (at STP and under the actual conditions). To calculate a change in volume, the equation is rearranged as follows:

$$V_2 = V_1 \left(\frac{P_1}{P_2} \right) \left(\frac{T_2}{T_1} \right)$$

V_2 is then used to find the density of the gas under nonstandard conditions.

$$d = \frac{m}{V_2}$$

If you *visualize* how the changes in pressure and temperature affect the volume of the gas, this can serve as a check to be sure you have not accidentally confused the pressure or temperature value that belongs in the numerator with the one that belongs in the denominator.

Example: What is the density of HCl gas at 2 atm and 45°C?

Solution: At STP, a mole of gas occupies 22.4 liters. Since the increase in pressure to 2 atm decreases volume, 22.4 L must be multiplied by $\left(\dfrac{1\,atm}{2\,atm}\right)$. And since the increase in temperature increases volume, the temperature factor will be $\left(\dfrac{318\,K}{273\,K}\right)$.

$$V_2 = \left(\frac{22.4\,L}{mol}\right)\left(\frac{1\,atm}{2\,atm}\right)\left(\frac{318\,K}{273\,K}\right) = \frac{13.0\,L}{mol}$$

$$d = \left(\frac{36\,g/mol}{13.0\,L/mol}\right) = 2.77\,g/L$$

2. MOLAR MASS

Sometimes the identity of a gas is unknown, and the molar mass must be determined in order to identify it. Using the equation for density derived from the ideal gas law, the molar mass of a gas can be determined experimentally as follows. The pressure and temperature of a gas contained in a bulb of a given volume are measured, and the weight of the bulb plus sample is found. Then, the bulb is evacuated, and the empty bulb is weighed. The weight of the bulb plus sample minus the weight of the bulb yields the weight of the sample. Finally, the density of the sample is determined by dividing the weight of the sample by the volume of the bulb. The density at STP is calculated. The molecular weight is then found by multiplying the number of grams per liter by 22.4 liters per mole.

Example: What is the molar mass of a 2 L sample of gas that weighs 8 g at a temperature of 15°C and a pressure of 1.5 atm?

$$d = \frac{8\,g}{2\,L} \text{ at } 15°C \text{ and } 1.5\,atm$$

$$V_{STP} = (2\,L)\left(\frac{273\,K}{288\,K}\right)\left(\frac{1.5\,atm}{1\,atm}\right) = 2.84\,L$$

$$\frac{8\,g}{2.84\,L} = 2.82\,g/L \text{ at STP}$$

$$\left(\frac{2.82\,g}{L}\right)\left(\frac{22.4\,L}{mol}\right) = 63.2\,g/mol$$

REAL GASES

In general, the ideal gas law is a good approximation of the behavior of real gases, but all real gases deviate from ideal gas behavior to some extent, particularly when the gas atoms or molecules are forced into close proximity under high pressure and at low temperature so that molecular volume and intermolecular attractions become significant.

> **REMEMBER**
>
> At high temperature and low pressure, deviations from ideality are usually small; good approximations can still be made from the ideal gas law.

A. Deviations Due to Pressure

As the pressure of a gas increases, the particles are pushed closer and closer together. As the condensation pressure for a given temperature is approached, intermolecular attraction forces become more and more significant until the gas condenses into the liquid state.

At moderately high pressure (a few hundred atmospheres), a gas's volume is less than would be predicted by the ideal gas law due to intermolecular attraction. At extremely high pressure, the size of the particles becomes relatively large compared to the distance between them, and this causes the gas to take up a larger volume than would be predicted by the ideal gas law.

B. Deviations Due to Temperature

As the temperature of a gas is decreased, the average velocity of the gas molecules decreases, and the attractive intermolecular forces become increasingly significant. As the condensation temperature is approached for a given pressure, intermolecular attractions eventually cause the gas to condense to a liquid state.

As the temperature of a gas is reduced towards its condensation point (which is the same as its boiling point), intermolecular attraction causes the gas to have a smaller volume than would be predicted by the ideal gas law. The closer the temperature of a gas is to its boiling point, the less ideal is its behavior.

DALTON'S LAW OF PARTIAL PRESSURES

When two or more gases are found in one vessel without chemical interaction, each gas will behave independently of the other(s). Therefore, the pressure exerted by each gas in the mixture will be equal to the pressure that gas would exert if it were the only one in the container. The pressure exerted by each individual gas is called the **partial pressure** of that gas. In 1801, John Dalton derived an expression, now known as **Dalton's Law of Partial Pressures,** which states that the total pressure of a gaseous mixture is equal to the sum of the partial pressures of the individual components. The equation is

$$P_T = P_A + P_B + P_C + \dots$$

The partial pressure of a gas is related to its mole fraction and can be determined using the following equations:

$$P_A = P_T x_A$$

where

$$x_A = \frac{n_A}{n_T} = \frac{\text{moles of A}}{\text{total moles}}$$

Example: A vessel contains 0.75 mol of nitrogen, 0.20 mol of hydrogen, and 0.05 mol of fluorine at a total pressure of 2.5 atm. What is the partial pressure of each gas?

First calculate the mole fraction of each gas.

$$x_{N_2} = \frac{0.75 \text{ mol}}{1.0 \text{ mol}} = 0.75 \quad x_{H_2} = \frac{0.20 \text{ mol}}{1.0 \text{ mol}} = 0.20 \quad x_{F_2} = \frac{0.05 \text{ mol}}{1.0 \text{ mol}} = 0.05$$

Then calculate the partial pressure.

$$P_A = x_A P_T$$

$$P_{N_2} = (2.5 \text{ atm})(0.75) \qquad P_{H_2} = (2.5 \text{ atm})(0.20) \qquad P_{F_2} = (2.5 \text{ atm})(0.05)$$
$$= 1.875 \text{ atm} \qquad\qquad = 0.5 \text{ atm} \qquad\qquad = 0.125 \text{ atm}$$

KINETIC MOLECULAR THEORY OF GASES

As indicated by the gas laws, all gases show similar physical characteristics and behavior. A theoretical model to explain the behavior of gases was developed during the second half of the 19th century. The combined efforts of Boltzmann, Maxwell, and others led to a simple explanation of gaseous molecular behavior based on the motion of individual molecules. This model is called the **Kinetic Molecular Theory of Gases**. Like the gas laws, this theory was developed in reference to ideal gases, although it can be applied with reasonable accuracy to real gases as well.

A. Assumptions of the Kinetic Molecular Theory

1. Gases are made up of particles whose volumes are negligible compared to the container volume.

2. Gas atoms or molecules exhibit no intermolecular attractions or repulsions.

3. Gas particles are in continuous, random motion, undergoing collisions with other particles and the container walls.

4. Collisions between any two gas particles are elastic, meaning that there is no overall gain or loss of energy.

5. The average kinetic energy of gas particles is proportional to the absolute temperature of the gas, and it is the same for all gases at a given temperature.

B. Applications of the Kinetic Molecular Theory of Gases

1. AVERAGE MOLECULAR SPEEDS

According to the kinetic molecular theory of gases, the average kinetic energy of a gas particle is proportional to the absolute temperature of the gas:

$$KE = \frac{1}{2}\,mv^2 = \frac{3}{2}\,kT$$

where k is the Boltzmann constant. The typical speed of a gas molecule is proportional to the square root of the absolute temperature.

A **Maxwell-Boltzmann distribution curve** shows the distribution of speeds of gas particles at a given temperature. Figure 7.3 shows a distribution curve of molecular speeds at two temperatures, T_1 and T_2, where $T_2 > T_1$. Notice that the bell-shaped curve flattens and shifts to the right as the temperature increases, indicating that at higher temperatures, more molecules are moving at high speeds.

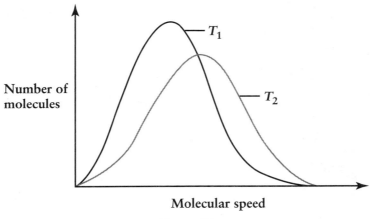

Number of molecules

Molecular speed

Figure 7.3

KEY CONCEPT

Like kinetic energy, the average molecular speed is constant at a given temperature.

2. GRAHAM'S LAW OF DIFFUSION AND EFFUSION

a. Diffusion

Diffusion occurs when gas molecules diffuse through a mixture. Diffusion accounts for the fact that an open bottle of perfume can quickly be smelled across a room. The kinetic molecular theory of gases predicted that heavier gas molecules diffuse more slowly than lighter ones because of their differing average speeds. In 1832, Thomas Graham showed mathematically that under isothermal and isobaric conditions, the rates at which two gases diffuse are inversely proportional to the square root of their molar masses. Thus,

$$\frac{r_1}{r_2} = \left(\frac{MM_2}{MM_1}\right)^{\frac{1}{2}} = \sqrt{\frac{MM_2}{MM_1}}$$

where r_1 and MM_1 represent the diffusion rate and molar mass of gas 1 and r_2 and MM_2 represent the diffusion rate and molar mass of gas 2.

b. Effusion

Effusion is the flow of gas particles under pressure from one compartment to another through a small opening. Graham used the kinetic molecular theory of gases to show that for two gases at the-same temperature, the rates of effusion are proportional to the average speeds. He then expressed the rates of effusion in terms of molar mass and found that the relationship is the same as that for diffusion:

$$\frac{r_1}{r_2} = \left(\frac{MM_2}{MM_1}\right)^{\frac{1}{2}}$$

8

Phases and Phase Changes

When the attractive forces between molecules (i.e., van der Waals forces) overcome the kinetic energy that keeps them apart, the molecules move closer together such that they can no longer move about freely, entering the **liquid** or **solid** phase. Because of their smaller volume relative to gases, liquids and solids are often referred to as the **condensed phases.**

LIQUIDS

In a liquid, atoms or molecules are held close together with little space between them. As a result, liquids have definite volumes and cannot easily be expanded or compressed. However, the molecules can still move around and are in a state of relative disorder. Consequently, the liquid can change shape to fit its container, and its molecules are able to **diffuse** and **evaporate.**

One of the most important properties of liquids is their ability to mix, both with each other and with other phases, to form **solutions.** The degree to which two liquids can mix is called their **miscibility.** Oil and water are almost completely **immiscible**; that is, their molecules tend to repel each other due to their polarity difference. Oil and water normally form separate layers when mixed, with oil on top because it is less dense. Under extreme conditions, such as violent shaking, two immiscible liquids can form a fairly homogeneous mixture called an **emulsion.** Although they look like solutions, emulsions are actually mixtures of discrete particles too small to be seen distinctly.

SOLIDS

In a solid, the attractive forces between atoms, ions, or molecules are strong enough to hold them rigidly together; thus, the particles' only motion is vibration about fixed positions, and the kinetic energy of solids is predominantly vibrational energy. As a result, solids have definite shapes and volumes.

A solid may be **crystalline** or **amorphous**. A crystalline solid, such as NaCl, possesses an ordered structure; its atoms exist in a specific, three-dimensional geometric arrangement with repeating patterns of atoms, ions, or molecules. An amorphous solid, such as glass, has no ordered three-dimensional arrangement, although the molecules are also fixed in place.

Most solids are crystalline in structure. The two most common forms of crystals are **metallic** and **ionic** crystals.

Ionic solids are aggregates of positively and negatively charged ions; there are no discrete molecules. The physical properties of ionic solids include high melting points, high boiling points, and poor electrical conductivity in the solid phase. These properties are due to the compounds' strong electrostatic interactions, which also cause the ions to be relatively immobile. Ionic structures are given by empirical formulas that describe the ratio of atoms in the lowest possible whole numbers. For example, the empirical formula $BaCl_2$ gives the ratio of barium to chloride within the crystal.

Metallic solids consist of metal atoms packed together as closely as possible. Metallic solids have high melting and boiling points as a result of their strong covalent attractions. Pure metallic structures (consisting of a single element) are usually described as layers of spheres of roughly similar radii.

The repeating units of crystals (both ionic and metallic) are represented by **unit cells**. There are many types of unit cells. We will now consider only the three cubic unit cells: **simple cubic, body-centered cubic,** and **face-centered cubic** (see Figure 8.1).

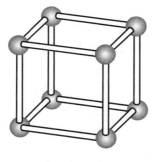
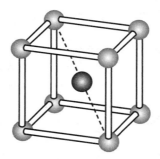
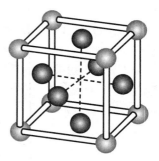

simple cubic

body-centered
cubic

face-centered
cubic

Figure 8.1

Atoms are represented as points but are actually adjoining spheres (see Figure 8.2). Each unit cell is surrounded by similar units. In the ionic unit cell, the spaces between points (anions) are filled with other ions (cations).

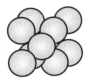

| simple cubic | body-centered cubic | face-centered cubic |

Figure 8.2

PHASE EQUILIBRIA

In an isolated system, phase changes (solid to liquid to gas) are reversible, and an equilibrium exists between phases. For example, at 1 atm and 0°C in an isolated system, an ice cube floating in water is in equilibrium. Some of the ice may absorb heat and melt, but an equal amount of water will release heat and freeze. Thus, the relative amounts of ice and water remain constant.

A. Gas-Liquid Equilibrium

The temperature of a liquid is related to the average kinetic energy of the liquid molecules; however, the kinetic energy of the molecules will vary. A few molecules near the surface of the liquid may have enough energy to leave the liquid phase and escape into the gaseous phase. This process is known as **evaporation** (or **vaporization**). Each time the liquid loses a high-energy particle, the temperature of the remaining liquid decreases; thus, evaporation is a cooling process. Given enough kinetic energy, the liquid will completely evaporate.

If a cover is placed on a beaker of liquid, the escaping molecules are trapped above the solution. These molecules exert a countering pressure, which forces some of the gas back into the liquid phase; this process is called **condensation.** Atmospheric pressure acts on a liquid in a similar fashion as a solid lid. As evaporation and condensation proceed, an equilibrium is reached in which the rates of the two processes become equal. Once this equilibrium is reached, the pressure that the gas exerts over the liquid is called the **vapor pressure** of the liquid. Vapor pressure increases as temperature increases, since more molecules have sufficient kinetic energy to escape into the gas phase. The temperature at which the vapor pressure of the liquid equals the external pressure is called the **boiling point.**

B. Liquid-Solid Equilibrium

The liquid and solid phases can also coexist in equilibrium (e.g., the ice-water mixture discussed above). Even though the atoms or molecules of a solid are confined to definite locations, each atom or molecule can undergo motions about some equilibrium position. These motions

BRIDGE

Note that ΔH will be positive for fusion, vaporization, or sublimation, as intermolecular attractions are being overcome. Note also that entropy increases for these same three phase transitions due to the increased disorder in the substance, and it is sensitive to pressure, which affects the motion of the particles.

As such, the equation $\Delta G = \Delta H - T\Delta S$ allows one to calculate the absolute temperature at which phase equilibria will exist at a given pressure.

(vibrations) increase when heat is applied. If atoms or molecules in the solid phase absorb enough energy in this fashion, the solid's three-dimensional structure breaks down, and the liquid phase begins. The transition from solid to liquid is called **fusion** or **melting**. The reverse process, from liquid to solid, is called **solidification**, **crystallization**, or **freezing**. The temperature at which these processes occur is called the **melting point** or **freezing point**, depending on the direction of the transition. Whereas pure crystals have distinct, very sharp melting points, amorphous solids, such as glass, tend to melt over a larger range of temperatures due to their less-ordered molecular distribution.

C. Gas-Solid Equilibrium

A third type of phase equilibrium is that between a gas and a solid. When a solid goes directly into the gas phase, the process is called **sublimation**. Dry ice (solid CO_2) sublimes; the absence of the liquid phase makes it a convenient refrigerant. The reverse transition, from the gaseous to the solid phase, is called **deposition.**

D. The Gibbs Function

The thermodynamic criterion for each of the above equilibria is that the change in Gibbs free energy must equal zero; $\Delta G = 0$. For an equilibrium between a gas and a solid,

$$\Delta G = G\,(g) - G\,(s),$$
$$\text{so } G\,(g) = G\,(s) \text{ at equilibrium.}$$

The same is true of the Gibbs functions for the other two equilibria.

PHASE DIAGRAMS

A. Single Component

REMEMBER

Every pure substance has a unique phase diagram.

A standard **phase diagram** depicts the phases and phase equilibria of a substance at defined temperatures and pressures. In general, the gas phase is found at high temperature and low pressure, the solid phase is found at low temperature and high pressure, and the liquid phase is found at high temperature and high pressure. A typical phase diagram is shown in Figure 8.3.

KEY CONCEPT

Note that while '*PT*' phase diagrams such as the one in Figure 8.3 are by far the most popular, any combination of the variables *P*, *V*, and *T* can be used to construct one.

The three phases are demarcated by lines indicating the temperatures and pressures at which two phases are in equilibrium. Line A represents freezing/melting, line B evaporation/condensation, and line C sublimation/deposition. The intersection of the three lines is called the **triple point**. At this temperature and pressure, unique for a given substance, all three phases are in equilibrium. The point at B is known as the **criti-**

cal point, the temperature and pressure above which no distinction between liquid and gas is possible.

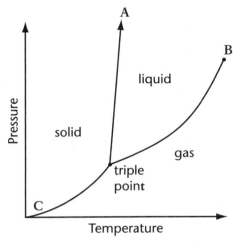

Figure 8.3

B. Multiple Components

The phase diagram for a mixture of two or more components (Figure 8.4) is complicated by the requirement that the composition of the mixture, as well as the temperature and pressure, must be specified. Consider a solution of two liquids, A and B. The vapor above the solution is a mixture of the vapors of A and B. The pressures exerted by vapor A and vapor B on the solution are the vapor pressures that each exerts above its individual liquid phase. **Raoult's Law** (described below) enables one to determine the relationship between the vapor pressure of vapor A and the concentration of liquid A in the solution.

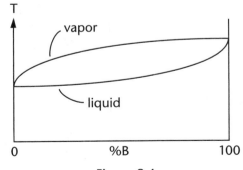

Figure 8.4

COLLIGATIVE PROPERTIES

Colligative properties are physical properties derived solely from the number of particles present, not the nature of those particles. These properties are usually associated with dilute solutions.

A. Freezing-Point Depression

Pure water (H_2O) freezes at 0°C; however, for every mole of solute particles dissolved in 1 L of water, the freezing point is lowered by 1.86°C. This is because the solute particles interfere with the process of crystal formation that occurs during freezing; the solute particles lower the temperature at which the molecules can align themselves into a crystalline structure.

The formula for calculating this **freezing-point depression** is

$$\Delta T_f = K_f m$$

where ΔT_f is the freezing-point depression, K_f is a proportionality constant characteristic of a particular solvent, and m is the molality of the solution (mol solute/kg solvent). The K_f for water—which you do not need to memorize—is $1.86°Cm^{-1}$. Each solvent has its own characteristic K_f.

B. Boiling-Point Elevation

A liquid boils when its vapor pressure equals the atmospheric pressure. If the vapor pressure of a solution is lower than that of the pure solvent, more energy (and consequently a higher temperature) will be required before its vapor pressure equals atmospheric pressure. The extent to which the boiling point of a solution is raised relative to that of the pure solvent is given by the following formula:

$$\Delta T_b = K_b m$$

where ΔT_b is the boiling-point elevation, K_b is a proportionality constant characteristic of a particular solvent, and m is the molality of the solution. The K_b for water is $0.51°Cm^{-1}$.

C. Osmotic Pressure

Consider a container separated into two compartments by a semipermeable membrane (which, by definition, selectively permits the passage of certain molecules). One compartment contains pure water, while the other contains water with dissolved solute. The membrane allows water but not solute to pass through. Because substances tend to flow, or **diffuse**, from higher to lower concentrations (which increases entropy), water will diffuse from the compartment containing pure water to the compartment containing the water-solute mixture. This net flow will cause the water level in the compartment containing the solution to rise above the level in the compartment containing pure water.

Because the solute cannot pass through the membrane, the concentrations of solute in the two compartments can never be equal. However, the pressure exerted by the water level in the solute-containing compartment will eventually oppose the influx of water; thus, the water level will rise only to the point at which it exerts a sufficient pressure to counterbalance the tendency of water to flow across the membrane. This pressure is defined as the **osmotic pressure (Π)** of the solution, and, it is given by this formula:

$$\Pi = MRT$$

where M is the molarity of the solution, R is the ideal gas constant, and T is the temperature on the Kelvin scale. This equation clearly shows that molarity and osmotic pressure are directly proportional (i.e., as the concentration of the solution increases, the osmotic pressure also increases). Thus, the osmotic pressure depends only on the amount of solute, not its identity.

D. Vapor-Pressure Lowering (Raoult's Law)

When solute B is added to pure solvent A, the vapor pressure of A above the solvent decreases (see Figure 8.4). If the vapor pressure of A above pure solvent A is designated by P°_A and the vapor pressure of A above the solution containing B is P_A, the vapor pressure decreases as follows:

$$\Delta P = P^\circ_A - P_A$$

In the late 1800s, the French chemist François Marie Raoult determined that this vapor pressure decrease is also equivalent to

$$\Delta P = x_B P^\circ_A$$

where x_B is the mole fraction of the solute B in solvent A. Since $x_B = 1 - x_A$ and $\Delta P = P^\circ_A - P_A$, substitution into the above equation leads to the common form of Raoult's Law:

$$P_A = x_A P^\circ_A$$

Similarly, the expression for the vapor pressure of the solute in solution (assuming it is volatile) is given by

$$P_B = x_B P^\circ_B$$

Raoult's Law holds only when the attraction between molecules of the different components of the mixture is equal to the attraction between the molecules of any one component in its pure state. When this condition does not hold, the relationship between mole fraction and vapor pressure will deviate from Raoult's Law. Solutions that obey Raoult's Law are called **ideal solutions**.

REAL WORLD CONNECTION

The molecular weight of a small, easily vaporized molecule can be determined via calculations based on the ideal gas law or by mass spectroscopy (see the Organic Chemistry section). Proteins, however, have molecular weights far above the limits of mass spec and will decompose upon heating long before they will enter the gas phase. Thus, their molecular weights are usually determined by application of colligative properties.

Suppose that we have a recently discovered protein and wish to determine its molecular weight. We can weigh out a small sample and dissolve it in a suitable solvent, hopefully water, then measure the freezing point or osmotic pressure. For example, let's say that we weigh out 1.000 grams of the unknown protein, dissolve it in 10.00 milliliters of water, and measure an osmotic pressure of 0.01250 atmospheres at 298 K.

The calculation of molecular weight is shown below:

$$P = MRT \Rightarrow M = \frac{P}{RT} =$$

$$\frac{0.0125}{(0.0821)(298)} = 5.11 \times 10^{-4}$$

$$\Rightarrow \frac{1.000\,g}{0.01000\,L} = \frac{5.11 \times 10^{-4}\,mol}{1.000\,L}$$

$$\Rightarrow 100.0\,g = 5.11 \times 10^{-4}\,mol$$

$$\Rightarrow 1.96\,g \times 10^5\,g/mol$$

Thus the molecular weight has been determined to be approximately 196,000 g/mol; as predicted, this is well above the limits of mass spectroscopy and unlikely to exist as a gas at any reasonable temperature and pressure.

9

Solutions

Solutions are **homogeneous** (everywhere the same) mixtures of substances that combine to form a single phase, generally the liquid phase. Many important chemical reactions, both in the laboratory and in nature, take place in solution (including almost all reactions in living organisms).

NATURE OF SOLUTIONS

A solution consists of a **solute** (e.g., NaCl, NH_3, or $C_{12}H_{22}O_{11}$) dispersed (dissolved) in a **solvent** (e.g., H_2O or benzene). The solvent is the component of the solution whose phase remains the same after mixing. If the two substances are already in the same phase, the solvent is the component present in greater quantity. Solute molecules move about freely in the solvent and can interact with other molecules or ions; consequently, chemical reactions occur easily in solution.

A. Solvation

The interaction between solute and solvent molecules is known as solvation or **dissolution;** when water is the solvent, the interaction is called **hydration**, and the resulting solution is known as an **aqueous solution.** Solvation is possible when the attractive forces between solute and solvent are stronger than those between the solute particles. For example, when NaCl dissolves in water, its component ions dissociate from one another and become surrounded by water molecules. Because water is polar, ion-dipole interactions can occur between the Na^+ and Cl^- ions and the water molecules. For nonionic solutes, solvation involves van der Waals forces between the solute and solvent molecules. The general rule is that like dissolves like; ionic and polar solutes are soluble in polar solvents, and nonpolar solutes are soluble in nonpolar solvents.

B. Solubility

The solubility of a substance is the maximum amount of that substance that can be dissolved in a particular solvent at a particular temperature. When this maximum amount of solute has been added, the solution is in equilibrium and is said to be **saturated;** if more solute is added, it will not dissolve. For example, at 18°C, a maximum of 83 g of glucose

($C_6H_{12}O_6$) will dissolve in 100 mL of H_2O. Thus, the solubility of glucose is 83 g/100 mL. If more glucose is added, it will remain in solid form, precipitating to the bottom of the container. A solution in which the proportion of solute to solvent is small is said to be **dilute,** and one in which the proportion is large is said to be **concentrated.**

C. Aqueous Solutions

The most common class of solutions is comprised of aqueous solutions, in which the solvent is water. The aqueous state is denoted by the symbol *aq.* In discussing the chemistry of aqueous solutions, it is useful to know how soluble various salts are in water; this information is given by the solubility rules below.

1. All salts of alkali metals are water soluble.

2. All salts of the ammonium ion (NH_4^+) are water soluble.

3. All chlorides, bromides, and iodides are water soluble, with the exceptions of Ag^+, Pb^{2+}, and Hg_2^{2+}.

4. All salts of the sulfate ion (SO_4^{2-}) are water soluble, with the exceptions of Ca^{2+}, Sr^{2+}, Ba^{2+}, and Pb^{2+}.

5. All metal oxides are insoluble, with the exception of the alkali metals and CaO, SrO, and BaO, all of which hydrolyze to form solutions of the corresponding metal hydroxides.

6. All hydroxides are insoluble, with the exception of the alkali metals and Ca^{2+}, Sr^{2+}, and Ba^{2+}.

7. All carbonates (CO_3^{2-}), phosphates (PO_4^{2-}), sulfides (S^{2-}), and sulfites (SO_3^{2-}) are insoluble, with the exception of the alkali metals and ammonium.

IONS

Ionic solutions are of particular interest to chemists because certain important types of chemical interactions—acid-base reactions and oxidation-reduction reactions, for instance—take place in ionic solutions.

A. Cations and Anions

Ionic compounds are made up of **cations** and **anions,** where a cation is a positive ion and an anion is a negative ion. The nomenclature of ionic compounds is based on the names of the component ions.

1. For elements (usually metals) that can form more than one positive ion, the charge is indicated by a Roman numeral in parentheses following the name of the element.

Fe^{2+} Iron (II) Cu^+ Copper (I)

Fe^{3+} Iron (III) Cu^{2+} Copper (II)

2. An older but still commonly used method is to add the endings **-ous** or **-ic** to the root of the Latin name of the element to represent the ions with lesser or greater charge, respectively.

Fe^{2+} Ferrous Cu^+ Cuprous

Fe^{3+} Ferric Cu^{2+} Cupric

3. Monatomic anions are named by dropping the ending of the name of the element and adding **-ide.**

H^- Hydride S^{2-} Sulfide

F^- Fluoride N^{3-} Nitride

O^{2-} Oxide P^{3-} Phosphide

4. Many polyatomic anions contain oxygen and are, therefore, called **oxyanions.** When an element forms two oxyanions, the name of the one with less oxygen ends in **-ite,** and the one with more oxygen ends in **-ate.**

NO_2^- Nitrite SO_3^{2-} Sulfite

NO_3^- Nitrate SO_4^{2-} Sulfate

5. When a series of oxyanions contains four oxyanions, prefixes are also used. **Hypo-** and **per-** are used to indicate less oxygen and more oxygen, respectively.

ClO^- Hypochlorite

ClO_2^- Chlorite

ClO_3^- Chlorate

ClO_4^- Perchlorate

6. Polyatomic anions often gain one or more H^+ ions to form anions of lower charge. The resulting ions are named by adding the word **hydrogen** or **dihydrogen** to the front of the anion's name. An older method uses the prefix **bi-** to indicate the addition of a single hydrogen ion.

HCO_3^- Hydrogen carbonate or bicarbonate

HSO_4^- Hydrogen sulfate or bisulfate

$H_2PO_4^-$ Dihydrogen phosphate

B. Ion Charges

Metals, which are found in the left part of the periodic table, generally form positive ions, whereas nonmetals, which are found in the right part of the periodic table, generally form negative ions. Note, however, the existence of anions that contain metallic elements (e.g., MnO_4^- [permanganate] and CrO_4^{2-} [chromate]). All elements in a given group tend to form monatomic ions with the same charge. Thus ions of alkali metals (Group IA) usually form cations with a single positive charge, the alkaline earth metals (Group IIA) form cations with a double positive charge, and the halides (Group VIIA) form anions with a single negative charge. Though other main group elements follow this trend, the intermediate electronegativity of such elements (making them less likely to form ionic compounds) and the transition from metallic to nonmetallic character complicates the picture.

C. Electrolytes

The electrical conductivity of aqueous solutions is governed by the presence and concentration of ions in solution. For example, pure water does not conduct an electrical current well, since the concentrations of hydrogen and hydroxide ions are very small. Solutes whose solutions are conductive are called electrolytes. A solute is considered a **strong electrolyte** if it dissociates completely into its constituent ions. Examples of strong electrolytes include ionic compounds, such as NaCl and KI, and molecular compounds with highly polar covalent bonds that dissociate into ions when dissolved, such as HCl in water. A **weak electrolyte**, on the other hand, ionizes or hydrolyzes incompletely in aqueous solution, and only some of the solute is present in ionic form. Examples include acetic acid and other weak acids, ammonia and other weak bases, and $HgCl_2$. Many compounds do not ionize at all in aqueous solution, retaining their molecular structure in solution, which usually limits their solubility. These compounds are called **nonelectrolytes** and include many nonpolar gases and organic compounds, such as oxygen and sugar.

CONCENTRATION

A. Units of Concentration

Concentration denotes the amount of solute dissolved in a solvent. The concentration of a solution is most commonly expressed as **percent composition by mass, mole fraction, molarity, molality,** or **normality.**

1. PERCENT COMPOSITION BY MASS

The percent composition by mass (%) of a solution is the mass of the solute divided by the mass of the solution (solute plus solvent), multiplied by 100.

Example: What is the percent composition by mass of a salt water solution if 100 g of the solution contains 20 g of NaCl?

Solution: $\dfrac{20 \text{ g NaCl}}{100 \text{ g}} \times 100 = 20\%$ NaCl solution

2. MOLE FRACTION

The mole fraction (x) of a compound is equal to the number of moles of the compound divided by the total number of moles of all species within the system. The sum of the mole fractions in a system will always equal 1.

Example: If 92 g of glycerol is mixed with 90 g of water, what will be the mole fractions of the two components? (MW of $H_2O = 18$; MW of $C_3H_8O_3 = 92$).

Solution:

$$90 \text{ g water} = 90 \text{ g} \times \frac{1 \text{ mol}}{18 \text{ g}} = 5 \text{ mol}$$

$$92 \text{ g glycerol} = 92 \text{ g} \times \frac{1 \text{ mol}}{92 \text{ g}} = 1 \text{ mol}$$

$$\text{Total mol} = 5 + 1 = 6 \text{ mol}$$

$$x_{\text{water}} = \frac{5 \text{ mol}}{6 \text{ mol}} = 0.833$$

$$x_{\text{glycerol}} = \frac{1 \text{ mol}}{6 \text{ mol}} = 0.167$$

$$x_{\text{water}} + x_{\text{glycerol}} = 0.833 + 0.167 = 1.000$$

3. MOLARITY

The molarity (m) of a solution is the number of moles of solute per liter of **solution.** Solution concentrations are usually expressed in terms of molarity. Molarity depends on the volume of the solution, not on the volume of solvent used to prepare the solution.

REMEMBER

For dilute solutions, the volume of the solution is approximately equal to the volume of solvent used.

Example: If enough water is added to 11 g of $CaCl_2$ to make 100 mL of solution, what is the molarity of the solution?

Solution: $\dfrac{11 \text{ g } CaCl_2}{110 \text{ g } CaCl_2 \text{ / mol } CaCl_2} = 0.10 \text{ mol } CaCl_2$

$$100 \text{ mL} \times \frac{1 \text{ L}}{1{,}000 \text{ mL}} = 0.10 \text{ L}$$

$$\text{molarity} = \frac{0.10 \text{ mol}}{0.10 \text{ L}} = 1.0 \text{ M}$$

4. MOLALITY

The molality (m) of a solution is the number of moles of solute per kilogram of **solvent**. For dilute aqueous solutions at 25°C, the molality is approximately equal to the molarity, because the density of water at this temperature is 1 kilogram per liter. But note that this is an approximation and true only for **dilute aqueous** solutions.

Example: If 10 g of NaOH are dissolved in 500 g of water, what is the molality of the solution?

Solution:

$$\frac{10\ \text{g NaOH}}{40\,\text{g NaOH}/\text{mol NaOH}} = 0.25\ \text{mol NaOH}$$

$$500\ \text{g} \times \frac{1\ \text{Kg}}{1,000\text{g}} = 0.50\ \text{Kg}$$

$$\text{molality} = \frac{0.25\ \text{mol}}{0.50\ \text{Kg}} = 0.50\ \text{mol}/\text{Kg} = 0.50m$$

5. NORMALITY

The normality (N) of a solution is equal to the number of gram equivalent weights of solute per liter of solution. A gram equivalent weight, or equivalent, is a measure of the reactive capacity of a molecule.

To calculate the normality of a solution, we must know for what purpose the solution is being used, because it is the concentration of the reactive species with which we are concerned. Normality is unique among concentration units in that it is reaction dependent. For example, a 1 molar solution of sulfuric acid would be 2 normal for acid-base reactions (because each mole of sulfuric acid is 2 moles of H^+ ions) but is only 1 normal for a sulfate precipitation reaction (because each mole of sulfuric acid only provides 1 mole of sulfate ions).

B. Dilution

A solution is diluted when solvent is added to a solution of high concentration to produce a solution of lower concentration. The concentration of a solution after dilution can be conveniently determined using this equation:

$$M_i V_i = M_f V_f$$

where M is molarity, V is volume, and the subscripts i and f refer to initial and final values, respectively.

Example: How many mL of a 5.5 M NaOH solution must be used to prepare 300 mL of a 1.2 M NaOH solution?

Solution: $5.5 \text{ M} \times V_i = 1.2 \text{M} \times 0.3 \text{ L}$

$$V_i = \frac{1.2 \text{M} \times 0.3 \text{ L}}{5.5 \text{ M}}$$

$$V_i = 0.065 \text{ L} = 65 \text{ mL}$$

SOLUTION EQUILIBRIA

The process of solvation, like other reversible chemical and physical changes, tends towards an equilibrium. Immediately after solute has been introduced into a solvent, most of the change taking place is dissociation, because no dissolved solute is initially present. However, according to Le Châtelier's Principle, as solute dissociates, the reverse reaction (precipitation of the solute) also begins to occur. Eventually an equilibrium is reached, with the rate of solute dissociation equal to the rate of precipitation, and the net concentration of the dissociated solute remains unchanged regardless of the amount of solute added.

An ionic solid introduced into a polar solvent dissociates into its component ions. The dissociation of such a solute in solution may be represented by

$$A_mB_n \ (s) \rightleftharpoons mA^{n+} \ (aq) + nB^{m-} \ (aq)$$

A. The Solubility Product Constant

A slightly soluble ionic solid exists in equilibrium with its saturated solution. In the case of AgCl, for example, the solution equilibrium is as follows:

$$AgCl \ (s) \rightleftharpoons Ag^+ \ (aq) + Cl^- \ (aq)$$

The **ion product**, I.P., of a compound in solution is defined as follows:

$$\text{I.P.} = [A^{n+}]m[B^{m-}]n$$

The same expression for a saturated solution at equilibrium defines the **solubility product constant, K$_{sp}$**.

$$K_{sp} = [A^{n+}]m[B^{m-}]n \text{ in a saturated solution}$$

However, I.P. is defined with respect to initial concentrations and does not necessarily represent either an equilibrium or a saturated solution, while K_{sp} does; at any point other than at equilibrium, the ion product is often referred to as Q_{sp}.

Each salt has its own distinct K_{sp} at a given temperature. If at a given temperature a salt's I.P. is equal to its K_{sp}, the solution is saturated, and the rate at which the salt dissolves equals the rate at which it precipitates out of solution. If a salt's I.P. exceeds its K_{sp}, the solution is supersaturated (holding more salt than it should be able to at a given temperature) and unstable. If the supersaturated solution is disturbed by adding more salt, other solid particles, or jarring the solution by a sudden decrease in temperature, the solid salt will precipitate until I.P. equals the K_{sp}. If I.P. is less than K_{sp}, the solution is unsaturated and no precipitate will form.

Example: The solubility of $Fe(OH)_3$ in an aqueous solution was determined to be 4.5×10^{-10} mol/L. What is the value of the K_{sp} for $Fe(OH)_3$?

Solution: The molar solubility (the solubility of the compound in mol/L) is given as 4.5×10^{-10} M. The equilibrium concentration of each ion can be determined from the molar solubility and the balanced dissociation reaction of $Fe(OH)_3$. The dissociation reaction is

$$Fe(OH)_3 \ (s) \rightleftharpoons Fe^{3+} \ (aq) + 3OH^- \ (aq)$$

Thus, for every mol of $Fe(OH)_3$ that dissociates, 1 mol of Fe^{3+} and 3 mol of OH^- are produced. Since the solubility is 4.5×10^{-10} M, the K_{sp} can be determined as follows:

$$K_{sp} = [Fe^{3+}][OH^-]^3$$
$$[OH^-] = 3[Fe^{3+}]; \qquad [Fe^{3+}] = 4.5 \times 10^{-10} M$$
$$K_{sp} = [Fe^{3+}](3[Fe^{3+}])^3 = 27[Fe^{3+}]^4$$
$$K_{sp} = (4.5 \times 10^{-10})[3(4.5 \times 10^{-10})]^3 = 27(4.5 \times 10^{-10})^4$$
$$K_{sp} = 1.1 \times 10^{-36}$$

Example: What are the concentrations of each of the ions in a saturated solution of $PbBr_2$, given that the K_{sp} of $PbBr_2$ is 2.1×10^{-6}? If 5 g of $PbBr_2$ are dissolved in water to make 1 L of solution at 25°C, would the solution be saturated, unsaturated, or supersaturated?

Solution: The first step is to write out the dissociation reaction:

$$PbBr_2 \ (s) \rightleftharpoons Pb^{2+} \ (aq) + 2Br^- \ (aq)$$
$$K_{sp} = [Pb^{2+}][Br^-]^2$$

Let x = the concentration of Pb^{2+}. Then $2x$ = the concentration of Br^- in the saturated solution at equilibrium (since $[Br^-]$ is two times $[Pb^{2+}]$).

$$(x)(2x)^2 = 4x^3$$
$$2.1 \times 10^{-6} = 4x^3$$

Solving for x, the concentration of Pb^{2+} in a saturated solution is 8.07×10^{-3} M, and the concentration of Br^- ($2x$) is 1.61×10^{-2} M.

Next, we convert 5 g of $PbBr_2$ into moles:

$$5\ g \times \frac{1\ mol\ PbBr_2}{367\ g} = 1.36 \times 10^{-2}\ mol$$

1.36×10^{-2} mol of $PbBr_2$ is dissolved in 1 L of solution, so the concentration of the solution 1.36×10^{-2} M. Since this is higher than the concentration of a saturated solution, this solution would be supersaturated.

B. Factors Affecting Solubility

The solubility of a substance varies depending on the temperature of the solution, the solvent, and, in the case of a gas-phase solute, the pressure. Solubility is also affected by the addition of other substances to the solution.

The solubility of a salt is considerably reduced when it is dissolved in a solution that already contains one of its ions, rather than in a pure solvent. For example, if a salt such as CaF_2 is dissolved in a solution already containing Ca^{2+} ions, the dissociation equilibrium will shift toward the production of the solid salt. This reduction in solubility, called the **common ion effect**, is another example of Le Châtelier's Principle.

Example: The K_{sp} of AgI in aqueous solution is 1×10^{-16} mol/L. If a 1×10^{-5} M solution of $AgNO_3$ is saturated with AgI, what will be the final concentration of the iodide ion?

Solution: The concentration of Ag^+ in the original $AgNO_3$ solution will be 1×10^{-5} mol/L. After AgI is added to saturation, the iodide concentration can be found by this formula:

$$1 \times 10^{-16} = [Ag^+][I^-]$$
$$= (1 \times 10^{-5})[I^-]$$
$$[I^-] = 1 \times 10^{-11}\ mol/L$$

> **REMEMBER**
>
> Every slightly soluble salt of general formula MX_2 will have $K_{sp} = 4x^3$, where x is the molar solubility.

> **REMEMBER**
>
> Every slightly soluble salt of general formula MX_2 will have $K_{sp} = 4x^3$, where x is the molar solubility.

If the AgI had been dissolved in pure water, the concentration of both Ag^+ and I^- would have been 1×10^{-8} mol/L. The presence of the common ion, silver, at a concentration 1,000 times higher than what it would normally be in a silver iodide solution, has reduced the iodide concentration to one thousandth of what it would have been otherwise. An additional 1×10^{-11} mol/L of silver will, of course, dissolve in solution along with the iodide ion, but this will not significantly affect the final silver concentration, which is much higher.

10

Acids and Bases

Many important reactions in chemical and biological systems involve two classes of compounds called **acids** and **bases.** Acids and bases cause color changes in certain compounds called **indicators**, which may be in solution or on paper. A particular common indicator is **litmus paper**, which turns red in acidic solution and blue in basic solution. A more extensive discussion of the chemical properties of acids and bases is outlined below.

DEFINITIONS

A. Arrhenius Definition

The first definitions of acids and bases were formulated by Svante Arrhenius towards the end of the 19th century. Arrhenius defined an acid as a species that produces H^+ (a proton) in an aqueous solution and a base as a species that produces OH^- (a hydroxide ion) in an aqueous solution. These definitions, though useful, fail to describe acidic and basic behavior in nonaqueous media.

B. Brønsted-Lowry Definition

A more general definition of acids and bases was proposed independently by Johannes Brønsted and Thomas Lowry in 1923. A Brønsted-Lowry acid is a species that donates protons, while a Brønsted-Lowry base is a species that accepts protons. For example, NH_3 and Cl^- are both Brønsted-Lowry bases because they accept protons. However, they cannot be called Arrhenius bases since in aqueous solution, they do not dissociate to form OH^-. The advantage of the Brønsted-Lowry concept of acids and bases is that it is not limited to aqueous solutions.

REMEMBER		
Definition	**Acid**	**Base**
Brønsted-Lowry	proton donor	proton acceptor
Lewis	e^- acceptor	e^- donor
Arrhenius	produces H^+	produces OH^-

Brønsted-Lowry acids and bases always occur in pairs, called **conjugate acid-base pairs.** The two members of a conjugate pair are related by the transfer of a proton. For example, H_3O^+ is the conjugate acid of the base H_2O, and NO_2^- is the conjugate base of HNO_2:

$$H_3O^+ \ (aq) \rightleftharpoons H_2O \ (aq) + H^+ \ (aq)$$
$$HNO_2 \ (aq) \rightleftharpoons NO_2^- \ (aq) + H^+ \ (aq)$$

C. Lewis Definition

At approximately the same time as Brønsted and Lowry, Gilbert Lewis also proposed definitions of acids and bases. Lewis defined an acid as an electron-pair acceptor and a base as an electron-pair donor. Lewis's are the most inclusive definitions. Just as every Arrhenius acid is a Brønsted-Lowry acid, every Brønsted-Lowry acid is also a Lewis acid (and likewise for bases). However, the Lewis definition encompasses some species not included within the Brønsted-Lowry definition. For example, BCl_3 and $AlCl_3$ can each accept an electron pair and are therefore Lewis acids, despite their inability to donate protons.

NOMENCLATURE OF ARRHENIUS ACIDS

The name of an acid is related to the name of the parent anion (the anion that combines with H^+ to form the acid). Acids formed from anions whose names end in -**ide** have the prefix **hydro-** and the ending -**ic**.

F^-	Fluoride	HF	Hydrofluoric acid
Br^-	Bromide	HBr	Hydrobromic acid

KEY CONCEPT

Some exceptions to the rules exist. For instance, MnO_4^- is called permanganate even though there are no "manganate" or "manganite" ions.

Acids formed from oxyanions are called **oxyacids**. If the anion ends in -**ite** (less oxygen), then the acid will end with -**ous acid**. If the anion ends in -**ate** (more oxygen), then the acid will end with -**ic acid**. Prefixes in the names of the anions are retained. Some examples:

ClO^-	Hypochlorite	HClO	Hypochlorous acid
ClO_2^-	Chlorite	HClO2	Chlorous acid
ClO_3^-	Chlorate	HClO3	Chloric acid
ClO_4^-	Perchlorate	HClO4	Perchloric acid
NO_2^-	Nitrite	HNO2	Nitrous acid
NO_3^-	Nitrate	HNO3	Nitric acid

PROPERTIES OF ACIDS AND BASES

A. Hydrogen Ion Equilibria (pH and pOH)

Hydrogen ion concentration, $[H^+]$, is generally measured as **pH**, where

$$pH = -\log[H^+] = \log(1/[H^+])$$

Likewise, hydroxide ion concentration, $[OH^-]$, is measured as **pOH**, where

$$pOH = -\log[OH^-] = \log(1/[OH^-])$$

In any aqueous solution, the H_2O solvent dissociates slightly:

$$H_2O(\ell) \rightleftharpoons H^+ (aq) + OH^- (aq)$$

This dissociation is an equilibrium reaction and is, therefore, described by a constant, K_w, **the water dissociation constant.**

$$K_w = [H^+][OH^-] = 10^{-14}$$

Rewriting this equation in logarithmic form gives this:

$$pH + pOH = 14$$

In pure H_2O, $[H^+]$ is equal to $[OH^-]$, since for every mole of H_2O that dissociates, one mole of H^+ and one mole of OH^- are formed. A solution with equal concentrations of H^+ and OH^- is neutral and has a pH of 7 ($-\log 10^{-7} = 7$). A pH below 7 indicates a relative excess of H^+ ions and, therefore, an acidic solution; a pH above 7 indicates a relative excess of OH^- ions and, therefore, a basic solution.

MATH NOTE: ESTIMATING P-SCALE VALUES

A useful skill for various problems involving acids and bases, as well as their corresponding buffer solutions, is the ability to convert pH, pOH, pK_a, and pK_b quickly into nonlogarithmic form and vice versa.

When the original value is a power of ten, the operation is relatively simple; changing the sign on the exponent gives the corresponding p-scale value directly. For example:

If $[H+] = 0.001$, or 10^{-3}, then pH = 3.

If $K_b = 1.0 \times 10^{-7}$, then $pK_b = 7$.

More difficulty arises (in the absence of a calculator) when the original value is not an exact power of 10; exact calculation would be excessively onerous, but a simple method of approximation exists. If the nonlogarithmic value is written in proper scientific notation, it will look like $n \times 10^{-m}$, where n is a number between 1 and 10. The log of this product can be written as $\log(n \times 10^{-m}) = -m + \log n$, and the negative log is thus $m - \log n$. Now, since n is a number between 1 and 10, its logarithm will be a fraction between 0 and 1. Thus, $m - \log n$ will be between $m - 1$ and m. Further, the larger n is, the larger the fraction $\log x$ will be and, therefore, the closer to $m - 1$ our answer will be.

Example: If $K_a = 1.8 \times 10^{-5}$, then $pK_a = 5 - \log 1.8$. Since 1.8 is small, its log will be small, and the answer will be closer to 5 than to 4. (The actual answer is 4.74.)

KEY CONCEPT

Recall that a fundamental property of logarithms is that the log of a product is equal to the sum of the logs: $\log(xy) = \log x + \log y$.

REMEMBER

Other important properties of logarithms include:

$\log x^n = n \log x$, and
$\log 10^x = x$.

From these two properties, one can derive the particularly useful relationship $-\log 10^{-x} = x$.

B. Strong Acids and Bases

Strong acids and bases are those that completely dissociate into their component ions in aqueous solution. For example, when NaOH is added to water, it dissociates completely:

$$NaOH(s) + \text{excess } H_2O(\ell) \rightarrow Na^+ (aq) + OH^- (aq)$$

Hence, in a 1 M solution of NaOH, complete dissociation gives 1 mole of OH^- ions per liter of solution.

$$pH = 14 - (-\log[OH^-]) = 14 + \log[1] = 14$$

Virtually no undissociated NaOH remains. Note that the $[OH^-]$ contributed by the dissociation of H_2O is considered to be negligible in this case. The contribution of OH^- and H^+ ions from the dissociation of H_2O can be neglected only if the concentration of the acid or base is greater than 10^{-7} M. For example, the pH of a 1×10^{-8} M HCl solution (HCl is a strong acid) might appear to be 8, since $-\log (1 \times 10^{-8}) = 8$. However, a pH of 8 is in the basic pH range, and an HCl solution is not basic. The discrepancy arises from the fact that at low HCl concentrations, H^+ from the dissociation of water does contribute significantly to the total $[H^+]$. The $[H^+]$ from the dissociation of water is less than 1×10^{-7} M due to the common ion effect. The total concentration of H^+ can be calculated from $K_w = (x + 1 \times 10^{-8})(x) = 1.0 \times 10^{-14}$, where $x = [H^+] = [OH^-]$ (both from the dissociation of water molecules).

Solving for x gives $x = 9.5 \times 10^{-8}$ M, so $[H^+]_{total} = (9.5 \times 10^{-8} + 1 \times 10^{-8})$ M $= 1.05 \times 10^{-7}$ M and pH $= -\log (1.05 \times 10^{-7}) = 6.98$, slightly less than 7, as should be expected for a very dilute, yet acidic, solution.

Strong acids commonly encountered in the laboratory include $HClO_4$ (perchloric acid), HNO_3 (nitric acid), H_2SO_4 (sulfuric acid), and HCl (hydrochloric acid). Commonly encountered strong bases include NaOH (sodium hydroxide), KOH (potassium hydroxide), and other soluble hydroxides of Group IA and IIA metals. Calculation of the pH and pOH of strong acids and bases assumes complete dissociation of the acid or base in solution: $[H^+]$ = normality of strong acid and $[OH^-]$ = normality of strong base.

C. Weak Acids and Bases

Weak acids and bases are those that only partially dissociate in aqueous solution. A weak monoprotic acid, HA, in aqueous solution will achieve the following equilibrium after dissociation (H_3O^+ is equivalent to H^+ in aqueous solution):

$$HA (aq) + H_2O (\ell) \rightleftharpoons H_3O^+ (aq) + A^- (aq)$$

The **acid dissociation constant, K_a,** is a measure of the degree to which an acid dissociates.

$$K_a = \frac{[H_3O^+][A^-]}{[HA]}$$

The weaker the acid, the smaller the K_a. Note that K_a does not contain an expression for the pure liquid, water.

A weak monovalent base, BOH, undergoes dissociation to give B^+ and OH^-. The **base dissociation constant, K_b,** is a measure of the degree to which a base dissociates. The weaker the base, the smaller its K_b. For a monovalent base, K_b is defined as follows:

$$K_b = \frac{[B^+][OH^-]}{[BOH]}$$

A **conjugate acid** is defined as the acid formed when a base gains a proton. Similarly, a **conjugate base** is formed when an acid loses a proton. For example, in the HCO_3^-/CO_3^{2-} conjugate acid/base pair, CO_3^{2-} is the conjugate base, and HCO_3^- is the conjugate acid:

$$HCO_3^- \, (aq) \rightleftharpoons H^+ \, (aq) + CO_3^{2-} \, (aq)$$

To find the K_a of the conjugate acid HCO_3^-, the reaction with water must be considered:

$$HCO_3^- \, (aq) + H_2O \, (\ell) \rightleftharpoons H_3O^+ \, (aq) + CO_3^{2-} \, (aq)$$

Likewise, for the K_b of CO_3^{2-},

$$CO_3^{2-} \, (aq) + H_2O \, (\ell) \rightleftharpoons HCO_3^- \, (aq) + OH^- \, (aq)$$

In a conjugate acid/base pair formed from a weak acid, the conjugate base is generally stronger than the conjugate acid. Thus, for HCO_3^- and CO_3^{2-}, the reaction of CO_3^{2-} (the conjugate base) in water to produce HCO_3^- (the conjugate acid) and OH^- occurs to a greater extent (i.e., is more favorable) than the reverse reaction.

The equilibrium constants for these reactions are as follows:

$$K_a = \frac{[H^+][CO_3^{2-}]}{[HCO_3^-]} \text{ and } K_b = \frac{[HCO_3^-][OH^-]}{[CO_3^{2-}]}$$

Adding the two reactions shows that the net reaction is simply the dissociation of water:

$$H_2O \, (\ell) \rightleftharpoons H^+ \, (aq) + OH^- \, (aq)$$

> **KEY CONCEPT**
>
> As a weak acid or base, the effect on pH will always be less than that of a strong acid or base of the same concentration. For example, before calculating the pH of a 0.01 M solution of acetic acid, $K_a = 1.8 \times 10^{-5}$, recognize that it will be higher than that of a 0.01 M solution of a strong acid like HCl; since the pH of 0.01 M HCl is 2, the pH of 0.01 M acetic acid must be greater than 2.

The equilibrium constant for this net reaction is $K_w = [H^+][OH^-]$, which is the product of K_a and K_b. Thus, if the dissociation constant either for an acid or for its conjugate base is known, then the dissociation constant for the other can be determined, using this equation:

$$K_a \times K_b = K_w = 1 \times 10^{-14}$$

Thus K_a and K_b are inversely related. In other words, if K_a is large (the acid is strong), then K_b will be small (the conjugate base will be weak), and vice versa.

D. Applications of K_a and K_b

To calculate the concentration of H^+ in a 2.0 M aqueous solution of acetic acid, CH_3COOH ($K_a = 1.8 \times 10^{-5}$), first write the equilibrium reaction:

$$CH_3COOH \ (aq) \rightleftharpoons H^+ \ (aq) + CH_3COO^- \ (aq)$$

Next, write the expression for the acid dissociation constant:

$$K_a = \frac{[H^+][CH_3COO^-]}{[CH_3COOH]} = 1.8 \times 10^{-5}$$

Since acetic acid is a weak acid, the concentration of CH_3COOH at equilibrium is equal to its initial concentration, 2.0 M, less the amount dissociated, x. Likewise $[H^+] = [CH_3COO^-] = x$, since each molecule of CH_3COOH dissociates into one H^+ ion and one CH_3COO^- ion. Thus, the equation can be rewritten as follows:

$$K_a = \frac{[x][x]}{[2.0 - x]} = 1.8 \times 10^{-5}$$

We can approximate that $2.0 - x \approx 2.0$, since acetic acid is a weak acid and only slightly dissociates in water. This simplifies the calculation of x:

$$K_a = \frac{[x][x]}{[2.0]} = 1.8 \times 10^{-5}$$

$$x = 6.0 \times 10^{-3} \ M$$

The fact that $[x]$ is so much less than the initial concentration of acetic acid (2.0 M) validates the approximation; otherwise, it would have been necessary to solve for x using the quadratic formula. (A rule of thumb is that the approximation is valid as long as x is less than 5 percent of the initial concentration.)

SALT FORMATION

Acids and bases may react with each other, forming a salt and (often, but not always) water, in what is termed a **neutralization reaction**. For example:

$$HA + BOH \rightarrow BA + H_2O$$

The salt may precipitate out or remain ionized in solution, depending on its solubility and the amount produced. Neutralization reactions generally go to completion. The reverse reaction, in which the salt ions react with water to give back the acid or base, is known as **hydrolysis.**

Four combinations of strong and weak acids and bases are possible:

1. strong acid + strong base: e.g., $HCl + NaOH \rightarrow NaCl + H_2O$

2. strong acid + weak base: e.g., $HCl + NH_3 \rightarrow NH_4Cl$

3. weak acid + strong base: e.g., $HClO + NaOH \rightarrow NaClO + H_2O$

4. weak acid + weak base: e.g., $HClO + NH_3 \rightleftharpoons NH_4ClO$

The products of a reaction between equal concentrations of a strong acid and a strong base are a salt and water. The acid and base neutralize each other, so the resulting solution is neutral (pH = 7), and the ions formed in the reaction do not react with water. The product of a reaction between a strong acid and a weak base is also a salt, but usually no water is formed since weak bases are usually not hydroxides. However, in this case, the cation of the salt will react with the water solvent, reforming the weak base. This reaction constitutes hydrolysis. For example:

$$HCl \ (aq) + NH_3 \ (aq) \rightleftharpoons NH_4^+ \ (aq) + Cl^- \ (aq) \qquad \text{Reaction I}$$

$$NH_4^+ \ (aq) + H_2O \ (aq) \rightleftharpoons NH_3 \ (aq) + H_3O^+ \ (aq) \quad \text{Reaction II}$$

NH_4^+ is the conjugate acid of a weak base (NH_3) and is, therefore, stronger than the conjugate base (Cl^-) of the strong acid HCl. NH_4^+ will thus react with OH^-, reducing the concentration of OH^-. There will thus be an excess of H^+, which will lower the pH of the solution.

On the other hand, when a weak acid reacts with a strong base, the solution is basic due to the hydrolysis of the salt to reform the acid with the concurrent formation of hydroxide ion from the hydrolyzed water molecules. The pH of a solution containing a weak acid and a weak base depends on the relative strengths of the reactants. For example, the acid HClO has a $K_a = 3.2 \times 10^{-8}$, and the base NH_3 has a $K_b = 1.8 \times 10^{-5}$. Thus, an aqueous solution of HClO and NH_3 is basic since K_a for HClO is less than K_b for NH_3.

POLYVALENCE AND NORMALITY

The relative acidity or basicity of an aqueous solution is determined by the relative concentrations of **acid** and **base equivalents.** An acid equivalent is equal to one mole of H^+ (or H_3O^+) ions; a base equivalent is equal to one mole of OH^- ions. Some acids and bases are polyvalent; that is, each mole of the acid or base liberates more than one acid or base equivalent. For example, the diprotic acid H_2SO_4 undergoes the following dissociation in water:

$$H_2SO_4 \ (aq) \rightarrow H^+ \ (aq) + HSO_4^- \ (aq)$$

$$HSO_4^- \ (aq) \rightleftharpoons H^+ \ (aq) + SO_4^{2-} \ (aq)$$

One mole of H_2SO_4 can thus produce 2 acid equivalents (2 moles of H^+). The acidity or basicity of a solution depends upon the concentration of acidic or basic equivalents that can be liberated. The quantity of acidic or basic capacity is directly indicated by the solution's normality. Since each mole of H_3PO_4 can liberate 3 moles (equivalents) of H^+, a 2 M H_3PO_4 solution would be 6 N (6 normal).

Another useful measurement is equivalent weight. For example, the gram molecular weight of H_2SO_4 is 98 g/mol. Since each mole liberates 2 acid equivalents, the gram equivalent weight of H_2SO_4 would be $\frac{98}{2} = 49g$; that is, the dissociation of 49 g of H_2SO_4 would release 1 acid equivalent. Common polyvalent acids include H_2SO_4, H_3PO_4, and H_2CO_3.

AMPHOTERIC SPECIES

An **amphoteric,** or **amphiprotic,** species is one that can act either as an acid or a base, depending on its chemical environment. In the Brønsted–Lowry sense, an amphoteric species can either gain or lose a proton. Water is the most common example. When water reacts with a base, it behaves as an acid:

$$H_2O + B^- \rightleftharpoons HB + OH^-$$

When water reacts with an acid, it behaves as a base:

$$HA + H_2O \rightleftharpoons H_3O^+ + A^-$$

The partially dissociated conjugate base of a polyprotic acid is usually amphoteric (e.g., HSO_4^- can either gain an H^+ to form H_2SO_4 or lose an H^+ to form SO_4^{2-}). The hydroxides of certain metals (e.g., Al, Zn, Pb, and Cr) are also amphoteric. Furthermore, species that can act as either oxidizing or reducing agents are considered to be amphoteric as well, since by accepting or donating electron pairs, they act as Lewis acids or bases, respectively.

TITRATION AND BUFFERS

Titration is a procedure used to determine the molarity of an acid or base. This is accomplished by reacting a known volume of a solution of unknown concentration with a known volume of a solution of known concentration. When the number of acid equivalents equals the number of base equivalents added, or vice versa, the **equivalence point** is reached. It is important to emphasize that, while a strong acid/strong base titration will have an equivalence point at pH 7, the equivalence point need not always occur at pH 7. Also, when titrating polyprotic acids or bases, there are several equivalence points, as each acidic or basic species is titrated separately.

The equivalence point in **a** titration is estimated in two common ways: either by using a graphical method, plotting the pH of the solution as a function of added titrant by using a **pH meter** (e.g., Figure 10.1), or by watching for a color change of an added **indicator**. Indicators are weak organic acids or bases that have different colors in their undissociated and dissociated states. Indicators are used in low concentrations and, therefore, do not significantly alter the equivalence point. The point at which the indicator actually changes color is not the equivalence point but is called the **end point**. If the titration is performed well, the volume difference (and therefore the error) between the end point and the equivalence point is usually small and may be either corrected for or ignored.

A. Strong Acid and Strong Base

Consider the titration of 10 mL of a 0.1 N solution of HCl with a 0.1 N solution of NaOH. Plotting the pH of the reaction solution versus the quantity of NaOH added gives the curve shown in Figure 10.1.

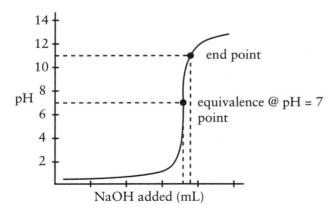

Figure 10.1. Titration of HCl with NaOH

Because HCl is a strong acid and NaOH is a strong base, the equivalence point of the titration will be at pH 7, and the solution will be neutral. Note that the end point shown is close to, but not exactly equal to, the equivalence point; selection of a better indicator—say, one that changes colors at pH 8—would have given a better approximation.

In the early part of the curve (when little base has been added), the acidic species predominates, so the addition of small amounts of base will not appreciably change either the [OH⁻] or the pH. Similarly, in the last part of the titration curve (when an excess of base has been added), the addition of small amounts of base will not change the [OH⁻] significantly, and the pH remains relatively constant. The addition of base most alters the concentrations of H⁺ and OH⁻ near the equivalence point, and thus the pH changes most drastically in that region.

> **REMEMBER**
>
> Any monoprotic strong acid titrated with a strong base will give a similar curve. The pH of the equivalence point is 7.

B. Weak Acid and Strong Base

Titration of a weak acid, HA, with a strong base produces the titration curve shown in Figure 10.2.

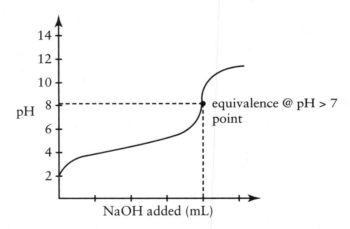

Figure 10.2. Titration of a Weak Acid, HA, with NaOH

> **REMEMBER**
>
> Any monoprotic weak acid titrated with a strong base will give a similar curve. The pH of the equivalence point depends on the identity of the weak acid.

Comparing Figure 10.2 with Figure 10.1 shows that the initial pH of the weak acid solution is greater than the initial pH of the strong acid solution. The pH changes most significantly early on in the titration, and the equivalence point is in the basic range.

C. Buffers

A **buffer solution** consists of a mixture of a weak acid and its salt (which consists of its conjugate base and a cation) or a mixture of a weak base and its salt (which consists of its conjugate acid and an anion). Two examples of buffers are a solution of acetic acid (CH_3COOH) and its salt, sodium acetate ($CH_3COO^-Na^+$), and a solution of ammonia (NH_3) and its salt, ammonium chloride ($NH_4^+Cl^-$). Buffer solutions have the useful property of resisting changes in pH when small amounts of acid or base are added.

Consider a buffer solution of acetic acid and sodium acetate:

$$CH_3COOH \rightleftharpoons H^+ + CH_3COO^-$$

When a small amount of NaOH is added to the buffer, the OH^- ions from the NaOH react with the H^+ ions present in the solution; subsequently, more acetic acid dissociates (equilibrium shifts to the right), restoring the $[H^+]$. Thus, an increase in $[OH^-]$ does not appreciably change pH. Likewise, when a small amount of HCl is added to the buffer, H^+ ions from the HCl react with the acetate ions to form acetic acid. Thus, $[H^+]$ is kept relatively constant, and the pH of the solution is relatively unchanged.

The **Henderson-Hasselbalch equation** is used to estimate the pH of a solution in the buffer region where the concentrations of the species and its conjugate are present in approximately equal concentrations. For a weak acid buffer solution,

$$pH = pK_a + \log \frac{[\text{conjugate base}]}{[\text{weak acid}]}$$

Note that when [conjugate base] = [weak acid] (in a titration, halfway to the equivalent point), the $pH = pK_a$ because the log 1 = 0. Likewise, for a weak base buffer solution,

$$pOH = pK_b + \log \frac{[\text{conjugate acid}]}{[\text{weak base}]}$$

and $pOH = pK_b$ when [conjugate acid] = [weak base].

D. Polyprotic Acids and Bases

The titration curve for a polyprotic acid or base looks different than that for a monoprotic acid or base. Figure 10.3 shows the titration of Na_2CO_3 with HCl in which the polyprotic acid H_2CO_3 is the ultimate product.

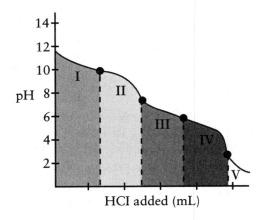

Figure 10.3. Titration of Na_2CO_3 with HCl

In region I, little acid has been added, and the predominant species is CO_3^{2-}. In region II, more acid has been added, and the predominant species are CO_3^{2-} and HCO_3^- in relatively equal concentrations. The flat part of the curve is the first buffer region, corresponding to the pK_a of HCO_3^- ($K_a = 5.6 \times 10^{-11}$ implies $pK_a = 10.25$).

Region III contains the equivalence point, at which all of the CO_3^{2-} is titrated to HCO_3^-. As the curve illustrates, a rapid change in pH occurs at the equivalence point; in the latter part of region III, the predominant species is HCO_3^-.

In region IV, the acid has neutralized approximately half of the HCO_3^-, and now H_2CO_3 and HCO_3^- are in roughly equal concentrations. This flat region is the second buffer region of the titration curve, corresponding to the pK_a of H_2CO_3 ($K_a = 4.3 \times 10^{-7}$ implies $pK_a = 6.37$). In region V, the equivalence point for the entire titration is reached, as all of the HCO_3^-, is converted to H_2CO_3. Again, a rapid change in pH is observed near the equivalence point as acid is added.

FLASHBACK

$-\log K_a = pK_a$

$-\log(5.6 \times 10^{-11}) = 11 - \log 5.6$

11

Redox Reactions and Electrochemistry

Electrochemistry is the study of the relationships between chemical reactions and electrical energy. **Electrochemical reactions** include spontaneous reactions that produce electrical energy and nonspontaneous reactions that use electrical energy to produce a chemical change. Both types of reactions always involve a transfer of electrons with conservation of charge and mass.

OXIDATION-REDUCTION REACTIONS

A. Oxidation and Reduction

The law of conservation of charge states that an electrical charge can be neither created nor destroyed. Thus, an isolated loss or gain of electrons cannot occur; **oxidation** (loss of electrons) and **reduction** (gain of electrons) must occur simultaneously, resulting in an electron transfer called a **redox reaction**. An **oxidizing agent** causes another atom in a redox reaction to undergo oxidation and is itself reduced. A **reducing agent** causes the other atom to be reduced and is itself oxidized.

B. Assigning Oxidation Numbers

It is important, of course, to know which atom is oxidized and which is reduced. **Oxidation numbers** are assigned to atoms in order to keep track of the redistribution of electrons during a chemical reaction. From the oxidation numbers of the reactants and products, it is possible to determine how many electrons are gained or lost by each atom. The oxidation number of an atom in a compound is assigned according to the following rules:

1. **The oxidation number of free elements is zero.** For example, the atoms in N2, P4, S8, and He all have oxidation numbers of zero.

> **REMEMBER**
>
> OIL RIG stands for "Oxidation Is Loss, Reduction Is Gain"— of electrons, that is.
>
> Alternatively, reduction is just what it sounds like: reduction of positive charge.

2. **The oxidation number for a monatomic ion is equal to the charge of the ion.** For example, the oxidation numbers for Na^+, Cu^{2+}, Fe^{3+}, Cl^-, and N^{3-} are +1, +2, +3, –1, and –3, respectively.

3. **The oxidation number of each Group IA element in a compound is +1.** The oxidation number of each Group IIA element in a compound is +2.

4. **The oxidation number of each Group VIIA element in a compound is –1, except when combined with an element of higher electronegativity.** For example, in HCl, the oxidation number of Cl is –1; in HOCl, however, the oxidation number of Cl is +1.

5. **The oxidation number of hydrogen is –1 in compounds with less electronegative elements than hydrogen (Groups IA and IIA).** Examples include NaH and CaH_2. The more common oxidation number of hydrogen is +1.

6. **In most compounds, the oxidation number of oxygen is –2.** This is not the case, however, in molecules such as OF_2. Here, because F is more electronegative than O, the oxidation number of oxygen is +2. Also, in peroxides such as BaO_2, the oxidation number of O is –1 instead of –2 because of the structure of the peroxide ion, $[O–O]^{2-}$. (Note that Ba, a Group IIA element, can not be a +4 cation.)

7. **The sum of the oxidation numbers of all the atoms present in a neutral compound is zero.** The sum of the oxidation numbers of the atoms present in a polyatomic ion is equal to the charge of the ion. Thus, for SO_4^{2-}, the sum of the oxidation numbers must be –2.

Example: Assign oxidation numbers to the atoms in the following reaction in order to determine the oxidized and reduced species and the oxidizing and reducing agents.

$$SnCl_2 + PbCl_4 \rightarrow SnCl_4 + PbCl_2$$

Solution: All these species are neutral, so the oxidation numbers of each compound must add up to zero. In $SnCl_2$, since there are two chlorines present and chlorine has an oxidation number of –1, Sn must have an oxidation number of +2. Similarly, the oxidation number of Sn in $SnCl_4$ is +4; the oxidation number of Pb is +4 in $PbCl_4$ and +2 in $PbCl_2$. Notice that the oxidation number of Sn goes from +2 to +4; it loses electrons and thus is oxidized, making it the reducing agent. Since the oxidation number of Pb has decreased from +4 to +2, it has gained electrons and been reduced. Pb is the oxidizing agent. The sum of the charges on both sides of the reaction is equal to zero, so charge has been conserved.

KEY CONCEPT

The conventions of formula writing put cation first and anion second. Thus NaH implies H^-, while HCl implies H^+.

REMEMBER

An oxidizing agent causes something else to oxidize. Conversely, a reducing agent causes something else to reduce.

C. Balancing Redox Reactions

By assigning oxidation numbers to the reactants and products, one can determine how many moles of each species are required for conservation of charge and mass, which is necessary to balance the equation. To balance a redox reaction, both the net charge and the number of atoms must be equal on both sides of the equation. The most common method for balancing redox equations is the half-reaction method, also known as the ion-electron method, in which the equation is separated into two half-reactions—the oxidation part and the reduction part. Each half-reaction is balanced separately, and they are then added to give a balanced overall reaction. Consider a redox reaction between $KMnO_4$ and HI in an acidic solution:

$$MnO_4^- + I^- \rightarrow I_2 + Mn^{2+}$$

Step 1: Separate the two half-reactions.

$$I^- \rightarrow I_2$$
$$MnO_4^- \rightarrow Mn^{2+}$$

Step 2: Balance the atoms of each half-reaction. First, balance all atoms except H and O. Next, in an acidic solution, add H_2O to balance the O atoms and then add H^+ to balance the H atoms. (In a basic solution, use OH^- and H_2O to balance the O's and H's.)

To balance the iodine atoms, place a coefficient of two before the I^- ion.

$$2\,I^- \rightarrow I_2$$

For the permanganate half-reaction, Mn is already balanced. Next, balance the oxygens by adding $4H_2O$ to the right side.

$$MnO_4^- \rightarrow Mn^{2+} + 4H_2O$$

Finally, add H^+ to the left side to balance the 4 H_2Os. These two half-reactions are now balanced.

$$MnO_4^- + 8\,H^+ \rightarrow Mn^{2+} + 4H_2O$$

Step 3: Balance the charges of each half-reaction. The reduction half-reaction must consume the same number of electrons as are supplied by the oxidation half. For the oxidation reaction, add 2 electrons to the right side of the reaction:

$$2\,I^- \rightarrow I_2 + 2e^-$$

For the reduction reaction, a charge of +2 must exist on both sides. Add 5 electrons to the left side of the reaction to accomplish this:

$$5 \ e^- + 8 \ H^+ + MnO_4^- \rightarrow Mn^{2+} + 4 \ H_2O$$

Next, both half-reactions must have the same number of electrons so that they will cancel. Multiply the oxidation half by 5 and the reduction half by 2.

$$5(2I^- \rightarrow I_2 + 2e^-)$$
$$2(5e^- + 8H^+ + MnO_4^- \rightarrow Mn^{2+} + 4 \ H_2O)$$

Step 4: Add the half-reactions:

$$10 \ I^- \rightarrow 5 \ I_2 + 10 \ e^-$$
$$16 \ H^+ + 2 \ MnO_4^- + 10 \ e^- \rightarrow 2 \ Mn^{2+} + 8 \ H_2O$$

The final equation is this:

$$10 \ I^- + 10 \ e^- + 16 \ H^+ + 2 \ MnO_4^- \rightarrow 5 \ I_2 + 2 \ Mn^{2+} + 10 \ e^- + 8 \ H_2O$$

To get the overall equation, cancel out the electrons and any H_2Os, H^+s, or OH^-s that appear on both sides of the equation.

$$10 \ I^- + 16 \ H^+ + 2 \ MnO_4^- \rightarrow 5 \ I_2 + 2 \ Mn^{2+} + 8 \ H_2O$$

Step 5: Finally, confirm that mass and charge are balanced. There is a +4 net charge on each side of the reaction equation, and the atoms are stoichiometrically balanced.

ELECTROCHEMICAL CELLS

Electrochemical cells are contained systems in which a redox reaction occurs. There are two types of electrochemical cells, galvanic cells (also known as voltaic cells) and electrolytic cells. Spontaneous reactions occur in galvanic cells, and nonspontaneous reactions in electrolytic cells. Both types contain electrodes at which oxidation and reduction occur. For all electrochemical cells, the electrode at which oxidation occurs is called the anode, and the electrode where reduction occurs is called the cathode.

A. Galvanic Cells

A redox reaction occurring in a **galvanic cell** has a negative ΔG and is therefore a **spontaneous reaction**. Galvanic cell reactions supply energy and are used to do work. This energy can be harnessed by placing the oxidation and reduction half-reactions in separate containers called half-cells. The half-cells are then connected by an apparatus that allows for the flow of electrons.

REMEMBER

A way to remember which electrode is which is AN OX and a RED CAT. Another easy way to remember this is by the spelling of the words: oxidAtion and reduCtion.

A common example of a galvanic cell is the Daniell cell shown in Figure 11.1.

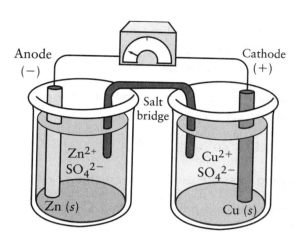

Figure 11.1. Daniell Cell

In the Daniell cell, a zinc bar is placed in an aqueous $ZnSO_4$ solution, and a copper bar is placed in an aqueous $CuSO_4$ solution. The anode of this cell is the zinc bar where Zn (s) is oxidized to Zn^{2+} (aq). The cathode is the copper bar, and it is the site of the reduction of Cu^{2+} (aq) to Cu (s). The half-cell reactions are written as follows:

$$Zn\ (s) \rightarrow Zn^{2+}\ (aq) + 2e^-\ \text{(anode)}$$
$$Cu^{2+}\ (aq) + 2e \rightarrow Cu\ (s)\ \text{(cathode)}$$

If the two half-cells were not separated, the Cu^{2+} ions would react directly with the zinc bar, and no useful electrical work would be obtained. To complete the circuit, the two solutions must be connected. Without connection, the electrons from the zinc oxidation half reaction would not be able to get to the copper ions; thus, a wire (or other conductor) is necessary. If only a wire were provided for this electron flow, the reaction would soon cease anyway, because an excess negative charge would build up in the solution surrounding the cathode, and an excess positive charge would build up in the solution surrounding the anode. This charge gradient is dissipated by the presence of a salt bridge, which permits the exchange of cations and anions. The salt bridge contains an inert electrolyte, usually KCl or NH_4NO_3, whose ions will not react with the electrodes or with the ions in solution. At the same time, the anions from the salt bridge (e.g., Cl^-) diffuse from the salt bridge of the Daniell cell into the $ZnSO_4$ solution to balance out the charge of the newly created Zn^{2+} ions, and the cations of the salt bridge (e.g., K^+) flow into the $CuSO_4$ solution to balance out the charge of the SO_4^{2-} ions left in solution when the Cu^{2+} ions deposit as copper metal.

During the course of the reaction, electrons flow from the zinc bar (anode) through the wire and the voltmeter toward the copper bar (cathode). The anions (Cl^-) flow externally (via the salt bridge) into the $ZnSO_4$, and the cations (K^+) flow into the $CuSO_4$. This flow depletes the salt bridge and, along with the finite quantity of Cu^{2+} in the solution, accounts for the relatively short lifetime of the cell.

A cell diagram is a shorthand notation representing the reactions in an electrochemical cell. A cell diagram for the Daniell cell is as follows:

$$Zn\ (s)\ \Big|\ Zn^{2+}(x\text{M}\ SO_4{}^{2-})\ \Big|\Big|\ Cu^{2+}(y\text{M}\ SO_4{}^{2-})\ \Big|\ Cu\ (s)$$

The following rules are used in constructing a cell diagram:

1. The reactants and products are always listed from left to right in the form:

$$\text{anode}\ \Big|\ \text{anode solution}\ \Big|\Big|\ \text{cathode solution}\ \Big|\ \text{cathode}$$

2. A single vertical line indicates a phase boundary.

3. A double vertical line indicates the presence of a salt bridge or some other type of barrier.

B. Electrolytic Cells

A redox reaction occurring in an **electrolytic cell** has a positive ΔG and is therefore **nonspontaneous**. In **electrolysis**, electrical energy is required to induce reaction. The oxidation and reduction half-reactions are usually placed in one container.

Michael Faraday was the first to define certain quantitative principles governing the behavior of electrolytic cells. He theorized that the amount of chemical change induced in an electrolytic cell is directly proportional to the number of moles of electrons that are exchanged during a redox reaction. The number of moles exchanged can be determined from the balanced half-reaction. In general, for a reaction which involves the transfer of n electrons per atom,

$$M^{n+} + n\ e^- \rightarrow M\ (s)$$

One mole of M (s) will be produced if n moles of electrons are supplied.

The number of moles of electrons needed to produce a certain amount of M (s) can now be related to a measurable electrical property. One electron carries a charge of 1.6×10^{-19} coulombs (C). The charge carried by one mole of electrons can be calculated by multiplying this number by Avogadro's number, as follows:

$$(1.6 \times 10^{-19})(6.022 \times 10^{23}) = 96{,}487\ \text{C/mol}\ e^-$$

This number is called **Faraday's constant**, and one **faraday (F)** is equivalent to the amount of charge contained in one mole of electrons (1 F = 96,487 coulombs, or J/V).

An example of an electrolytic cell, in which molten NaCl is electrolyzed to form Cl_2 (g) and Na (l), is given in Figure 11.2.

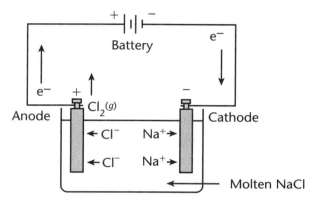

Figure 11.2. Example of an Electrolytic Cell

In this cell, Na^+ ions migrate towards the cathode, where they are reduced to Na (ℓ). Similarly, Cl^- ions migrate towards the anode, where they are oxidized to Cl_2 (g). This cell is used in industry as the major means of sodium and chlorine production. Note that sodium is a liquid at the temperature of molten NaCl; it is also less dense than the molten salt and thus is easily removed as it floats to the top of the reaction vessel.

C. Electrode Charge Designations

The anode of an **electrolytic cell** is considered **positive**, since it is attached to the positive pole of the battery and so attracts anions from the solution. The anode of a **galvanic cell,** on the other hand, is considered **negative**, because the **spontaneous** oxidation reaction that takes place at the galvanic cell's anode is the original source of that cell's negative charge (i.e., is the source of electrons). In spite of this difference in designating charge, oxidation takes place at the anode in both types of cells, and electrons always flow through the wire from the anode to the cathode.

In a galvanic cell, charge is spontaneously created as electrons are released by the oxidizing species at the anode; since this is the source of electrons, the anode of a galvanic cell is considered the negative electrode.

In an electrolytic cell, electrons are forced through the cathode, where they encounter the species which is to be reduced. Here it is the cathode that is providing electrons, and thus the cathode of an electrolytic cell

KEY CONCEPT

In an electrolytic cell, the anode is positive, and the cathode is negative. In a galvanic cell, the anode is negative, and the cathode is positive. However, in both types of cells, reduction occurs at the cathode, and oxidation occurs at the anode.

is considered the negative electrode. Alternatively, one can think of the cathode as the electrode attached to the negative pole of the battery (or other power source) used for the electrolysis.

In either case, a simple mnemonic is that the CAThode attracts the CATions. In the Daniell cell, for example, the electrons created at the anode as the zinc oxidizes travel through the wire to the copper half-cell, where they attract copper(II) cations to the cathode.

One common topic in which this distinction arises is electrophoresis, a technique often used to separate amino acids based on their isoelectronic points, or pI's (see Organic Chemistry). The positively charged amino acids (i.e., those that are protonated at the pH of the solution) will migrate towards the cathode; negatively charged amino acids (i.e., those that are deprotonated at the solution pH) migrate instead towards the anode.

REDUCTION POTENTIALS AND THE ELECTROMOTIVE FORCE

A. Reduction Potentials

Sometimes when electrolysis is carried out in an aqueous solution, water, rather than the solute, is oxidized or reduced. For example, if an aqueous solution of NaCl is electrolyzed, water may be reduced at the cathode to produce H_2 (g) and OH^- ions, instead of Na^+ being reduced to Na (s), as occurs in the absence of water. The species in a reaction that will be oxidized or reduced can be determined from the **reduction potential** of each species, defined as the tendency of a species to acquire electrons and be reduced. Each species has its own intrinsic reduction potential; the more positive the potential, the greater the species' tendency to be reduced.

A reduction potential is measured in volts (V) and is defined relative to the **standard hydrogen electrode (SHE)**, which is arbitrarily given a potential of 0.00 volts. **Standard reduction potential, ($E°$)**, is measured under **standard conditions**: 25°C, a 1 M concentration for each ion participating in the reaction, a partial pressure of 1 atm for each gas that is part of the reaction, and metals in their pure state. The relative reactivities of different half-cells can be compared to predict the direction of electron flow. A higher $E°$ means a greater tendency for reduction to occur, while a lower $E°$ means a greater tendency for oxidation to occur.

Example: Given the following half-reactions and $E°$ values, determine which species would be oxidized and which would be reduced.

$$Ag^+ + e \rightarrow Ag\ (s) \qquad E° = +0.80\ V$$
$$Tl^+ + e- \rightarrow Tl\ (s) \qquad E° = -0.34\ V$$

Solution: Ag^+ would be reduced to Ag (s) and Tl (s) would be oxidized to Tl^+, since Ag^+ has the higher $E°$. Therefore, the reaction equation would be

$$Ag^+ + Tl\ (s) \rightarrow Tl^+ + Ag\ (s)$$

which is the sum of the two spontaneous half-reactions.

It should be noted that reduction and oxidation are opposite processes. Therefore, to obtain the oxidation potential of a given half-reaction, the reduction half-reaction and the sign of the reduction potential are both reversed. For instance, from the example above, the oxidation half-reaction and oxidation potential of Tl (s) are as follows:

$$Tl\ (s) \rightarrow Tl^+ + e^- \qquad E° = +0.34\ V$$

B. The Electromotive Force

Standard reduction potentials are also used to calculate the **standard electromotive force (emf or $E°_{cell}$)** of a reaction, the difference in potential between two half-cells. The emf of a reaction is determined by adding the standard reduction potential of the reduced species and the standard oxidation potential of the oxidized species. When adding standard potentials, do *not* multiply by the number of moles oxidized or reduced.

$$emf = E°_{red} + E°_{ox} \qquad \text{(Equation 1)}$$

The standard emf of a galvanic cell is positive, while the standard emf of an electrolytic cell is negative.

Example: Given that the standard reduction potentials for Sm^{3+} and $[RhCl_6]^{3-}$ are –2.41 V and +0.44 V, respectively, calculate the emf of the following reaction:

$$Sm^{3+} + Rh + 6\ Cl^- \rightarrow [RhCl_6]^{3-} + Sm$$

Solution: First, determine the oxidation and reduction half-reactions. As written, the Rh is oxidized, and the Sm^{3+} is reduced. Thus, the Sm^{3+} reduction potential is used as is, while the reverse reaction for Rh, $[RhCl_6]^{3-} \rightarrow Rh + 6\ Cl^-$, applies, and the oxidation potential of $[RhCl_6]^{3-}$ must be used. Then, using Equation 1, the emf can be calculated to be $(-2.41 \text{ V}) + (-0.44 \text{ V}) = -2.85 \text{ V}$. The cell is thus electrolytic as written. From this result, it is evident that the reaction would proceed spontaneously to the left, in which case the Sm would be oxidized, while $[RhCl_6]^{3-}$ would be reduced.

THERMODYNAMICS OF REDOX REACTIONS

A. Emf and Gibbs Free Energy

The thermodynamic criterion for determining the spontaneity of a reaction is ΔG, Gibbs free energy, the maximum amount of useful work produced by a chemical reaction. In an electrochemical cell, the work done is dependent on the number of coulombs and the energy available. Thus, ΔG and emf are related as follows:

$$\Delta G = -nFE_{cell} \quad \text{(Equation 2)}$$

where n is the number of moles of electrons exchanged, F is Faraday's constant, and E_{cell} is the emf of the cell. **Keep in mind that if Faraday's constant is expressed in coulombs (J/V), then ΔG must be expressed in J, not kJ.**

If the reaction takes place under standard conditions (25°C, 1 atm pressure, and all solutions at 1M concentration), then the ΔG is the standard Gibbs free energy and E_{cell} is the standard cell potential. The above equation then becomes

$$\Delta G° = -nFE°_{cel} \quad \text{(Equation 3)}$$

B. The Effect of Concentration on Emf

FLASHBACK

Recall that if ΔG is positive, the reaction is not spontaneous; if ΔG is negative, the reaction is spontaneous.

Thus far, only the calculations for the emf of cells in unit concentrations (all the ionic species present have a molarity of 1, and all gases are at a pressure of 1 atm) have been discussed. However, concentration does have an effect on the emf of a cell: emf varies with the changing concentrations of the species involved. It can also be determined by the use of the **Nernst equation:**

$$E_{cell} = E°_{cell} - (RT/nF)(\ln Q)$$

Q is the reaction quotient for a given reaction. For example, in this reaction,

$$a\,A + b\,B \rightarrow c\,C + d\,D$$

the reaction quotient would be

$$Q = \frac{[C]^c\,[D]^d}{[A]^a\,[B]^b}$$

The emf of a cell can be measured by a **voltmeter**. A **potentiometer** is a kind of voltmeter that draws no current and gives a more accurate reading of the difference in potential between two electrodes.

C. Emf and the Equilibrium Constant (Keq)

For reactions in solution, $\Delta G°$ can be determined in another manner, as follows:

$$\Delta G° = -RT \ln K_{eq} \quad \text{(Equation 4)}$$

where R is the gas constant 8.314 J/(K·mol), T is the temperature in K, and K_{eq} is the equilibrium constant for the reaction.

If Equations 3 and 4 are combined, then

$$\Delta G° = -nFE°_{cell} = -RT \ln K_{eq}$$

or simply

$$nFE°_{cell} = RT \ln K_{eq} \quad \text{(Equation 5)}$$

If the values for n, T, and K_{eq} are known, then the $E°_{cell}$ for the redox reaction can be readily calculated.

12

Nuclear Phenomena

The subject of this chapter is the nucleus and nuclear phenomena. It begins with a review of some of the standard terminology used in nuclear chemistry and physics. The concept of binding energy and the equivalent concept of the mass defect are then introduced. Briefly, an amount of energy, called the **binding energy**, is required to break up a given nucleus into its constituent protons and neutrons. That energy is converted to mass via Einstein's $E = mc2$, resulting in a larger mass for the constituent protons and neutrons than that of the original nucleus, the difference being called the **mass defect**. The remainder of the chapter is concerned with a brief discussion of nuclear reactions (**fission** and **fusion**) and an extended treatment of **radioactive decay**, which itself is presented in two distinct parts. The first deals with the four types of radioactive decay and a discussion of the reaction equations that describe them. The second covers the general problem of determining the number of nuclei that have not decayed as a function of time, along with the associated concept of the half-life of a decay process.

NUCLEI

At the center of an atom lies its nucleus, consisting of one or more **nucleons** (protons or neutrons) held together with considerably more energy than the energy needed to hold electrons in orbit around the nucleus. The radius of the nucleus is about 100,000 times smaller than the radius of the atom. Some common nuclear properties are the following:

A. Atomic Number (Z)

Z is always an integer and is equal to the **number of protons** in the nucleus. Each element has a unique number of protons; therefore, the atomic number *Z* identifies the element. *Z* is used as a presubscript to the chemical symbol in **isotopic notation**. The chemical symbols and the atomic numbers of all the elements are given in the periodic table.

ATOMIC NUMBERS OF SELECTED CHEMICAL ELEMENTS

Atomic number Z	Chemical symbol	Element name
1	H	hydrogen
2	He	helium
3	Li	lithium
.	.	.
.	.	.
92	U	uranium
.	.	.
.	.	.
.	.	.

B. Mass Number (A)

A is an integer equal to the total **number of nucleons** (neutrons and protons) in a nucleus. Let N represent the number of neutrons in a nucleus. The equation relating A, N, and Z is simply:

$$A = N + Z$$

In isotopic notation, A appears as a presuperscript to the chemical symbol.

Examples: $_1^1H$ —a single proton; the nucleus of ordinary hydrogen

$_2^4He$ —the nucleus of ordinary helium, consisting of 2 protons and 2 neutrons. It is also known as an alpha particle (α-particle).

$_{92}^{235}U$ —a fissionable form of uranium, consisting of 92 protons and 143 neutrons

C. Isotope

The nucleus of a given element can have different numbers of neutrons and, hence, different mass numbers. For a nucleus of a given element with a given number of protons (atomic number Z), the various nuclei with different numbers of neutrons are called **isotopes** of that element. The term *isotope* is also used in a generic sense to refer to any nucleus. The term **radionuclide** is another generic term used to refer to any radioactive isotope, especially those used in **nuclear medicine.**

Example: The three isotopes of hydrogen are these:

^1_1H —a single proton; the nucleus of ordinary hydrogen

^2_1H —a proton and a neutron together, often called a **deuteron**; the nucleus of one type of heavy hydrogen called **deuterium**

^3_1H —a proton and two neutrons together, often called a **triton**; the nucleus of a heavier type of heavy hydrogen called **tritium**

D. Atomic Mass and Atomic Mass Unit

Atomic mass is most commonly measured in **atomic mass units** (abbreviated amu or simply u). By definition, 1 amu is exactly one-twelfth the mass of the neutral carbon-12 atom (not just the nucleus—the atom includes the nucleus and all 6 electrons). In terms of more familiar mass units,

$$1 \text{ amu} = 1.66 \times 10^{-27} \text{ kg} = 1.66 \times 10^{-24} \text{ g}$$

E. Atomic Weight

Because isotopes exist, atoms of a given element can have different masses. The atomic weight refers to a weighted average of the **masses** (not the weights) of an element. The average is weighted according to the natural abundances of the various isotopic species of an element. The atomic weight can be measured in amu.

Example: 99.985499% of hydrogen occurs in the common ^1H isotope with a mass of 1.00782504 u. About 0.0142972% occurs as deuterium with a mass (including the electron) of 2.01410 u, and about 0.0003027% occurs as tritium with a mass of 3.01605 u. The atomic weight of hydrogen $A_r(H)$ is the sum of the mass of each isotope multiplied by its natural abundance (x):

$$A_r(H) = m_{1H}x_{1H} + m_{2H}x_{2H} + m_{3H}x_{3H}$$
$$= (1.00782504)(0.99985499)$$
$$+ (2.01410)(0.000142972)$$
$$+ (3.01605)(0.000003027)$$
$$= 1.00797 \text{ amu}$$

NUCLEAR BINDING ENERGY AND MASS DEFECT

Every nucleus (other than ^1_1H) has a smaller mass than the combined mass of its constituent protons and neutrons. The difference is called the **mass defect.** Scientists had difficulty explaining why this mass defect occurred until Einstein discovered the equivalence of matter and energy, embodied by the equation $E = mc^2$. The mass defect is a result of matter that has been converted to energy. This energy, called **binding energy,** holds the nucleons together in the nucleus. (Note: The binding energy per nucleon peaks at iron, which implies that iron is the most stable atom. In general, intermediate-sized nuclei are more stable than large and small nuclei.)

The mass defect and binding energy of ^4He are calculated in the following example.

Example: Measurements of the atomic mass of a neutron and a proton yield these results:

$$proton = 1.00728 \text{ amu}$$
$$neutron = 1.00867 \text{ amu}$$

A measurement of the atomic mass of a ^4He nucleus yields this:

$$^4He = 4.00260 \text{ amu}$$

^4He consists of 2 protons and 2 neutrons, which should theoretically give a ^4He mass of

$$Z(m_p) + N(m_n) = 2(1.00728) + 2(1.00867)$$
$$= 4.03190 \text{ amu}$$

What is the mass defect and binding energy of this nucleus?

Solution: The difference, $4.03190 - 4.00260 = 0.02930$ amu, is the mass defect (Δm) for ^4He and is interpreted as the conversion of mass into the binding energy of the nucleus. The rest energy of 1 amu is 932 MeV, so using $E = mc^2$, we find that $c^2 = 932$ MeV/amu. Therefore, the binding energy (B.E.) of ^4He is

$$B.E. = \Delta mc^2$$
$$= (0.02930)(932)$$
$$= 27.3 \text{ MeV}$$

NUCLEAR REACTIONS AND DECAY

Nuclear reactions, such as fusion, fission, and radioactive decay, involve either combining or splitting the nuclei of atoms. Since the binding energy per nucleon is greatest for intermediate-sized atoms, when small atoms combine or large atoms split, a great amount of energy is released.

A. Fusion

Fusion occurs when small nuclei combine into a larger nucleus. As an example, many stars, including the sun, power themselves by fusing four hydrogen nuclei to make one helium nucleus. By this method, the sun produces 4×10^{26} J every second. Here on earth, researchers are trying to find ways to use fusion as an alternative energy source.

B. Fission

Fission is a process in which a large nucleus splits into smaller nuclei. Spontaneous fission rarely occurs. However, by the absorption of a low-energy neutron, fission can be induced in certain nuclei. Of special interest are those fission reactions that release more neutrons, since these other neutrons will cause other atoms to undergo fission. This in turn releases more neutrons, creating a **chain reaction.** Such induced fission reactions power commercial nuclear electric-generating plants.

Example: A fission reaction occurs when uranium-235 (U-235) absorbs a low-energy neutron, briefly forming an excited state of U-236, which then splits into xenon-140, strontium-94, and x more neutrons. In isotopic notation form the reactions are

$$^{235}_{92}U + {}^{1}_{0}n \longrightarrow {}^{236}_{92}U \longrightarrow {}^{140}_{54}Xe + {}^{94}_{38}Sr + x\,{}^{1}_{0}n$$

How many neutrons are produced in the last reaction?

Solution: The question is asking "What is x?" By treating each arrow as an equal sign, the problem is simply asking to balance the last "equation." The mass numbers (A) on either side of each arrow must be equal. This is an application of **nucleon** or **baryon number conservation,** which says that the total number of neutrons plus protons remains the same, even if neutrons are converted to protons and vice versa, as they are in some decays. Since $235 + 1 = 236$, the first arrow is indeed balanced. To find the number of neutrons, solve for x in the last equation (arrow):

$$236 = 140 + 94 + x$$
$$x = 236 - 140 - 94$$
$$= 2$$

So two neutrons are produced in this reaction. These neutrons are free to go on and be absorbed by more ^{235}U and cause more fissioning, and the process continues in a chain reaction. Note that it really was not necessary to know that the intermediate state $^{236}_{92}U$ was formed.

Some radioactive nuclei may be induced to fission via more than one **decay channel** or **decay mode**. For example, a different fission reaction may occur when uranium-235 absorbs a slow neutron and then immediately splits into barium-139, krypton-94, and three more neutrons with no intermediate state:

$$^{236}_{92}U + {}^1_0n \longrightarrow {}^{139}_{56}Ba + {}^{94}_{36}Kr + 3{}^1_0n$$

C. Radioactive Decay

Radioactive decay is a naturally occurring spontaneous decay of certain nuclei accompanied by the emission of specific particles. It could be classified as a certain type of fission. Radioactive decay problems are of three general types:

1. The integer arithmetic of particle and isotope species

2. Radioactive half-life problems

3. The use of exponential decay curves and decay constants

1. ISOTOPE DECAY ARITHMETIC AND NUCLEON CONSERVATION

Let the letters X and Y represent nuclear isotopes, and let us further consider the three types of decay particles and how they affect the mass number and atomic number of the **parent isotope** $^A_Z X$ and the resulting **daughter isotope** $^{A'}_{Z'} Y$ in the decay:

$$^A_Z X \longrightarrow {}^{A'}_{Z'} Y + \text{emitted decay particle}$$

a. **Alpha decay** is the emission of an α-particle, which is a ^4He nucleus that consists of two protons and two neutrons. The alpha particle is very massive (compared to a beta particle) and doubly charged. Alpha particles interact with matter very easily; hence, they do not penetrate shielding (such as lead sheets) very far.

The emission of an α-particle means that the daughter's atomic number Z will be 2 less than the parent's atomic number, and the daughter's mass number will be 4 less than the parent's mass number. This can be expressed in two simple equations:

REMEMBER

An α-particle is a helium nucleus with 2 protons and 2 neutrons (i.e., ^4He).

α **decay**

$$Z_{daughter} = Z_{parent} - 2$$

$$A_{daughter} = A_{parent} - 4$$

The generic alpha decay reaction is then:

$$^A_Z X \longrightarrow ^{A-4}_{Z-2} Y + \alpha$$

Example: Suppose a parent X alpha decays into a daughter Y such that

$$^{238}_{92} X \longrightarrow ^{A'}_{Z'} Y + \alpha$$

What are the mass number (A') and atomic number (Z') of the daughter isotope Y?

Solution: Since $\alpha = ^4_2 He$, balancing the mass numbers and atomic numbers is all that needs to be done:

$$238 = A' + 4$$

$$A' = 234$$

$$92 = Z' + 2$$

$$Z' = 90$$

So $A' = 234$ and $Z' = 90$. Note that it was not necessary to know the chemical species of the isotopes to do this problem. However, it would have been possible to look at the periodic table and see that $Z = 92$ means X is uranium-238 ($^{238}_{92} U$) and that $Z = 90$ means Y is thorium-234 ($^{234}_{90} Th$).

b. **Beta decay** is the emission of a β-particle, which is an electron given the symbol e⁻ or β⁻. Electrons do not reside in the nucleus but are emitted by the nucleus when a neutron in the nucleus decays into a proton and a β⁻ (and an antineutrino). Since an electron is singly charged and about 1,836 times lighter than a proton, the beta radiation from radioactive decay is more penetrating than alpha radiation. In some cases of induced decay, a positively charged antielectron known as a **positron** is emitted. The positron is given the symbol e⁺ or β⁺.

β⁻ decay means that a neutron disappears and a proton takes its place. Hence, the parent's mass number is unchanged, and the parent's atomic number is increased by 1. In other words, the daughter's A is the same as the parent's, and the daughter's Z is one more than the parent's.

> **REMEMBER**
>
> A β⁻-particle is also called a β-particle and is just an electron.

In positron decay, a proton (instead of a neutron as in β^- decay) splits into a positron and a neutron. Therefore, a β^+ decay means that the parent's mass number is unchanged and the parent's atomic number is decreased by 1. In other words, the daughter's A is the same as the parent's, and the daughter's Z is one less than the parent's. In equation form:

β^- decay

$$Z_{daughter} = Z_{parent} + 1$$
$$A_{daughter} = A_{parent}$$

β^+ decay

$$Z_{daughter} = Z_{parent} - 1$$
$$A_{daughter} = A_{parent}$$

The generic negative beta decay reaction is as follows:

$$^A_Z X \longrightarrow {}^A_{Z+1} Y + \beta^-$$

The generic positive beta decay reaction is

$$^A_Z X \longrightarrow {}^A_{Z-1} Y + \beta^+$$

Example: Suppose a cobalt-60 nucleus beta-decays:

$$^{60}Co \longrightarrow {}^{A'}_{Z'} Y + e^-$$

What is the element Y, and what are A' and Z'?

Solution: Again, balance mass numbers:

$$60 = A' + 0$$
$$A' = 60$$

Now balance the atomic numbers, taking into account that cobalt has 27 protons (you learn this by consulting the periodic table) and that there is one more proton on the right-hand side:

$$27 = Z' - 1$$
$$Z' = 28$$

By looking at the periodic table, one finds that $Z' = 28$ is nickel:

$$Y = {}^{60}_{28}\text{Ni}$$

c. **Gamma decay** is the emission of γ–particles, which are high-energy photons. They carry no charge and simply lower the energy of the emitting (parent) nucleus without changing the mass number or the atomic number. In other words, the daughter's A is the same as the parent's, and the daughter's Z is the same as the parent's.

γ **decay**

$Z_{\text{parent}} = Z_{\text{daughter}}$

$A_{\text{parent}} = A_{\text{daughter}}$

The generic gamma decay reaction is thus

$$_{Z}^{A}\text{X}^{*} \longrightarrow {}_{Z}^{A}\text{X} + \gamma$$

Example: Suppose a parent isotope $_{Z}^{A}\text{X}$ emits a β^+ and turns into an excited state of the isotope $_{Z'}^{A'}\text{Y}^{*}$, which then γ decays to $_{Z''}^{A''}\text{Y}$, which in turn α decays to $_{Z'''}^{A'''}\text{W}$. If W is ^{60}Fe, what is $_{Z}^{A}\text{X}$?

Solution: Since the final daughter in this chain of decay is given, it will be necessary to work backward through the reactions. By looking at the periodic table, one finds that W = Fe means $Z''' = 26$; hence, the last reaction is the following α decay:

$$_{Z''}^{A''}\text{Y} \longrightarrow {}_{26}^{60}\text{Fe} + {}_{2}^{4}\text{He}$$

By balancing the atomic numbers, you find

$$Z'' = 26 + 2 = 28$$

A balancing of the mass numbers implies

$$A'' = 60 + 4 = 64$$

The second-to-last reaction is a γ decay, which simply releases energy from the nucleus but does not alter the atomic number or the mass number of the parent. That is, $Z' = Z'' = 28$, and $A' = A'' = 64$. So the second reaction is

$$^{64}_{28}Y\text{*} \longrightarrow {}^{64}_{28}Y + \gamma$$

The first reaction was a β^+ decay that must have looked like this:

$$^A_ZX \longrightarrow {}^{64}_{28}Y\text{*} + e^+$$

Again, balance the atomic numbers:

$$Z = 28 + 1 = 29$$

You carry out a balancing of mass numbers by taking into account that a proton has disappeared on the left and reappeared as a neutron on the right, leaving mass number unchanged:

$$A = 64 + 0 = 64$$

By looking at the periodic table, you find that $Z = 29$ means that X is Cu. Since $A = 64$, that means that the solution is

$$^A_ZX = {}^{64}_{29}Cu$$

While the problem did not ask for it, it is possible again to look at the periodic table to find that $Z' = Z'' = 28$ means $Y\text{*} = Y = Ni$. The total chain of decays can be written as follows:

$$^{64}_{29}Cu \longrightarrow {}^{64}_{28}Ni\text{*} + \beta^+$$

$$^{64}_{28}Ni\text{*} \longrightarrow {}^{64}_{28}Ni + \gamma$$

$$^{64}_{28}Ni \longrightarrow {}^{60}_{26}Fe + \alpha$$

d. Electron capture

Certain unstable radionuclides are capable of capturing an inner (K or L shell) electron that combines with a proton to form a neutron. The atomic number is now one less than the original, but the mass number remains the same. Electron capture is a rare process that is perhaps best thought of as an inverse β^- decay.

2. RADIOACTIVE DECAY HALF-LIFE ($T1/2$)

In a collection of a great many identical radioactive isotopes, the **half-life** ($T_{1/2}$) of the sample is the time it takes for half of the sample to decay.

Example: If the half-life of a certain isotope is 4 years, what fraction of a sample of that isotope will remain after 12 years?

Solution: If 4 years is one half-life, then 12 years is three half-lives. During the first half-life—the first 4 years—half of the sample will have decayed. During the second half-life (years 4 to 8), half of the remaining half will decay, leaving one-fourth of the original. During the third and final period (years 8 to 12), half of the remaining fourth will decay, leaving one-eighth of the original sample. Thus, the fraction remaining after 3 half-lives is $(1/2)^3$ or $(1/8)$.

> **REMEMBER**
>
> (fraction of original nuclei remaining after n half-lives) = $(1/2)^n$.

3. EXPONENTIAL DECAY

Let n be the number of radioactive nuclei that have not yet decayed in a sample. It turns out that the **rate** at which the nuclei decay ($\Delta n/\Delta t$) is proportional to the number that remain (n). This suggests the following equation:

$$\frac{\Delta n}{\Delta t} = -\lambda n$$

where λ is known as the **decay constant.** The solution of this equation tells us how the number of radioactive nuclei changes with time.

The solution is known as an **exponential decay:**

$$n = n_0 e^{-\lambda t}$$

where n_0 is the number of undecayed nuclei at time $t = 0$. (The decay constant is related to the half-life by $\lambda = \dfrac{\ln 2}{T_{1/2}} = \dfrac{0.693}{T_{1/2}}$.)

Example: If at time $t = 0$ there is a 2 mole sample of radioactive isotopes of decay constant 2 (hour)$^{-1}$, how many nuclei remain after 45 minutes?

Solution: Since 45 minutes is 3/4 of an hour, the exponent is

$$\lambda t = (2)\frac{3}{4} = \frac{6}{4} = \frac{3}{2}$$

The exponential factor will be a number smaller than 1:

$$e^{-\lambda t} = e^{-3/2} = 0.22$$

> **KEY CONCEPT**
>
> (number of nuclei that have decayed in time t) = $(n_0 - n)$, where $n = n_0 e^{-\lambda t}$.

So only 0.22 or 22 percent of the original two-mole sample will remain. To find n_0, we can multiply the number of moles we have by the number of particles per mole (Avogadro's number):

$$n_0 = 2(6.02 \times 10^{23}) = 1.2 \times 10^{24}$$

From the equation that describes exponential decay, you can calculate the number that remain after 45 minutes:

$$n = n_0 e^{-\lambda t}$$
$$= (1.2 \times 10^{24})(0.22)$$
$$= 2.6 \times 10^{23} \text{ particles}$$

ORGANIC CHEMISTRY

Nomenclature

Nomenclature, the set of accepted conventions for naming compounds, is crucial to a discussion of organic chemistry. The rules of nomenclature presented in this chapter are for general cases only. More specific examples will be discussed in the chapters dealing with particular types of compounds.

You may see specific nomenclature questions such as "Name the following compound," or "Which structure represents the following named compound?" But more importantly, nomenclature represents the basic language of organic chemistry. If you don't know it, you may feel as though you're taking a test in a foreign language—which, in a way, you would be!

ALKANES

Alkanes are the simplest organic molecules, consisting only of carbon and hydrogen atoms held together by single bonds.

A. Straight-Chain Alkanes

The names of the four simplest alkanes are

CH_4	CH_3CH_3	$CH_3CH_2CH_3$	$CH_3CH_2CH_2CH_3$
methane	ethane	propane	butane

The names of the longer-chain alkanes consist of prefixes derived from the Greek root for the number of carbon atoms, with the ending **-ane**.

C_5H_{12} = **pent**ane	C_9H_{20} = **non**ane
C_6H_{14} = **hex**ane	$C_{10}H_{22}$ = **dec**ane
C_7H_{16} = **hept**ane	$C_{11}H_{24}$ = **undec**ane
C_8H_{18} = **oct**ane	$C_{12}H_{26}$ = **dodec**ane

These prefixes are applicable to more complex organic molecules and should be memorized.

REMEMBER

You must memorize the nomenclature prefixes for the four simplest carbon chains:
- Meth-
- Eth-
- Prop-
- But-

KEY CONCEPT

All straight-chain alkanes have the general formula $C_nH_{2n} + 2$ (where n is an integer).

BRIDGE

Straight-chain alkanes are fat soluble (i.e., nonpolar).

B. Branched-Chain Alkanes

The International Union of Pure and Applied Chemistry (IUPAC) has proposed a set of simple rules for naming complex molecules. This basic system can be used to name all classes of organic compounds. Throughout these notes, the IUPAC names will be listed as the primary name, and common names will appear in parentheses.

REMEMBER

1. Identify the longest backbone.
2. Number it, keeping numbers for the substituents as low as possible.
3. Name substituents.
4. Assign numbers.
5. Put the whole name together, remembering to alphabetize substituents.

1. FIND THE LONGEST CHAIN IN THE COMPOUND.

The longest continuous carbon chain within the compound is taken as the backbone. If there are two or more chains of equal length, the most highly substituted chain takes precedence. The longest chain may not be obvious from the structural formula as it is drawn. For example, the backbone shown in Figure 1.1 is an octane (it contains eight carbon atoms).

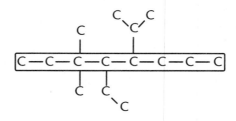

Figure 1.1

2. NUMBER THE CHAIN.

Number the chain from one end in such a way that the lowest set of numbers is obtained for the substituents.

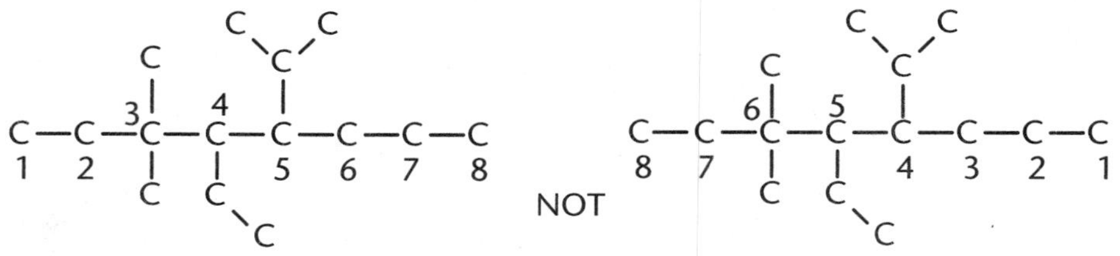

Figure 1.2

3. NAME THE SUBSTITUENTS.

Substituents are named according to their appropriate prefix with the ending **-yl**. More complex substituents are named as derivatives of the longest chain in the group.

CH_3–	CH_3CH_2–	$CH_3CH_2CH_2$–
methyl	ethyl	*n*-propyl

The prefix *n*- in the above example indicates an unbranched ("normal") compound. There are special names for some common branched alkanes, and these are usually used in the naming of substituents.

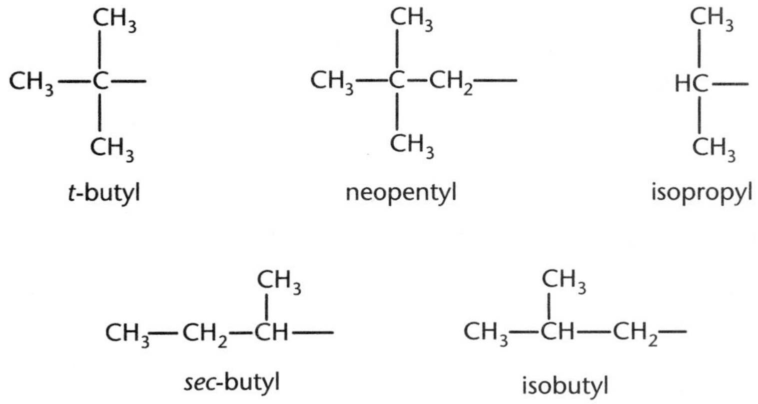
t-butyl
neopentyl
isopropyl
sec-butyl
isobutyl

Figure 1.3

> **KEY CONCEPT**
>
> You should memorize these common structures.

If there are two or more equivalent groups, the prefixes **di-**, **tri-**, **tetra-**, etc. are used.

4. **ASSIGN A NUMBER TO EACH SUBSTITUENT.**

   Each substituent is assigned a number to identify its point of attachment to the principal chain. If the prefixes **di-**, **tri-**, **tetra-**, etc. are used, a number is still necessary for each individual group.

5. **COMPLETE THE NAME.**

   List the substituents in alphabetical order with their corresponding numbers. Prefixes such as di-, tri-, etc. as well as the hyphenated prefixes (*tert*- [or *t*-], *sec*-, *n*-) are ignored in alphabetizing. In contrast, **cyclo-**, **iso-**, and **neo-** are considered part of the group name and are alphabetized. Commas should be placed between numbers, and dashes should be placed between numbers and words. Figure 1.4 shows an example.

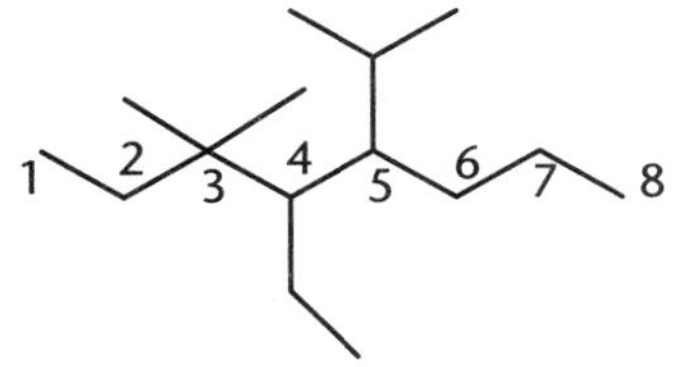

4-ethyl-5-isopropyl-3,3-dimethyl octane

Figure 1.4

You may also need to indicate the isomer you are describing—e.g., *cis* or *trans*, *R* or *S*, etc.

C. Cycloalkanes

Alkanes can form rings. These are named according to the number of carbon atoms in the ring with the prefix **cyclo-**.

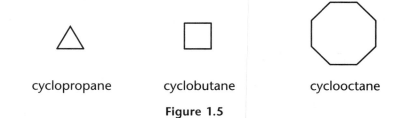

cyclopropane   cyclobutane   cyclooctane

Figure 1.5

Substituted cycloalkanes are named as derivatives of the parent cycloalkane. The substituents are named, and the carbon atoms are numbered around the ring *starting from the point of greatest substitution*. Again, the goal is to provide the lowest series of numbers, as in rule number 2 above.

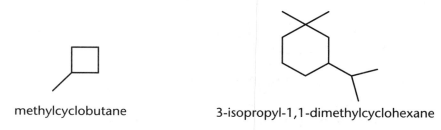

methylcyclobutane   3-isopropyl-1,1-dimethylcyclohexane

Figure 1.6

MORE COMPLICATED MOLECULES

Organic molecules that are more complicated than simple alkanes can also be named using this five-step process, with a few additional considerations.

MULTIPLE BONDS

A. Alkenes

Alkenes (or **olefins**) are compounds containing carbon-carbon double bonds. The nomenclature rules are essentially the same as for alkanes, except that the ending **-ene** is used rather than **-ane**. (Exceptions: The common names *ethylene* and *propylene,* are used preferentially over the IUPAC names *ethene* and *propene*).

When identifying the carbon backbone, select the longest chain that contains the double bond (or the greatest number of double bonds, if more than one is present).

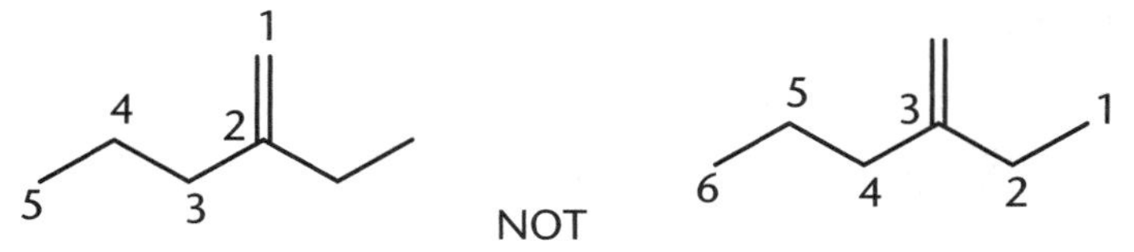

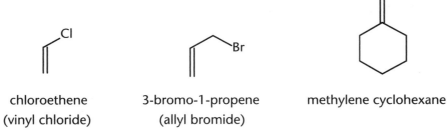

Figure 1.7

Number the backbone so that the double bond receives the lowest number possible. Remember that multiple double bonds must be named using the prefixes di-, tri-, etc. and that each must receive a number. Also, you may need to name the configurational isomer (*cis/trans*, *Z/E*).

Substituents are named as they are for alkanes, and their positions are specified by the number of the backbone carbon atom to which they are attached.

Frequently, an alkene group must be named as a substituent. In these cases, the systematic names may be used, but common names are more popular. **Vinyl**- derivatives are monosubstituted ethylenes (**ethenyl-**), and **allyl**-derivatives are propylenes substituted at the C3 position (**2-propenyl**). **Methylene** refers to the –CH$_2$ group.

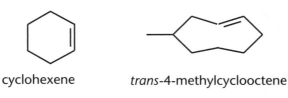

| chloroethene | 3-bromo-1-propene | methylene cyclohexane |
| (vinyl chloride) | (allyl bromide) | |

Figure 1.8

B. Cycloalkenes

Cycloalkenes are named like cycloalkanes but with the suffix **-ene** rather than **-ane**. If there is only one double bond and no other substituents, a number is not necessary.

cyclohexene   *trans*-4-methylcyclooctene

Figure 1.9

REMEMBER

Straight-chain alkynes have the general formula C_nH_{2n-2} (n is an integer).

C. Alkynes

Alkynes are compounds that possess carbon-carbon triple bonds. The suffix **-yne** replaces *-ane* in the parent alkane. The position of the triple bond is indicated by a number when necessary. The common name for ethyne is **acetylene,** and this name is used almost exclusively. Regardless of how they are drawn, triple bonds are linear.

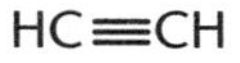

HC≡CH
ethyne
(acetylene)

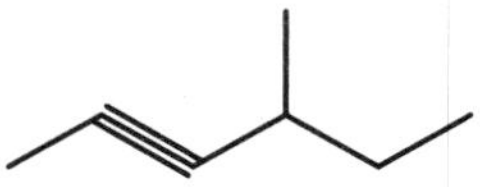

4-methyl-2-hexyne

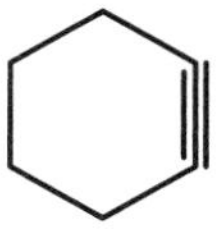

cyclohexyne

Figure 1.10

SUBSTITUTED ALKANES

A. Haloalkanes

Compounds that contain a halogen (F, Cl, Br, or I) substituent are named haloalkanes. The substituents are numbered and listed alphabetically in the compound name in the same way as alkyl groups. Notice that the presence of the halide does not dramatically affect the numbering of the chain, and we still proceed so that substituents receive the lowest possible numbers. Figure 1.11 shows two examples.

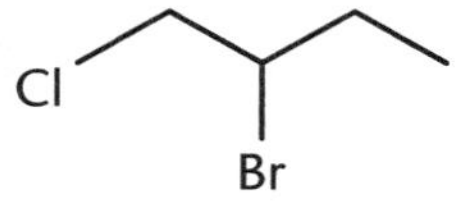

2-bromo-1-chlorobutane

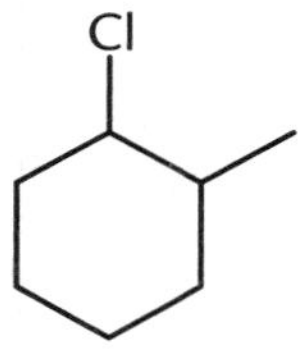

1-chloro-2-methylcyclohexane

Figure 1.11

Alternatively, the haloalkane may be named as an **alkyl halide.** In this system, chloroethane is called **ethyl chloride**. Other examples are shown in Figure 1.12.

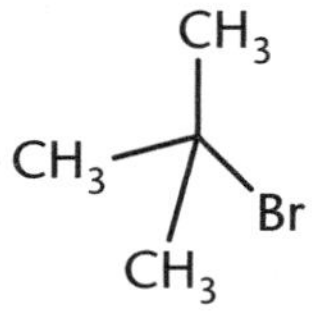

2-bromo-2-methylpropane
(*t*-butyl bromide)

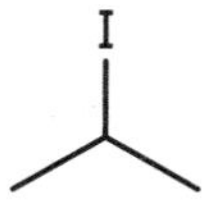

2-iodopropane
(isopropyl iodide)

Figure 1.12

B. Alcohols

In the IUPAC system, **alcohols** are named by replacing the *-e* of the corresponding alkane with **-ol**. The chain is numbered so that the carbon attached to the hydroxyl group (–OH) receives the lowest number possible.

In compounds that possess a multiple bond and a hydroxyl group, numerical priority is given to the carbon attached to the –OH.

KEY CONCEPT

–OH has priority over a multiple bond when numbering the chain.

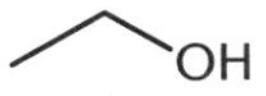

ethanol

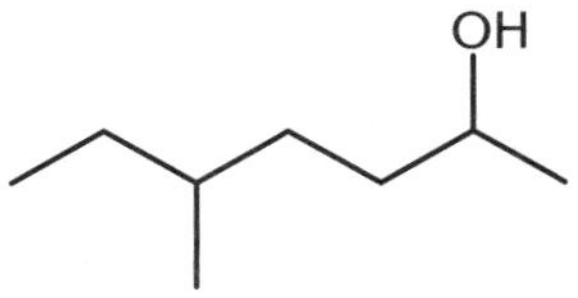

5-methyl-2-heptanol

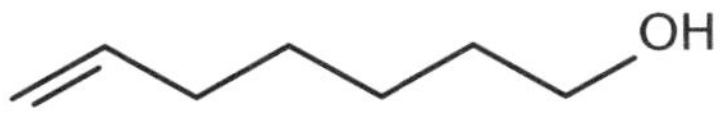

hept-6-en-1-ol

Figure 1.13

A common system of nomenclature exists for alcohols in which the name of the alkyl group is combined with the word *alcohol*. These common names are used for simple alcohols. For example, methanol may be named "methyl alcohol," while 2-propanol may also be named "isopropyl alcohol."

Molecules with two hydroxyl groups are called **diols** (or **glycols**) and are named with the suffix **-diol**. Two numbers are necessary to locate the two functional groups. Diols with hydroxyl groups on adjacent carbons are referred to as **vicinal**, and diols with hydroxyl groups on the same carbon are **geminal**. Geminal diols (also called **hydrates**) are not commonly observed because they spontaneously lose water **(dehydrate)** to produce carbonyl compounds (containing C=O).

C. Ethers

In the IUPAC system, **ethers** are named as derivatives of alkanes, and the larger alkyl group is chosen as the backbone. The ether functionality is specified as an **alkoxy-** prefix, indicating the presence of an ether (*-oxy-*), and the corresponding smaller alkyl group (*alk-*). The chain is numbered to give the ether the lowest position. Common names for ethers are frequently used. They are derived by naming the two alkyl groups in alphabetical order and adding the word *ether*. The generic term *ether* refers to diethyl ether, a commonly used solvent.

KEY CONCEPT

Ethers may have the prefix *alkoxy–* or be given a common name (e.g., ethyl methyl ether).

For **cyclic ethers**, numbering of the ring begins at the oxygen and proceeds to provide the lowest numbers for the substituents. Three-membered rings are termed **oxiranes** by IUPAC, although they are commonly called **epoxides**.

KEY CONCEPT

Cyclic ethers with three members are *epoxides.*

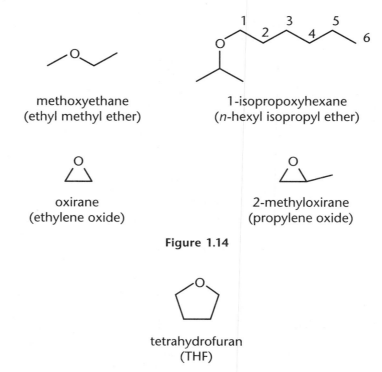

methoxyethane
(ethyl methyl ether)

1-isopropoxyhexane
(*n*-hexyl isopropyl ether)

oxirane
(ethylene oxide)

2-methyloxirane
(propylene oxide)

Figure 1.14

tetrahydrofuran
(THF)

Figure 1.15

D. Aldehydes and Ketones

Aldehydes are named according to the longest chain containing the aldehyde functional group. The suffix **-al** replaces the *-e* of the corresponding alkane. The carbonyl carbon receives the lowest number, although numbers are not always necessary since, by definition, an aldehyde is terminal and receives the number 1.

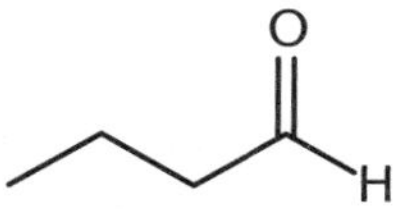

n-butanal

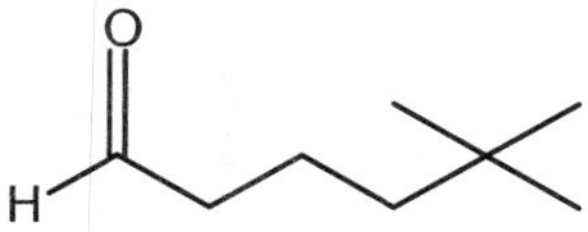

5,5-dimethylhexanal

Figure 1.16

The common names *formaldehyde*, *acetaldehyde*, and *propionaldehyde* are used almost exclusively instead of the IUPAC names *methanal*, *ethanal*, and *propanal*, respectively.

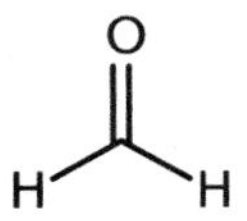

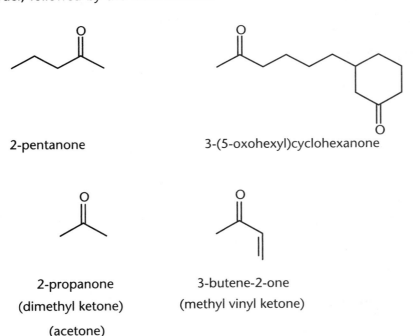

methanal
(formaldehyde)

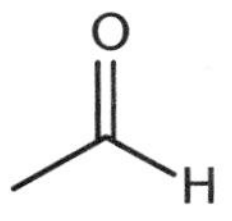

ethanal
(acetaldehyde)

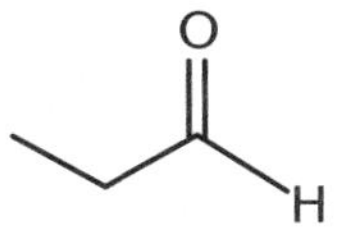

propanal
(propionaldehyde)

Figure 1.17

Ketones are named analogously, with **-one** as a suffix. The carbonyl group has to be assigned the lowest possible number. In complex molecules, the carbonyl group can be named as a prefix with the term **oxo-**. Alternatively, the individual alkyl groups may be listed in alphabetical order, followed by the word **ketone**.

KEY CONCEPT

The carbonyl in a ketone should receive the lowest number possible, unless there is a higher-priority group.

2-pentanone

3-(5-oxohexyl)cyclohexanone

2-propanone
(dimethyl ketone)
(acetone)

3-butene-2-one
(methyl vinyl ketone)

Figure 1.18

A commonly used alternative to the numerical designation of substituents is to term the carbon atom adjacent to the carbonyl carbon as α and the carbon atoms successively along the chain as β, γ, δ, etc. This system is encountered with dicarbonyl compounds and halocarbonyl compounds.

E. Carboxylic Acids

Carboxylic acids are named with the ending **-oic** and the word **acid** replacing the -e ending of the corresponding alkane. Carboxylic acids are terminal functional groups and, like aldehydes, are numbered one (1). The common names formic acid (methanoic acid), acetic acid (ethanoic acid), and propionic acid (propanoic acid) are used almost exclusively.

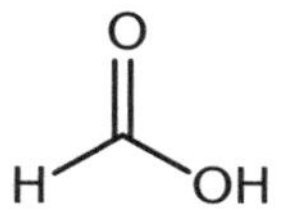

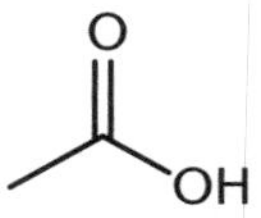

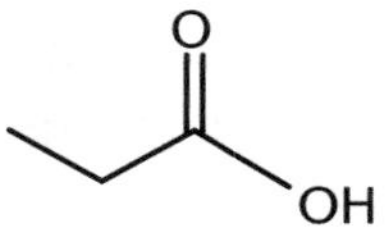

| methanoic acid | ethanoic acid | propanoic acid |
| (formic acid) | (acetic acid) | (propionic acid) |

Figure 1.19

F. Amines

The longest chain attached to the nitrogen atom is taken as the backbone. For simple compounds, name the alkane and replace the final e with *amine*. More complex molecules are often named using the prefix *amino-*.

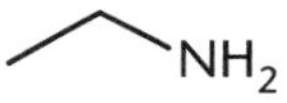

ethanamine 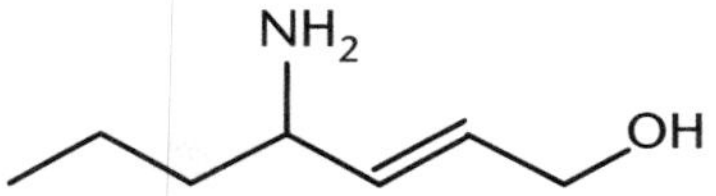   4-aminohept-2-en-1-ol

Figure 1.20

To specify the location of an additional alkyl group that is attached to the nitrogen, the prefix N- is used, as shown in Figure 1.21.

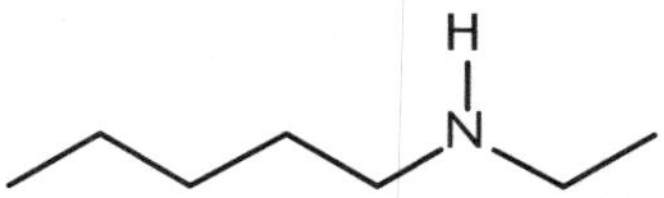

N-ethylpentanamine
(ethylpentylamine)

Figure 1.21

SUMMARY OF FUNCTIONAL GROUPS

Table 1.1 lists the major functional groups you need to know.

Table 1.1

Functional Group	Structure	IUPAC Prefix	IUPAC Suffix
Carboxylic acid	R—C(=O)OH	carboxy-	-oic acid
Ester	R—C(=O)OR	alkoxycarbonyl-	-oate
Acyl halide	R—C(=O)X	halocarbonyl-	-oyl halide
Amide	R—C(=O)NH$_2$	amido-	-amide
Nitril/Cyanide	RC≡N	cyano-	-nitrile
Aldehyde	R—C(=O)H	oxo-	-al
Ketone	R—C(=O)—R	oxo-	-one
Alcohol	ROH	hydroxy-	-ol
Thiol	RSH	sulfhydryl-	-thiol
Amine	RNH$_2$	amino-	-amine
Imine	R$_2$C=NR'	imino-	-imine
Ether	ROR	alkoxy-	-ether
Sulfide	R$_2$S	alkylthio-	
Halide	-I, -Br, -Cl, -F	halo-	
Nitro	RNO$_2$	nitro-	
Azide	RN$_3$	azido-	
Diazo	RN$_2^+$	diazo-	

KEY CONCEPTS

More complex molecules can also be named with the same five steps, with a few additional considerations:

1. Multiple bonds should be on the main carbon backbone whenever possible.

2. –OH is a high-priority functional group, placed above multiple bonds in numbering.

3. Haloalkanes, ethers, and ketones are often given common names (e.g., methyl chloride, ethyl methyl ether, diethyl ketone).

4. Aldehydes and carboxylic acids are terminal functional groups. If present, they define C1 of the carbon chain (taking precedence over hydroxy, –OH, or multiple bonds).

5. Remember to specify the isomer, if relevant (such as *cis* or *trans*, *R* or *S*, etc.).

Isomers

2

Isomers are chemical compounds that have the same molecular formula but differ in structure—that is, in their atomic connectivity, rotational orientation, or three-dimensional position of their atoms. Isomers may be extremely similar, sharing most or all of their physical and chemical properties, or they may be very different.

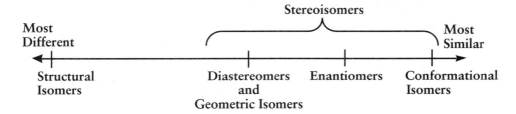

Note that geometric isomers are actually a class of diastereomers.

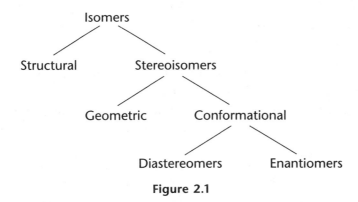

Figure 2.1

STRUCTURAL ISOMERISM

Structural isomers are compounds that share only their molecular formula. Because their atomic connections may be completely different, they often have very different chemical and physical properties (such as melting point, boiling point, solubility, etc.). For example, five different structures exist for compounds with the formula C_6H_{14}.

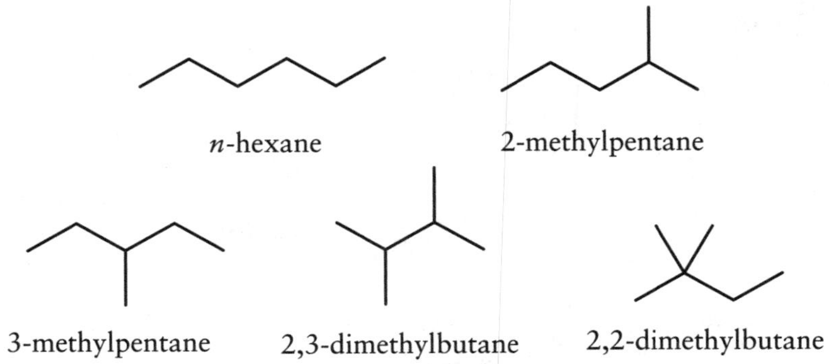

n-hexane   2-methylpentane

3-methylpentane   2,3-dimethylbutane   2,2-dimethylbutane

Figure 2.2

All have the same formula, but they differ in their carbon framework and in the number and type of atoms bonded to each other.

STEREOISOMERISM

Like structural isomers, stereoisomers have the same chemical formula. In addition, they also have the same atomic connectivity. The only difference among stereoisomers is how the atoms are arranged in space. Geometric isomers, enantiomers, diastereomers, *meso* compounds, and conformational isomers all fall under the category of stereoisomers.

A. Geometric Isomers

KEY CONCEPT

Geometric isomers differ in their arrangement of atoms around a double bond. They may have different physical properties, such as melting and boiling points. However, they tend to have quite similar chemical reactivity.

Geometric isomers are compounds that differ in the position of substituents attached to a double bond. For simple geometric isomers, if two substituents are on the same side, the double bond is called *cis*. If they are on opposite sides, it is a *trans* double bond.

For compounds with polysubstituted double bonds, the situation can be confusing, and an alternative method of naming is employed. The highest-priority substituent attached to each double-bonded carbon has to be determined: The higher the atomic number, the higher the priority, and if the atomic numbers are equal, priority is determined by the substituents of these atoms. The alkene is called (*Z*) (from German *zusammen*, meaning together) if the two highest-priority substituents on each carbon lie on the same side of the double bond and (*E*) (from German *entgegen*, meaning opposite) if they are on opposite sides.

REMEMBER

Z = *z*ame *z*ide (same side)

E = *e*pposite (opposite sides)

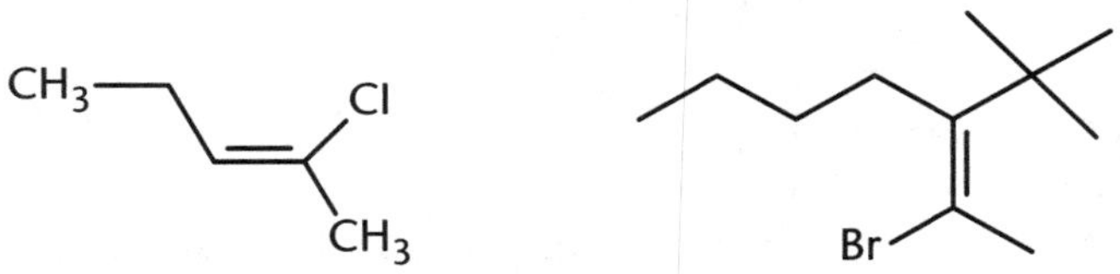

(*Z*)-2-chloro-2-pentene   (*E*)-2-bromo-3-*t*-butyl-2-heptene

Figure 2.3

B. Chirality

An object that is not superimposable upon its mirror image is called **chiral**. Familiar chiral objects are your right and left hands. Although essentially identical, they differ in their ability to fit into a right-handed glove. They are mirror images of each other yet cannot be superimposed. **Achiral** objects are mirror images that can be superimposed; for example, the letter *A* is identical to its mirror image and therefore achiral.

Figure 2.4

In organic chemistry, chirality is most frequently encountered when carbon atoms have four different substituents. Such a carbon atom is called *asymmetric* because it lacks a plane or point of symmetry. For example, the C–1 carbon atom in 1-bromo-1-chloroethane has four different substituents. The molecule is chiral because it is not superimposable on its mirror image. Chiral objects that are nonsuperimposable mirror images are called **enantiomers** and are a specific type of stereoisomer.

KEY CONCEPT

A carbon must have four different substituents to be a chiral center.

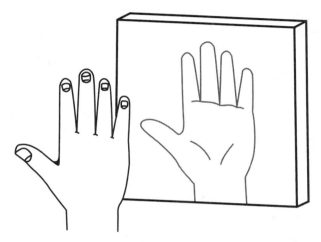

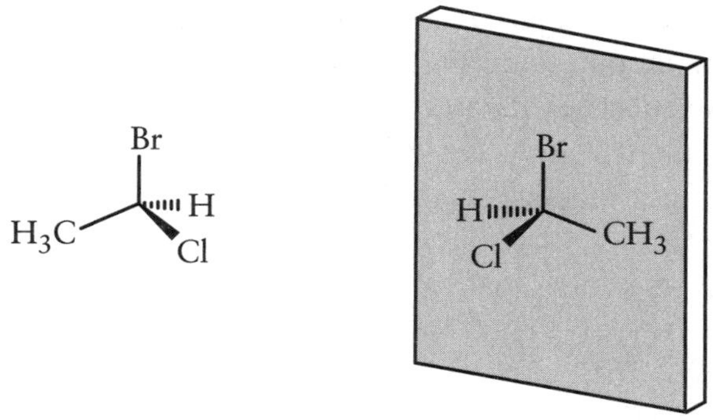

Figure 2.5

REMEMBER

Rotating a molecule in space does not change its chirality.

A carbon atom with only three different substituents, such as 1,1-dibro-moethane, has a plane of symmetry and is therefore achiral. A simple 180° rotation along the *y*-axis allows the compound to be superimposed upon its mirror image.

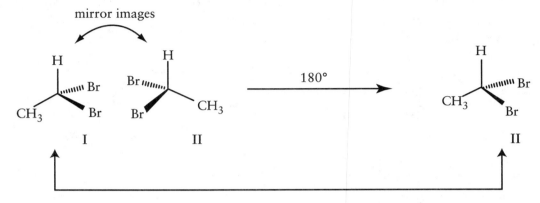

Superimposable

Figure 2.6

1. RELATIVE AND ABSOLUTE CONFIGURATION

The **configuration** is the spatial arrangement of the atoms or groups of a stereoisomer. The **relative configuration** of a chiral molecule is its configuration in relation to another chiral molecule. The **absolute configuration** of a chiral molecule describes the spatial arrangement of these atoms or groups. There is a set sequence to determine the absolute configuration of a molecule at a single chiral center.

Step 1:

Assign priority to the four substituents, looking only at the first atom that is directly attached to the chiral center. Higher atomic number takes precedence over lower atomic number. If the atomic numbers are equal, then priority is determined by the substituents attached to these atoms. See the example in Figure 2.7.

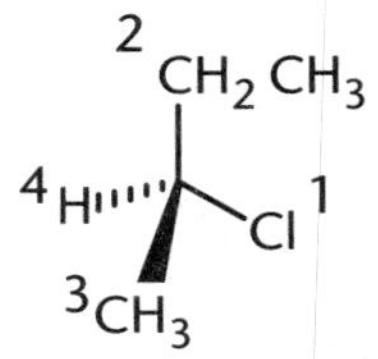

Figure 2.7

Step 2:

Orient the molecule in space so that the line of sight proceeds down the bond from the asymmetric carbon atom (the chiral center) to the substituent with lowest priority. The three substituents with highest priority should radiate from the asymmetric atom like the spokes of a wheel.

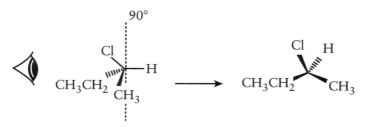

Figure 2.8

Step 3:

Proceeding from highest priority (#1) on down, determine the order of substituents around the wheel as either clockwise or counterclockwise. If the order is clockwise, the asymmetric atom is called **R** (from Latin *rectus,* meaning right). If it is counterclockwise, it is called **S** (from Latin *sinister,* meaning left).

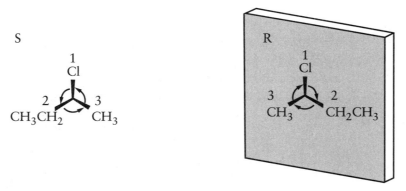

Figure 2.9

Step4:

Provide a full name for the compound. The terms *R* and *S* are put in parentheses and separated from the rest of the name by a dash. If there is more than one asymmetric carbon, location is specified by a number preceding the *R* or *S* within the parentheses, without a dash.

2. FISCHER PROJECTIONS

A three-dimensional molecule can be conveniently represented in two dimensions in a **Fischer projection**. In this system, horizontal lines indicate bonds that project out from the plane of the page, while vertical lines indicate bonds behind the plane of the page. The point of intersection of the lines represents a carbon atom. They can be interconverted by interchanging any two pairs of substituents or by rotating the projection in the plane of the page by 180°. If only one pair of substituents is interchanged, or if the molecule is rotated by 90°, the mirror image of the original compound is obtained.

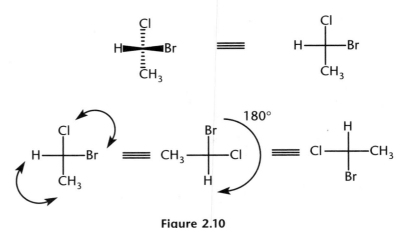

Figure 2.10

This provides another way to determine the chirality at a chiral center. If the lowest-priority substituent is on the vertical axis, it is already pointing away from you. Simply picture moving from #1 → #2 → #3, and you'll be able to name the center.

However, if the lowest-priority substituent is on the horizontal axis, it is pointing towards you, so the situation is trickier. Here are some ways to handle this situation:

1) Go ahead and imagine rotating from #1 → #2 → #3. Obtain a designation (R or S). The *true* designation will be the opposite of what you have just obtained.

2) Alternatively, make a single switch—move the low-priority substituent so that it is on the vertical axis. Obtain the designation (R or S). Again, the *true* designation will be the opposite of what you have just obtained.

3) Another approach is to make two switches or interconversions—that is, move the low-priority atom to the vertical axis and "trade" some other pair of atoms at the same time. This new molecule has the same configuration as the molecule you started with. So you can go ahead and determine the correct designation right away.

3. OPTICAL ACTIVITY

Enantiomers have identical chemical and physical properties with one exception: **optical activity**. A compound is optically active if it has the ability to rotate plane-polarized light. Ordinary light is unpolarized. It consists of waves vibrating in all possible planes perpendicular to its direction of motion. A polarizer allows light waves oscillating only in a particular direction to pass, producing plane-polarized light.

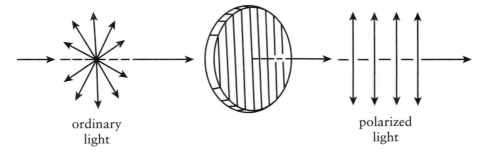

ordinary   polarized
light   light

Figure 2.11

If plane-polarized light is passed through an optically active compound, the orientation of the plane is rotated by an angle α. The enantiomer of this compound will rotate light by the same amount but in the opposite direction. A compound that rotates the plane of polarized light to the right, or clockwise (from the point of view of an observer seeing the light approach), is **dextrorotatory** and is indicated by (+). A compound that rotates light toward the left, or counterclockwise, is **levorotatory** and is labeled (−). The direction of rotation cannot be determined from the structure of a molecule and must be determined experimentally.

The amount of rotation depends on the number of molecules that a light wave encounters. This depends on two factors: the concentration of the optically active compound and the length of the tube through which the light passes. Chemists have set standard conditions of 1 g/mL for concentration and 1 dm for length to compare the optical activities of different compounds. Rotations measured at different concentrations and tube lengths can be converted to a standardized **specific rotation** (α) using the following equation:

$$\text{specific rotation } ([\alpha]) = \frac{\text{observed rotation } (\alpha)}{\text{concentration (g/mL)} \times \text{length (dm)}}$$

A **racemic mixture**, or **racemic modification**, is a mixture of equal concentrations of both the (+) and (−) enantiomers. The rotations cancel each other and no optical activity is observed.

> **BRIDGE**
>
> This equation can be rewritten as
>
> $$\alpha = [\alpha] \times \text{conc} \times \text{length}$$
>
> Notice how similar this equation is to Beer's Law (spectroscopy).

C. Other Chiral Compounds

1. DIASTEREOMERS

For any molecule with n chiral centers, there are $2n$ possible stereo-isomers. Thus, if a compound has two chiral carbon atoms, it has four possible stereoisomers (see Figure 2.12).

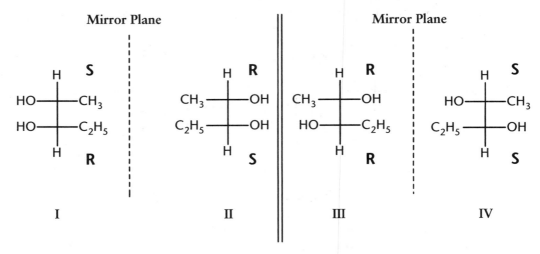

Figure 2.12

I and II are mirror images of each other and are therefore enantiomers. Similarly, III and IV are enantiomers. However, I and III are not. They are stereoisomers that are not mirror images, so they are called **diastereomers**. Notice that other combinations of nonmirror image stereoisomers are also diastereomeric. Hence I and IV, II and III, I and III, and II and IV are all pairs of diastereomers.

2. *MESO* COMPOUNDS

The criterion for optical activity of a molecule containing a single chiral center is that it has no plane of symmetry. The same applies to a molecule with two or more chiral centers. If a plane of symmetry exists, the molecule is not optically active, even though it possesses chiral centers. Such a molecule is called a *meso* compound. Figure 2.13 shows some examples.

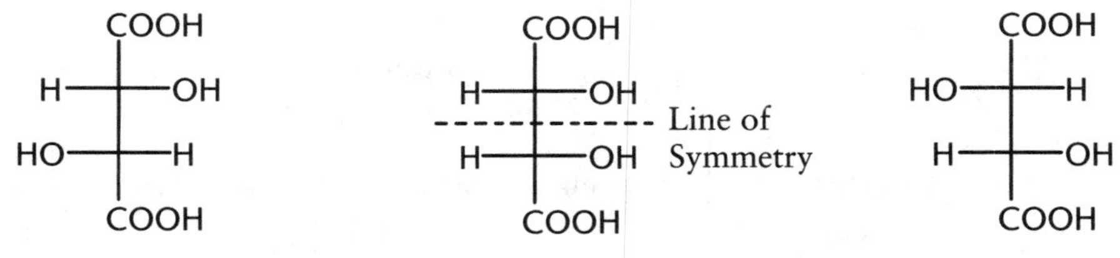

COOH	COOH	COOH

L-tartaric acid   *Meso*-tartaric acid   *D*-tartaric acid

Figure 2.13

D- and *L*-tartaric acid are both optically active, but *meso*-tartaric acid has a plane of symmetry and is not optically active. Although *meso*-tartaric acid has two chiral carbon atoms, the lack of optical activity is a function of the molecule as a whole.

BRIDGE

See carbohydrates chapter for explanation of *D* versus *L* configurations.

D. Conformational Isomerism

Conformational isomers are compounds that differ only by rotation about one or more single bonds. Essentially, these isomers represent the same compound in a slightly different position—analogous to a person who may be either standing up or sitting down. These different conformations can be seen when the molecule is depicted in a **Newman projection,** in which the line of sight extends along a carbon-carbon bond axis. The conformations are encountered as the molecule is rotated about this axis. The classic example for demonstrating conformational isomerism in a straight chain is *n*-butane. In this Newman projection, the line of sight extends through the C2–C3 bond axis.

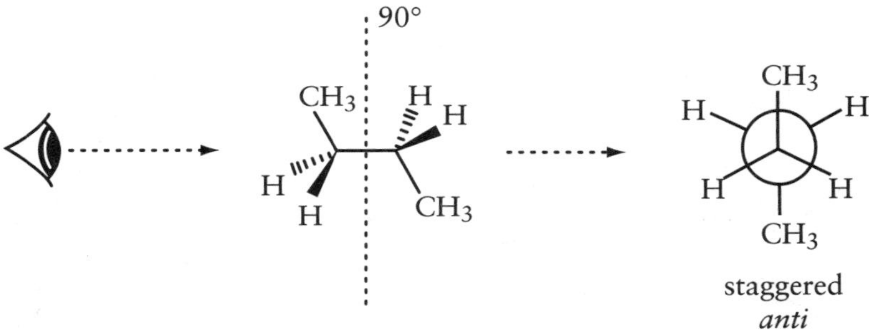

Figure 2.14

1. STRAIGHT-CHAIN CONFORMATIONS

The most stable conformation is when the two methyl groups (C1 and C4) are oriented 180° from each other. There is no overlap of atoms along the line of sight (besides C2 and C3), so the molecule is said to be in a **staggered** conformation. Specifically, it is called the *anti* conformation, because the two methyl groups are antiperiplanar to each other. This particular orientation is very stable and thus represents an energy minimum because all atoms are far apart, minimizing repulsive steric interactions.

REMEMBER

It's "gauche" (or inappropriate) for one methyl group to stand too close to another group!

The other type of staggered conformation, called *gauche,* occurs when the two methyl groups are 60° apart. To convert from the *anti* to the *gauche* conformation, the molecule must pass through an **eclipsed** conformation, in which the two methyl groups are 120° apart and overlap with the H atoms on the adjacent carbon. When the two methyl groups overlap with each other, the molecule is said to be **totally eclipsed** and is in its highest energy state.

REMEMBER

Groups are "eclipsed" when they are completely in line with one another—think of a solar eclipse!

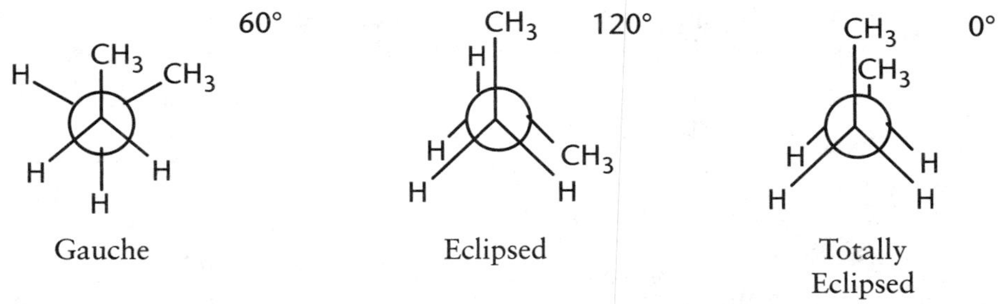

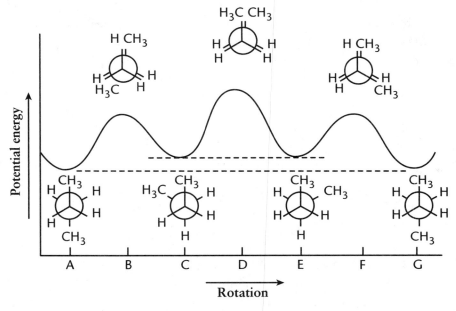

Figure 2.15

A plot of potential energy versus the degree of rotation about the C2–C3 bond shows the relative minima and maxima the molecule encounters throughout its various conformations.

KEY CONCEPT

Notice that the *anti* isomer has the lowest energy, while the totally eclipsed isomer has the highest energy.

Figure 2.16

It is important to note that these barriers are rather small (3–4 kcal/mol) and are easily overcome at room temperature. Very low temperatures will slow conformational interconversion. If the molecules do not possess sufficient energy to cross the energy barrier, they may not rotate at all.

2. CYCLIC CONFORMATIONS

a. Strain energies

In cycloalkanes, ring strain arises from three factors: angle strain, torsional strain, and nonbonded strain. **Angle strain** results when bond angles deviate from their ideal values, **torsional strain** results when cyclic molecules must assume conformations that have eclipsed interactions, and **nonbonded strain** (van der Waals repulsion) results when atoms or groups compete for the same space. To alleviate these three types of strain, cycloalkanes attempt to adopt nonplanar conformations. Cyclobutane puckers into a slight V shape; cyclopentane adopts what is called the **envelope** conformation; and cyclohexane exists mainly in three conformations called the **chair**, the **boat**, and the **twist** or **skew-boat** (see Figure 2.17).

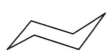

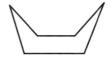

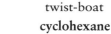

| puckered **cyclobutane** | envelope conformation **cyclopentane** | chair **cyclohexane** | boat **cyclohexane** | twist-boat **cyclohexane** |

Figure 2.17. Conformations of Cyclic Hydrocarbons

b. Cyclohexane

i. Unsubstituted

The most stable conformation of cyclohexane is the chair conformation. In this conformation, all three types of strain are eliminated. The hydrogen atoms that are perpendicular to the plane of the ring are called axial, and those parallel are called equatorial. The axial-equatorial orientations alternate around the ring.

The boat conformation is adopted when the chair "flips" and converts to another chair. In such a process, hydrogen atoms that were equatorial become axial, and vice versa, in the new chair. In the boat conformation, all of the atoms are eclipsed, creating a high-energy state. To avoid this strain, the boat can twist into a slightly more stable form called the twist or skew-boat conformation.

ii. Monosubstituted

The interconversion between the two chairs can be slowed or even prevented if a sterically bulky group is attached to the ring. The equatorial position is favored over the axial position because of steric repulsion with other axial substituents.

Hence, a large group, such as *t*-butyl, can lock the molecule in one conformation.

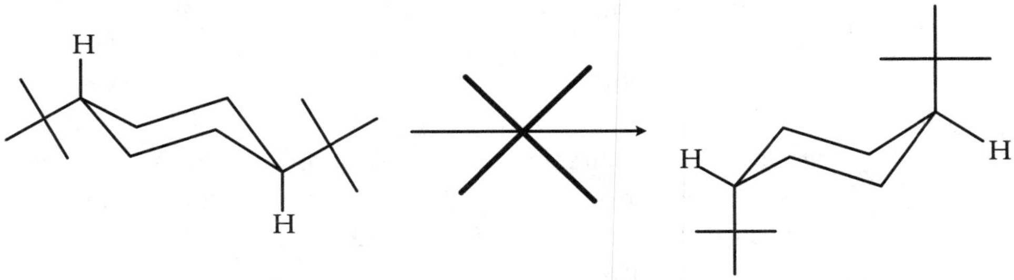

Figure 2.18

iii. Disubstituted

Different isomers can exist for disubstituted cycloalkanes. If both substituents are located on the same side of the ring, the molecule is called **cis**; if the two groups are on opposite sides of the ring, it is called **trans**.

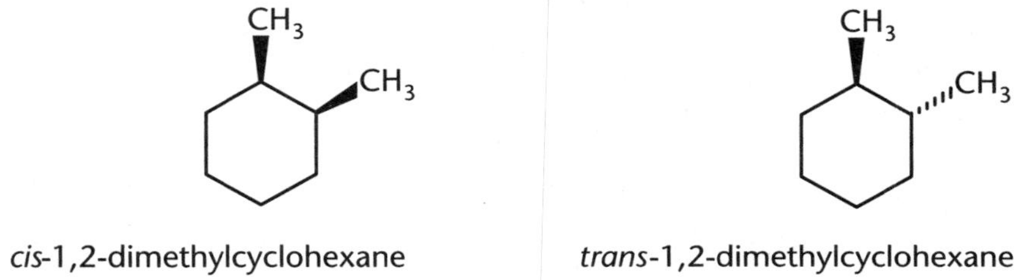

cis-1,2-dimethylcyclohexane   trans-1,2-dimethylcyclohexane

Figure 2.19

In *trans*-1,4-dimethylcyclohexane, both of the methyl groups are equatorial in one chair conformation and axial in the other, but in either case, they point in opposite directions relative to the plane of the ring.

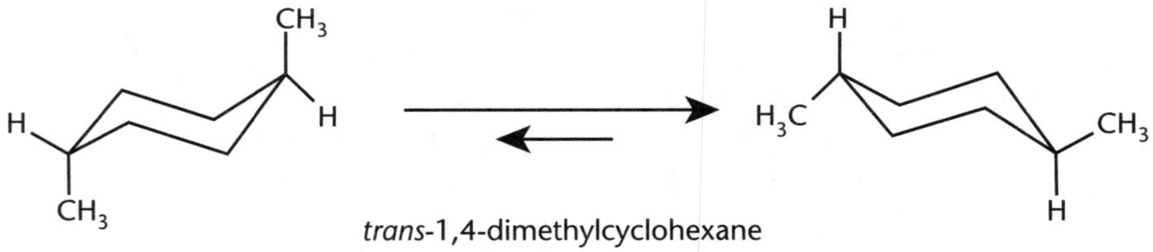

trans-1,4-dimethylcyclohexane

Figure 2.20

Bonding

3

As we discussed in General Chemistry, there are two types of chemical bonds: **ionic**, in which an electron is transferred from one atom to another, and **covalent**, in which pairs of electrons are shared between two atoms. In organic chemistry, it is important to understand the details of covalent bonding, as these play a crucial role in determining the properties and reactions of organic compounds.

ATOMIC ORBITALS

The first three quantum numbers, n, ℓ, and m, describe the size, shape, and number of the atomic orbitals an element possesses. The number n, which can equal 1, 2, 3, . . . , corresponds to the energy levels in an atom and is essentially a measure of size. Within each electron shell, there can be several types of orbitals (s, p, d, f, g, . . . corresponding to the quantum numbers $\ell = 0, 1, 2, 3, 4, . . .$).

Each type of atomic orbital has a specific shape. An s-orbital is spherical and symmetrical, centered around the nucleus. A p-orbital is composed of two lobes located symmetrically about the nucleus and contains a **node** (an area where the probability of finding an electron is zero). A d-orbital is composed of four symmetrical lobes and contains two nodes. Both d- and f-orbitals are complex in shape and are rarely encountered in organic chemistry (refer to General Chemistry).

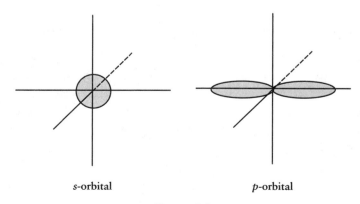

s-orbital   *p*-orbital

Figure 3.1

MOLECULAR ORBITALS

A. Single Bonds

Two atomic orbitals can be combined to form what is called a **molecular orbital (MO)**. Molecular orbitals are obtained mathematically by adding the wave functions of the atomic orbitals. If the signs of the wave functions are the same, a lower-energy **bonding orbital** is produced. If the signs are different, a higher-energy **antibonding orbital** is produced. This is represented schematically by the addition of two s-orbitals. Two p-orbitals or one p- and one s-orbital can also be combined in a similar fashion.

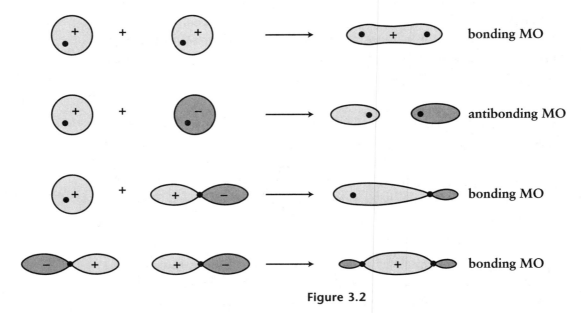

Figure 3.2

When a molecular orbital is formed by head-to-head overlap, as in Figure 3.2, the resulting bond is called a **sigma (σ) bond**. All single bonds are sigma bonds, accommodating two electrons. Shorter single bonds are stronger than longer single bonds.

B. Double and Triple Bonds

When two p-orbitals overlap in a parallel fashion, a bonding MO is formed called a **pi (π) bond**. When both a sigma and a pi bond exist between two atoms, a **double bond** is formed. When a sigma bond and two pi bonds exist, a **triple bond** is formed. As can be seen in Figure 3.3, the overlap of the p-orbitals involved in a π bond hinder rotation about double and triple bonds.

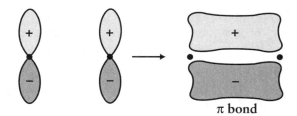

π bond

Figure 3.3

A pi bond cannot exist independently of a sigma bond. Only after the formation of a sigma bond will the *p*-orbitals of adjacent carbons be parallel, because without the bond, the three *p*-orbitals are orthogonal to one another.

In general, pi bonds are weaker than sigma bonds; it is possible to break one bond of a double bond, leaving a single bond intact.

HYBRIDIZATION

The carbon atom has the electron configuration $1s^2 2s^2 2p^2$ and, therefore, needs four electrons to complete its octet. A typical molecule formed by carbon is methane, CH_4. Experimentation shows that the four sigma bonds in methane are equal. This is inconsistent with an asymmetrical distribution of valence electrons: two electrons in the $2s$-orbital, one in the p_x-orbital, one in the p_y-orbital, and none in the p_z-orbital.

A. sp^3

The theory of **orbital hybridization** was developed to account for this discrepancy. Hybrid orbitals are formed by mixing different types of atomic orbitals. If one *s*-orbital and three *p*-orbitals are mathematically combined, the result is four sp^3-hybrid orbitals that have a new shape.

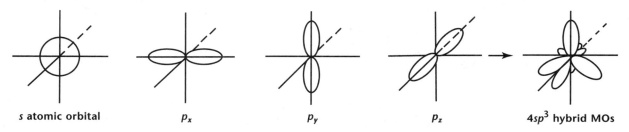

s atomic orbital p_x p_y p_z $4sp^3$ hybrid MOs

Figure 3.4

These four orbitals will point towards the vertices of a tetrahedron, minimizing repulsion. This explains the preferred tetrahedral geometry adopted by carbon.

BRIDGE

VSEPR theory, which determines the shape of molecules, is discussed in General Chemistry.

The hybridization is accomplished by promoting one of the $2s$ electrons into the $2p_z$-orbital (see Figure 3.5). This produces four valence orbitals, each with one electron, which can be mathematically mixed to provide the hybrids.

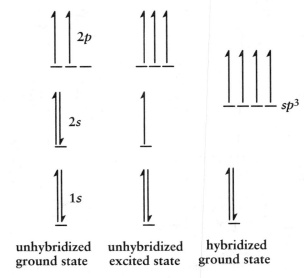

unhybridized   unhybridized   hybridized
ground state   excited state   ground state

Figure 3.5

B. sp^2

Although carbon is most often found with sp^3 hybridization, there are other possibilities. If one s-orbital and two p-orbitals are mixed, three sp^2 hybrid orbitals are obtained.

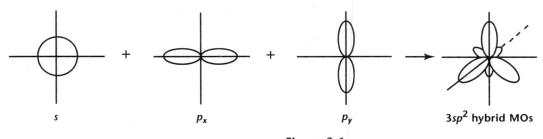

Figure 3.6

This occurs, for example, in ethylene. The third p-orbital of each carbon atom is left unhybridized and participates in the pi bond. The three sp^2 orbitals are 120° apart, allowing maximum separation. These orbitals participate in the formation of the C=C and C–H single bonds.

C. *sp*

If two *p*-orbitals are used to form a triple bond, and the remaining *p*-orbital is mixed with an *s*-orbital, two *sp* hybrid orbitals are obtained. They are oriented 180° apart, explaining the linear structure of molecules like acetylene.

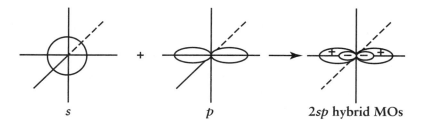

s   +   *p*   →   2*sp* hybrid MOs

Figure 3.7

BONDING SUMMARY

Tables 3.1 and 3.2 summarizes the major features of bonding in organic molecules.

Table 3.1

Bond Order	Component Bonds	Hybridization	Angles	Examples
single	sigma	sp^3	109.5°	C–C; C–H
double	sigma pi	sp^2	120°	C=C; C=O
triple	sigma pi pi	sp	180°	C≡C; C≡N

Table 3.2

	Hybridization	Bond Length	Bond Energy
C–C	sp^3	Largest	Lowest
C=C	sp^2	Medium	Medium
C≡C	sp	Shortest	Highest

4

Alkanes

Alkanes are fully saturated hydrocarbons, compounds consisting only of hydrogen and carbon atoms joined by single bonds. Their general formula is C_nH_{2n+2}, which means they have the maximum possible number of hydrogen atoms attached to each carbon atom.

FLASHBACK

Refer to nomenclature chapter for the general rules of naming alkanes.

NOMENCLATURE

Once again, be sure that you are familiar with common, frequently encountered names, such as those shown in Figure 4.1.

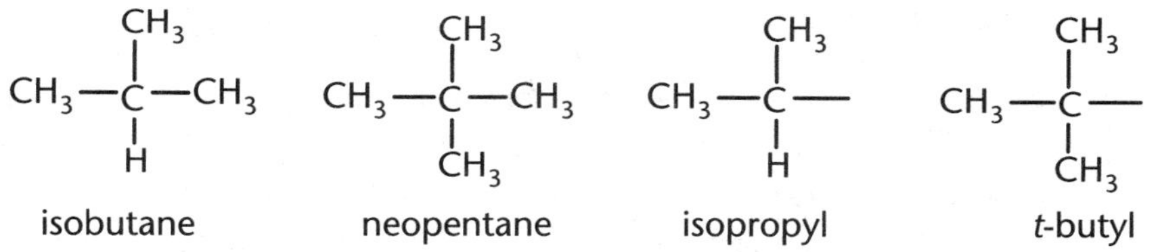

Figure 4.1

Carbon atoms can be characterized by the number of other carbon atoms to which they are directly bonded. A **primary** carbon atom (written as **1°**) is bonded to only one other carbon atom. A **secondary (2°)** carbon is bonded to two, a **tertiary (3°)** to three, and a **quaternary (4°)** to four other carbon atoms. In addition, hydrogen atoms attached to 1°, 2°, or 3° carbon atoms are referred to as 1°, 2°, or 3°, respectively.

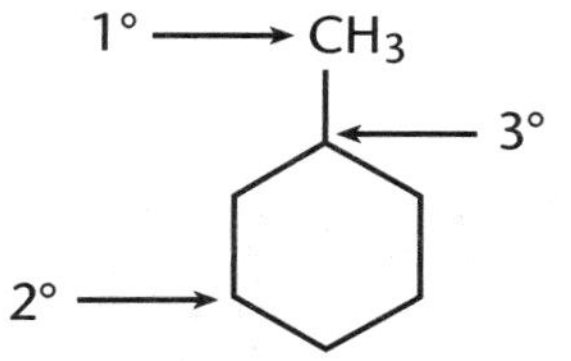

Figure 4.2

PHYSICAL PROPERTIES

REMEMBER

↑ chain length ↑ b.p.

↑ m.p.

↑ density

↑ branching ↓ b.p.

↓ m.p.

↓ density

The physical properties of alkanes vary in a regular manner. In general, as the molecular weight increases, the melting point, boiling point, and density also increase. At room temperature, the straight-chain compounds C_1 through C_4 are gases, C_5 through C_{16} are liquids, and the longer-chain compounds are waxes and harder solids. Branched molecules have slightly lower boiling and melting points than their straight-chain isomers. Greater branching reduces the surface area of a molecule, decreasing the weak intermolecular attractive forces (van der Waals forces). Hence, the molecules are held together less tightly, effectively lowering the boiling point. In addition, branched molecules are more difficult to pack into a tight, three-dimensional structure. This difficulty is reflected in the lower melting points of branched alkanes.

REACTIONS

A. Free Radical Halogenation

One frequently encountered reaction of alkanes is **halogenations**, in which one or more hydrogen atoms are replaced by halogen atoms (Cl, Br, or I) via a **free-radical substitution** mechanism. These reactions involve three steps:

1. **Initiation**—Diatomic halogens are homolytically cleaved by either heat or light ($h\nu$), resulting in the formation of free radicals. Free radicals are neutral species with unpaired electrons (such as Cl• or $R_3C•$). They are extremely reactive and readily attack alkanes.

$$\text{Initiation: } X_2 \xrightarrow[\text{or } \Delta]{h\nu} 2X•$$

2. **Propagation**—A propagation step is one in which a radical produces another radical that can continue the reaction. A free radical reacts with an alkane, removing a hydrogen atom to form HX and creating an alkyl radical. The alkyl radical can then react with X_2 to form an alkyl halide, generating X•.

$$\text{Propagation:} \quad X• + RH \rightarrow HX + R•$$
$$R• + X_2 \rightarrow RX + X•$$

3. **Termination**—Two free radicals combine with one another to form a stable molecule.

$$\text{Termination:} \quad 2X• \rightarrow X_2$$
$$X• + R• \rightarrow RX$$
$$2R• \rightarrow R_2$$

A single free radical can initiate many reactions before the reaction chain is terminated.

Larger alkanes have many hydrogens that the free radical can attack. Bromine radicals react fairly slowly and primarily attack the hydrogens on the carbon atom that can form the most stable free radical (i.e., the most substituted carbon atom).

$$\bullet CR_3 > \bullet CR_2H > \bullet CRH_2 > \bullet CH_3$$
$$3° > 2° > 1° > \text{methyl}$$

REMEMBER

Free radicals, as well as carbocations, follow the same patterns of stability:

3° > 2° > 1° > methyl

Thus, a tertiary radical is the most likely to be formed in a free-radical bromination reaction.

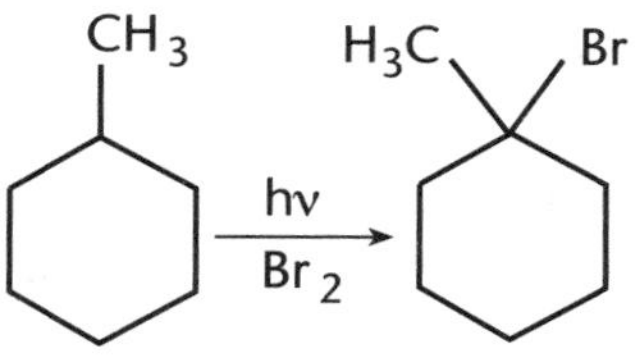

Figure 4.3

Free-radical chlorination is a more rapid process and, thus, depends not only on the stability of the intermediate but on the number of hydrogens present. Free-radical chlorination reactions are likely to replace primary hydrogens because of their abundance, despite the relative instability of primary radicals. Unfortunately, free-radical chlorination reactions produce mixtures of products and are preparatively useful only when just one type of hydrogen is present.

B. Combustion

The reaction of alkanes with molecular oxygen, to form carbon dioxide, water, and heat, is a process of great practical importance. It is an unusual reaction because heat, not a chemical species, is generally the desired product. The reaction mechanism is very complex and is believed to proceed through a radical process. The equation for the complete **combustion** of propane is

$$C_3H_8 + 5O_2 \rightarrow 3CO_2 + 4H_2O + \text{heat}$$

Combustion is often incomplete, producing significant quantities of carbon monoxide instead of carbon dioxide. This frequently occurs, for example, in the burning of gasoline in an internal combustion engine.

C. Pyrolysis

Pyrolysis occurs when a molecule is broken down by heat. Pyrolysis, also called **cracking**, is most commonly used to reduce the average molecular weight of heavy oils and to increase the production of the more desirable volatile compounds. In the pyrolysis of alkanes, the C–C bonds are cleaved, producing smaller-chain alkyl radicals. These radicals can recombine to form a variety of alkanes:

$$CH_3CH_2CH_3 \xrightarrow{\Delta} CH_3\bullet + \bullet CH_2CH_3$$

$$2\ CH_3\bullet \longrightarrow CH_3CH_3$$

$$2\ \bullet CH_2CH_3 \longrightarrow CH_3CH_2CH_2CH_3$$

Figure 4.4

Alternatively, in a process called **disproportionation**, a radical transfers a hydrogen atom to another radical, producing an alkane and an alkene:

$$CH_3\bullet + \bullet CH_2CH_3 \rightarrow CH_4 + CH_2 = CH_2$$

Figure 4.5

SUBSTITUTION REACTIONS OF ALKYL HALIDES

Alkyl halides and other substituted carbon atoms can take part in reactions known as **nucleophilic substitutions**. **Nucleophiles** ("nucleus lovers") are electron-rich species that are attracted to positively polarized atoms.

A. Nucleophiles

1. BASICITY

If the nucleophiles have the same attacking atom (for example, oxygen), then nucleophilicity is roughly correlated to basicity. In other words, the stronger the base, the stronger the nucleophile. For example, nucleophilic strength decreases in this order:

$$RO^- > HO^- > RCO_2^- > ROH > H_2O$$

2. SIZE AND POLARIZABILITY

If the attacking atoms differ, nucleophilic ability doesn't necessarily correlate to basicity. In a protic solvent, large atoms tend to be better nucleophiles, as they can shed their solvent molecules and are more polarizable. Hence, nucleophilic strength decreases in this order:

$$CN^- > I^- > RO^- > HO^- > Br^- > Cl^- > F^- > H_2O$$

REMEMBER

In protic solvents (solvents capable of hydrogen bonding), larger atoms are better nucleophiles. In aprotic solvents, more basic atoms are better nucleophiles.

In aprotic solvents, however, the nucleophiles are "naked"; they are not solvated. In this situation, nucleophilic strength is related to basicity. For example, in DMSO, the order of nucleophilic strength is the same as base strength:

$$F^- > Cl^- > Br^- > I^-$$

Note that this is the opposite of what happens in polar solvents.

B. Leaving Groups

The ease with which nucleophilic substitution takes place is also dependent on the leaving group. The best leaving groups are those that are weak bases, as these can accept an electron pair and dissociate to form a stable species. In the case of the halogens, therefore, this is the opposite of base strength:

$$I^- > Br^- > Cl^- > F^-$$

> **REMEMBER**
>
> Weak bases make good leaving groups.

C. S$_N$1 Reactions

S$_N$1 is the designation for **unimolecular nucleophilic substitution** reaction. It is called unimolecular because the rate of the reaction is dependent upon only one species. Generally, the rate-determining step is the dissociation of this species to form a stable, positively charged ion called a **carbocation** or **carbonium ion**.

1. MECHANISM OF S$_N$1 REACTIONS

S$_N$1 reactions involve two steps: the dissociation of a molecule into a carbocation and a good leaving group, followed by the combination of the carbocation with a strong nucleophile.

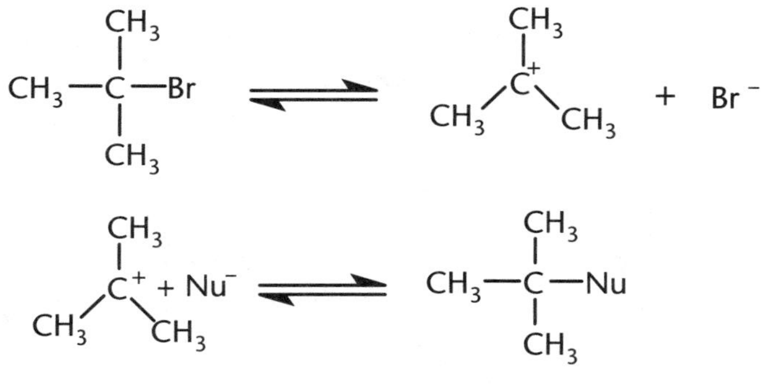

Figure 4.6

In the first step, a carbocation is formed. Carbocations are stabilized by polar solvents that have lone electron pairs to donate (e.g., water, acetone). Carbocations are also stabilized by charge delocalization.

More highly substituted cations are therefore more stable. The order of stability for carbocations is as follows:

tertiary > secondary > primary > methyl

To get the desired product, the original substituent should be a better leaving group than the nucleophile, so that at equilibrium, RNu is the main product. Conditions are usually chosen so that the second step of the reaction is essentially irreversible.

2. RATE OF S_N1 REACTIONS

BRIDGE

The kinetics of unimolecular reactions are first order. See General Chemistry.

The rate at which a reaction occurs can never be greater than the rate of its slowest step. Such a step is termed the **rate-limiting** or **rate-determining step** of the reaction, because it limits the speed of the reaction. In an S_N1 reaction, the slowest step is the dissociation of the molecule to form a carbocation, a step that is energetically unfavorable. The formation of a carbocation is, therefore, the rate-limiting step of an S_N1 reaction. The only reactant in this step is the original molecule, so the rate of the entire reaction, under a given set of conditions, depends only on the concentration of this original molecule (a so-called **first-order reaction**). The rate is *not* dependent on the concentration or the nature of the nucleophile, because it plays no part in the rate-limiting step.

The rate of an S_N1 reaction can be increased by anything that accelerates the formation of the carbocation. The most important factors are as follows:

a. Structural factors: Highly substituted alkyl halides allow for distribution of the positive charge over a greater number of carbon atoms and thus form the most stable carbocations.

b. Solvent effects: Highly polar solvents are better at surrounding and isolating ions than are less polar solvents. Polar protic solvents, such as water, work best since solvation stabilizes the intermediate state.

c. Nature of the leaving group: Weak bases dissociate more easily from the alkyl chain and thus make better leaving groups, increasing the rate of carbocation formation.

D. S$_N$2 Reactions

The formation of a carbocation is not always favorable. Under certain conditions, substitution can proceed by a different mechanism, which does not involve a carbocation. An S$_N$2 (**bimolecular nucleophilic substitution**) reaction involves a nucleophile pushing its way into a compound while simultaneously displacing the leaving group. Its rate-determining, and only, step involves two molecules: the **substrate** and the nucleophile.

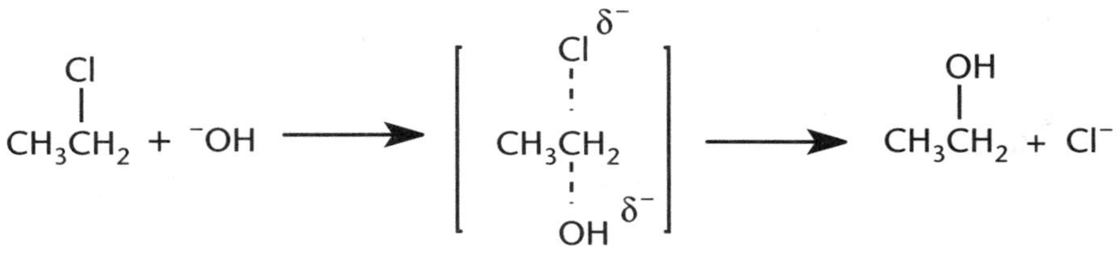

Figure 4.7

1. MECHANISM OF S$_N$2 REACTIONS

In S$_N$2 reactions, the nucleophile actively displaces the leaving group. For this to occur, the nucleophile must be strong, and the reactant cannot be sterically hindered. The nucleophile attacks the reactant from the backside of the leaving group, forming a trigonal bipyramidal **transition state**. As the reaction progresses, the bond to the nucleophile strengthens while the bond to the leaving group weakens. The leaving group is displaced as the bond to the nucleophile becomes complete.

2. RATE OF S$_N$2 REACTIONS

The single step of an S$_N$2 reaction involves *two* reacting species: the substrate (the molecule with a leaving group, usually an alkyl halide) and the nucleophile. The concentrations of both therefore play a role in determining the rate of an S$_N$2 reaction; the two species must "meet" in solution, and raising the concentration of either will make such a meeting more likely. Since the rate of the S$_N$2 reaction depends on the concentration of two reactants, it follows **second-order kinetics**.

E. S$_N$1 Versus S$_N$2

Certain reaction conditions favor one substitution mechanism over the other. It is also possible for both to occur in the same flask. Sterics, nucleophilic strength, leaving group ability, reaction conditions, and solvent effects are all important in determining which reaction will occur.

KEY CONCEPT

An intermediate is distinct from a transition state. An intermediate is a well-defined species with a finite lifetime. On the other hand, a transition state is a theoretical structure used to define a mechanism.

BRIDGE

The kinetics of second-order reactions such as S$_N$2 are discussed in General Chemistry.

STEREOCHEMISTRY OF SUBSTITUTION REACTIONS

A. S$_N$1 Stereochemistry

S$_N$1 reactions involve carbocation intermediates, which are approximately planar and therefore achiral.

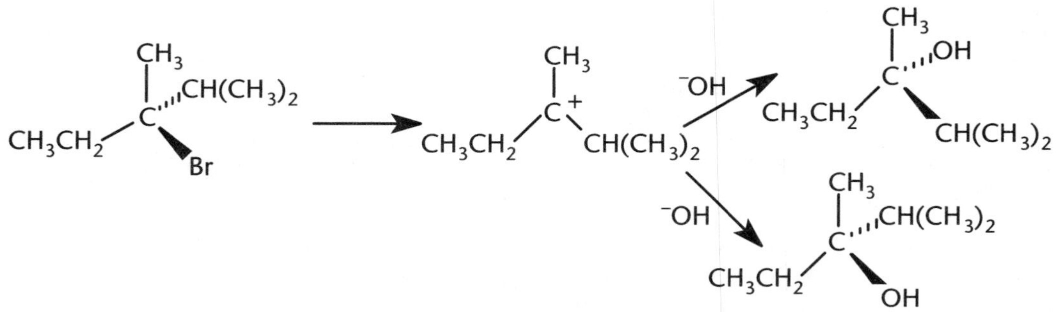

Figure 4.8

FLASHBACK

Refer to the isomer chapter for further discussion of optical activity.

If the original compound is optically active because of the reacting chiral center, then a racemic mixture will be produced. Therefore, S$_N$1 reactions result in a loss of optical activity.

B. S$_N$2 Stereochemistry

The single step of an S$_N$2 reaction involves a chiral transition state. Since the nucleophile attacks from one side of the central carbon and the leaving group departs from the opposite side, the reaction "flips" the bonds attached to the carbon.

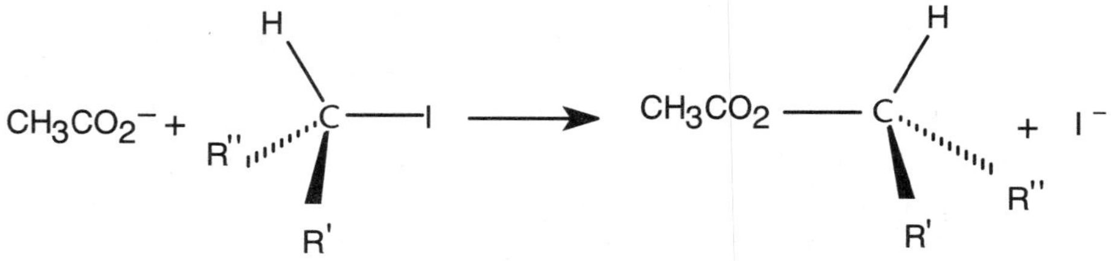

Figure 4.9

If the reactant is chiral, optical activity is usually retained; however, in the case of S$_N$2 reactions, an inversion of configuration occurs.

Figure 4.10 summarizes S$_N$^{1} and S$_N$^{2} reactions.

S_N1	S_N2
· 2 steps	· 1 step
· Favored in polar protic solvents.	· Favored in polar aprotic solvents.
· 3° > 2° > 1° > methyl	· 1° > 2° > 3°
· Rate = k[RX]	· Rate = k[Nu][RX]
· Racemic products	· Optically active/ inverted products
· Favored with the use of bulky nucleophiles.	

Figure 4.10

5

Alkenes and Alkynes

ALKENES

Alkenes are hydrocarbons that contain carbon-carbon double bonds. The general formula for a straight-chain alkene with one double bond is C_nH_{2n}. The degree of unsaturation (the number N of double bonds or rings) of a compound of molecular formula C_nH_m can be determined according to this equation:

$$N = \frac{1}{2}(2n + 2 - m)$$

Double bonds are considered functional groups, and alkenes are more reactive than their corresponding alkanes.

A. Nomenclature

Alkenes, also called **olefins,** may be described by the terms *cis, trans, E,* and *Z.* The common names *ethylene, propylene,* and *isobutylene* are often used over the IUPAC names.

FLASHBACK

Refer to the nomenclature chapter for the general rules of naming alkenes.

$CH_2\!=\!CH_2$

ethene
(ethylene)

$CH_3CH\!=\!CH_2$

propene
(propylene)

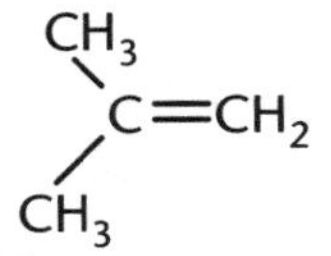

2-methyl-1-propene
(isobutylene)

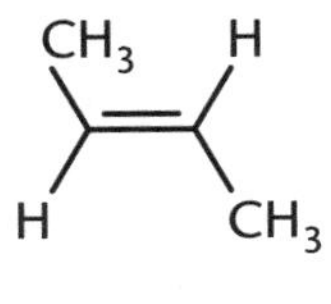

trans-2-butene

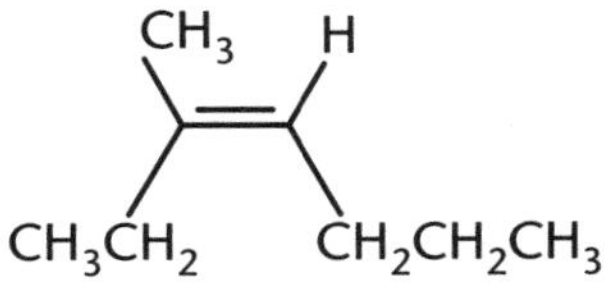

(Z)-3-methyl-3-heptene

Figure 5.1

B. Physical Properties

The physical properties of alkenes are similar to those of alkanes. For example, the melting and boiling points increase with increasing molecular weight and are similar in value to those of the corresponding alkanes. Terminal alkenes (or 1-alkenes) usually boil at a lower temperature than internal alkenes, and they can be separated by fractional distillation. *Trans*-alkenes generally have higher melting points than *cis*-alkenes because their higher symmetry allows better packing in the solid state. They also tend to have lower boiling points than *cis*-alkenes because they are less **polar**.

Polarity is a property that results from the asymmetrical distribution of electrons in a particular molecule. In alkenes, this distribution creates dipole moments that are oriented from the electropositive alkyl groups toward the electronegative alkene. In *trans*-2-butene, the two dipole moments are oriented in opposite directions and cancel each other. The compound possesses no net dipole moment and is not polar. On the other hand, *cis*-2-butene has a net dipole moment, resulting from addition of the two smaller dipoles. The compound is polar, and the additional intermolecular forces tend to raise the boiling point.

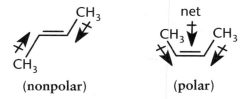

(nonpolar)   (polar)

Figure 5.2

The net dipole of alkene compound can grossly be assessed by the distribution of electrons across the molecule.

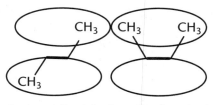

(no net dipole)   (net dipole exists)

Figure 5.3

C. Synthesis

Alkenes can be synthesized in a number of different ways. The most common method involves **elimination reactions** of either alcohols or alkyl halides. In these reactions the carbon skeleton loses HX (where X is a halide), or a molecule of water, to form a double bond:

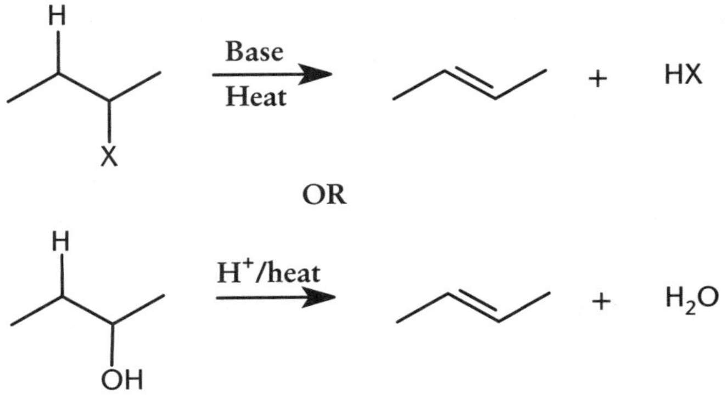

Figure 5.4

Elimination occurs by two distinct mechanisms, unimolecular and bimolecular, which are referred to as **E1** and **E2**, respectively.

1. UNIMOLECULAR ELIMINATION

Unimolecular elimination, abbreviated E1, is a two-step process proceeding through a carbocation intermediate. The rate of reaction is dependent on the concentration of only one species, namely the substrate. The elimination of a leaving group and a proton results in the production of a double bond. In the first step, the leaving group departs, producing a carbocation. In the second step, a proton is removed by a base.

E1 is favored by the same factors that favor S_N1: highly polar solvents, highly branched carbon chains, good leaving groups, and weak nucleophiles in low concentration. These mechanisms are therefore competitive, and directing a reaction toward either E1 or S_N1 alone is difficult, although high temperatures tend to favor E1.

2. BIMOLECULAR ELIMINATION

Bimolecular elimination, termed E2, occurs in one step. Its rate is dependent on the concentration of two species, the substrate and the base. A strong base, such as the ethoxide ion ($C_2H_5O^-$), removes a proton, while a halide ion *anti* to the proton leaves, resulting in the formation of a double bond.

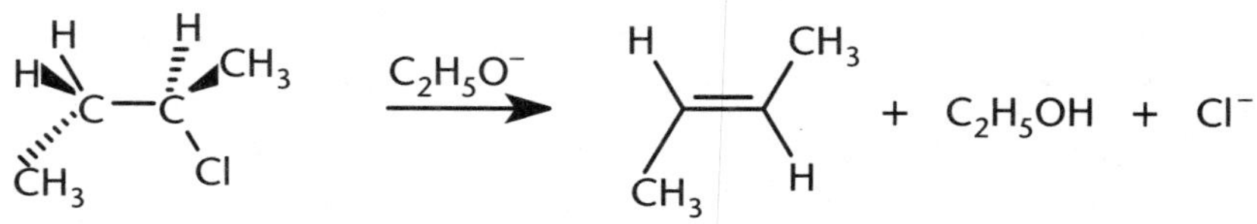

Figure 5.5

Often there are two possible products. In such cases, the more substituted double bond is formed preferentially.

Controlling E2 versus S_N2 is easier than controlling E1 versus S_N1.

- Steric hindrance does not greatly affect E2 reactions. Therefore, highly substituted carbon chains, which form the most stable alkenes, undergo E2 most easily and S_N2 rarely.

- A strong base favors E2 over S_N2. S_N2 is favored over E2 by weak Lewis bases (strong nucleophiles).

Other factors, such as the polarity of the solvent and branching of the carbon chain, can be modified to reduce the competition between E1 and S_N1 reactions.

D. Reactions

1. REDUCTION

Catalytic hydrogenation is the reductive process of adding molecular hydrogen to a double bond with the aid of a metal catalyst. Typical catalysts are platinum, palladium, and nickel (usually Raney nickel, a special powdered form), but occasionally rhodium, iridium, or ruthenium is used.

The reaction takes place on the surface of the metal. One face of the double bond is coordinated to the metal surface, and thus the two hydrogen atoms are added to the same face of the double bond. This type of addition is called *syn* addition.

REMEMBER

Reactions where one stereo-isomer is favored are termed stereospecific reactions.

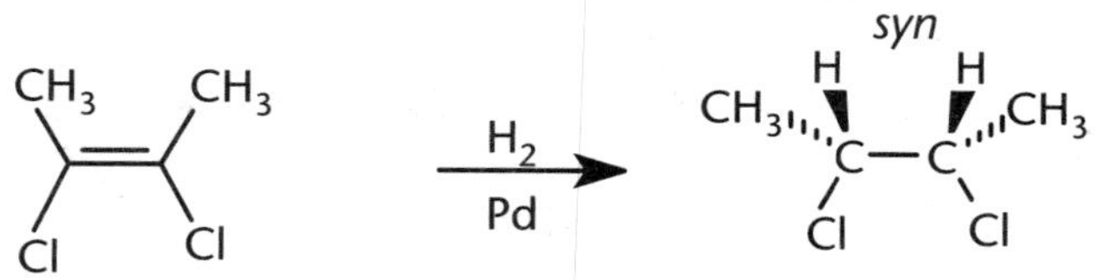

Figure 5.6

2. ELECTROPHILIC ADDITIONS

The π bond is somewhat weaker than the σ bond and can therefore be broken without breaking the σ bond. As a result, one can *add* compounds to double bonds while leaving the carbon skeleton intact.

Though many different **addition reactions** exist, most operate via the same essential mechanism.

The electrons of the π bond are particularly exposed and are thus easily attacked by molecules that seek to accept an electron pair (Lewis acids). Because these groups are electron seeking, they are more often termed **electrophiles** (literally, "lovers of electrons").

a. Addition of HX

The electrons of the double bond act as a Lewis base and react with electrophilic HX molecules. The first step yields a carbocation intermediate after the double bond reacts with a proton. In the second step, the halide ion combines with the carbocation to give an alkyl halide. In cases where the alkene is asymmetrical, the initial protonation proceeds to produce the *most stable carbocation*. The proton will add to the less substituted carbon atom (the carbon atom with the most protons), since alkyl substituents stabilize carbocations. This phenomenon is called **Markovnikov's Rule**. An example is shown in Figure 5.7:

> **KEY CONCEPT**
>
> Markovnikov's Rule refers to the addition of something (e.g., halide, hydroxyl group) to the most substituted carbon in the double bond.

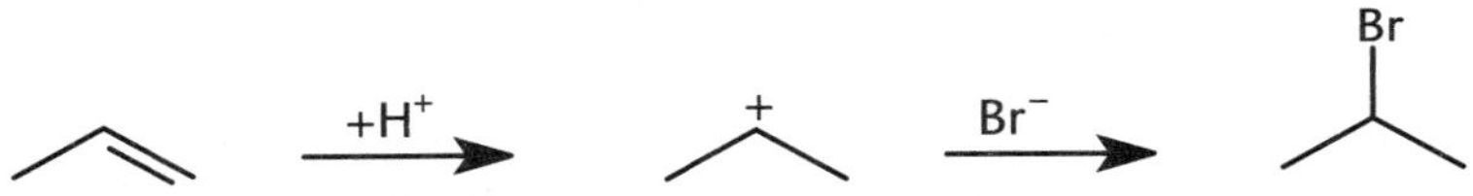

Figure 5.7

b. Addition of X_2

The addition of halogens to a double bond is a rapid process. It is frequently used as a diagnostic tool to test for the presence of double bonds. The double bond acts as a nucleophile and attacks an X_2 molecule, displacing X^-. The intermediate carbocation forms a **cyclic halonium ion,** which is then attacked by X^-, giving the dihalo compound. Note that this addition is *anti*, because the X^- attacks the cyclic halonium ion in a standard S_N2 displacement.

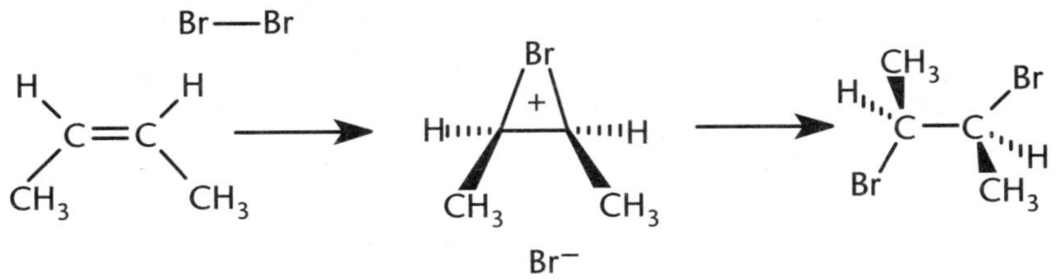

Anti addition

Figure 5.8

If the reaction is carried out in a nucleophilic solvent, the solvent molecules can compete in the displacement step, producing, for example, a **halo alcohol** (rather than the **dihalo** compound).

c. **Addition of H₂O**

Water can be added to alkenes under acidic conditions. The double bond is protonated according to Markovnikov's Rule, forming the most stable carbocation. This carbocation reacts with water, forming a protonated alcohol, which then loses a proton to yield the alcohol. The reaction is performed at low temperature because the reverse reaction is an acid-catalyzed **dehydration** favored by high temperatures.

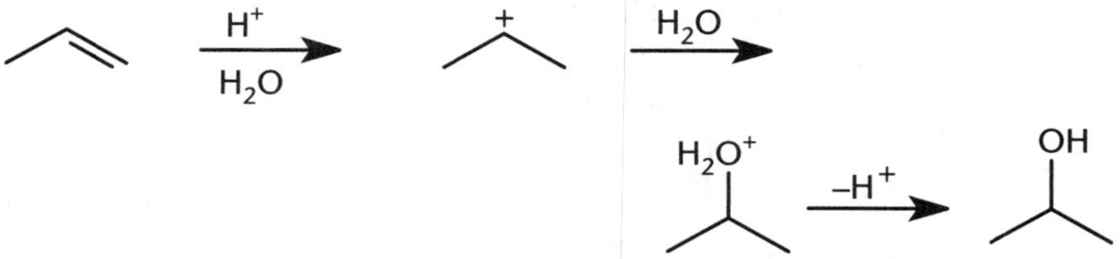

Figure 5.9

Direct addition of water is generally not useful in the laboratory because yields vary greatly with reaction conditions; therefore, this reaction is generally carried out indirectly using mercuric acetate, $Hg(CH_3COO)_2$.

3. **FREE RADICAL ADDITIONS**

An alternate mechanism exists for the addition of HX to alkenes, which proceeds through **free-radical intermediates** and occurs when peroxides, oxygen, or other impurities are present. Free-radical additions disobey the Markovnikov Rule because X• adds first to the double bond, producing the most stable free radical, whereas H⁺ adds first in standard electrophilic additions, producing the most stable carbocation. The reaction is useful for HBr but is not practical for HCl or HI, because the energetics are unfavorable.

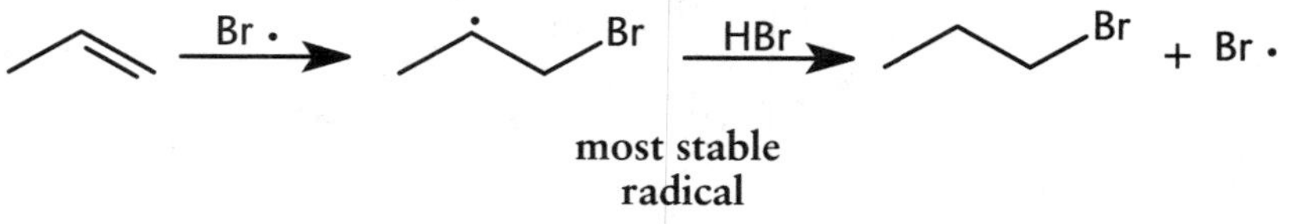

most stable
radical

Figure 5.10

> **REMEMBER**
>
> When peroxides are present, expect free-radical reactions that do not follow Markovnikov's Rule.

4. HYDROBORATION

Diborane (B_2H_6) adds readily to double bonds. The boron atom is a Lewis acid and attaches to the less sterically hindered carbon atom. The second step is an oxidation-hydrolysis with peroxide and aqueous base, producing the alcohol with overall anti-Markovnikov, *syn* orientation.

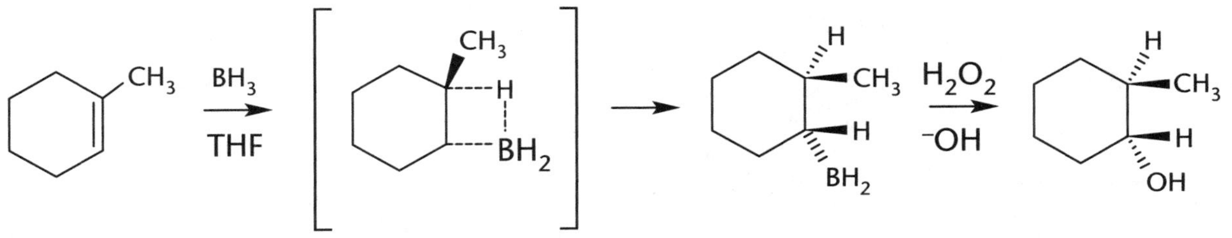

Figure 5.11

5. OXIDATION

a. Potassium permanganate

Alkenes can be oxidized with $KMnO_4$ to provide different types of products, depending upon the reaction conditions. Cold, dilute, aqueous $KMnO_4$ reacts to produce 1,2 diols (vicinal diols), which are also called glycols, with *syn* orientation, as shown in Figure 5.12.

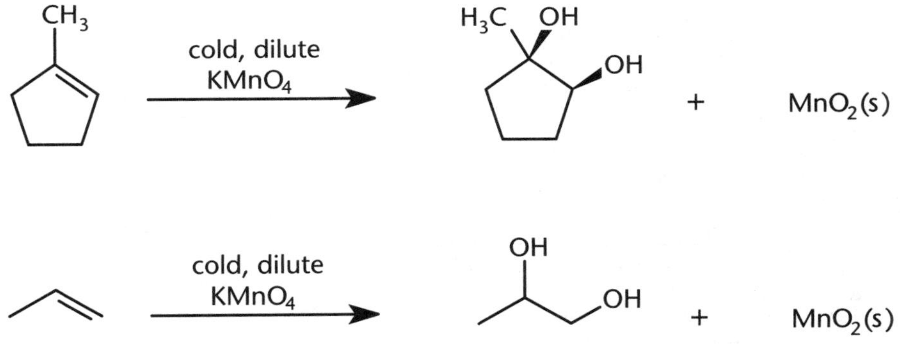

Figure 5.12

BRIDGE

As we see in General Chemistry, the reaction $Mn^{7+} + 3e^- \rightarrow Mn^{4+}$, is a reduction in the electrochemical sense. By default, the organic compound is oxidized. Note that in aqueous solutions, another reaction, $Mn^{7+} + 5e^- \rightarrow Mn^{2+}$, is more likely.

If a *hot, basic* solution of potassium permangenate is added to the alkene and then acidified, nonterminal alkenes are cleaved to form two molar equivalents of carboxylic acid, and terminal alkenes are cleaved to form a carboxylic acid and carbon dioxide. If the nonterminal double-bonded carbon is disubstituted, however, a ketone will be formed, as shown in Figure 5.13.

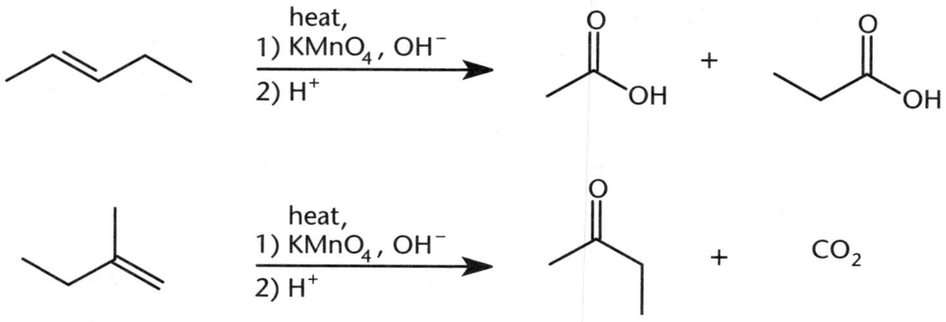

Figure 5.13

b. Ozonolysis

Treatment of alkenes with ozone followed by reduction with zinc and water results in cleavage of the double bond in the manner shown in Figure 5.14.

> **REMEMBER**
>
> 1) $KMnO_4^-$, OH, 2) H^+, heat → : 1. cleavage 2. oxidation
>
> 1) O_3, CH_2Cl_2, 2) Zn/H_2O → : 1. cleavage only

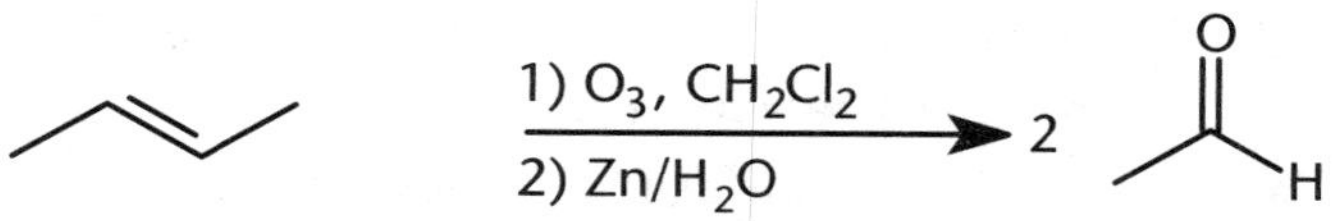

Figure 5.14

If the reaction mixture is reduced with sodium borohydride, $NaBH_4$, the corresponding alcohols are produced, as shown in Figure 5.15.

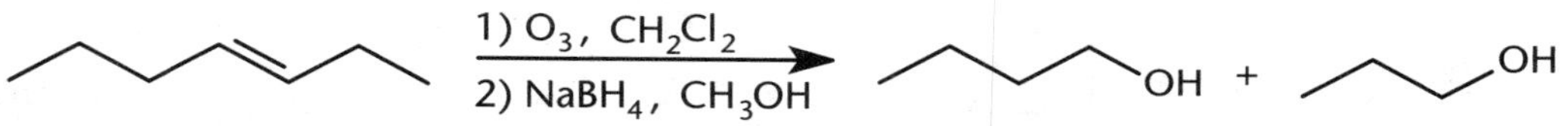

Figure 5.15

c. Peroxycarboxylic acids

Alkenes can be oxidized with peroxycarboxylic acids. Peroxyacetic acid (CH_3CO_3H) and *m*-chloroperoxybenzoic acid (MCPBA) are commonly used. The products formed are **oxiranes** (also called **epoxides**), as shown in Figure 5.16.

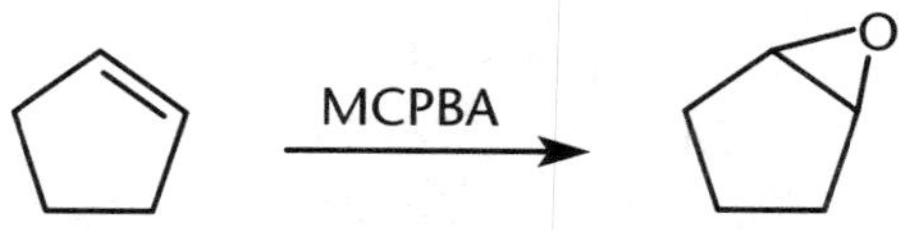

Figure 5.16

6. POLYMERIZATION

Polymerization is the creation of long, high-molecular-weight chains **(polymers)**, composed of repeating subunits (called **monomers**). Polymerization usually occurs through a radical mechanism, although anionic and even cationic polymerizations are commonly observed. A typical example is the formation of polyethylene from ethylene (ethene), which requires high temperatures and pressures (see Figure 5.17).

$$CH_2{=}CH_2 \xrightarrow[\text{high pressure}]{\text{R} \bullet,\ \text{heat}} RCH_2CH_2(CH_2CH_2)_nCH_2CH_2R$$

Figure 5.17

ALKYNES

Alkynes are hydrocarbon compounds that possess one or more carbon-carbon triple bonds.

A. Nomenclature

The suffix **-yne** is used, and the position of the triple bond is specified when necessary. A common exception to the IUPAC rules is ethyne, which is called *acetylene*. Frequently, compounds are named as derivatives of acetylene.

FLASHBACK

Refer to the nomenclature chapter for the general rules of naming of alkynes.

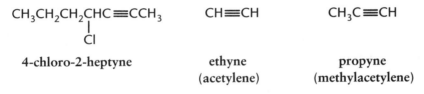

| 4-chloro-2-heptyne | ethyne (acetylene) | propyne (methylacetylene) |

Figure 5.18

B. Physical Properties

The physical properties of the alkynes are similar to those of the analogous alkenes and alkanes. In general, the shorter-chain compounds are gases, boiling at somewhat higher temperatures than the corresponding alkenes. Internal alkynes, like alkenes, boil at higher temperatures than terminal alkynes.

Asymmetrical distribution of electron density causes alkynes to have dipole moments that are larger than those of alkenes but still small in magnitude. Thus, solutions of alkynes can be slightly polar.

Terminal alkynes are fairly acidic, having pK_a's of approximately 25. This property is exploited in some of the reactions of alkynes, which will be discussed later.

C. Synthesis

Triple bonds can be made by the elimination of two molecules of HX from a geminal or vicinal dihalide, as shown in Figure 5.19.

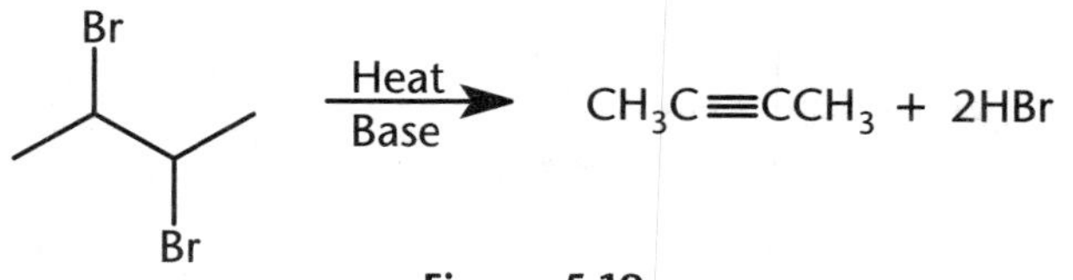

$$CH_3C{\equiv}CCH_3 + 2HBr$$

Figure 5.19

This reaction is not always practical and requires high temperatures and a strong base. A more useful method adds an already existing triple bond into a particular carbon skeleton. A terminal triple bond is converted to a nucleophile by removing the acidic proton with strong base, producing an **acetylide ion**. This ion will perform nucleophilic displacements on alkyl halides at room temperature, as shown in Figure 5.20.

$$CH{\equiv}CH \xrightarrow{\ n\text{-BuLi}\ } CH{\equiv}C^-Li^+ \xrightarrow{\ CH_3Cl\ } CH{\equiv}CCH_3$$

Figure 5.20

D. Reactions

1. REDUCTION

Alkynes, just like alkenes, can be hydrogenated with a catalyst to produce alkanes. A more useful reaction stops the reduction after addition of just one equivalent of H_2, producing alkenes. This partial hydrogenation can take place in two different ways. The first uses **Lindlar's catalyst**, which is palladium on barium sulfate ($BaSO_4$) with quinoline, a poison that stops the reaction at the alkene stage. Because the reaction occurs on a metal surface, the product alkene is the *cis* isomer. The other method uses sodium in liquid ammonia below –33°C (the boiling point of ammonia) and produces the *trans* isomer of the alkene via a free radical mechanism (see Figure 5.21).

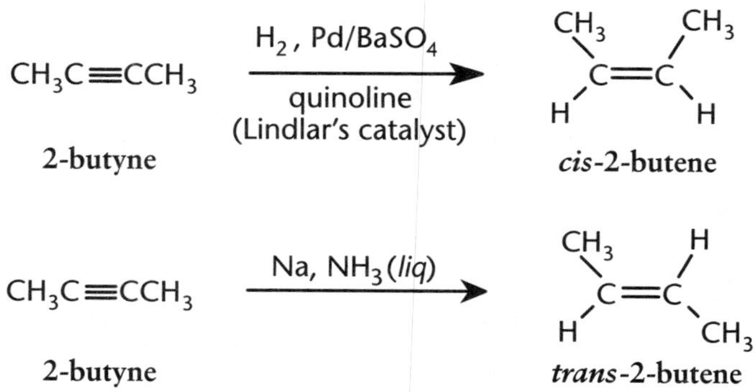

$$CH_3C{\equiv}CCH_3 \xrightarrow[\substack{\text{quinoline} \\ \text{(Lindlar's catalyst)}}]{H_2,\ Pd/BaSO_4}$$

2-butyne

cis-2-butene

$$CH_3C{\equiv}CCH_3 \xrightarrow{\ Na,\ NH_3\,(liq)\ }$$

2-butyne

trans-2-butene

Figure 5.21

2. ADDITION

a. Electrophilic

Electrophilic addition to alkynes occurs in the same manner as it does to alkenes. The reaction occurs according to Markovnikov's Rule. The addition can generally be stopped at the intermediate alkene stage, or it can be carried further. The examples in Figure 5.22 are illustrative.

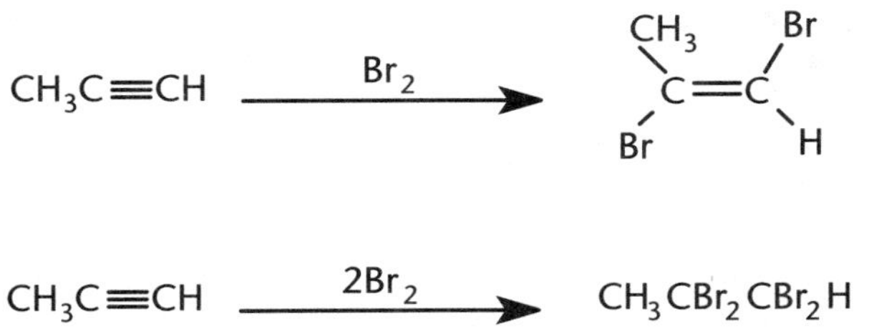

$$CH_3C\equiv CH \xrightarrow{Br_2} \underset{Br}{\overset{CH_3}{}}C=C\underset{H}{\overset{Br}{}}$$

$$CH_3C\equiv CH \xrightarrow{2Br_2} CH_3CBr_2CBr_2H$$

Figure 5.22

b. Free radical

Radicals add to triple bonds as they do to double bonds—with anti-Markovnikov orientation. The reaction product is usually the *trans* isomer, because the intermediate vinyl radical can isomerize to its more stable form.

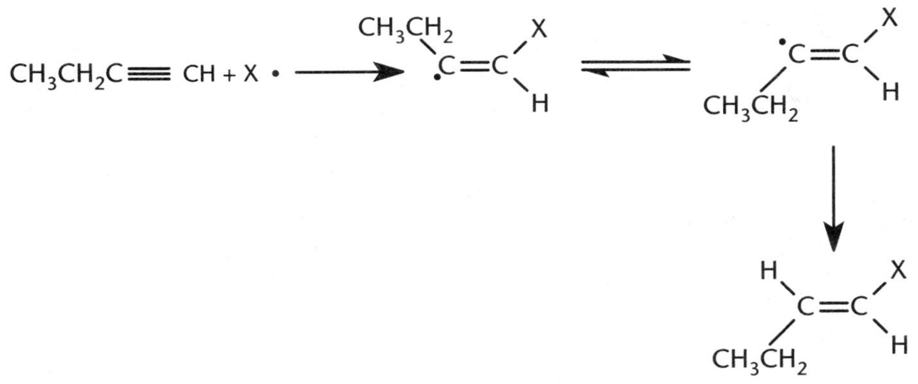

Figure 5.23

3. HYDROBORATION

Addition of boron to triple bonds occurs by the same method as addition of boron to double bonds. Addition is *syn,* and the boron atom adds first. The boron atom can be replaced with a proton from acetic acid to produce a *cis* alkene, as shown in Figure 5.24.

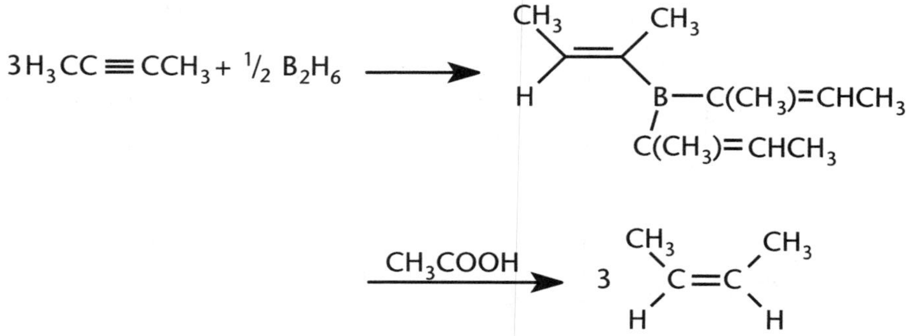

Figure 5.24

With terminal alkynes, a disubstituted borane is used to prevent further boration of the vinylic intermediate to an alkane. The vinylic borane intermediate can be oxidatively cleaved with hydrogen peroxide (H_2O_2), creating an intermediate vinyl alcohol, which rearranges to the more stable carbonyl compound (via **keto-enol tautomerism;**) keto-enol tautomerisms will be discussed in the Aldehydes and Ketones chapter.

Free Radical (Hx)	anti-Markovnikov	1. Add X 2. Add H
Ions (Hx)	Markovnikov	1. Add H$^+$ 2. Add X$^-$

Figure 5.25

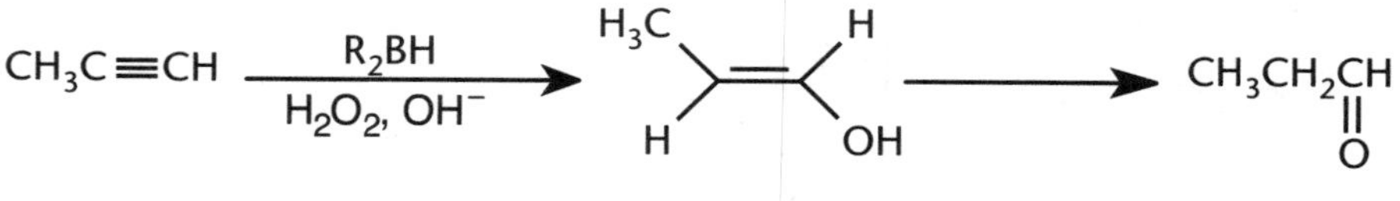

Figure 5.26

4. OXIDATION

Alkynes can be oxidatively cleaved with either basic potassium permangenate (followed by acidification) or ozone.

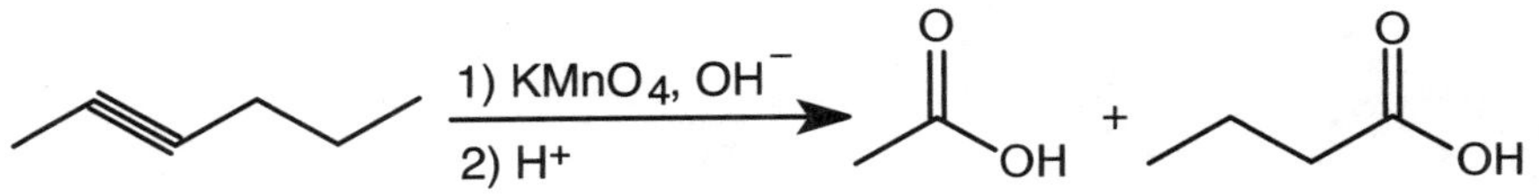

Figure 5.27

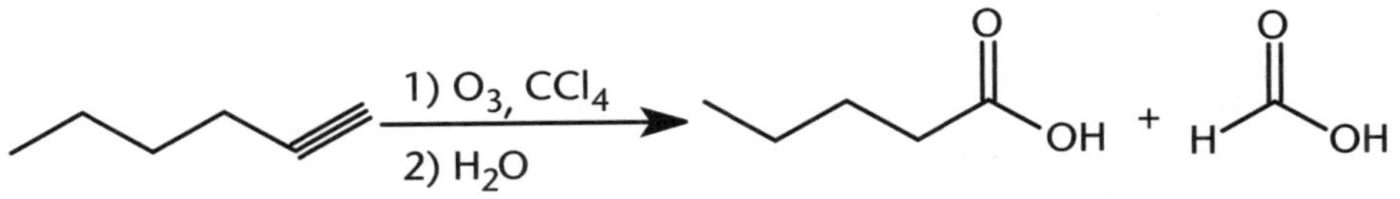

Figure 5.28

6

Aromatic Compounds

The terms **aromatic** and **aliphatic,** meaning "fragrant" and "fatty," respectively, were used originally to distinguish types of organic compounds. The terms persist with new definitions. *Aromatic* now describes any unusually stable ring system. These compounds are cyclic, conjugated polyenes that possess $4n + 2$ pi electrons and adopt planar conformations to allow maximum overlap of the conjugated pi orbitals. *Aliphatic* describes all compounds that are not aromatic.

The criterion of $4n + 2$ pi electrons is known as **Hückel's Rule,** and it is an important indicator of aromaticity. In general, if a cyclic conjugated polyene follows Hückel's Rule, then it is an aromatic compound. Neutral compounds, anions, and cations may all be aromatic. Some typical aromatic compounds and ions are shown in Figure 6.1.

> **REMEMBER**
>
> *n* can be any nonnegative integer; thus, $4n + 2$ can be 2, 6, 10, 14, 18, etc.

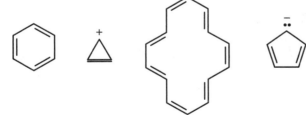

Figure 6.1

A cyclic, conjugated polyene that possesses $4n$ electrons is said to be **antiaromatic** (a cyclic, conjugated polyene that is destabilized). Some typical antiaromatic compounds are shown in Figure 6.2.

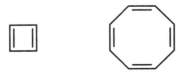

Figure 6.2

NOMENCLATURE

Aromatic compounds are referred to as **aryl** compounds, or **arenes,** and are represented by the symbol **Ar.** Aliphatic compounds are called **alkyl** and are represented by the symbol **R.** Common names exist for many mono- and disubstituted aromatic compounds.

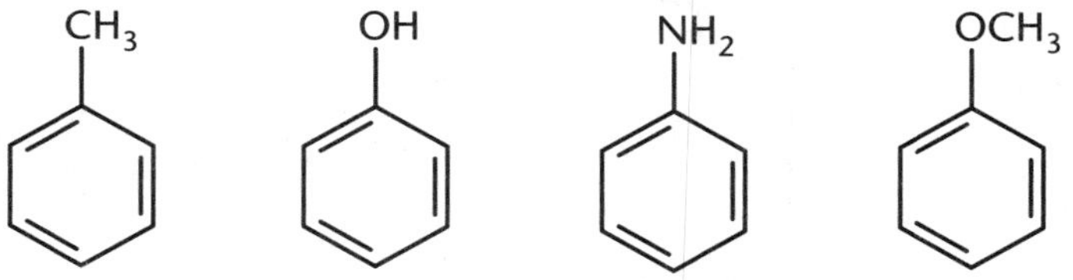

| toluene | phenol | aniline | anisole |

Figure 6.3

The benzene group is called a **phenyl** group **(Ph)** when named as a substituent. The term **benzyl** refers to a toluene molecule substituted at the methyl position.

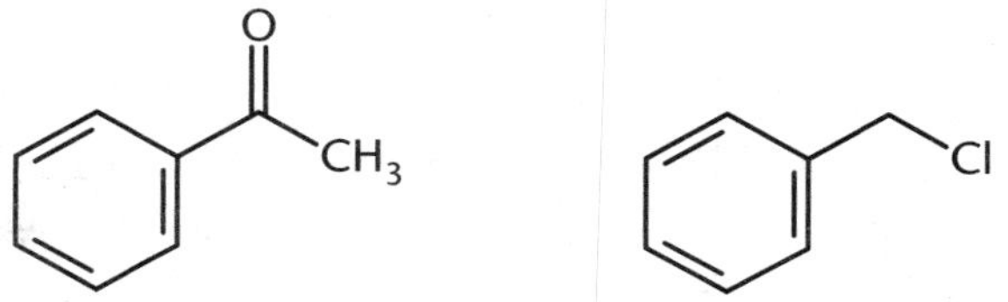

methyl phenyl ketone   benzyl chloride

Figure 6.4

Substituted benzene rings are named as alkyl benzenes, with the subst ituents numbered to produce the lowest sequence. A 1,2-disubstituted compound is called *ortho-* or *o-*; a 1,3-disubstituted compound is called *meta-* or *m-*; and a 1,4-disubstituted compound is called *para-* or *p-*.

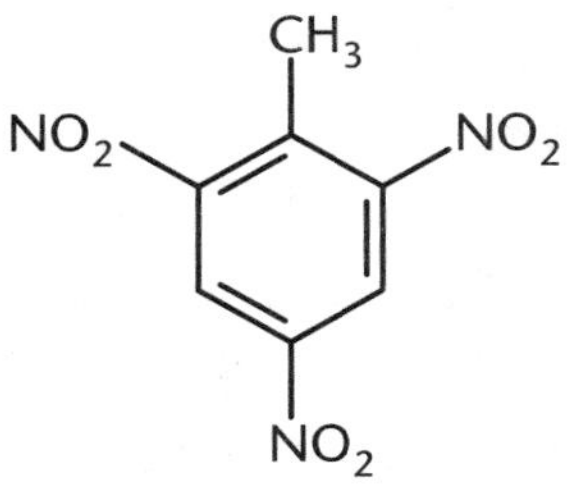

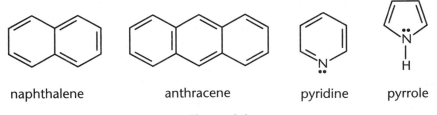

2,4,6-trinitrotoluene (TNT) 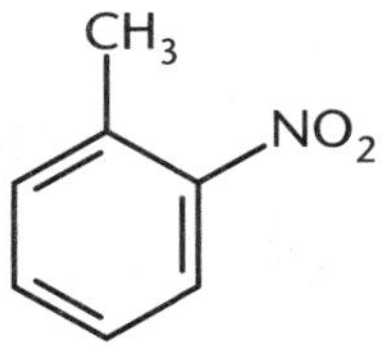   o-nitrotoluene 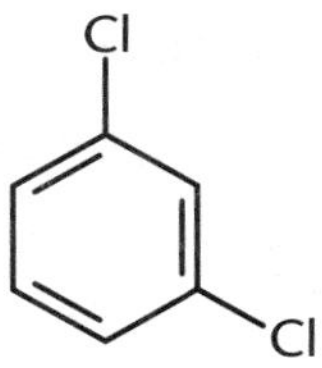   m-dichlorobenzene

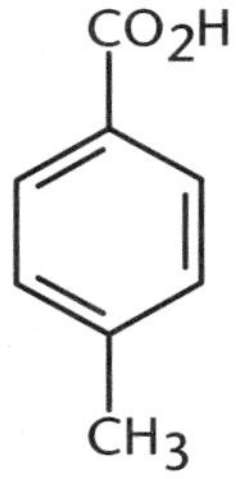

p-methylbenzoic acid

Figure 6.5

There are many polycyclic and heterocyclic aromatic compounds.

naphthalene   anthracene   pyridine   pyrrole

Figure 6.6

KEY CONCEPT

The nonbonding electron pair in pyridine is in a nitrogen sp^2 orbital. This orbital is perpendicular to the p-orbitals around the ring and, therefore, is not involved in the conjugated pi system. On the other hand, the nonbonding pair in pyrrole is in a nitrogen sp^3 orbital parallel to the ring p-orbitals and, therefore, can participate in the delocalized pi system.

PROPERTIES

The physical properties of aromatic compounds are generally similar to those of other hydrocarbons. By contrast, chemical properties are significantly affected by aromaticity. The characteristic planar shape of benzene permits the ring's six pi orbitals to overlap, delocalizing the electron density. All six carbon atoms are sp^2 hybridized, and each of the six orbitals overlaps equally with its two neighbors. As a result, the delocalized electrons form two "pi electron clouds," one above and one below the plane of the ring. This delocalization stabilizes the molecule, making it fairly unreactive: In particular, benzene does not undergo addition reactions as do alkenes. The same holds true for other aromatic compounds, since the definition of an aromatic compound includes the condition that it have a delocalized pi electron system.

REACTIONS

A. Electrophilic Aromatic Substitution

The most important reaction of aromatic compounds is electrophilic aromatic substitution. In this reaction, an electrophile replaces a proton on an aromatic ring, producing a substituted aromatic compound. The most common examples are halogenation, sulfonation, nitration, and acylation.

1. HALOGENATION

Aromatic rings react with bromine or chlorine in the presence of a Lewis acid, such as $FeCl_3$, $FeBr_3$, or $AlCl_3$, to produce monosubstituted products in good yield. Reaction of fluorine and iodine with aromatic rings is less useful, as fluorine tends to produce multisubstituted products and iodine's lack of reactivity requires special conditions for the reaction to proceed.

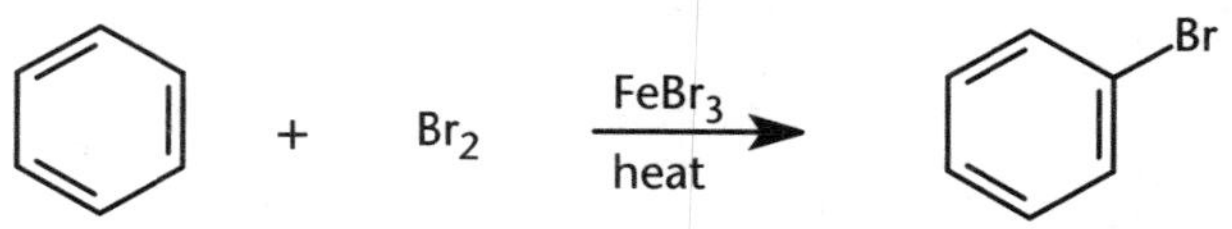

Figure 6.7

2. SULFONATION

Aromatic rings react with fuming sulfuric acid (a mixture of sulfuric acid and sulfur trioxide) to form sulfonic acids.

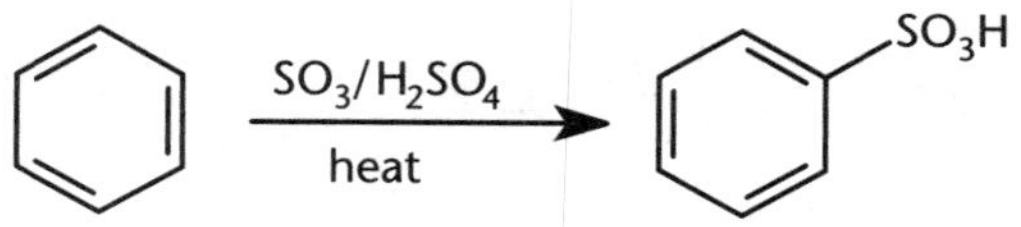

Figure 6.8

3. NITRATION

The nitration of aromatic rings is another synthetically useful reaction. A mixture of nitric and sulfuric acids is used to create the nitronium ion, NO_2^+, a strong electrophile. This reacts with aromatic rings to produce nitro compounds.

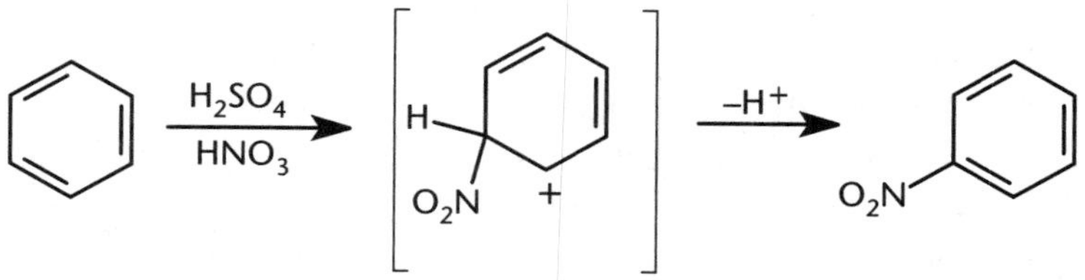

Figure 6.9

4. ACYLATION (FRIEDEL-CRAFTS REACTION)

In a Friedel-Crafts acylation reaction, a carbocation electrophile, usually an acyl group, is incorporated into the aromatic ring. These reactions are usually catalyzed by Lewis acids, such as $AlCl_3$.

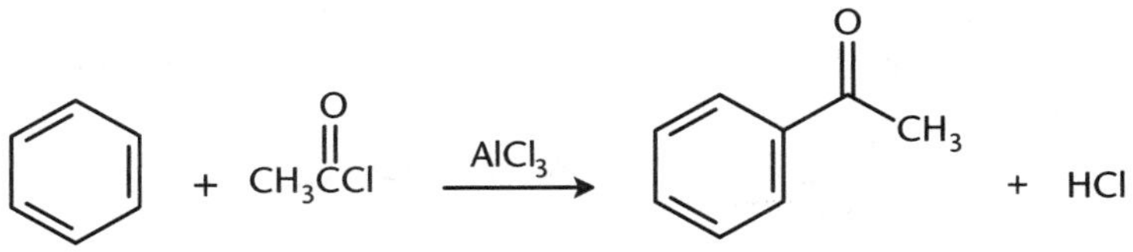

Figure 6.10

5. SUBSTITUENT EFFECTS

Substituents on an aromatic ring strongly influence the susceptibility of the ring to electrophilic aromatic substitution, and they also strongly affect what position on the ring an incoming electrophile is most likely to attack. Substituents can be grouped into three different classes according to whether substitution is enhanced (**activating**) or inhibited (**deactivating**) and where the reaction is likely to take place with respect to the group already present. These effects depend on whether the group tends to donate or withdraw electron density and how it does so; the specifics of these mechanisms will not be discussed here. Arranged in order of decreasing strength of the substituent effect, the three classes are listed below:

a. Activating, *ortho/para*-directing substituents (electron donating): NH_2, NR_2, OH, NHCOR, OR, OCOR, and R.

b. Deactivating, *ortho/para*-directing substituents (weakly electron withdrawing): F, Cl, Br, and I.

c. Deactivating, *meta*-directing substituents (electron withdrawing): NO_2, SO_3H, and carbonyl compounds, including COOH, COOR, COR, and CHO.

For example, when toluene undergoes electrophilic aromatic substitution, the methyl group directs substitution to occur at the *ortho* and *para* positions, as shown in Figure 6.11.

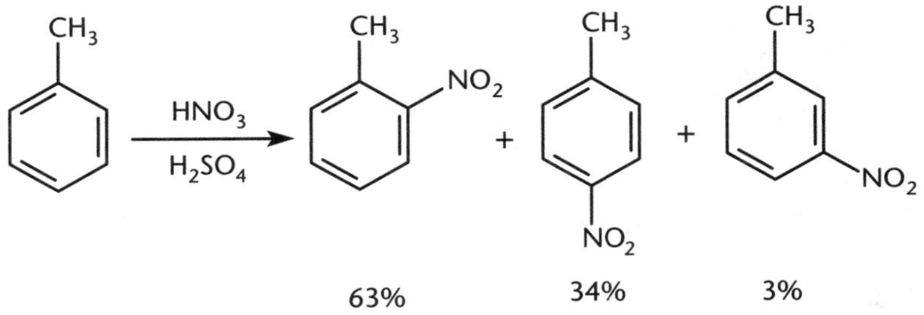

63%   34%   3%

Figure 6.11

B. REDUCTION

1. CATALYTIC REDUCTION

Benzene rings can be reduced by catalytic hydrogenation under vigorous conditions (elevated temperature and pressure) to yield cyclohexane. Ruthenium or rhodium on carbon are the most common catalysts; platinum or palladium may also be used.

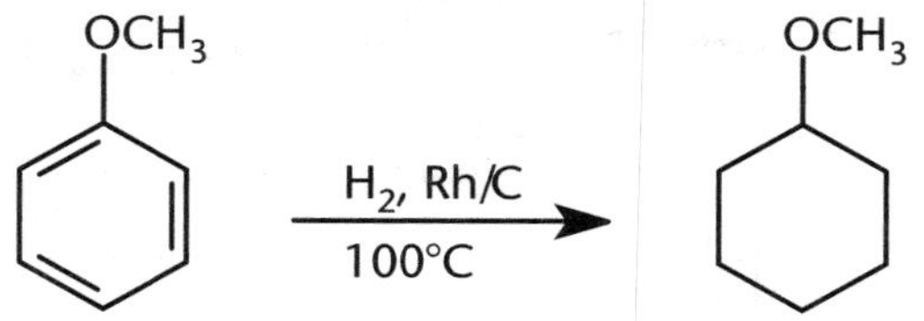

Figure 6.12

7

Alcohols and Ethers

ALCOHOLS

Alcohols are compounds with the general formula **ROH**. The functional group **–OH** is called the **hydroxyl** group. An alcohol can be thought of as a substituted water molecule, with an alkyl group R replacing one H atom.

A. Nomenclature

Alcohols are named in the IUPAC system by replacing the **-e** ending of the root alkane with the ending **-ol**. The carbon atom attached to the hydroxyl group must be included in the longest chain and receive the lowest possible number. Figure 7.1 shows some examples.

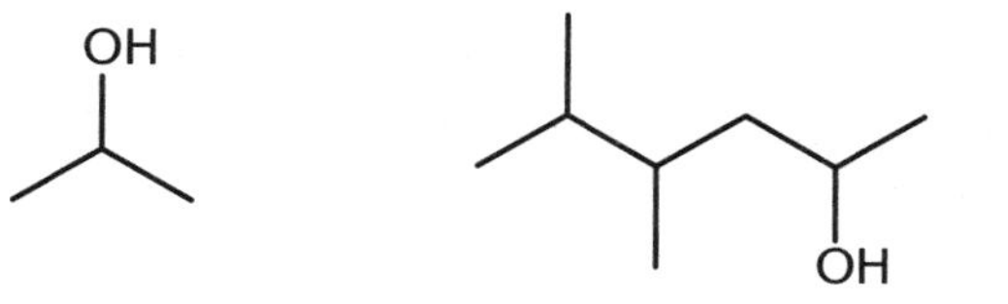

REMEMBER

The –OH group has high priority, so its C must be in the carbon backbone with the lowest number possible.

2-propanol   4,5-dimethyl-2-hexanol

Figure 7.1

Alternatively, the alkyl group can be named as a derivative, followed by the word *alcohol*.

ethyl alcohol   isobutyl alcohol

Figure 7.2

Compounds of the general formula ArOH, with a hydroxyl group attached to an aromatic ring, are called **phenols** (see chapter 6).

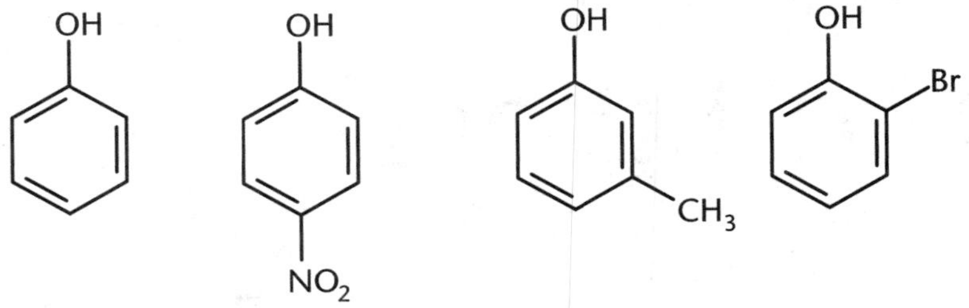

phenol | *p*-nitrophenol | *m*-cresol (*m*-methylphenol) | *o*-bromophenol

Figure 7.3

B. Physical Properties

The boiling points of alcohols are significantly higher than those of the analogous hydrocarbons due to **hydrogen bonding**. Hydrogen bonding results in both elevated boiling points and better solubility in water.

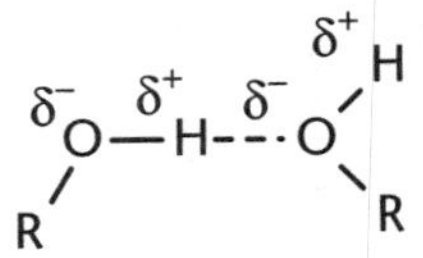

Figure 7.4

REMEMBER

Hydrogen bonds form because chemistry is FON!
(Fluorine, Oxygen, Nitrogen)

Molecules with more than one hydroxyl group show greater degrees of hydrogen bonding, as is evident from the boiling points shown in Figure 7.5.

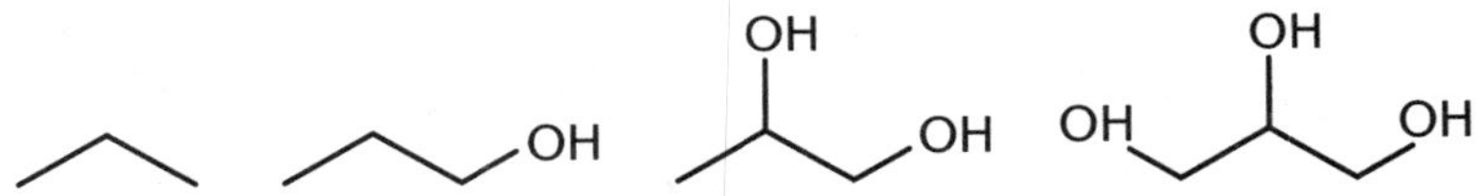

boiling point (°C): –42.1 | 97.4 | 189.0 | 290.0

Figure 7.5

KEY CONCEPT

Alcohols are weakly acidic:
$ROH \rightleftharpoons RO^- + H^+$

Hydrogen bonding can also occur when hydrogen atoms are attached to other highly electronegative atoms, such as nitrogen and fluorine. HF has particularly strong hydrogen bonds, because the high electronegativity of fluorine causes the HF bond to be highly polarized.

The hydroxyl hydrogen atom is weakly acidic, and alcohols can dissociate into protons and alkoxy ions just as water dissociates into protons and hydroxide ions. pK_a values of several compounds are listed in Table 7.1.

Table 7.1

Dissociation		pK$_a$	
$H_2O \rightleftharpoons HO^- + H^+$		15.7	
$CH_3OH \rightleftharpoons$	$CH_3O^- + H^+$		15.5
$C_2H_5OH \rightleftharpoons C_2H_5O^- + H^+$		15.9	
$i\text{-PrOH} \rightleftharpoons i\text{-PrO}^- + H^+$		17.1	
$t\text{-BuOH} \rightleftharpoons$	$t\text{-BuO}^- + H^+$		18.0
$CF_3CH_2OH \rightleftharpoons CF_3CH_2O^- + H^+$		12.4	
$PhOH \rightleftharpoons PhO^- + H^+$		≈ 10.0	

BRIDGE

$pK_a = -\log K_a$

Strong acids have high K$_a$'s and small pK$_a$'s. Thus, phenol, which has the smallest pK$_a$, is the most acidic (see General Chemistry).

The hydroxyl hydrogens of phenols are more acidic than those of alcohols due to resonance structures that distribute the negative charge throughout the ring, thus stabilizing the anion. As a result, these compounds form intermolecular hydrogen bonds and have relatively high melting and boiling points. Phenol is slightly soluble in water (presumably due to hydrogen bonding), as are some of its derivatives. Phenols are much more acidic than aliphatic alcohols and can form salts with inorganic bases such as NaOH.

The presence of other substituents on the ring has significant effects on the acidity, boiling points, and melting points of phenols. As with other aromatic compounds, electron-withdrawing substituents increase acidity, and electron-donating groups decrease acidity.

KEY CONCEPT

Acidity decreases as more alkyl groups are attached because the electron-donating alkyl groups destabilize the alkoxide anion. Electron-withdrawing groups stabilize the alkoxy anion, making the alcohol more acidic.

C. Review

1. KEY REACTION FOR MECHANISMS FOR ALCOHOLS AND ETHERS

As you read about synthesis of (and from) alcohols and ethers, you'll see the same basic reaction mechanisms recurring over and over. Rather than memorizing each reaction individually, try to think of them in broad categories. Focus on how the basic mechanism works and on how this particular reaction exemplifies it. The "Big Three" mechanisms for alcohols and ethers are:

REMEMBER

Charge likes to be spread out as widely as possible!

↑ acidity   resonance
                e⁻ withdrawing
↓ acidity   e⁻ donating

a. S$_N$1, S$_N$2: nucleophilic substitution

Example:

$$CH_3Br + OH^- \longrightarrow CH_3OH + Br^-$$

b. **Electrophilic addition to a double bond**

Example:

$$H_2O \quad + \quad \text{(alkene)} \longrightarrow \text{(alcohol)}$$

c. **Nucleophilic addition to a carbonyl**

Example:

$$CH_3MgBr \quad + \quad \text{(aldehyde)} \longrightarrow \text{(alcohol)}$$

REMEMBER

In general, more bonds to oxygen means more oxidized.

Also, when thinking about alcohols, you should keep in mind their place on the oxidation-reduction continuum:

OXIDATION

1° alcohols ⟷ aldehydes ⟷ carboxylic acids

2° alcohols ⟷ ketones

REDUCTION

As you read about the individual reactions in which alcohols participate, try to fit them into this framework (possible for most reactions, though not all).

D. Synthesis

Alcohols can be prepared from a variety of compounds. Methanol, also called wood alcohol, is obtained from the destructive distillation of wood. It is toxic and can cause blindness if ingested. Ethanol, or grain alcohol, is produced from the fermentation of sugars and can be metabolized by the body; however, in large enough quantities, it too is toxic.

1. ADDITION REACTIONS

Alcohols can be prepared via several reactions that involve addition of water to double bonds (discussed in the Alkenes chapter). Alcohols can also be prepared from the addition of organometallic compounds to carbonyl groups.

2. SUBSTITUTION REACTIONS

Both S_N1 and S_N2 reactions can be used to produce alcohols under the proper conditions (discussed in "Substitution Reactions in Alkyl Halides").

3. REDUCTION REACTIONS

Alcohols can be prepared from the reduction of aldehydes, ketones, carboxylic acids, or esters. Lithium aluminum hydride ($LiAlH_4$, or LAH) and sodium borohydride ($NaBH_4$) are the two most frequently used reducing reagents. LAH is more powerful and more difficult to work with, whereas $NaBH_4$ is more selective and easier to handle. For example, LAH will reduce carboxylic acids and esters, while $NaBH_4$ will not.

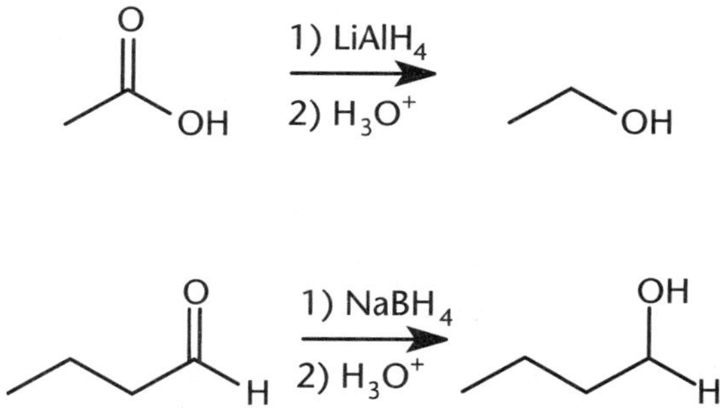

Figure 7.6

4. PHENOL SYNTHESIS

Phenols can be synthesized from arylsulfonic acids with hot NaOH. However, this reaction is useful only for phenol or its alkylated derivatives, as most functional groups are destroyed by the harsh reaction conditions.

A more versatile method of synthesizing phenols is via hydrolysis of diazonium salts.

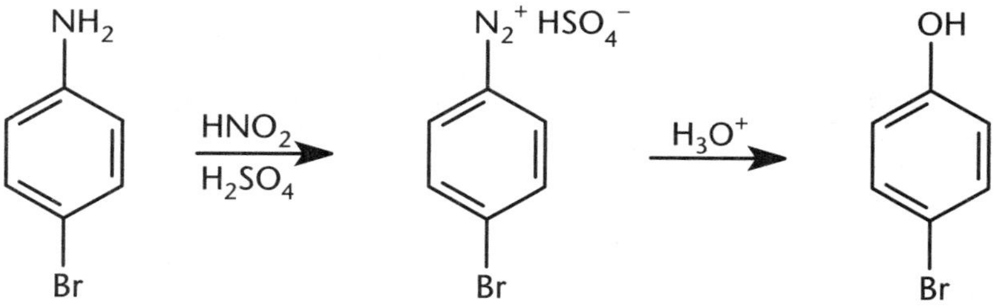

Figure 7.7

KEY CONCEPT

Think of electrophilic addition of H_2O to a double bond, only this time it's in reverse—elimination.

E. Reactions

1. ELIMINATION REACTIONS

Alcohols can be **dehydrated** in a strongly acidic solution (usually H_2SO_4) to produce alkenes. The mechanism of this dehydration reaction is E1, and it proceeds via the protonated alcohol.

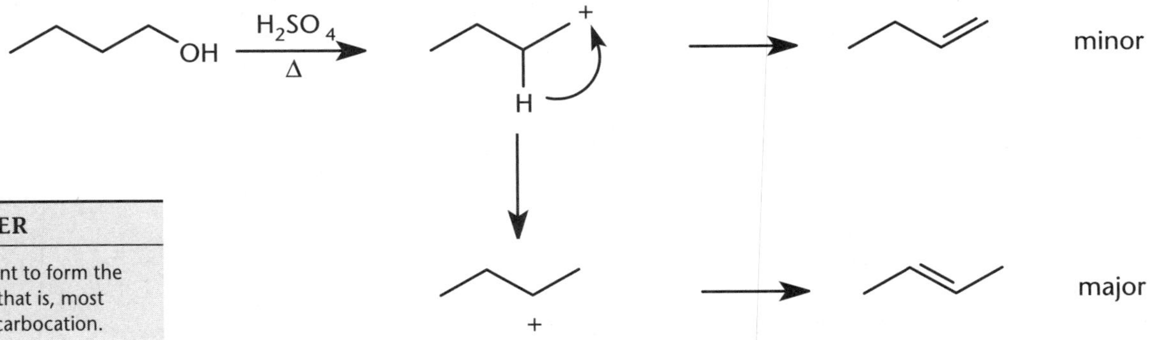

REMEMBER

In E1, you want to form the most stable (that is, most substituted) carbocation.

Figure 7.8

Notice from Figure 7.8 that two products are obtained, with the more stable alkene being the major product. This occurs via movement of a proton to produce the more stable 2° carbocation. This type of rearrangement is commonly encountered with carbocations.

KEY CONCEPT

Alcohols can participate in S_N1/S_N2 reactions, but only if you turn the –OH into a better leaving group by one of the following methods:

— Protonate it.
— Convert to a tosylate.
— Form an inorganic ester.

2. SUBSTITUTION REACTIONS

The displacement of hydroxyl groups in substitution reactions is rare because the hydroxide ion is a poor leaving group. If such a transformation is desired, the hydroxyl group must be made into a good leaving group. Protonating the alcohol makes water the leaving group, which is good for S_N1 reactions; even better, the alcohol can be converted into a tosylate (*p*-toluenesulfonate) group, which is an excellent leaving group for S_N2 reactions (see Figures 7.9a and 7.9b).

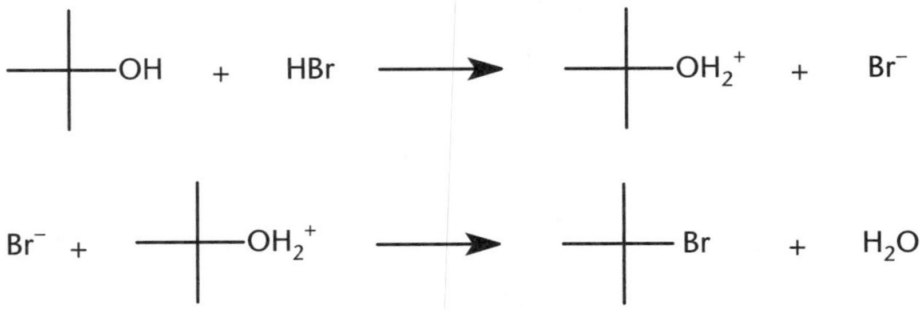

Figure 7.9a

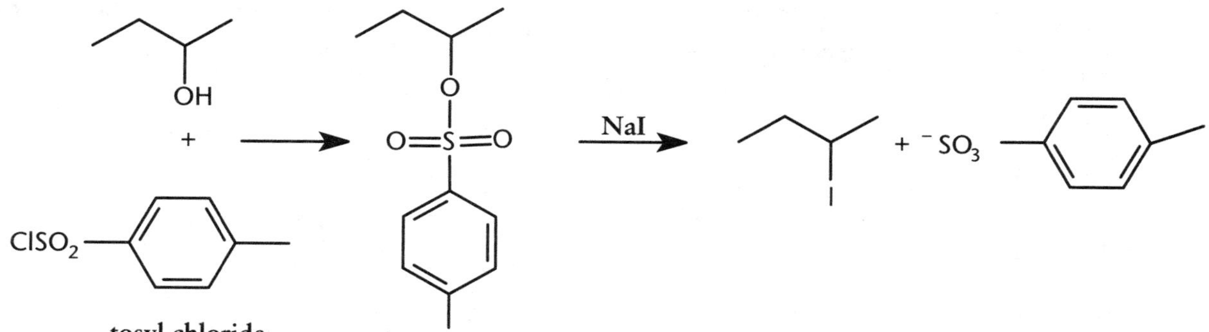

Figure 7.9b

A common method of converting alcohols into alkyl halides involves the formation of inorganic esters, which readily undergo S_N2 reactions. Alcohols react with thionyl chloride to produce an intermediate inorganic ester (a chlorosulfite) and HCl. The chloride ion of HCl displaces SO_2 and regenerates Cl⁻, forming the desired alkyl chloride.

$$CH_3OH + SOCl_2 \longrightarrow CH_3OSOCl + HCl$$

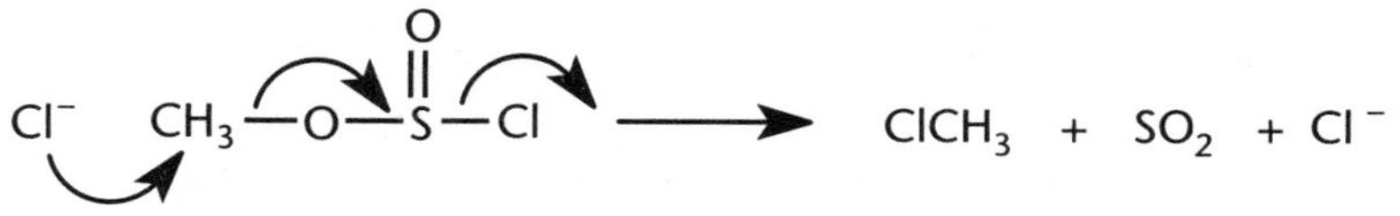

Figure 7.10

An analogous reaction, where the alcohol is treated with PBr_3 instead of thionyl chloride, produces alkyl bromides.

Phenols readily undergo electrophilic aromatic substitution reactions; because it has lone pairs that it can donate to the ring, the –OH group is a strongly activating, *ortho/para*-directing ring substituent.

> **KEY CONCEPT**
>
> Phenols are good substrates for electrophilic aromatic substitution; the –OH is activating and *ortho/para* directing.

3. OXIDATION REACTIONS

The oxidation of alcohols generally involves some form of chromium (VI) as the oxidizing agent, which is reduced to chromium (III) during the reaction. PCC (pyridinium chlorochromate, $C_5H_6NCrO_3Cl$) is commonly used as a mild oxidant. It converts primary alcohols to aldehydes without overoxidation to the acid. (In contrast, $KMnO_4$ is a very strong oxidizing agent that will take the alcohol all the way to the carboxylic acid.) It can also be used to form ketones from 2° alcohols. Tertiary alcohols cannot be oxidized for valence reasons.

> **REMEMBER**
>
> When you see a transition metal (such as Cr or Mn) with lots of oxygen (Cr_2O_7, CrO_3, MnO_4), think OXIDATION.

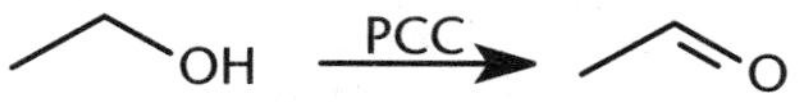

Figure 7.11

REMEMBER

Alcohols can be formed by and can participate in many of the key reaction mechanisms you've already seen:

1) S_N1, S_N2 (although –OH must be made into a better leaving group);
2) addition of H_2O to a double bond (including electrophilic addition) and reverse reactions such as E1;
3) nucleophilic addition to a carbonyl;

4) oxidation/reduction reactions.

Another reagent used to oxidize secondary alcohols is alkali (either sodium or potassium) dichromate salt. This will also oxidize 1° alcohols to carboxylic acids.

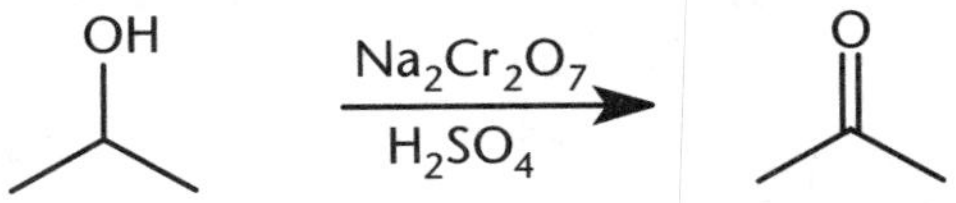

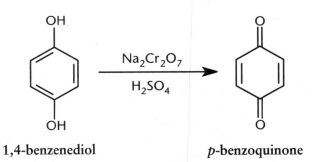

Figure 7.12

A stronger oxidant is chromium trioxide, CrO_3. This is often dissolved with dilute sulfuric acid in acetone; the mixture is called **Jones reagent**. It oxidizes primary alcohols to carboxylic acids and secondary alcohols to ketones.

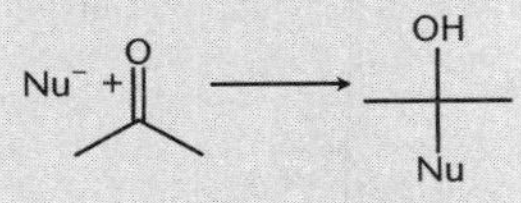

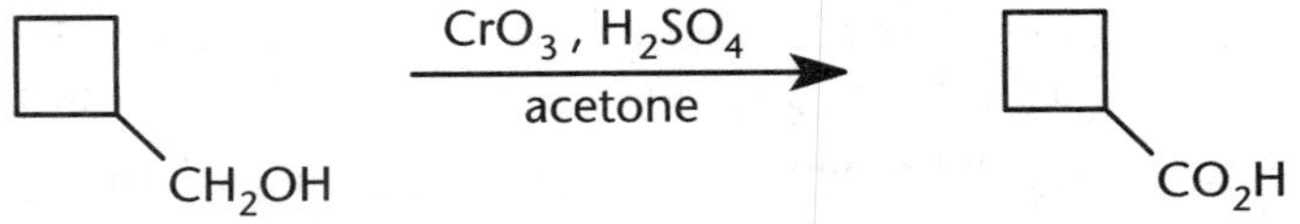

Figure 7.13

Treatment of phenols with oxidizing reagents produces compounds called quinones (2,5-cyclohexadiene-1,4-diones).

1,4-benzenediol *p*-benzoquinone

Figure 7.14

ETHERS

An ether is a compound with two alkyl (or aryl) groups bonded to an oxygen atom. The general formula for an ether is **ROR**. Ethers can be thought of as disubstituted water molecules. The most familiar ether is diethyl ether, once used as a medical anesthetic and still often used that way in the laboratory.

A. Nomenclature

Ethers are named according to IUPAC rules as **alkoxyalkanes,** with the smaller chain as the prefix and the larger chain as the suffix. There is a common system of nomenclature in which ethers are named as alkyl

alkyl ethers. In this system, methoxyethane would be named ethyl methyl ether. The alkyl substituents are alphabetized.

O

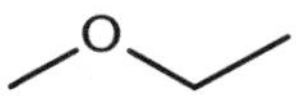

methoxyethane
(ethyl methyl ether)

O

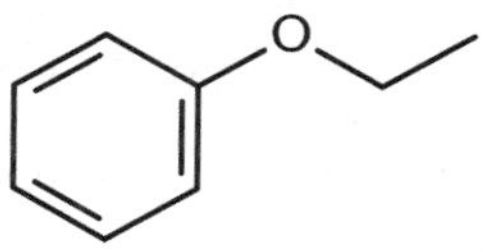

ethoxybenzene
(ethyl phenyl ether)

Figure 7.15

Exceptions to these rules occur for cyclic ethers, for which many common names also exist.

O

oxirane
(epoxide)

O

oxyethane

O

oxacyclopentane
(tetrahydrofuran)

Figure 7.16

REMEMBER

Remember that smaller rings have more angle strain, making them less stable.

B. Physical Properties

Ethers do not undergo hydrogen bonding because they have no hydrogen atoms bonded to the oxygen atoms. Ethers therefore boil at relatively low temperatures compared to alcohols; in fact, they boil at approximately the same temperatures as alkanes of comparable molecular weight.

Ethers are only slightly polar and, therefore, only slightly soluble in water. They are rather inert to most organic reagents and are frequently used as solvents.

C. Synthesis

The Williamson ether synthesis produces ethers from the reaction of metal alkoxides with primary alkyl halides or tosylates. The alkoxides behave as nucleophiles and displace the halide or tosylate via an S_N2 reaction, producing an ether.

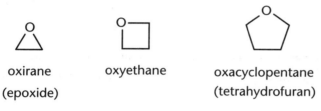

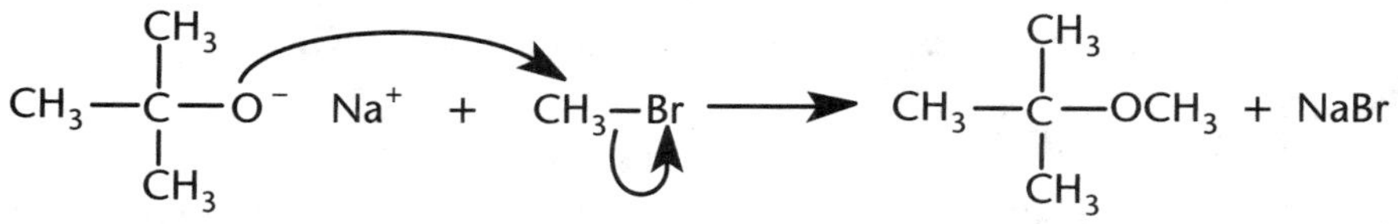

CH3
CH3—C—O⁻ Na+ + CH3—Br
CH3
CH3
CH3—C—OCH3 + NaBr
CH3

Figure 7.17

BRIDGE

Look! It's S_N2 again! Therefore, you need a strong nucleophile (alkoxides are good) and an unhindered substrate (*not* bulky or highly substituted).

It is important to remember that alkoxides will attack only nonhindered halides. Thus, to synthesize a methyl ether, an alkoxide must attack a methyl halide; the reaction cannot be accomplished with methoxide ion attacking a hindered alkyl halide substrate.

The Williamson ether synthesis can also be applied to phenols. Relatively mild reaction conditions are sufficient, due to the phenols' acidity.

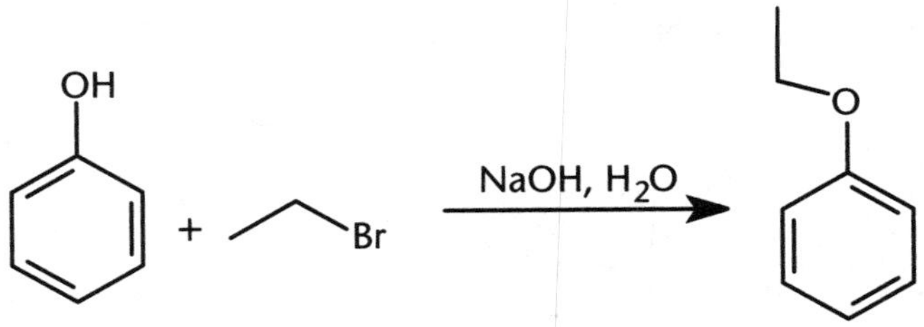

Figure 7.18

BRIDGE

More S_N2! This time, however, it's intramolecular—the nucleophile and leaving group are part of the same molecule.

Cyclic ethers are prepared in a number of ways. Oxiranes can be synthesized by means of an internal S_N2 displacement.

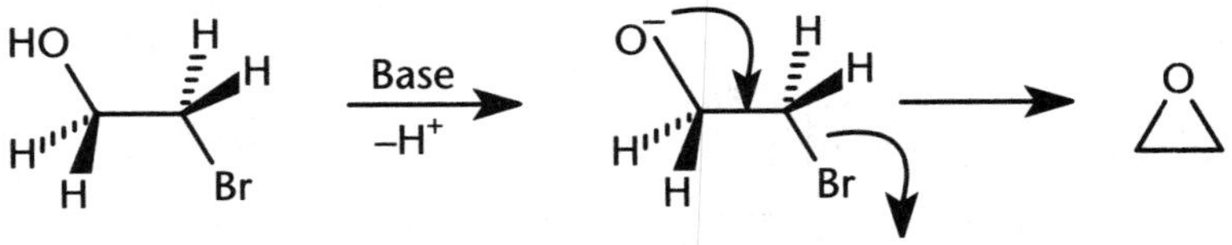

Figure 7.19

Oxidation of an alkene with a **peroxy acid** (general formula RCOOOH) such as MCPBA (*m*-chloroperoxybenzoic acid) will also produce an oxirane.

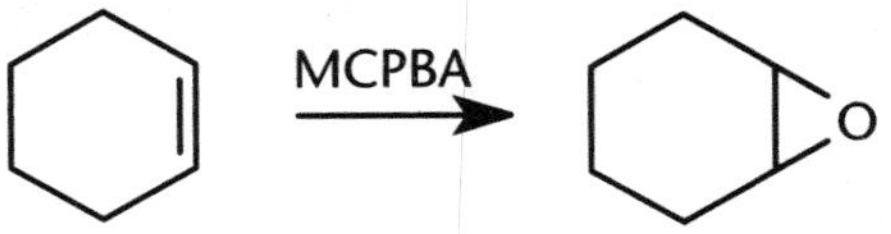

Figure 7.20

D. Reactions

1. PEROXIDE FORMATION

Ethers react with the oxygen in air to form highly explosive compounds called **peroxides** (general formula ROOR).

REMEMBER

Remember, strong bases are poor leaving groups. Without protonation, the leaving group would be an alkoxide (strongly basic), and the reaction would be unlikely to proceed.

2. CLEAVAGE

Cleavage of straight-chain ethers will take place only under vigorous conditions: usually at high temperatures in the presence of HBr or HI. Cleavage is initiated by protonation of the ether oxygen. The reaction then proceeds by an S_N1 or S_N2 mechanism, depending on the conditions and the structure of the ether. Although not shown in Figure 7.21, the alcohol products usually react with a second molecule of hydrogen halide to produce an alkyl halide.

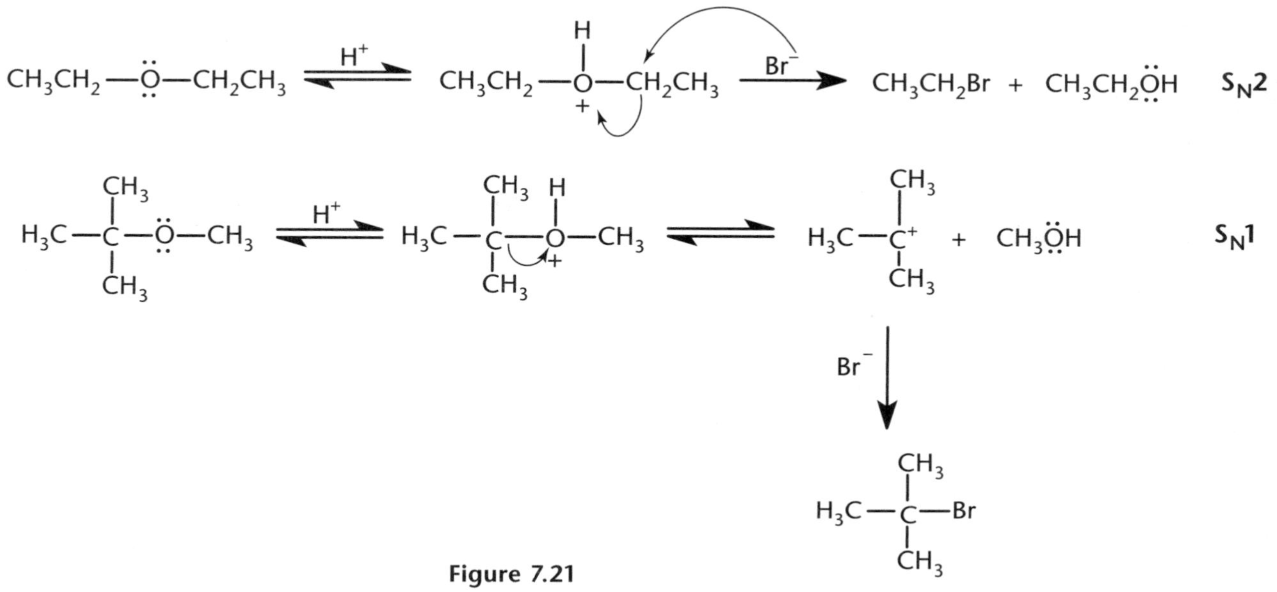

Figure 7.21

Since epoxides are highly strained cyclic ethers, they are susceptible to S_N2 reactions. Unlike straight-chain ethers, these reactions can be catalyzed by acid or base. In symmetrical epoxides, either carbon can be nucleophilically attacked, but in asymmetrical epoxides, the most substituted carbon is nucleophilically attacked in the presence of acid, and the least substituted carbon is attacked in the presence of base (see Figure 7.22).

KEY CONCEPT

Cleavage of straight-chain ethers s acid-catalyzed. Cleavage of cyclic ethers can be acid- or base-catalyzed.

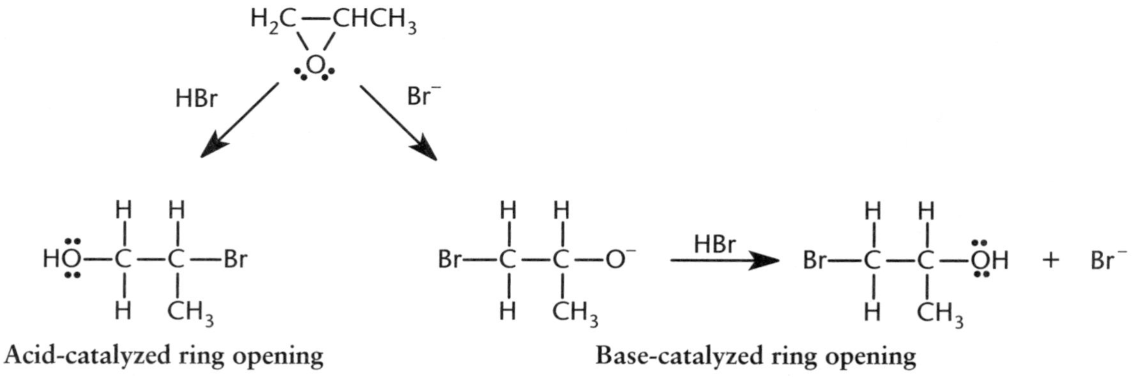

Acid-catalyzed ring opening   Base-catalyzed ring opening

Figure 7.22

Base-catalyzed cleavage has the most S_N2 character, so it occurs at the least hindered (least substituted) carbon. The basic environment provides the best nucleophile.

In contrast, acid-catalyzed cleavage is thought to have some S_N1 character as well as some S_N2 character. The epoxide O can be protonated, making it a better leaving group. This gives the carbons a bit of positive charge. Since substitution stabilizes this charge (remember, 3° carbons make the best carbocations), the more substituted C becomes a good target for nucleophilic attack.

Don't let epoxides intimidate you; the same basic principles and reaction mechanisms apply, just as we've seen with more simple compounds.

8

Aldehydes and Ketones

Aldehydes and **ketones** are compounds that contain the **carbonyl group, C=O,** a double bond between a carbon atom and an oxygen atom. A ketone has two alkyl or aryl groups bonded to the carbonyl, whereas an aldehyde has one alkyl group and one hydrogen (or, in the case of formaldehyde, two hydrogens) bonded to the carbonyl. The carbonyl group is one of the most important functional groups in organic chemistry. In addition to aldehydes and ketones, it is also found in carboxylic acids, esters, amides, and more complicated compounds.

NOMENCLATURE

In the IUPAC system, aldehydes are named with the suffix **-al**. The position of the aldehyde group does not need to be specified: It must occupy the terminal (C1) position. Common names exist for the first five aldehydes: formaldehyde, acetaldehyde, propionaldehyde, butyraldehyde, and valeraldehyde (see Figure 8.1).

> **REMEMBER**
>
> An aldehyde is a terminal functional group; it defines C1.

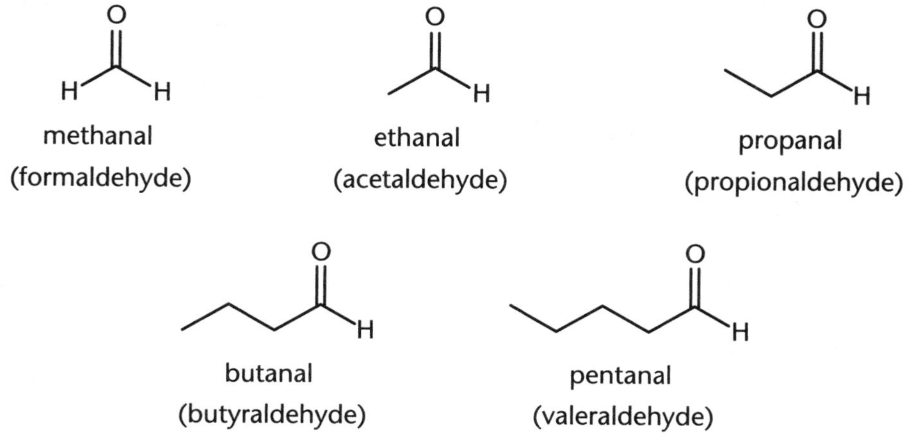

methanal
(formaldehyde)

ethanal
(acetaldehyde)

propanal
(propionaldehyde)

butanal
(butyraldehyde)

pentanal
(valeraldehyde)

Figu're 8.1

In more complicated molecules, the suffix **-carbaldehyde** can be used. In addition, the aldehyde can be named as a functional group with the prefix **formyl-**.

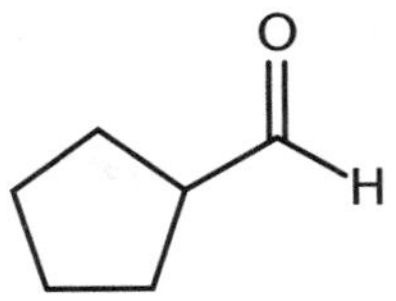

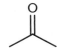

cyclopentanecarbaldehyde

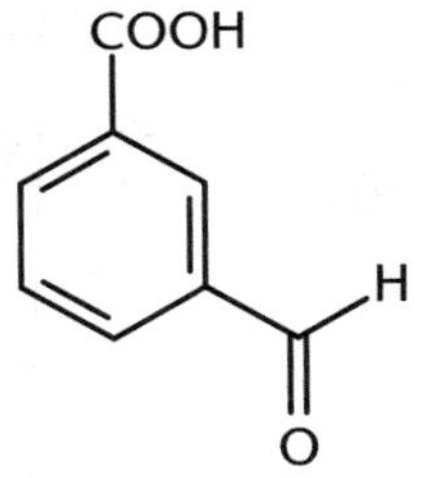

m-formylbenzoic acid

Figure 8.2

Ketones are named with the suffix **-one**. The location of the carbonyl group must be specified with a number, except in cyclic ketones, where it is assumed to occupy the number 1 position. The common system of naming **ketones** lists the two alkyl groups followed by the word *ketone*. When it is necessary to name the carbonyl as a substituent, the prefix **oxo-** is used.

2-propanone
(dimethyl ketone)
(acetone)

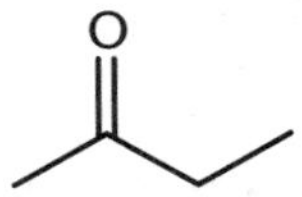

2-butanone
(ethyl methyl ketone)

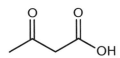

3-oxobutanoic acid

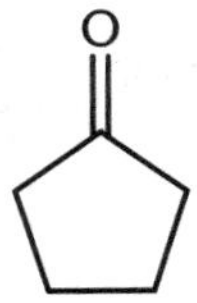

cyclopentanone

Figure 8.3

PHYSICAL PROPERTIES

The physical properties of aldehydes and ketones are governed by the presence of the carbonyl group. The dipole moments associated with the polar carbonyl groups align, causing an elevation in boiling point relative to the alkanes. This elevation is less than that in alcohols, since no hydrogen bonding is involved.

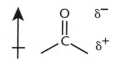

Figure 8.4

SYNTHESIS

There are numerous methods of preparing aldehydes and ketones; four of the most common are described below.

A. Oxidation of Alcohols

An aldehyde can be obtained from the oxidation of a primary alcohol; a ketone can be obtained from a secondary alcohol. These reactions are usually performed with PCC, sodium or potassium dichromate, or chromium trioxide (Jones reagent).

B. Ozonolysis of Alkenes

Double bonds can be oxidatively cleaved to yield aldehydes and/or ketones, typically with ozone.

C. Friedel-Crafts Acylation

This reaction produces ketones of the form R–CO–Ar.

REACTIONS

A. Enolization and Reactions of Enols

Protons alpha to carbonyl groups are relatively acidic ($pK_a \approx 20$) due to resonance stabilization of the conjugate base. A hydrogen atom that detaches itself from the alpha carbon has a finite probability of reattaching itself to the oxygen instead of the carbon. Therefore, aldehydes and ketones exist in solution as a mixture of two isomers, the familiar **keto** form and the **enol** form, representing the unsaturated alcohol (**ene** = the double bond, **ol** = the alcohol, so **ene** + **ol** = **enol**). The two isomers, which differ only in the placement of a proton, are called **tautomers**.

The equilibrium between the tautomers lies far to the keto side. The process of interconverting from the keto to the enol tautomer is called **enolization**. Tautomers are structural isomers, *not* resonance structures.

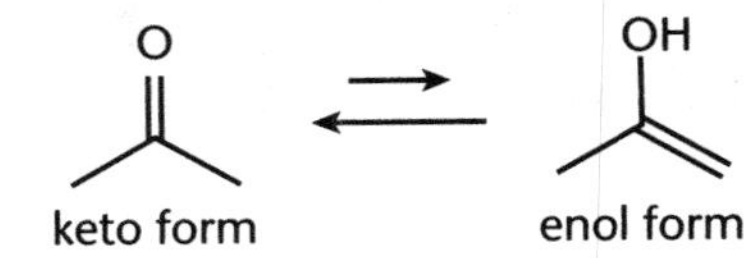
O
OH
keto form
(more stable)
enol form

Figure 8.5

Enols are the necessary intermediates in many reactions of aldehydes and ketones. The enolate carbanion, which is nucleophilic, can be created with a strong base, such as lithium diisopropyl amide (LDA) or potassium hydride (KH). This nucleophilic carbanion reacts via S_N2 with α,β-unsaturated carbonyl compounds in reactions called **Michael additions**.

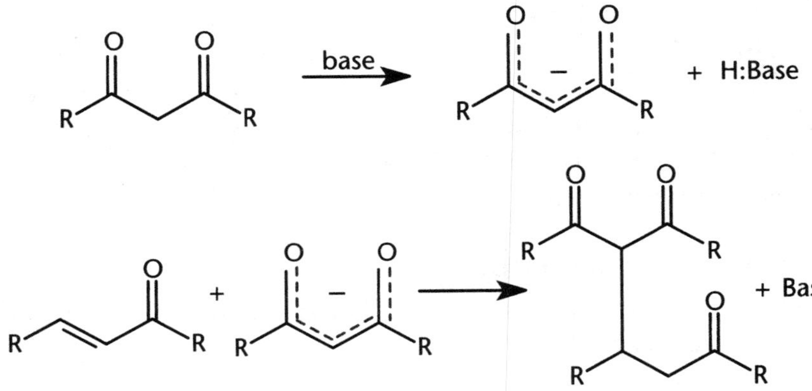
base
+ H:Base
+ Base

Figure 8.6

B. Addition Reactions

General Reaction Mechanism: Nucleophilic Addition to a Carbonyl

Many of the reactions of aldehydes and ketones share this general reaction mechanism. Rather than memorizing them all individually, focus on understanding the basic pattern. Then, you can learn how each reaction exemplifies it.

As shown in Figure 8.4, the C=O bond is polarized, with a partial positive charge on C and a partial negative charge on O. This makes the carbon ripe for nucleophilic attack.

REMEMBER

The carbonyl carbon is a good target for nucleophilic attack.

The nucleophile attacks, forming a bond to the C, which causes the pi bond in the C=O to break. This generates a tetrahedral intermediate. If no good leaving group is present, the double bond cannot re-form, and the final product is nearly identical to the intermediate, except that usually the O^- will accept a proton to become a hydroxyl (–OH).

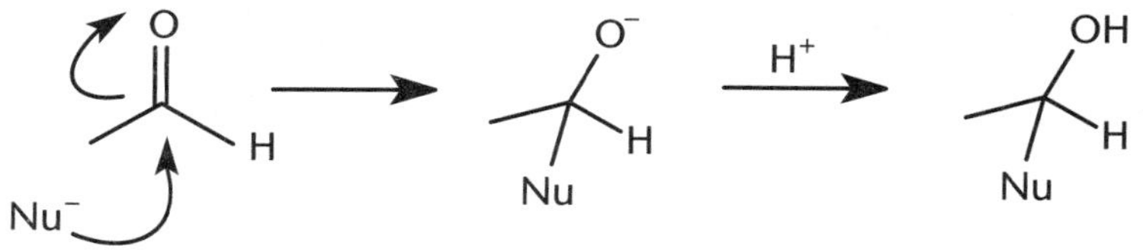

Figure 8.7

REMEMBER

When H_2O is the nucleophile, hydration occurs.

Although Figure 8.7 only shows nucleophilic addition to an aldehyde, this mechanism applies to ketones as well.

1. HYDRATION

In the presence of water, aldehydes and ketones react to form *gem* diols (1,1-diols). In this case, water acts as the nucleophile attacking at the carbonyl carbon. This hydration reaction proceeds slowly; the rate may be increased by the addition of a small amount of acid or base.

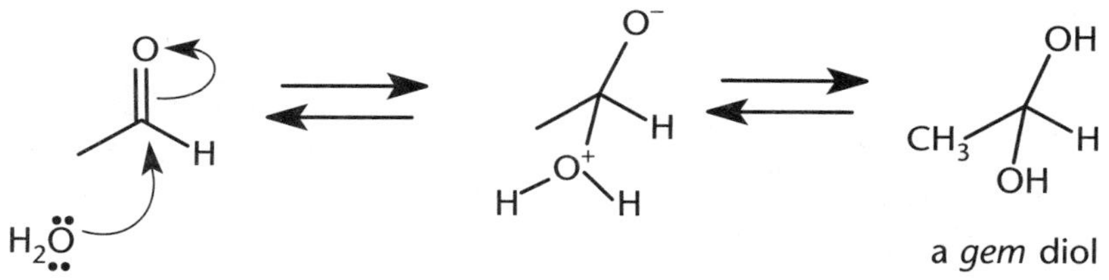

a *gem* diol

Figure 8.8

2. ACETAL AND KETAL FORMATION

A reaction similar to hydration occurs when aldehydes and ketones are treated with alcohols. When one equivalent of alcohol (the nucleophile in this reaction) is added to an aldehyde or ketone, the product is a **hemiacetal** or a **hemiketal,** respectively. When two equivalents of alcohol are added, the product is an **acetal** or a **ketal,** respectively. The reaction mechanism is the same as for hydration and is catalyzed by anhydrous acid. Acetals and ketals, which are comparatively inert, are frequently used as protecting groups for carbonyl functionalities. They can easily be converted back to the carbonyl with aqueous acid.

REMEMBER

When ROH is the nucleophile, hemiacetals (or hemiketals) and acetals (or ketals) are formed.

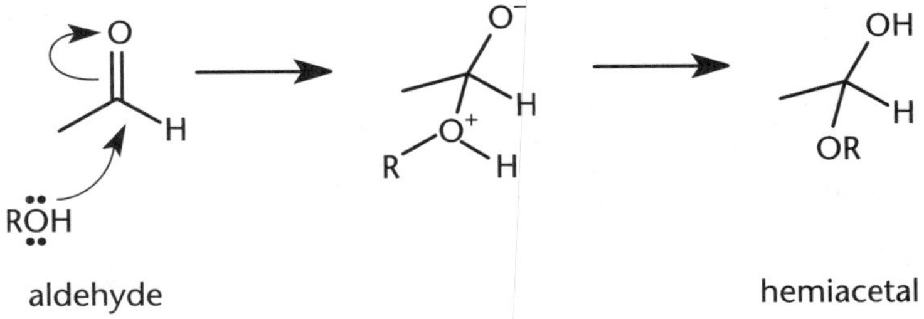

Figure 8.9

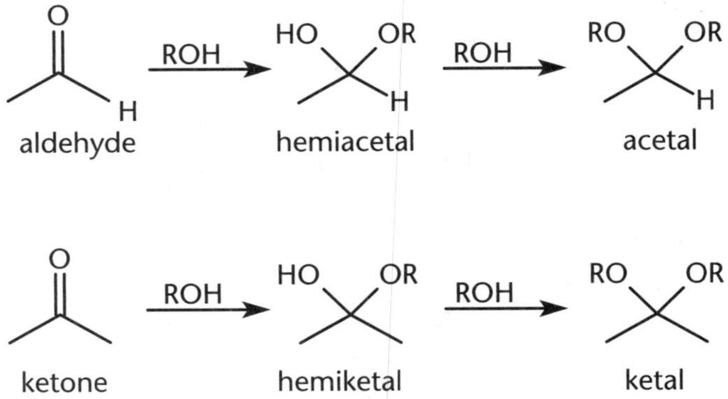

Figure 8.10

3. REACTION WITH HCN

> **REMEMBER**
>
> When CN^- is the nucleophile, cyanohydrins are formed.

Aldehydes and ketones react with HCN (hydrogen cyanide) to produce stable compounds called **cyanohydrins**. HCN dissociates and the nucleophilic cyanide anion attacks the carbonyl carbon atom. Protonation of the oxygen produces the cyanohydrin. The cyanohydrin gains its stability from the newly formed C–C bond. (In contrast, when a carbonyl reacts with HCl, a weak C–Cl bond is formed, and the resulting chlorohydrin is unstable.)

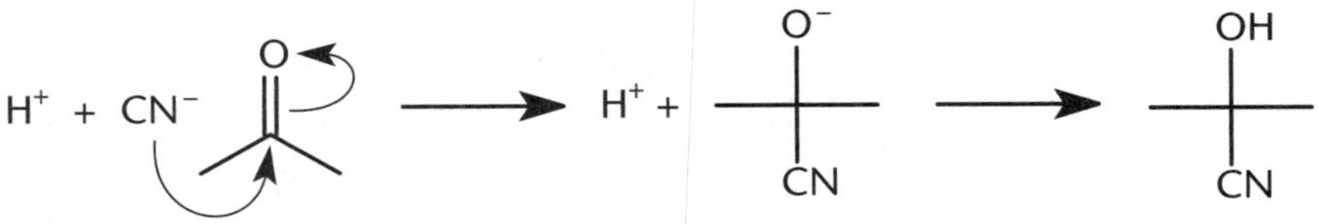

Figure 8.11

4. CONDENSATIONS WITH AMMONIA DERIVATIVES

Ammonia and some of its derivatives are nucleophiles and can add to carbonyl compounds. In the simplest case, ammonia adds to the carbon atom and water is lost, producing an **imine,** a compound with a nitrogen atom double-bonded to a carbon atom. (A reaction in which water is lost between two molecules is called a **condensation reaction.**)

In this case, the first part of the reaction follows the mechanism of nucleophilic addition described above. However, after formation of a tetrahedral intermediate, this reaction proceeds further: The C=O double bond reforms, and a leaving group is kicked off. This mechanism is called nucleophilic *substitution* on a carbonyl.

Some common ammonia derivatives that react with aldehydes and ketones are hydroxylamine (H_2NOH), hydrazine (H_2NNH_2), and semicarbazide ($H_2NNHCONH_2$); these form oximes, hydrazones, and semicarbazones, respectively.

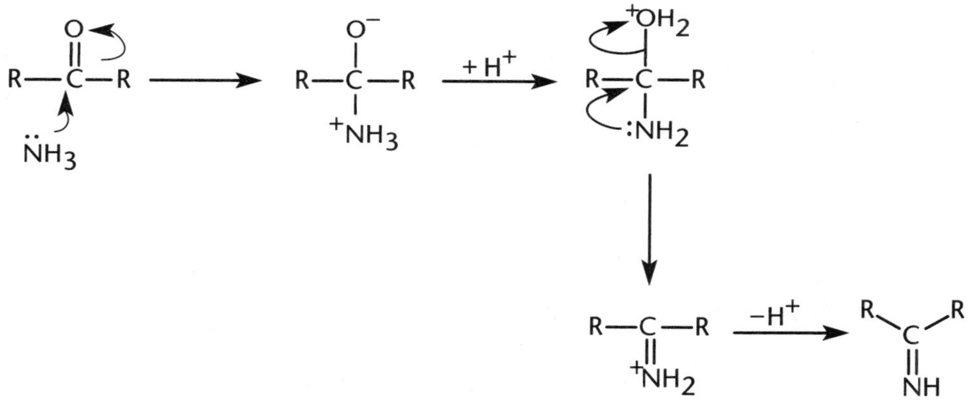

Figure 8.12

Don't worry too much about protons coming and going; there should be plenty in the solution, so you can transiently put them where needed to facilitate this reaction.

REMEMBER

Nitrogen-containing compounds can be nucleophiles too.

Examples of other potential nucleophiles and their respective products are shown in Figure 8.13.

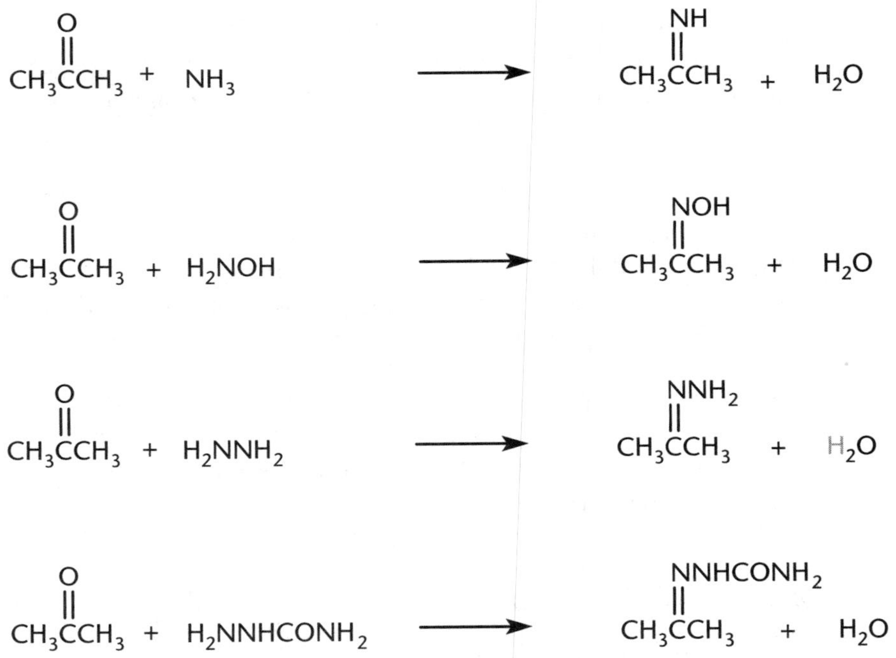

$$
\underset{\substack{O \\ \parallel \\ CH_3CCH_3}}{} + NH_3 \longrightarrow \underset{\substack{NH \\ \parallel \\ CH_3CCH_3}}{} + H_2O
$$

$$
\underset{\substack{O \\ \parallel \\ CH_3CCH_3}}{} + H_2NOH \longrightarrow \underset{\substack{NOH \\ \parallel \\ CH_3CCH_3}}{} + H_2O
$$

$$
\underset{\substack{O \\ \parallel \\ CH_3CCH_3}}{} + H_2NNH_2 \longrightarrow \underset{\substack{NNH_2 \\ \parallel \\ CH_3CCH_3}}{} + H_2O
$$

$$
\underset{\substack{O \\ \parallel \\ CH_3CCH_3}}{} + H_2NNHCONH_2 \longrightarrow \underset{\substack{NNHCONH_2 \\ \parallel \\ CH_3CCH_3}}{} + H_2O
$$

Figure 8.13

C. The Aldol Condensation

KEY CONCEPT

In the aldol condensation, aldehydes act as nucleophile and target (substrate).

The aldol condensation is an important reaction that basically follows the mechanism of nucleophilic addition to a carbonyl that was described above. In this case, an aldehyde acts both as nucleophile (enol form) and target (keto form.) When acetaldehyde (ethanal) is treated with base, an enolate ion is produced. This enolate ion, being nucleophilic, can react with the carbonyl group of another acetaldehyde molecule. The product is 3-hydroxybutanal, which contains both an alcohol and an aldehyde functionality. This type of compound is called an **aldol**, from **ald**ehyde and alcoh**ol**. With stronger base and higher temperatures, condensation occurs, producing an α,β-unsaturated aldehyde. This type of condensation reaction has become known as the **aldol condensation**.

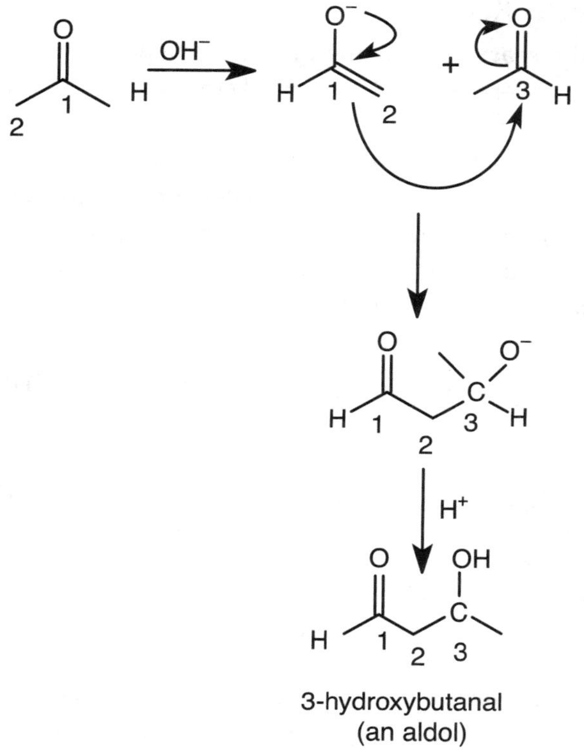

3-hydroxybutanal
(an aldol)

Figure 8.14a

When heated, this molecule can undergo elimination and lose H_2O to form a double bond, as shown in Figure 8.14b.

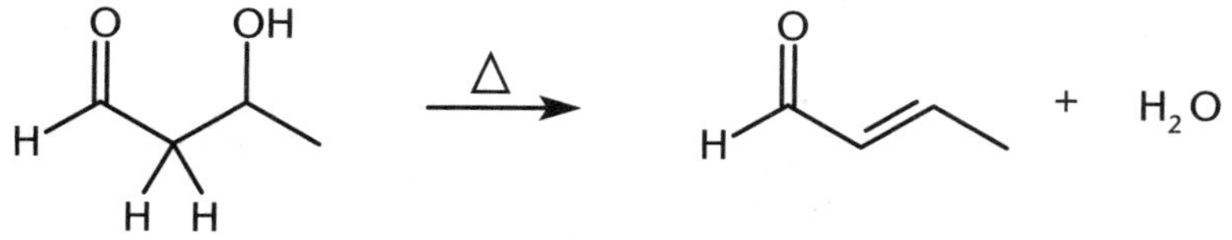

Figure 8.14b

The aldol condensation is most useful when only one type of aldehyde or ketone is present, since mixed condensations usually result in a mixture of products.

D. The Wittig Reaction

KEY CONCEPT

The Wittig reaction ultimately converts C=O to C=C.

The **Wittig reaction** is a method of forming carbon-carbon double bonds by converting aldehydes and ketones into alkenes. The first step involves the formation of a phosphonium salt from the S_N2 reaction of an alkyl halide with the nucleophile triphenylphosphine, $(C_6H_5)_3P$. The phosphonium salt is then deprotonated (losing the proton α to the phosphorus) with a strong base, yielding a neutral compound called an **ylide** (pronounced "ill-id") or **phosphorane**. (The phosphorus atom may be drawn as pentavalent, utilizing the low-lying 3*d* atomic orbitals.)

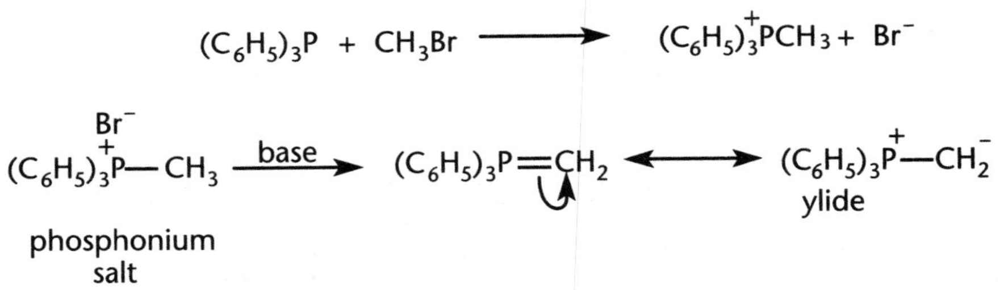

Figure 8.15

KEY CONCEPT

The ylide can act as a nucleophile and attack the carbonyl.

Notice that an ylide is a type of carbanion and has nucleophilic properties. When combined with an aldehyde or ketone, an ylide attacks the carbonyl carbon, giving an intermediate called a **betaine**, which forms a four- membered ring intermediate called an oxaphosphetane. This decomposes to yield an alkene and triphenylphosphine oxide.

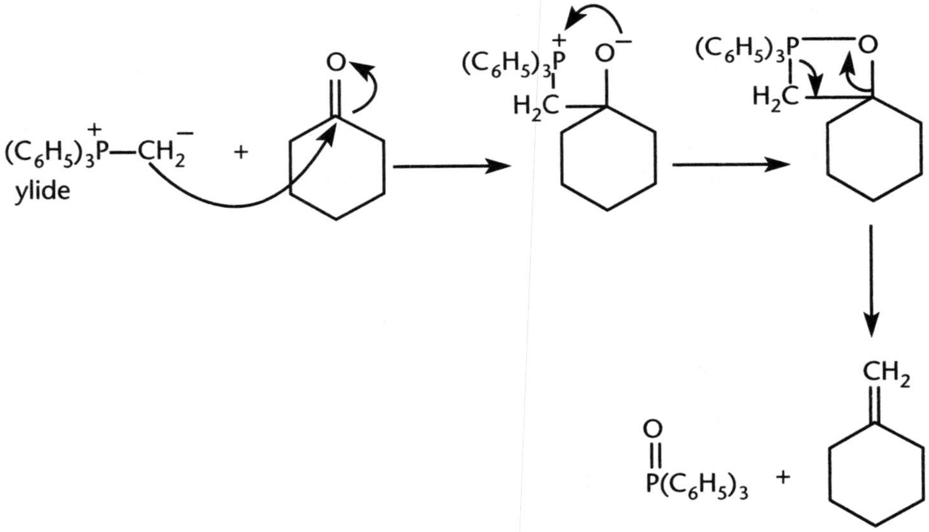

Figure 8.16

The decomposition reaction is driven by the strength of the phosphorus-oxygen bond that is formed.

E. Oxidation and Reduction

Aldehydes and ketones occupy the middle of the oxidation-reduction continuum. They are more oxidized than alcohols but less oxidized than carboxylic acids.

Aldehydes can be oxidized with a number of different reagents, such as $KMnO_4$, CrO_3, Ag_2O, or H_2O_2. The product of oxidation is a carboxylic acid.

$$CH_3\overset{O}{\overset{\|}{C}}H \xrightarrow[\text{or } Ag_2O]{\substack{KMnO_4, \\ CrO_3,}} CH_3\overset{O}{\overset{\|}{C}}-OH$$

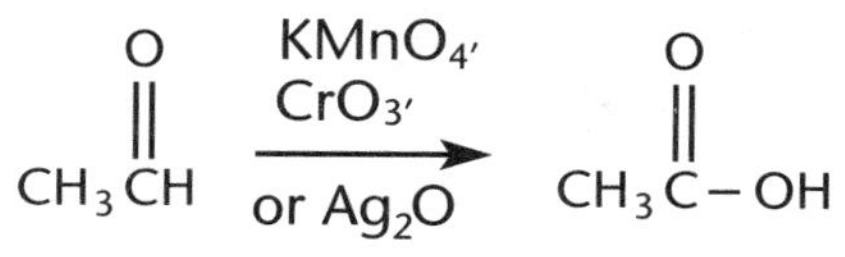

Figure 8.17

A number of reagents will reduce aldehydes and ketones to alcohols. The most common is lithium aluminum hydride (LAH); sodium borohydride ($NaBH_4$) is often used when milder conditions are needed.

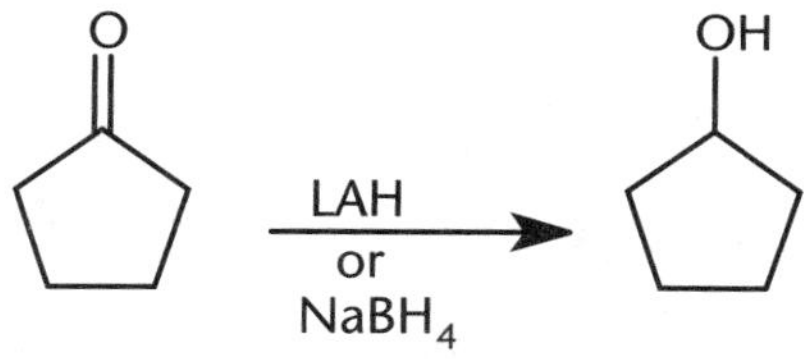

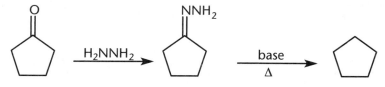

Figure 8.18

Aldehydes and ketones can be completely reduced to alkanes by two common methods. In the **Wolff-Kishner** reduction (see Figure 8.19), the carbonyl is first converted to a hydrazone, which releases molecular nitrogen (N_2) when heated and forms an alkane (the protons being abstracted from the solvent). The Wolff-Kishner reaction is performed in basic solution and, therefore, is only useful when the product is stable under basic conditions.

Figure 8.19

An alternative reduction not subject to this restriction is the **Clemmensen reduction** (see Figure 8.20), where an aldehyde or ketone is heated with amalgamated zinc in hydrochloric acid.

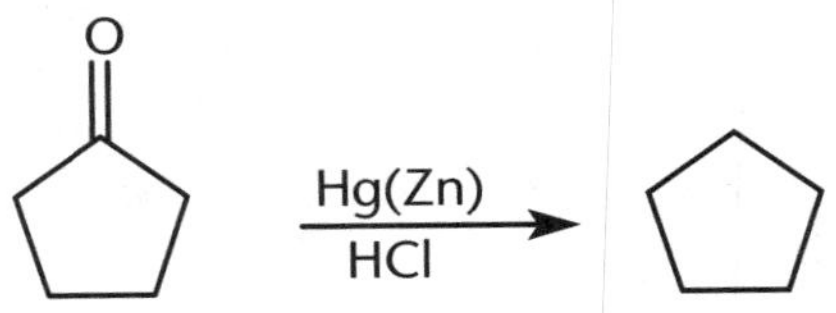

Figure 8.20

9

Carboxylic Acids

Carboxylic acids are compounds that contain hydroxyl groups attached to carbonyl groups. This functionality is known as a **carboxyl group**. The hydroxyl hydrogen atoms are acidic, with pK_a values in the general range of 3 to 6. Carboxylic acids occur widely in nature and are synthesized by all living organisms.

NOMENCLATURE

In the IUPAC system of nomenclature, carboxylic acids are named by adding the suffix **-oic acid** to the alkyl root. The chain is numbered so that the carboxyl group receives the lowest possible number. Additional substituents are named in the usual fashion.

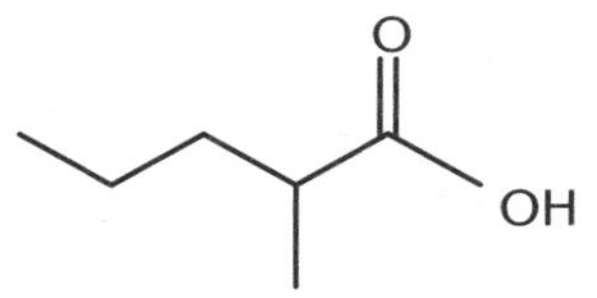

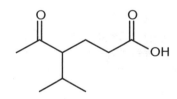

2-methylpentanoic acid   4-isopropyl-5-oxohexanoic acid

Figure 9.1

REMEMBER

This is a very high priority group! It determines C1 of the carbon backbone, as well as the suffix (-oic acid).

Carboxylic acids were among the first organic compounds discovered. Their original names continue today in the common system of nomenclature. For example, formic acid (from Latin *formica*, meaning ant) was found in ants and butyric acid (from Latin *butyrum*, meaning butter) in rancid butter. The common and IUPAC names of the first three carboxylic acids are listed in Figure 9.2.

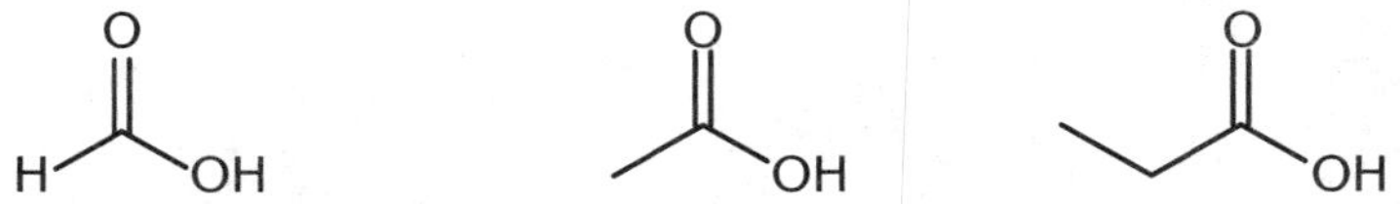

methanoic acid (formic acid) | ethanoic acid (acetic acid) | propanoic acid (propionic acid)

Figure 9.2

REMEMBER

Salts have the suffix *-ate* (e.g., sodium hexanoate).

Cyclic carboxylic acids are usually named as cycloalkane carboxylic acids. The carbon atom to which the carboxyl group is attached is numbered 1. Salts of carboxylic acids are named beginning with the cation, followed by the name of the acid with the ending **-ate** replacing **-ic acid**. Typical examples are shown in Figure 9.3.

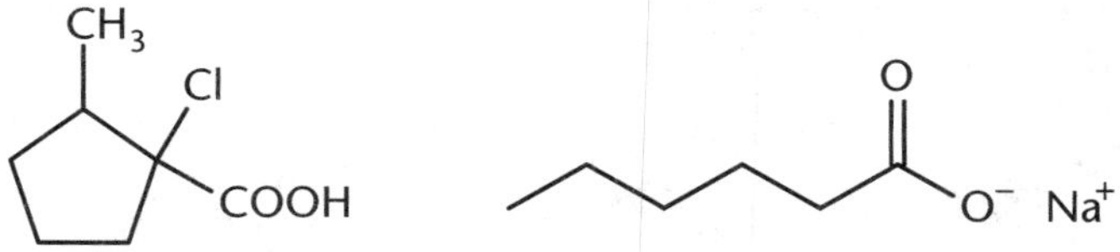

1-chloro-2-methylcyclo-pentane carboxylic acid | sodium hexanoate

Figure 9.3

Dicarboxylic acids—compounds with two carboxyl groups—are common in biological systems. The first six straight-chain terminal dicarboxylic acids are oxalic, malonic, succinic, glutaric, adipic, and pimelic acids. Their IUPAC names are ethanedioic acid, propanedioic acid, butanedioic acid, pentanedioic acid, hexanedioic acid, and heptanedioic acid.

PHYSICAL PROPERTIES

A. Hydrogen Bonding

Carboxylic acids are polar and can form hydrogen bonds. As a result, carboxylic acids can form dimers: pairs of molecules connected by hydrogen bonds. The boiling points of carboxylic acids are, therefore, even higher than those of the corresponding alcohols. The boiling points follow the usual trend of increasing with molecular weight.

B. Acidity

The acidity of carboxylic acids is due to the resonance stabilization of the carboxylate anion (the conjugate base). When the hydroxyl proton dissociates from the acid, the negative charge left on the carboxylate group is delocalized between the two oxygen atoms.

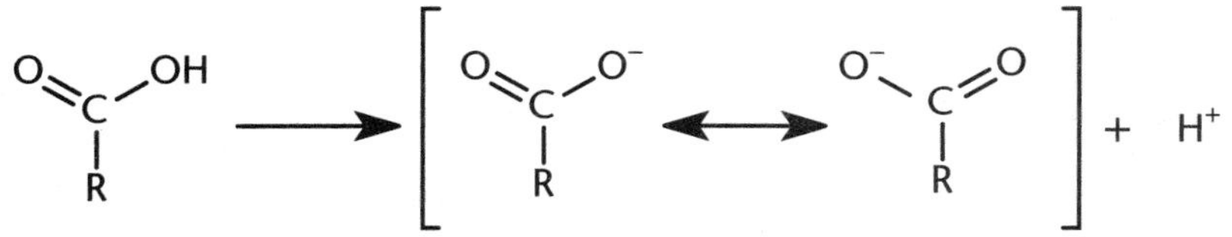

Figure 9.4

Substituents on carbon atoms adjacent to a carboxyl group can influence acidity. Electron-withdrawing groups, such as –Cl or –NO$_2$, further delocalize the negative charge and increase acidity. Electron-donating groups, such as –NH$_2$ or –OCH$_3$, destabilize the negative charge, making the compound less acidic.

In dicarboxylic acids, one –COOH group (which is electron withdrawing) influences the other, making the compound more acidic than the analogous monocarboxylic acid. The second carboxyl group is then influenced by the carboxylate anion. Ionization of the second group will create a doubly charged species in which the two negative charges repel each other. Since this is unfavorable, the second proton is less acidic than that of a monocarboxylic acid.

β-dicarboxylic acids are notable for the high acidity of the α-hydrogens located between the two carboxyl groups (pK$_a$ ~ 10). Loss of this acidic hydrogen atom produces a carbanion that is stabilized by the electron-withdrawing effect of the two carboxyl groups (the same effect seen in β-ketoacids, RC=OCH$_2$ COOH).

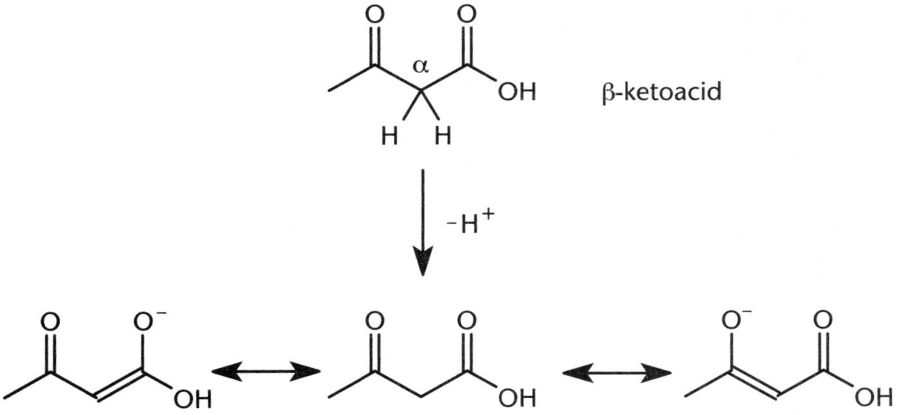

Figure 9.5

Similarly, the β-dicarboxylic acid also has acidic α hydrogens.

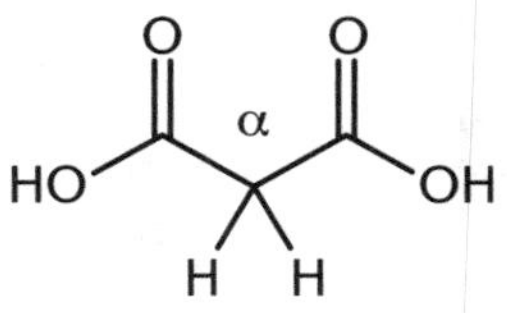

Figure 9.6

SYNTHESIS

A. Oxidation Reactions

Carboxylic acids can be prepared via oxidation of aldehydes, primary alcohols, and certain alkylbenzenes. The oxidant is usually potassium permanganate, $KMnO_4$. Note that secondary and tertiary alcohols cannot be oxidized to carboxylic acids because of valence limitations.

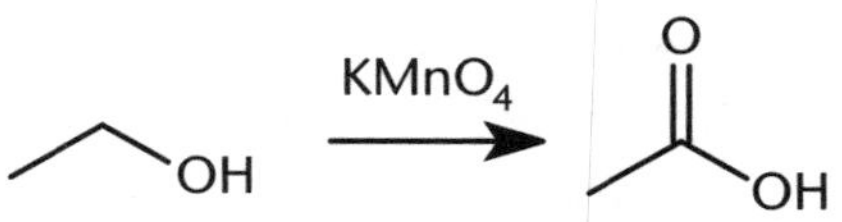

Figure 9.7

B. Carbonation of Organometallic Reagents

Organometallic reagents, such as Grignard reagents, react with carbon dioxide (CO_2) to form carboxylic acids. This reaction is useful for the conversion of tertiary alkyl halides into carboxylic acids, which cannot be accomplished through other methods. Note that this reaction adds one carbon atom to the chain.

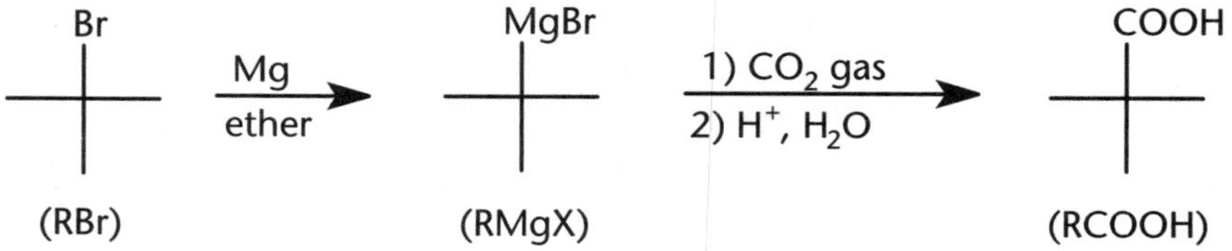

Figure 9.8

C. Hydrolysis of Nitriles

REMEMBER

Both carbonation and hydrolysis *increase* the chain length by one carbon.

Nitriles, also called cyanides, are compounds containing the functional group –CN. The cyanide anion CN^- is a good nucleophile and will displace primary and secondary halides in typical S_N2 fashion.

Nitriles can be hydrolyzed under either acidic or basic conditions. The products are carboxylic acids and ammonia (or ammonium salts).

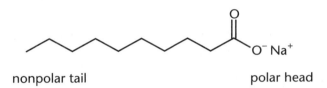

Figure 9.9

This allows for the conversion of alkyl halides into carboxylic acids. As in the carbonation reaction, an additional carbon atom is introduced. For instance, if the desired product is acetic acid, a possible starting material would be methyl iodide.

REACTIONS

A. Soap Formation

When long-chain carboxylic acids react with sodium or potassium hydroxide, they form salts. These salts, called soaps, are able to solubilize nonpolar organic compounds in aqueous solutions because they possess both a nonpolar "tail" and a polar carboxylate "head," as shown in Figure 9.10.

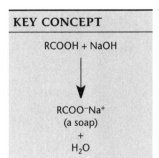

nonpolar tail   polar head

Figure 9.10

When placed in aqueous solution, soap molecules arrange themselves into spherical structures called **micelles**. The polar heads face outward, where they can be solvated by water molecules, and the nonpolar hydrocarbon chains are inside the sphere, protected from the solvent. Nonpolar molecules, such as grease, can dissolve in the hydrocarbon interior of the spherical micelle, while the micelle as a whole is soluble in water because of its polar shell (see Figure 9.11).

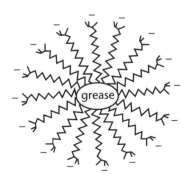

Figure 9.11

B. Nucleophilic Substitution

Many of the reactions that carboxylic acids (and their derivatives) participate in can be described by a single mechanism: nucleophilic substitution.
This mechanism is very similar to nucleophilic addition to a carbonyl,
shown in the preceding chapter. The key difference: Nucleophilic substitution concludes with re-formation of the C=O double bond and elimination
of a leaving group.

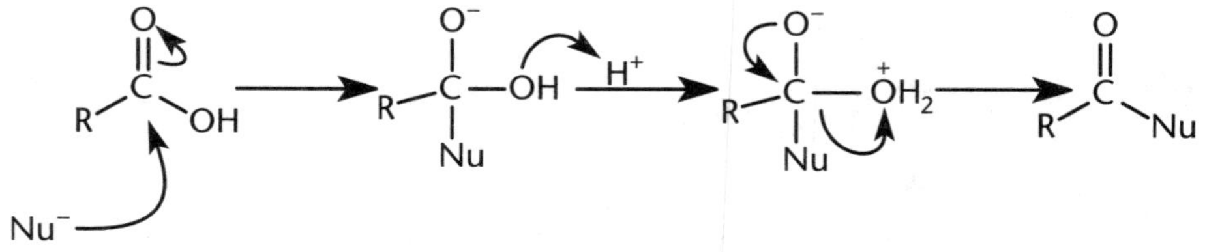

Figure 9.12

1. REDUCTION

Carboxylic acids occupy the most oxidized side of the oxidation-
reduction continuum. Carboxylic acids are reduced with lithium
aluminum hydride (LAH) to the corresponding alcohols. Aldehyde
intermediates that may be formed in the course of the reaction are
also reduced to the alcohol. The reaction occurs by nucleophilic addition of hydride to the carbonyl group.

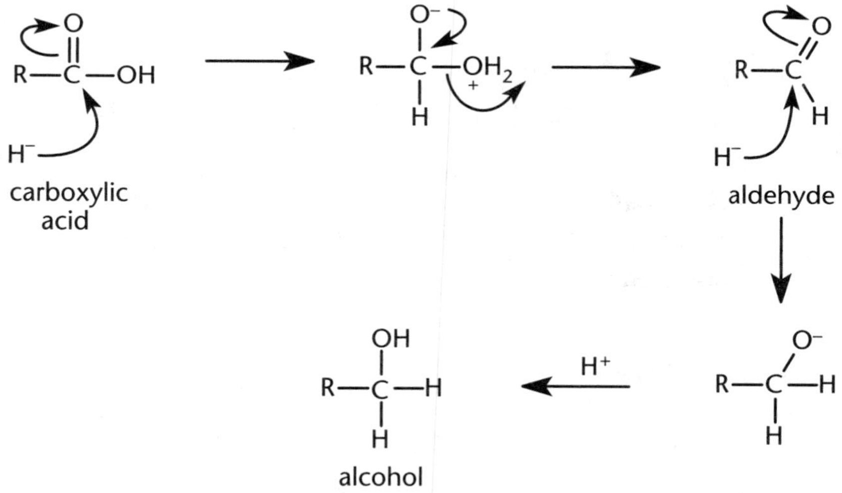

Figure 9.13

2. ESTER FORMATION

Carboxylic acids react with alcohols under acidic conditions to form esters and water. In acidic solution, the O on the C=O can become protonated. This accentuates the polarity of the bond, putting even more positive charge on the C and making it even more susceptible to nucleophilic attack. This condensation reaction occurs most rapidly with primary alcohols.

KEY CONCEPT

Protonating the C=O makes the C even more ripe for nucleophilic attack.

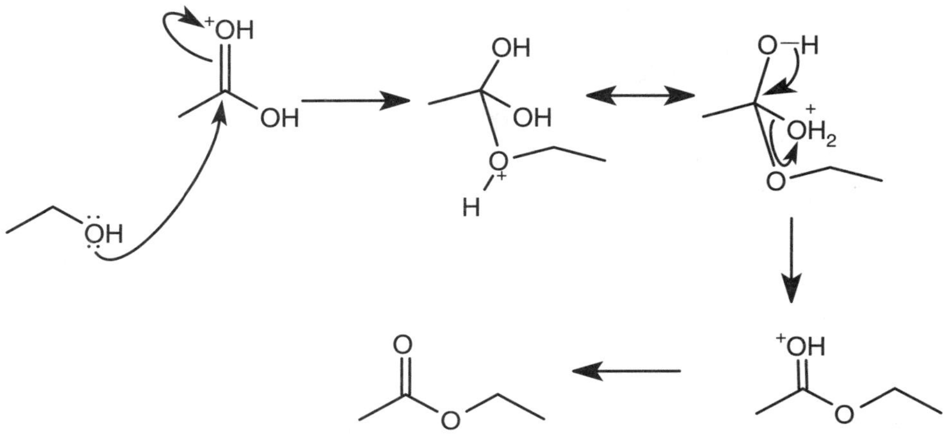

Figure 9.14

3. ACYL HALIDE FORMATION

Acyl halides, also called acid halides, are compounds with carbonyl groups bonded to halides. Several reagents can accomplish this transformation; *thionyl chloride*, $SOCl_2$, is the most common.

REMEMBER

Acid chlorides are among the highest-energy (least stable and most reactive) members of the carbonyl family.

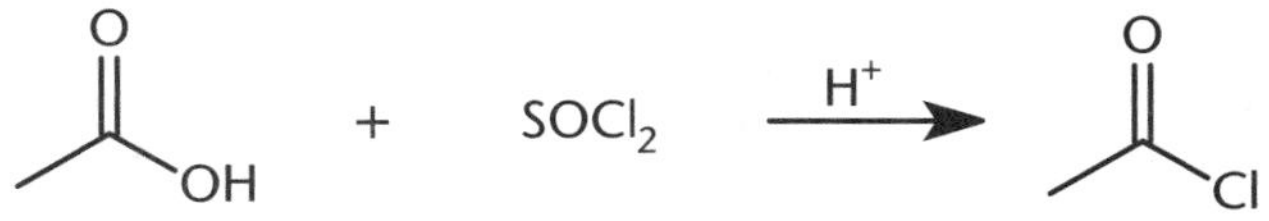

Figure 9.15

Acid chlorides are very reactive, as the greater electron-withdrawing power of the Cl^- makes the carbonyl carbon more susceptible to nucleophilic attack than the carbonyl carbon of a carboxylic acid. Thus, acid chlorides are frequently used as intermediates in the conversion of carboxylic acids to esters and amides.

C. Decarboxylation

Carboxylic acids can undergo decarboxylation reactions, resulting in the loss of carbon dioxide.

1,3-dicarboxylic acids and other β-keto acids may spontaneously decarboxylate when heated. The carboxyl group is lost and replaced with a hydrogen. The reaction proceeds through a six-membered ring transition state. The enol initially formed tautomerizes to the more stable keto form (see Figure 9.16).

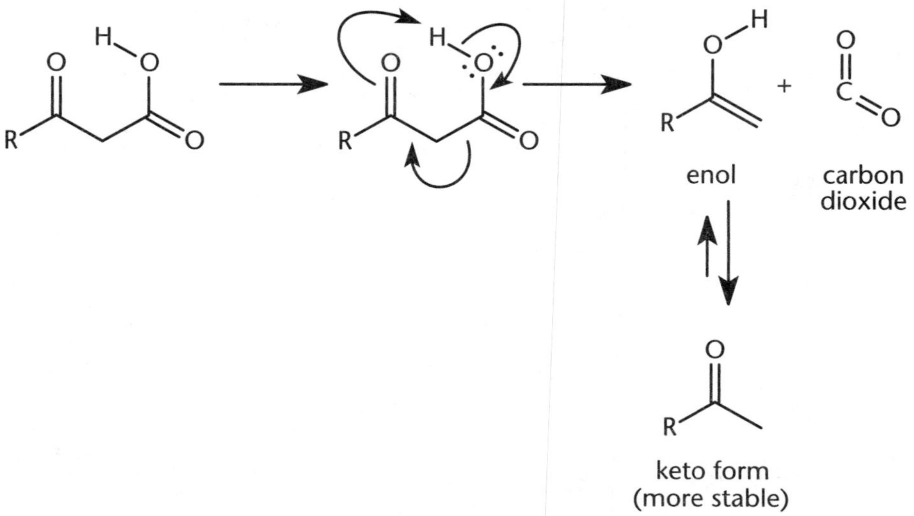

enol   carbon dioxide

keto form
(more stable)

Figure 9.16

10

Carboxylic Acid Derivatives

Carboxylic acids can be converted into several types of derivatives: **acyl halides, anhydrides, amides,** and **esters**. These are compounds in which the **–OH** of the carboxyl group has been replaced with **–X, –OCOR, –NH$_2$,** or **–OR,** respectively. They readily undergo nucleophilic substitution reactions, including hydrolysis (H_2O as nucleophile), which produces the original carboxylic acid. They also undergo other additions and substitutions, including various interconversions between different acid derivatives. In general, the acyl halides are the most reactive of the carboxylic acid derivatives, followed by the anhydrides, the esters, and the amides.

REMEMBER

Order of reactivity:
acyl halides > anhydrides > esters > amides.

ACYL HALIDES

A. Nomenclature

Acyl halides are also called **acid** or **alkanoyl halides**. (The acyl group is RCO–.) They are the most reactive of the carboxylic acid derivatives. They are named in the IUPAC system by changing the *-ic acid* ending of the carboxylic acid to **-yl halide**. Some typical examples are ethanoyl chloride (also called acetyl chloride), benzoyl chloride, and *n*-butanoyl bromide.

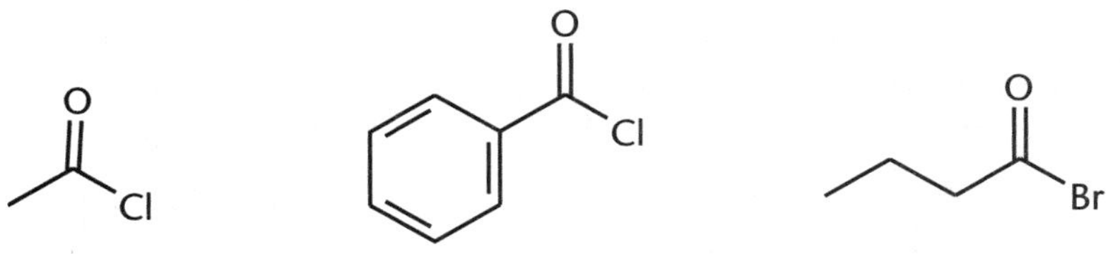

ethanoyl chloride (acetyl chloride) | benzoyl chloride | *n*-butanoyl bromide

Figure 10.1

REMEMBER

The most common acyl halide is acyl chloride, made with RCOOH + $SOCl_2$.

B. Synthesis

The most common acyl halides are the acid chlorides, although acid bromides and iodides are occasionally encountered. They are prepared by reaction of the carboxylic acid with thionyl chloride, $SOCl_2$, producing SO_2 and HCl as side products. Alternatively, PCl_3 or PCl_5 (or PBr_3, to make an acid bromide) will accomplish the same transformation.

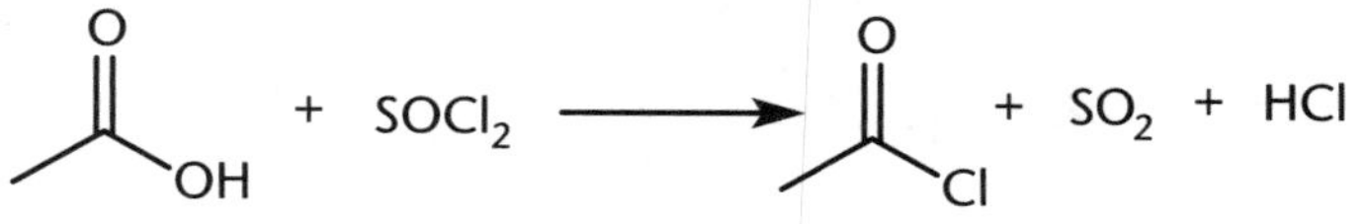

Figure 10.2

REMEMBER

Hydrolysis = hydro + lysis, or cleavage by water.

C. Reactions: Nucleophilic Acyl Substitution

The following reactions of acyl halides proceed via the mechanism of nucleophilic substitution on a carbonyl.

1. HYDROLYSIS

KEY CONCEPT

1. Hydrolysis regenerates the carboxylic acid.
2. All carboxylic acid derivatives are susceptible to hydrolysis.

The simplest reaction of acid halides is their conversion back to carboxylic acids. They react very rapidly with water to form the corresponding acid, along with HCl, which is responsible for their irritating odor.

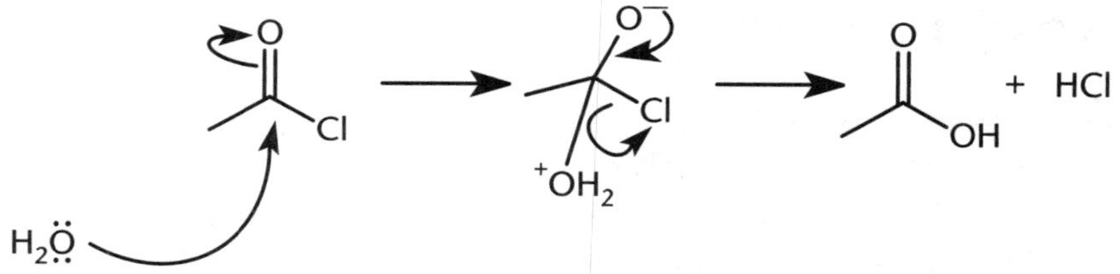

Figure 10.3

2. CONVERSION INTO ESTERS

Acyl halides can be converted into esters by reaction with alcohols. The same type of nucleophilic attack found in hydrolysis leads to the formation of a tetrahedral intermediate, with the hydroxyl oxygen as the nucleophile. Chloride is displaced, and HCl is released as the side-product.

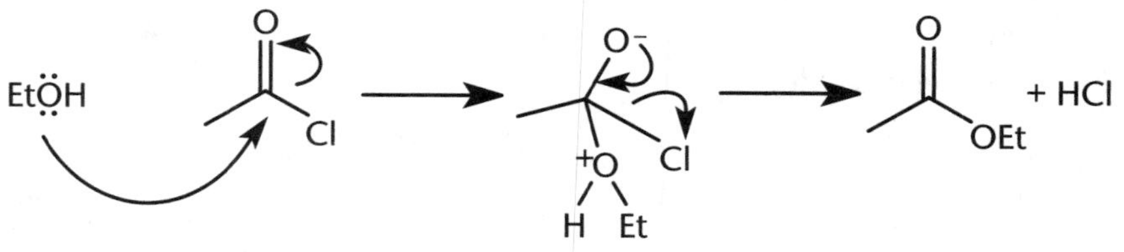

Figure 10.4

3. CONVERSION INTO AMIDES

Acyl halides can be converted into amides (compounds of the general formula $RCONR_2$) by an analogous reaction with amines. Nucleophilic amines, such as ammonia, attack the carbonyl group, displacing chloride. The side product is ammonium chloride, formed from excess ammonia and HCl.

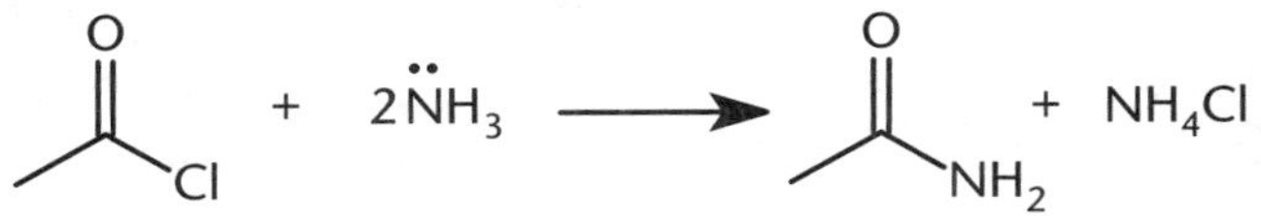

Figure 10.5

D. Other Reactions

1. FRIEDEL-CRAFTS ACYLATION

Aromatic rings can be acylated in a Friedel-Crafts reaction. The mechanism is electrophilic aromatic substitution, and the attacking reagent is an acylium ion, formed by reaction of an acid chloride with $AlCl_3$ or another Lewis acid. The product is an alkyl aryl ketone.

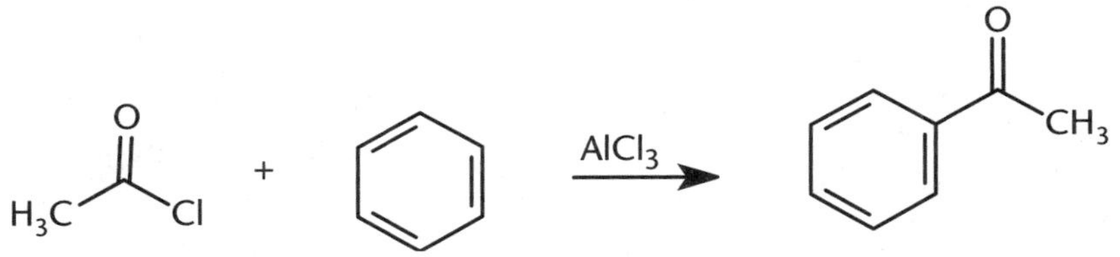

Figure 10.6

2. REDUCTION

Acid halides can be reduced to alcohols or selectively reduced to the intermediate aldehydes. Catalytic hydrogenation in the presence of a "poison" like quinoline accomplishes the latter transformation. (Compare with Lindlar's catalyst.)

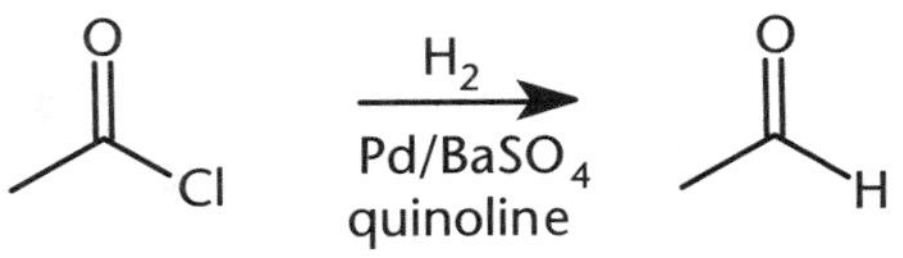

Figure 10.7

ANHYDRIDES

A. Nomenclature

KEY CONCEPT

Anhydride means "without water." Anhydrides are formed by two acid molecules condensing (losing water).

Anhydrides, also called **acid anhydrides**, are the condensation dimers of carboxylic acids with the general formula RCOOCOR. They are named by substituting the word **anhydride** for the word *acid* in an alkanoic acid. The most common and important anhydride is acetic anhydride, the dimer of acetic acid. Other common anhydrides, such as succinic, maleic, and phthalic anhydrides, are **cyclic anhydrides** arising from intramolecular condensation or dehydration of diacids (Figure 10.9).

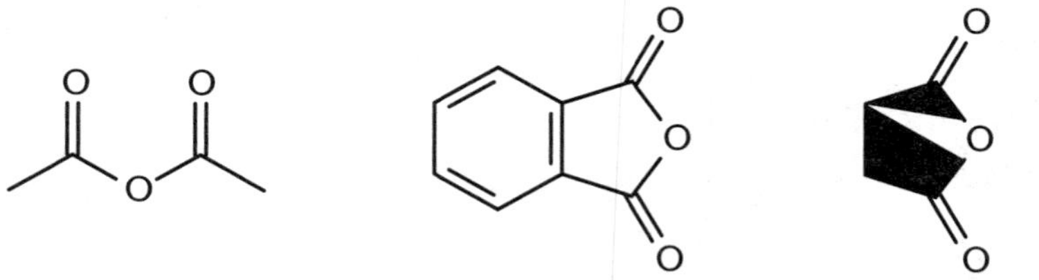

acetic anhydride (ethanoic anhydride) phthalic anhydride succinic anhydride

Figure 10.8

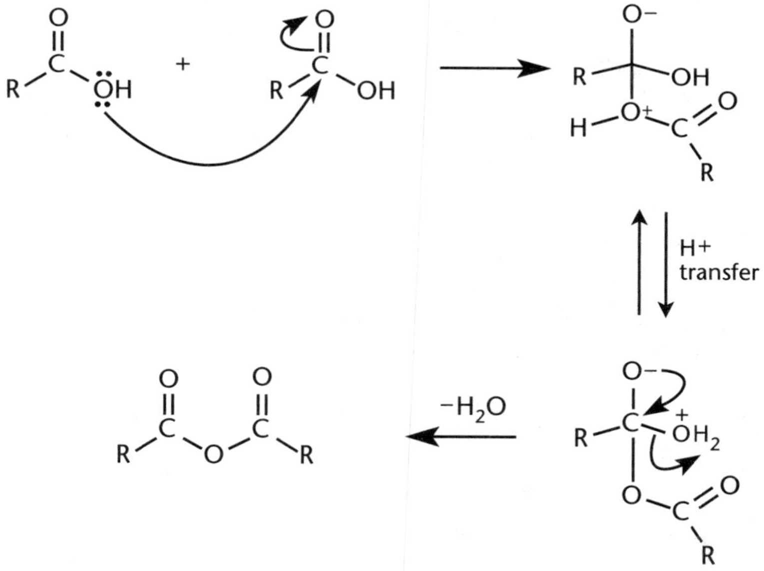

Figure 10.9. Condensation of Two Carboxylic Acid Molecules to Form an Anhydride

B. Synthesis

Anhydrides can be synthesized by reaction of an acid chloride with a carboxylate salt.

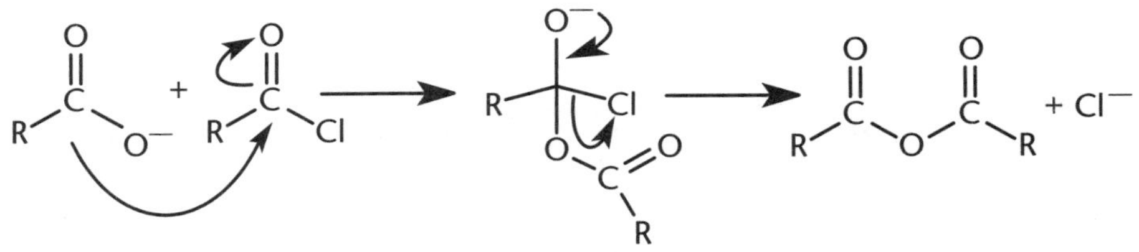

**Figure 10.10. Reaction of Acid Chloride
with Carboxylate Anion to Form an Anhydride**

Certain cyclic anhydrides can be formed simply by heating carboxylic acids. The reaction is driven by the increased stability of the newly formed ring; hence, only five- and six-membered ring anhydrides are easily made. In this case, the hydroxyl of one –COOH moiety acts as a nucleophile, attacking the carbonyl on the other –COOH moiety.

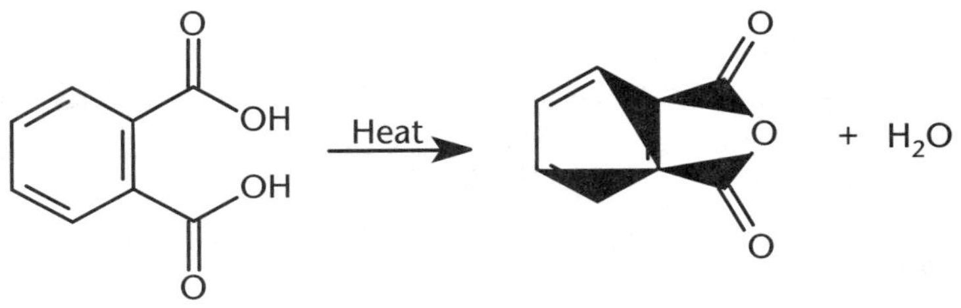

o-phtalic acid   phthalic anhydride

Figure 10.11

C. Reactions

Anhydrides react under the same conditions as acid chlorides, but since they are somewhat more stable, they are a bit less reactive. The reactions are slower and produce a carboxylic acid as the side product instead of HCl. Cyclic anhydrides are also subject to these reactions, which cause ring opening at the anhydride group along with formation of the new functional groups.

1. HYDROLYSIS

Anhydrides are converted into carboxylic acids when exposed to water. Note that in the reaction shown in Figure 10.12, the leaving group is actually a carboxylic acid.

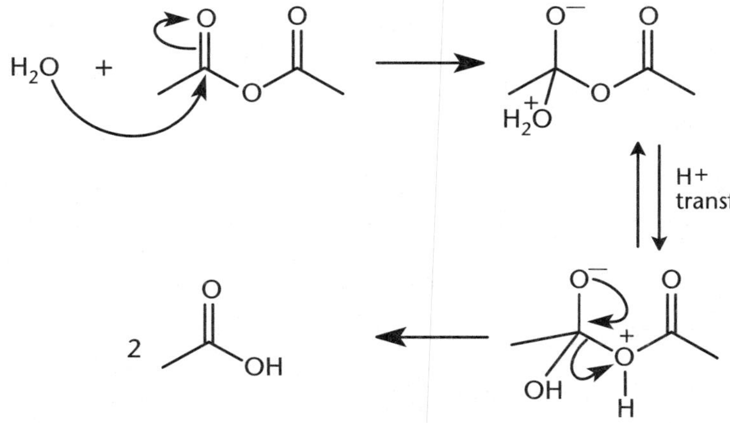

Figure 10.12

2. CONVERSION INTO AMIDES

Anhydrides are cleaved by ammonia, producing amides and ammonium carboxylates. Thus, as shown in Figure 10.13, even though the leaving group is actually a carboxylic acid, the final products are an amide and the ammonium salt of a carboxylate anion.

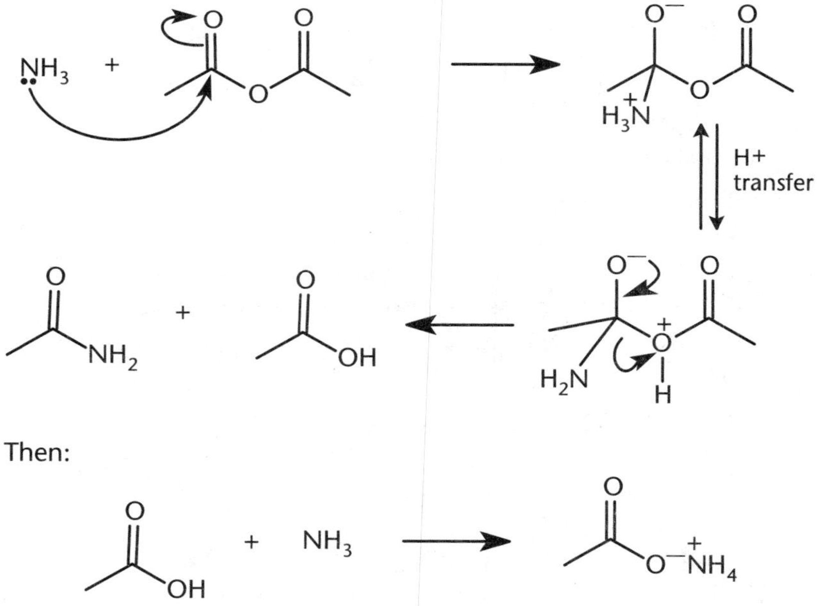

Then:

Figure 10.13

3. **CONVERSION INTO ESTERS AND CARBOXYLIC ACIDS**

Anhydrides react with alcohols to form esters and carboxylic acids.

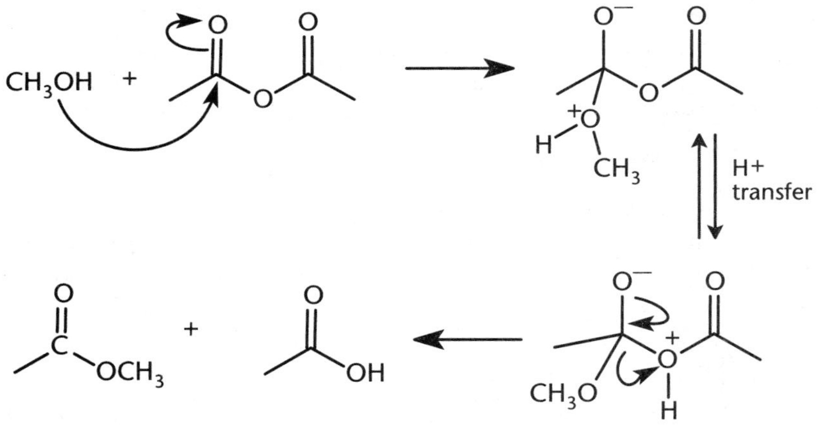

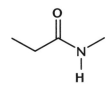

Figure 10.14

4. **ACYLATION**

Friedel-Crafts acylation occurs readily with $AlCl_3$ or other Lewis acid catalysts.

REMEMBER

This reaction proceeds via electrophilic aromatic substitution.

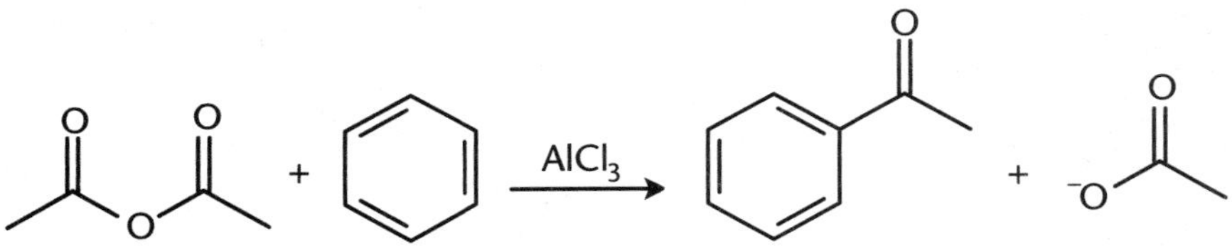

Figure 10.15

AMIDES

A. Nomenclature

Amides are compounds with the general formula $RCONR_2$. They are named by replacing the *-oic* acid ending with **-amide**. Alkyl substituents on the nitrogen atom are listed as prefixes, and their location is specified with the letter *N*, as in the example in Figure 10.16.

BRIDGE

The peptide bond is actually an amide linkage.

N-methylpropanamide

Figure 10.16

B. Synthesis

Amides are generally synthesized by the reaction of acid chlorides with amines or by the reaction of acid anhydrides with ammonia (see above). Note that loss of hydrogen is required; thus, only primary and secondary amines will undergo this reaction.

C. Reactions

1. HYDROLYSIS

Amides can be hydrolyzed under acidic conditions, via nucleophilic substitution, to produce carboxylic acids or basic conditions to form carboxylates, as shown in Figure 10.17.

> **KEY CONCEPT**
>
> Under acidic conditions, the carbonyl oxygen becomes protonated, making the carbon more susceptible to nucleophilic attack.

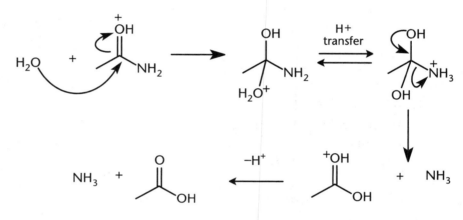

Figure 10.17

2. HOFMANN REARRANGEMENT

> **KEY CONCEPT**
>
> Hofmann rearrangement:
>
> amides
>
> ↓
>
> primary amines
> (with loss of a carbon)

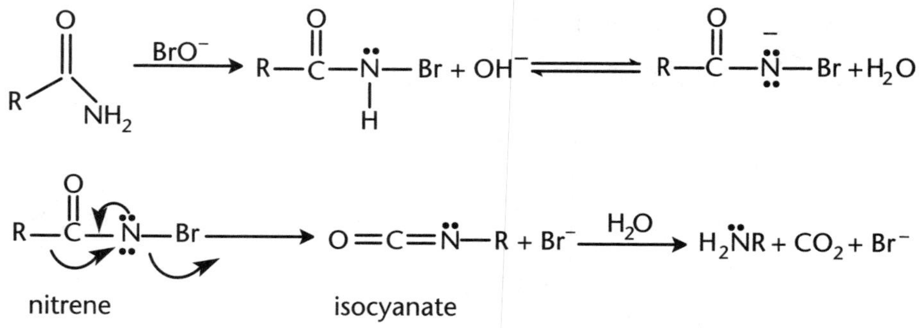

The **Hofmann rearrangement** converts amides to primary amines with the loss of the carbonyl carbon. The mechanism involves the formation of a **nitrene**, the nitrogen analog of a carbene. The nitrene is attached to the carbonyl group and rearranges to form an **isocyanate**, which under the reaction condition is hydrolyzed to the amine.

Figure 10.18

3. REDUCTION

Amides can be reduced with LAH to the corresponding amine. Notice in Figure 10.19 that this differs from the product of the Hofmann rearrangement in that no carbon atom is lost.

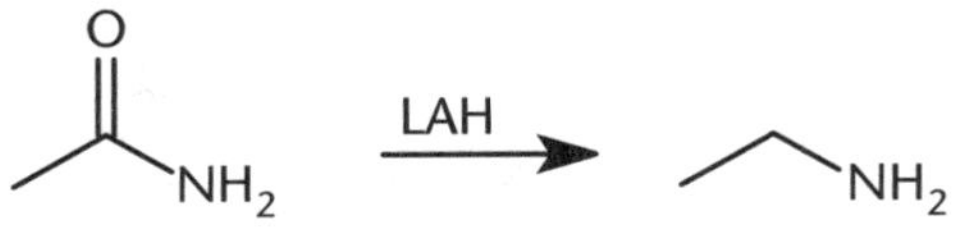

Figure 10.19

ESTERS

A. Nomenclature

Esters are the dehydration products of carboxylic acids and alcohols. They are commonly found in many fruits and perfumes. They are named in the IUPAC system as **alkyl** or **aryl alkanoates**. For example, ethyl acetate, derived from the condensation of acetic acid and ethanol, is called ethyl ethanoate according to IUPAC nomenclature.

B. Synthesis

Mixtures of carboxylic acids and alcohols will condense into esters, liberating water, under acidic conditions. Esters can also be obtained from reaction of acid chlorides or anhydrides with alcohols (see above). Phenolic (aromatic) esters are produced in the same way, although the aromatic acid chlorides are less reactive than aliphatic acid chlorides so that base must generally be added as a catalyst.

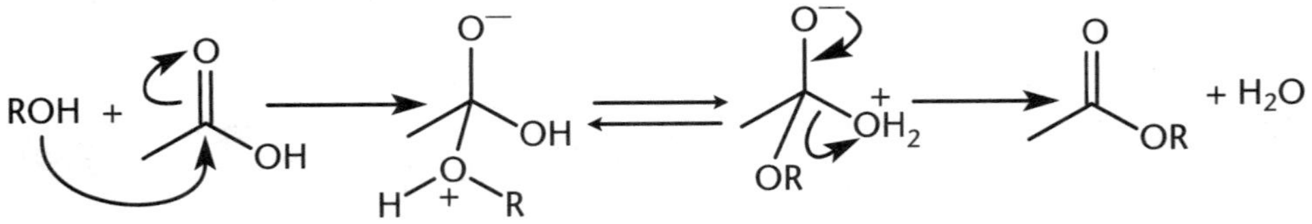

Figure 10.20

527

C. Reactions

1. HYDROLYSIS

Esters, like the other derivatives of carboxylic acids, can be hydrolyzed, yielding carboxylic acids and alcohols. Hydrolysis can take place under either acidic or basic conditions. Figure 10.21 shows this reaction under acidic conditions.

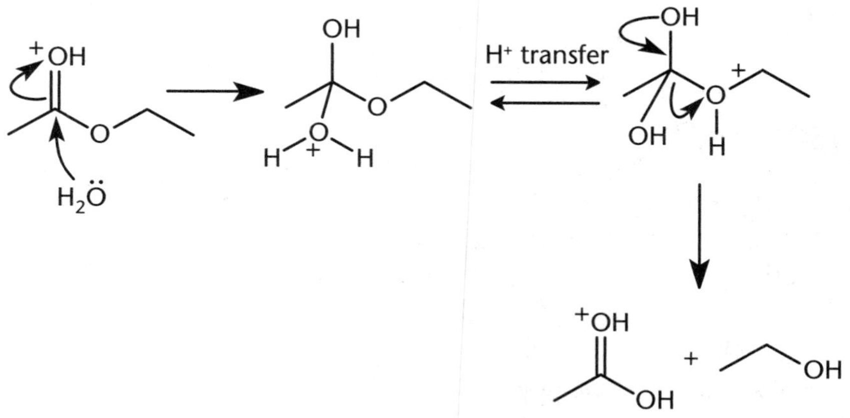

Figure 10.21

The reaction proceeds similarly under basic conditions, except that the oxygen on the C=O is not protonated, and the nucleophile is OH⁻.

Triacylglycerols, also called fats, are esters of long-chain carboxylic acids, often called fatty acids, and glycerol (1,2,3-propanetriol). **Saponification** is the process whereby fats are hydrolyzed under basic conditions to produce soaps. (Note: Acidification of the soap retrieves triacylglycerol.)

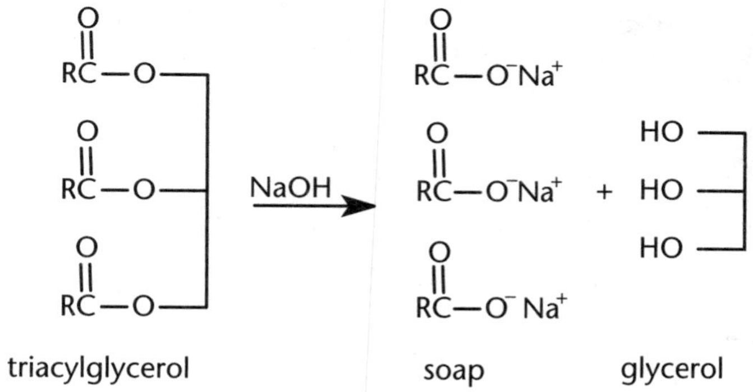

<table>
<tr><td>

BRIDGE

Triacylglycerols are actually esters, with glycerol as the alcohol (ROH) and free fatty acids as RCOOH.

</td></tr>
</table>

triacylglycerol   soap   glycerol

Figure 10.22

2. CONVERSION INTO AMIDES

Nitrogen bases, such as ammonia, will attack the electron-deficient carbonyl carbon atom, displacing alkoxide to yield an amide and an alcohol side-product. In Figure 10.23, ammonia is the nucleophile.

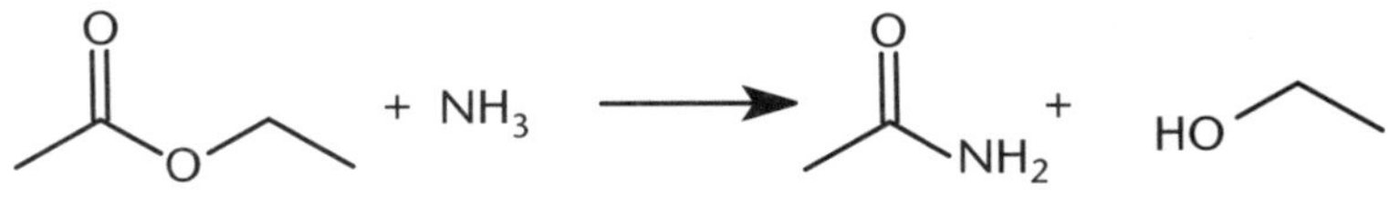

Figure 10.23

3. TRANSESTERIFICATION

Alcohols can act as nucleophiles and displace the alkoxy groups on esters. This process, which transforms one ester into another, is called **transesterification**.

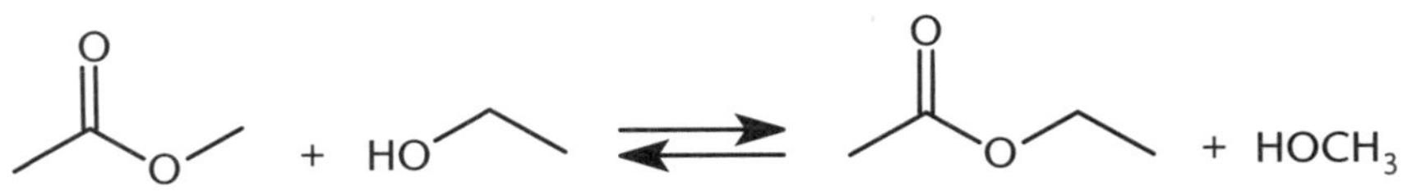

Figure 10.24

4. GRIGNARD ADDITION

Grignard reagents add to the carbonyl groups of esters to form ketones; however, these ketones are more reactive than the initial esters and are readily attacked by more Grignard reagent. Two equivalents of Grignard reagent can thus be used to produce tertiary alcohols with good yield. (The intermediate ketone can be isolated only if the alkyl groups are sufficiently bulky to prevent further attack.) This reaction proceeds via nucleophilic substitution followed by nucleophilic addition.

KEY CONCEPT

Grignard reagents, RMgX, are essentially equivalent to R⁻ nucleophiles.

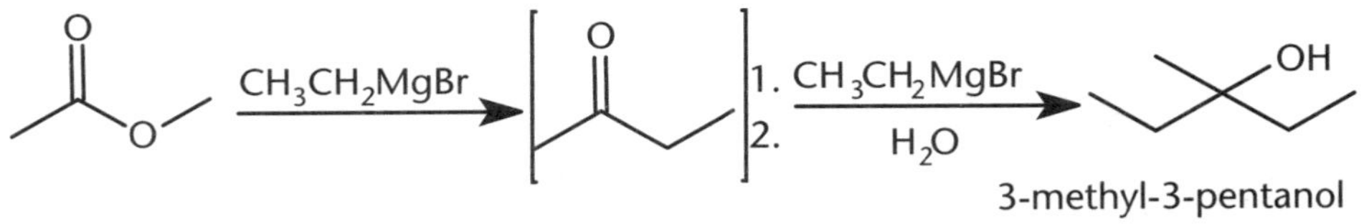

3-methyl-3-pentanol

Figure 10.25

REAL-WORLD ANALOGY

The Claisen condensation is the mechanism by which the long hydrocarbon chains of lipids are synthesized in biological systems. Acetyl coenzyme A performs the function of ethyl acetate, and long chains are built up by units of 2 carbon atoms. This is why long-chain compounds with 14, 16, and 18 carbon atoms are more common in living organisms than those with the odd chain-lengths of 15 and 17.

5. CONDENSATION REACTIONS

An important reaction of esters is the **Claisen condensation**. In the simplest case, two moles of ethyl acetate react under basic conditions to produce a β-keto ester, ethyl 3-oxobutanoate, or acetoacetic ester by its common name. (The Claisen condensation is also called the **acetoacetic ester condensation**.) The reaction proceeds by addition of an enolate anion to the carbonyl group of another ester, followed by displacement of ethoxide ion. This mechanism is analogous to that of the aldol condensation.

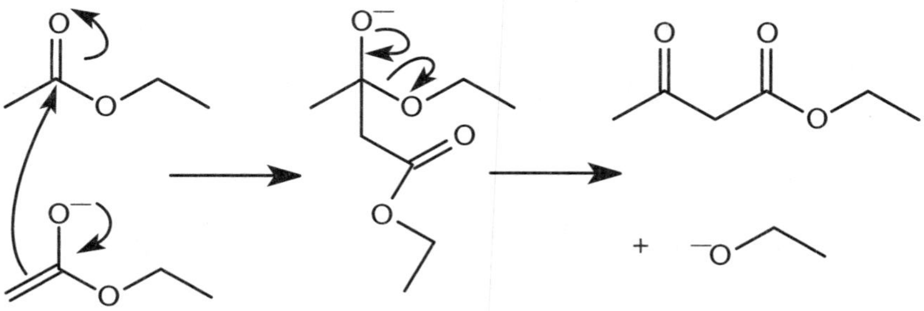

Figure 10.26

REMEMBER

LAH is essentially equivalent to a H⁻ nucleophile.

6. REDUCTION

Esters may be reduced to primary alcohols with LAH but not with $NaBH_4$. This allows for selective reduction in molecules with multiple functional groups.

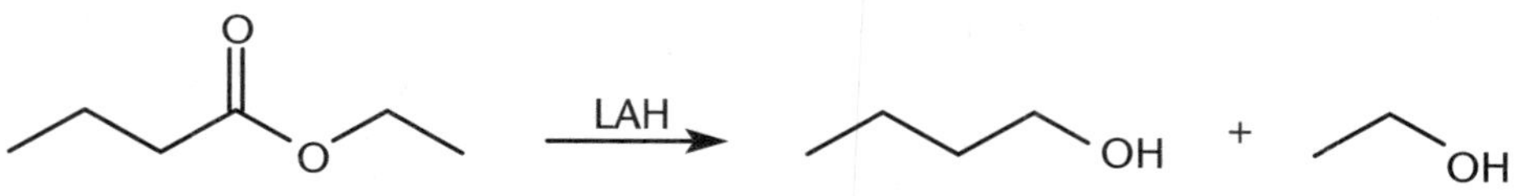

Figure 10.27

D. Phosphate Esters

While phosphoric acid derivatives are not carboxylic acid derivatives, they form esters similar to those in the previous section.

where R = H or hydrocarbon

phosphoric acid   phosphoric ester

Figure 10.28

Phosphoric acid and the mono- and diesters are acidic (more so than carboxylic acids) and usually exist as anions. Like all esters, under acidic conditions, they can be cleaved into the parent acid (in Figure 10.28, H_3PO_4) and alcohols.

Phosphate esters are found in living systems in the form of **phospholipids** (phosphoglycerides), in which glycerol is attached to two carboxylic acids and one phosphoric acid.

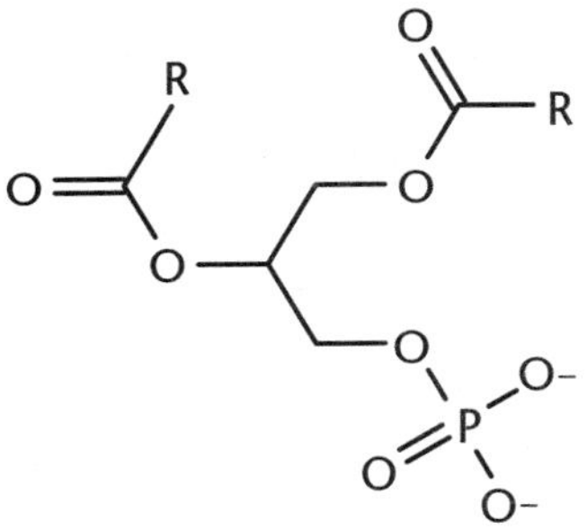

phosphatidic acid
diacylglycerol phosphate
(a phosphoglyceride)

Figure 10.29

Phospholipids are the main component of cell membranes, and phospholipid/carbohydrate polymers form the backbone of nucleic acids, the hereditary material of life. The nucleic acid derivative **adenosine triphosphate (ATP)** can give up and regain one or more phosphate groups. ATP facilitates many biological reactions by releasing phosphate groups to other compounds, thereby increasing their reactivities.

BRIDGE

Remember phosphodiester bonds? They hold the backbone of DNA together, connecting nucleotides with covalent linkages.

SUMMARY OF REACTIONS

- The most important derivatives of carboxylic acids are acyl halides, anhydrides, esters, and amides. These are listed from most reactive (least stable) to least reactive (most stable).

Acyl Halides

- Can be formed by adding $RCOOH + SOCl_2$, PCl_3 or PCl_5, or PBr_3.
- Undergo many different nucleophilic substitutions; H_2O yields carboxylic acid, ROH yields an ester, and NH_3 yields an amide.
- Can participate in Friedel-Crafts acylation to form an alkyl aryl ketone.
- Can be reduced to alcohols or, selectively, to aldehydes.

Anhydrides

- Can be formed by RCOOH + RCOOH (condensation) or $RCOO^-$ + RCOCl (substitution).
- Undergo many nucleophilic substitution reactions, forming products that include carboxylic acids, amides, and esters.
- Can participate in Friedel-Crafts acylation.

Esters

- Formed by RCOOH + ROH or, better, by acid chlorides or anhydrides + ROH.
- Hydrolyze to yield acids + alcohols; adding ammonia yields an amide.
- Reaction with Grignard reagent (2 moles) produces a tertiary alcohol.
- In Claisen condensation, analogous to the aldol, the ester acts both as nucleophile and target.
- Are very important in biological processes, particularly phosphate esters, which can be found in membranes, nucleic acids, and metabolic reactions.

Amides

- Can be formed by acid chlorides + amines or acid anhydrides + ammonia.
- Hydrolysis yields carboxylic acids or carboxylate anions.
- Can be transformed to primary amines via Hofmann rearrangement or reduction.

11

Amines and Nitrogen-Containing Compounds

NOMENCLATURE

Amines are compounds of the general formula NR_3. They are classified according to the number of alkyl (or aryl) groups to which they are bound. A **primary (1°)** amine is attached to one alkyl group, a **secondary (2°)** amine to two, and a **tertiary (3°)** amine to three. A nitrogen atom attached to four alkyl groups is called a **quaternary ammonium compound**. The nitrogen carries a positive charge; thus, these compounds generally exist as salts.

In the common system, amines are generally named as alkylamines. The groups are designated individually or by using the prefixes *di-* or *tri-* if they are the same. In the IUPAC system, amines are named by substituting the suffix **-amine** for the final *e* of the name of the alkane to which the nitrogen is attached. *N* is used to label substituents attached to the nitrogen in secondary or tertiary amines. The prefix **amino-** is used for naming compounds containing an OH or a CO_2H group. Aromatic amines are named as derivatives of aniline ($C_6H_5NH_2$), the IUPAC name for which is benzenamine. Table 11.1 shows some examples.

Formula:	$CH_3CH_2NH_2$	$CH_3CH_2N(CH_3)_2$	$H_2NCH_2CH_2CH_2OH$
IUPAC:	ethanamine	*N,N*-dimethylethanamine	2-aminoethanol
Common:	ethylamine	dimethylethylamine	ethanolamine

Table 11.1

There are many other nitrogen-containing organic compounds. **Amides** are the condensation products of carboxylic acids and amines. **Carbamates** are compounds with the general formula RNHC(O)OR′. They are also called **urethanes** and can form polymers called **polyurethanes**. Carbamates are derived from compounds called **isocyanates** (general formula RNCO) by the addition of an alcohol. **Enamines** are the nitrogen analogs of enols, with an amine group attached to one carbon of a double bond. **Imines** are nitrogen compounds that contain nitrogen-carbon double bonds. **Nitriles**, or **cyanides**, are compounds with a triple bond between a carbon atom and a nitrogen atom. They are named with either the prefix **cyano-** or the suffix **-nitrile**. **Nitro** compounds contain the nitro group, NO$_2$. **Diazo** compounds contain an N$_2$ functionality. They tend to lose N$_2$ to form carbenes. **Azides** are compounds with an N$_3$ functionality. When azides lose nitrogen (N$_2$), they form **nitrenes**, the nitrogen analogs of carbenes. Examples of these various compounds are shown in Figure 11.1.

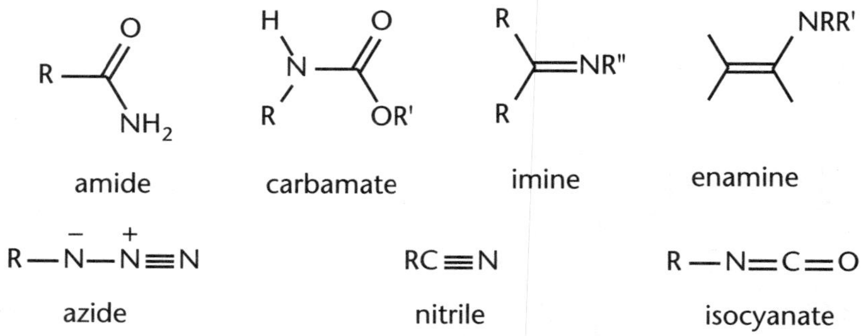

Figure 11.1

PROPERTIES

The boiling points of amines are between those of alkanes and alcohols. For example, ammonia boils at −33°C, whereas methane boils at −161°C and methanol at 64.5°C. As molecular weight increases, so do boiling points. Primary and secondary amines can form hydrogen bonds, while tertiary amines cannot; therefore, tertiary amines have lower boiling points. Since nitrogen is not as electronegative as oxygen, the hydrogen bonds of amines are not as strong as those of alcohols.

The nitrogen atom in an amine is approximately sp^3 hybridized. Nitrogen must bond to only three substituents in order to complete its octet; a lone pair occupies the last sp^3 orbital. This lone pair is very important to the chemistry of amines; it is associated with their basic and nucleophilic properties.

Nitrogen atoms bonded to three different substituents are chiral because of the geometry of the orbitals. However, these enantiomers cannot be isolated, because they interconvert rapidly in a process called **nitrogen inversion**: an inversion of the sp^3 orbital occupied by the lone pair. The activation energy for this process is only 6 kcal/mol, and only at very low temperatures is it significantly slowed or stopped.

KEY CONCEPT

Certain amines can be optically active if inversion is hindered by structure.

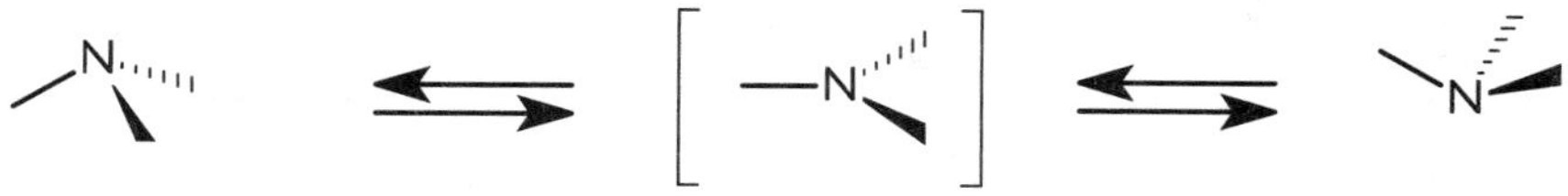

Figure 11.2

Amines are bases and readily accept protons to form ammonium ions. The pK_b values of alkyl amines are around 4, making them slightly more basic than ammonia (pK_b = 4.76) but less basic than hydroxide (pK_b = –1.7). Aromatic amines such as aniline (pK_b = 9.42) are far less basic than aliphatic amines, because the electron-withdrawing effect of the ring reduces the basicity of the amino group. The presence of other substituents on the ring alters the basicity of anilines: Electron-donating groups (such as –OH, $–CH_3$, and $–NH_2$) increase basicity, while electron-withdrawing groups (such as NO_2) reduce basicity.

Amines also function as very weak acids. The pK_as of amines are around 35, and a very strong base is required for deprotonation. For example, the proton of diisopropylamine may be removed with butyllithium, forming the sterically hindered base lithium diisopropylamide, LDA.

REAL-WORLD ANALOGY

An interesting property of several nitrogen-containing compounds, such as nitroglycerin and nitrous oxide, is their ability to act as relaxants. Nitroglycerine is given sublingually to relieve coronary artery spasms in people with chest pain, and nitrous oxide (laughing gas) is a common dental anesthetic. Nitroglycerine has the additional property of rapidly decomposing to form gas and is thus fairly explosive.

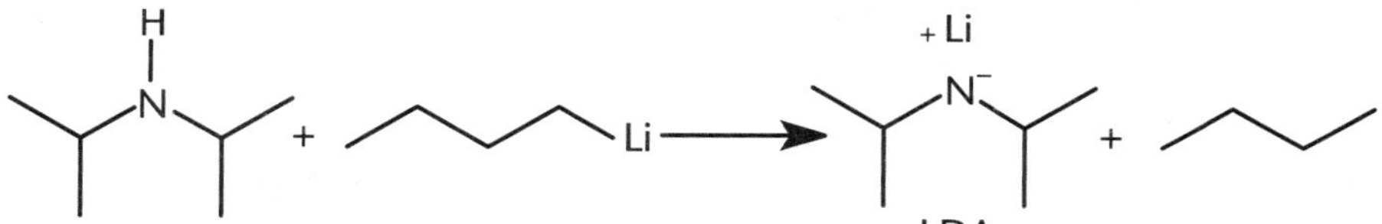

LDA

Figure 11.3

SYNTHESIS

A. Alkylation Of Ammonia

1. DIRECT

Alkyl halides react with ammonia to produce alkylammonium halide salts. Ammonia functions as a nucleophile and displaces the halide atom. When the salt is treated with base, the alkylamine product is formed.

$$CH_3Br + NH_3 \longrightarrow CH_3\overset{+}{N}H_3Br^- \xrightarrow{NaOH} CH_3NH_2 + NaBr + H_2O$$

$$CH_3NH_2 + CH_3Br \longrightarrow CH_3-\underset{\underset{CH_3}{|}}{NH} + CH_3Br \longrightarrow CH_3-\underset{\underset{CH_3}{|}}{N}-CH_3$$

$$\longrightarrow (CH_3)_4N^+$$

Figure 11.4

KEY CONCEPT

Alkylation of ammonia proceeds to completion and forms of quarternary ammonium salts.

This reaction often leads to side products, because the alkylamine formed is nucleophilic and can react with the alkyl halide to form more complex products.

2. GABRIEL SYNTHESIS

The **Gabriel synthesis** converts a primary alkyl halide to a primary amine. The use of a disguised form of ammonia prevents side-product formation.

FLASHBACK

Addition of ammonia to an alkyl halide and the Gabriel synthesis are both S_N2 reactions. With its unshared electron pair, ammonia is a very good nucleophile, while the halides are all good leaving groups.

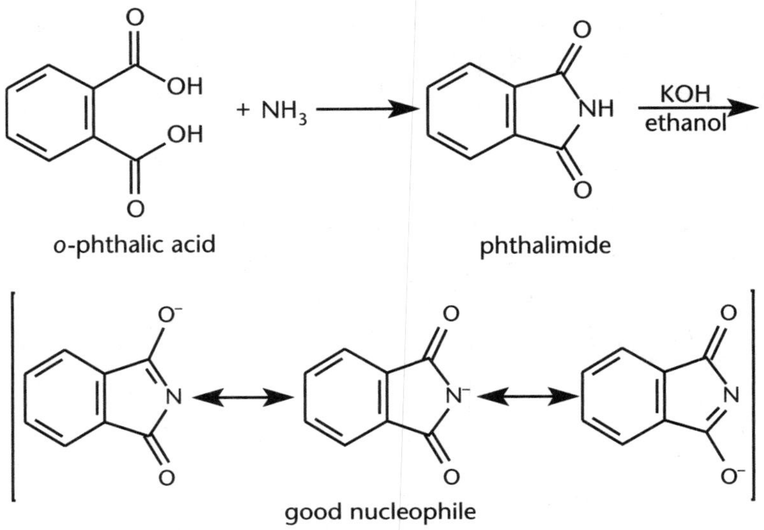

Figure 11.5

Phthalimide, the condensation product of phthalic acid and ammonia, acts as a good nucleophile when deprotonated. It displaces halide ions, forming *N*-alkylphthalimides, which do not react with other alkyl halides. When the reaction is complete, the *N*-alkylphthalimide can be hydrolyzed with aqueous base to produce the alkylamine.

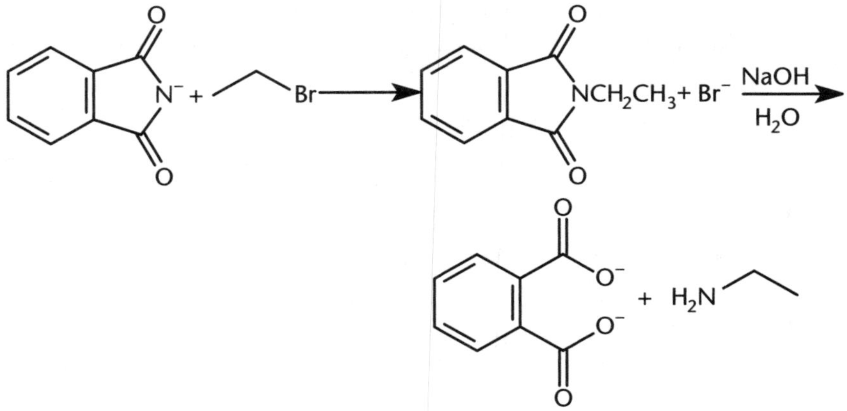

Figure 11.6

B. Reduction

Amines can be obtained from other nitrogen-containing functionalities via reduction reactions.

1. FROM NITRO COMPOUNDS

Nitro compounds are easily reduced to primary amines. The most common reducing agent is iron or zinc and dilute hydrochloric acid, although many other reagents can be used. This reaction is especially useful for aromatic compounds, because nitration of aromatic rings is facile.

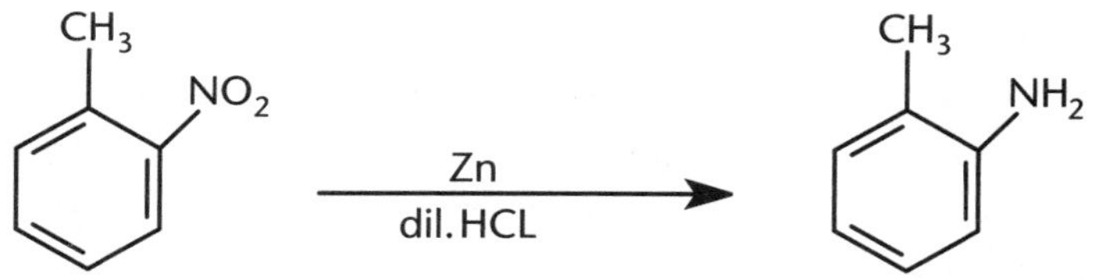

Figure 11.7

2. FROM NITRILES

Nitriles can be reduced with hydrogen and a catalyst, or with lithium aluminum hydride (LAH), to produce primary amines.

$$CH_3CH_2C \equiv N \xrightarrow{\text{LAH}} CH_3CH_2CH_2NH_2$$

Figure 11.8

3. FROM IMINES

Amines can be synthesized by **reductive amination**, a process whereby an aldehyde or ketone is reacted with ammonia, a primary amine, or a secondary amine to form a primary, secondary, or tertiary amine, respectively. When the amine reacts with the aldehyde or the ketone, an imine is produced. Consequently, it will undergo hydride reduction in much the same way that a carbonyl does. When the imine is reduced with hydrogen in the presence of a catalyst, an amine is produced.

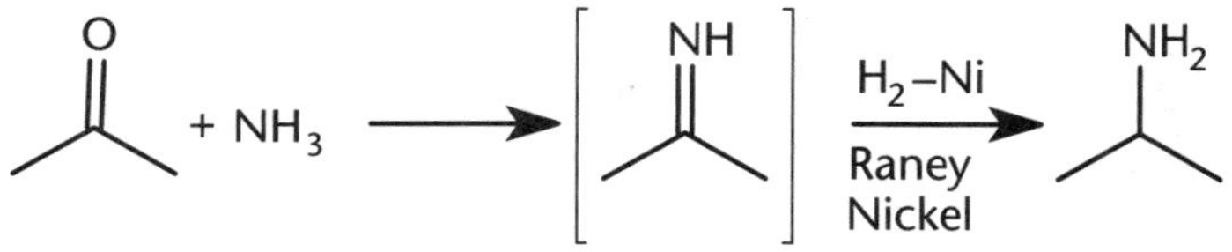

| acetone | imine isopropylimine | amine isopropylamine (aminoisopropane) |

Figure 11.9

> **REMEMBER**
>
> Amines can be formed by
>
> 1) S_N2 reactions
>   - ammonia reacting with alkyl halides
>   - Gabriel synthesis
> 2) Reduction of
>   - amides
>   - aniline and its derivatives
>   - nitriles
>   - imines
>
> Amines can be destroyed (converted to alkenes) by exhaustive methylation.

4. **FROM AMIDES**

Amides can be reduced with LAH to form amines.

KEY CONCEPT

An imine is a nitrogen double-bonded to a carbon and has about the same polarity as a carbonyl functionality.

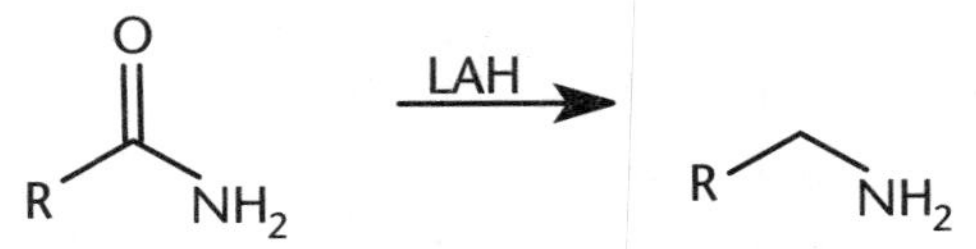

Figure 11.10

REACTIONS

A. Exhaustive Methylation

Exhaustive methylation is also known as **Hofmann elimination**. In this process, an amine is converted to a quaternary ammonium iodide by treatment with excess methyl iodide. Treatment with silver oxide and water converts this to the ammonium hydroxide, which, when heated, undergoes elimination to form an alkene and an amine. The predominant alkene formed is the least substituted, in contrast with normal elimination reactions where the predominant alkene product is the most substituted.

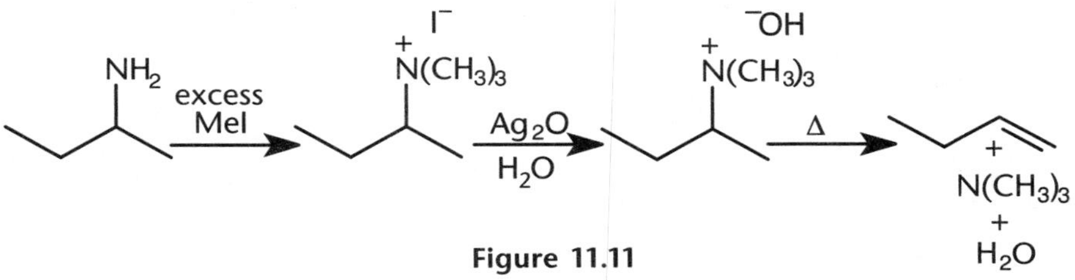

Figure 11.11

Purification and Separation

Much of organic chemistry is concerned with the isolation and purification of the desired reaction product. A reaction itself may be completed in a matter of minutes, but separating the product from the reaction mixture is often a difficult and time-consuming process. Many techniques have been developed to accomplish this objective: to obtain a pure compound separated from solvents, reagents, and other products.

BASIC TECHNIQUES

A. Extraction

One way of separating out a desired product is through **extraction**, the transfer of a dissolved compound (here, the desired product) from one solvent into another in which it is more soluble. Most impurities will be left behind in the first solvent. The two solvents should be immiscible (form two layers that do not mix because of mutual insolubility). The two layers are temporarily mixed together so that solute can pass from one to the other. For example, a solution of isobutyric acid in diethyl ether can be extracted with water. Isobutyric acid is more soluble in water than in ether, so when the two solvents are placed together, isobutyric acid transfers to the water phase.

The water (**aqueous**) and ether (**organic**) phases are separated in a specialized piece of glassware called a separatory funnel (see Figure 12.1). Once separated, the isobutyric acid can be isolated from the aqueous phase in pure form. Some isobutyric acid will remain dissolved in the ether phase, so the extraction should be repeated several times with fresh solvent (water). More product can be obtained with successive extractions (i.e., it is more effective to perform three successive extractions of 10 mL each than to perform one extraction of 30 mL). Once the compound has been isolated in its purified form in a solvent, it can then be obtained by evaporation of the solvent.

> **KEY CONCEPT**
>
> Think of the aqueous and organic layers as being like oil and water in salad dressing: You can shake the mixture to increase their interaction, but ultimately they will separate again.

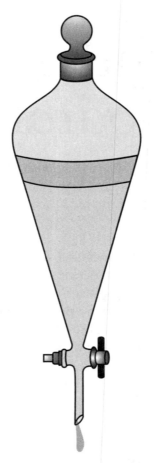

Figure 12.1. Separatory Funnel

An extraction carried out to remove unwanted impurities rather than to isolate a pure product is called a **wash**.

B. Filtration

Filtration is used to isolate a solid from a liquid. In this technique, a liquid/solid mixture is poured onto a paper filter that allows only the solvent to pass through. The result of this process is the separation of the solid (often referred to as the residue) from the liquid or **filtrate**. The two basic types of filtration are **gravity filtration** and **vacuum filtration**. In gravity filtration, the solvent's own weight pulls it through the filter. Frequently, however, the pores of the filter become clogged with solid, slowing the rate of filtration. For this reason, in gravity filtration it is generally desirable for the substance of interest to be in solution (dissolved in the solvent), while impurities remain undissolved and can be filtered out. This allows the desired product to flow more easily and rapidly through the apparatus. To ensure that the product remains dissolved, gravity filtration is usually carried out with hot solvent.

In vacuum filtration (see Figure 12.2), the solvent is forced through the filter by a vacuum on the other side. Vacuum filtration is used to isolate relatively large quantities of solid, usually when the solid is the desired product.

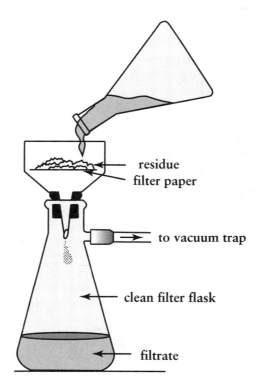

residue
filter paper

to vacuum trap

clean filter flask

filtrate

Vacuum filtration

Figure 12.2. Vacuum Filtration

C. Recrystallization

Recrystallization is a process in which impure crystals are dissolved in a minimum amount of hot solvent. As the solvent is cooled, the crystals re-form, leaving the impurities in solution. For recrystallization to be effective, the solvent must be chosen carefully. It must dissolve the solid while it is hot, but not while it is cold. In addition, it must dissolve the impurities at both temperatures so that they remain in solution. Solvent choice is usually a matter of trial and error, although some generalizations can be made. An estimate of polarity is useful, since polar solvents dissolve polar compounds, while nonpolar solvents dissolve nonpolar compounds. A solvent with intermediate polarity is generally desirable in recrystallization. In addition, the solvent should have a low enough freezing point that the solution may be sufficiently cooled.

KEY CONCEPT

Ideally, the desired product should have solubility that depends on temperature—it should be more soluble at high temperature, less so at low. In contrast, impurities should be equally soluble at various temperatures.

In some instances, a mixed solvent system may be used. Here the crude compound is dissolved in a solvent in which it is highly soluble. Another solvent, in which the compound is less soluble, is then added in drops, just until solid begins to precipitate. The solution is heated a bit more to redissolve the precipitate and then slowly cooled to induce crystal formation.

D. Sublimation

Sublimation occurs when a heated solid turns directly into a gas without an intervening liquid stage. It is used as a method of purification because the impurities found in most reaction mixtures will not sublime easily. The vapors are made to condense on a **cold finger**, a piece of glassware packed with dry ice or with cold water running through it (see Figure 12.3). Most sublimations are performed under vacuum, because at higher pressures more compounds will pass through a liquid phase rather than subliming; low pressure also reduces the temperature required for sublimation and thus the danger that the compound will decompose. The optimal conditions depend on the compound to be purified, since each compound has a different phase diagram.

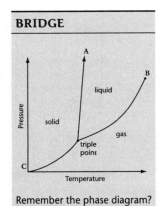

BRIDGE

Remember the phase diagram?

To make a solid sublime, you must either

a) raise the temperature at a low enough pressure; or

b) lower the pressure at a very cold temperature.

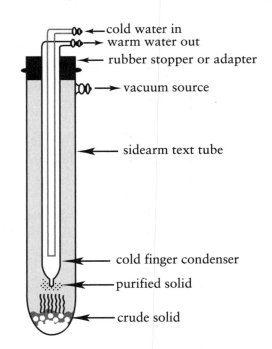

Figure 12.3. Sublimation

E. Centrifugation

Particles in a solution settle, or **sediment**, at different rates depending upon their mass, their density, and their shape. Sedimentation can be accelerated by **centrifuging** the solution. A centrifuge is an apparatus in which test tubes containing the solution are spun at high speed, which subjects them to centrifugal force (see Figure 12.4). Compounds of greater mass and density settle toward the bottom of the test tubes, while lighter compounds remain near the top. This method of separation is effective for many different types of compounds and is frequently used in biochemistry to separate cells, organelles, and biological macromolecules.

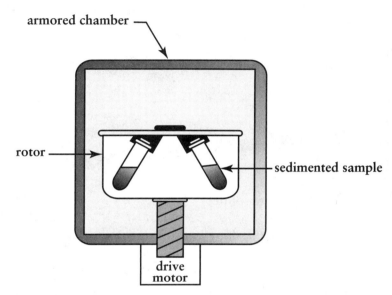

Figure 12.4. Centrifuge

DISTILLATION

Distillation is the separation of one liquid from another through vaporization and condensation. A mixture of two (or more) miscible liquids is slowly heated; the compound with the lowest boiling point is preferentially vaporized, condenses on a water-cooled distillation column, and is separated from the other, higher-boiling compound(s). (Immiscible liquids can be separated in a separatory funnel and thus do not require distillation.)

A. Simple

Simple distillation is used to separate liquids that boil *below* 150°C and at least 25°C apart. The apparatus consists of a distilling flask containing the two liquids, a distillation column consisting of a thermometer and a condenser, and a receiving flask to collect the distillate.

B. Vacuum

Vacuum distillation is used to separate liquids that boil *above* 150°C and at least 25°C apart (see Figure 12.5). The entire system is operated under reduced pressure, lowering the boiling points of the liquids and thus preventing their decomposition due to excessive temperature.

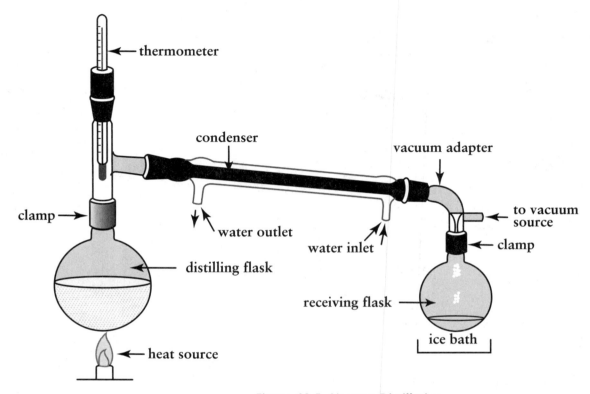

Figure 12.5. Vaccum Distillation

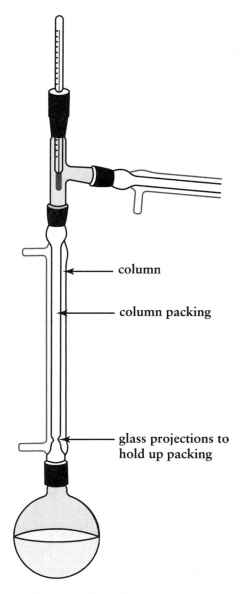

← column

← column packing

← glass projections to
hold up packing

Figure 12.6. Fractional Distillation

C. Fractional

Fractional distillation is used to separate liquids that boil less than 25°C apart (see Figure 12.6). A fractionating column is used to connect the distilling flask to the distillation column. It is filled with inert objects, such as glass beads, that have a large surface area. The vapors condense on these surfaces, re-evaporate, and then condense further up the column. Each time the liquid evaporates, the vapors contain a greater proportion of the lower-boiling component. Eventually, near the top of the fractionating column, the vapor is composed solely of one component, which will condense on the distillation column and collect in the receiving flask.

KEY CONCEPT

CHROMATOGRAPHY

A. General Principles

Chromatography is a technique that allows scientists to separate, identify, and isolate individual compounds from a complex mixture based on their differing chemical properties. First, the sample is placed, or loaded, onto a solid medium called the **stationary phase** or **adsorbant**. Then, the **mobile phase**, a liquid (or gas for gas chromatography), is run through the stationary phase, to displace (or **elute**) adhered substances. Different compounds will adhere to the stationary phase with different strengths and, therefore, migrate with different speeds. This causes separation of the compounds within the stationary phase, allowing each compound to be isolated.

Several forms of media are used as the stationary phase, which separate compounds based on different chemical properties. How quickly a compound travels through the stationary phase depends on a variety of factors. Commonly, the key is polarity. For instance, thin-layer chromatography (TLC) often uses silica gel, which is highly polar. Thus, polar compounds bind tightly, eluting poorly into the less polar organic solvent. Size or charge may also play a role, as in column chromatography (described in detail below). Newer techniques, such as affinity chromatography, take advantage of unique properties of a substance (such as its strong binding to a specific antibody or to a known receptor or ligand) to bind it tightly to the stationary phase.

Compounds can be distinguished from each other because they travel across the stationary phase (adsorbant) at different rates. In practice, a substance can be identified based on

- how far it travels in a given amount of time (as in TLC); or how rapidly it travels a given distance (e.g., how quickly it elutes off the column, as in gas or column chromatography).

The four most commonly used types of chromatography are **thin-layer chromatography**, **column chromatography**, **gas chromatography**, and **high-pressure** (or **performance**) **liquid chromatography**.

B. Thin-Layer Chromatography

The adsorbant in thin-layer chromatography is either a piece of paper or a thin layer of silica gel or alumina on a plastic or glass sheet (see Figure 12.7). The mixture to be separated is placed on the adsorbant; this is called **spotting**, because a small, well-defined spot is desirable. The TLC plate is then **developed**—placed upright in a developing chamber (usually a beaker with a lid or a wide-mouthed jar), containing **eluant** (solvent) approximately 1/4-inch deep (this value depends on the size of the plate). It is imperative that the initial spots on the plate be above the level of the solvent, or else they will simply elute off the plate into the solvent rather than moving neatly up the plate itself. The solvent creeps up the plate by capillary action, moving different compounds at different rates. When the **solvent front** nears the top of the plate, the plate is removed from the chamber and allowed to dry.

Chromatography is often done with silica gel as the adsorbant because it is very polar and hydrophilic. The mobile phase, usually an organic solvent of weak to moderate polarity, is then used to "run" the sample through the gel. Nonpolar compounds move very quickly, while polar molecules are stuck tightly to the gel. The more polar the solvent, the faster the sample will migrate. Reverse-phase chromatography is just the opposite. Here the stationary phase is very nonpolar, so polar molecules run very quickly, while non-polar molecules stick more tightly.

The spots of individual compounds (usually white) are not usually visible on the white TLC plate. They are **visualized** by placing the TLC plate under UV light, which will show any compounds that are UV-sensitive, or by allowing iodine, I_2, to stain the spots. Other chemical staining agents include phosphomolybdic acid and vanillin. Note that these compounds destroy the product (usually by oxidation), so it cannot be recovered for further study.

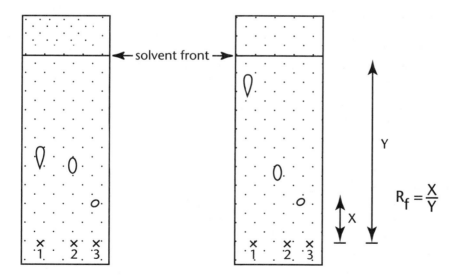

Figure 12.7. Thin-Layer Chromatograms

The distance a compound travels, divided by the distance the solvent travels, is called the **R_f value**. This value is relatively constant for a particular compound in a particular solvent and can, therefore, be used for identification.

TLC is most frequently used for qualitative identification (i.e., determining the identity of a compound). It can also be used on a larger scale as a means of purification. **Preparative** or **prep TLC** uses a large TLC plate upon which a sizeable streak of a mixture is placed. As the plate develops, the streak splits into bands of individual compounds, which can then be scraped off. Rinsing with a polar solvent will recover the pure compounds from the silica.

C. Column Chromatography

The principle behind column chromatography is the same as for TLC. Column chromatography, however, uses silica gel or alumina as an adsorbant (not paper), and this adsorbant is in the form of a column (not a layer), allowing much more separation (see Figure 12.8). In TLC, the solvent and compounds move up the plate (by capillary action), whereas in column chromatography, they move down the column (by gravity). Sometimes the solvent is forced through the column with nitrogen gas; this is called **flash column chromatography.**

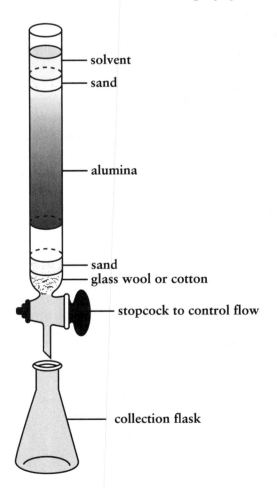

solvent
sand

alumina

sand
glass wool or cotton

stopcock to control flow

collection flask

Figure 12.8. Column Chromatography

The solvent drips out the end of the column, and fractions are collected in flasks or test tubes. These fractions contain bands corresponding to the different compounds, and when the solvents are evaporated, the compounds can be isolated.

Column chromatography is particularly useful in biochemistry, because it can be used to separate macromolecules such as proteins or nucleic acids. Several techniques exist:

1) In *ion exchange chromatography*, the beads in the column are coated with charged substances, so they will attract or bind compounds with an opposing charge. For instance, a positively charged column will attract and hold negative substances while letting those with positive charge pass through.

2) In *size-exclusion chromatography*, the column contains beads with many tiny pores. Very small molecules can enter the beads, which slows down their progress, while large molecules move around/between the beads and thus travel through the column faster.

3) In *affinity chromotography*, columns can be "customized" to bind a substance of interest. For example, to purify substance A, a scientist might use a column of beads coated with something that binds A very tightly, such as a receptor for A, A's biological target, or even a specific antibody. Substance A will bind to the column very tightly. It can later be eluted by washing with free receptor (or target or antibody), which will compete with the bead-bound receptor and ultimately free substance A from the column.

D. Gas Chromatography

Gas chromatography (GC) is another method of qualitative separation. In gas chromatography, also called **vapor-phase chromatography** (VPC), the eluant that passes through the adsorbant is a gas, usually helium or nitrogen. The adsorbant is inside a 30-foot column that is coiled and kept inside an oven to control its temperature (see Figure 12.9). The mixture to be separated is injected into the column and vaporized. The gaseous compounds travel through the column at different rates, because they adhere to the adsorbant to different degrees, and will separate by the time they reach the end of the column. At this point, they are registered by a detector, which records the presence of a compound as a peak.

KEY CONCEPT

Again, note that there is a stationary phase (here, a 30-foot column) and a mobile phase or eluant (here, a gas).

REMEMBER

To identify a compound or distinguish two different compounds, look at their "retention times"—that is, how *long* it took for each to travel through the column.

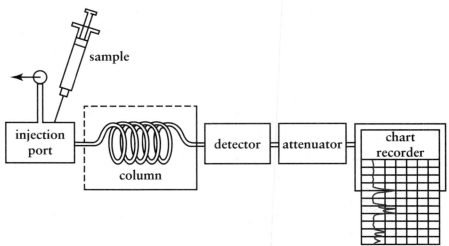

Figure 12.9. Gas Chromatography

GC can be used on a larger scale for quantitative separation; it is then called preparative or prep GC. This is, however, very tedious and difficult to perform.

E. HPLC

HPLC stands for either high-pressure or high-performance liquid chromatography. The eluant is a liquid that travels through a column similar to a GC column, but it is under pressure. In the past, very high pressures were used. Now they are much lower; hence, the change from high *pressure* to high *performance*.

In HPLC, a sample is injected into the column, and separation occurs as it flows through. The compounds pass through a detector and are collected as the solvent flows out the end of the apparatus. The eluant may vary, as in thin-layer or column chromatography.

ELECTROPHORESIS

KEY CONCEPT

In most forms of electrophoresis, the size of a macromolecule is usually the most important factor—small molecules move faster, while large ones move more slowly and may in fact take hours to leave the well.

When a molecule is placed in an electric field, it will move towards either the cathode or the anode, depending on its size and charge. **Electrophoresis** employs this phenomenon to separate macromolecules (usually biological macromolecules) such as proteins or DNA. The migration velocity, v, of a molecule is directly proportional to the electric field strength, E, and to the net charge on the molecule, z, and it is inversely proportional to a frictional coefficient, f, which depends on the mass and shape of the migrating molecules.

$$V = \frac{EZ}{f}$$

Therefore, in a constant electric field, highly charged molecules will move most rapidly, as will small molecules.

A. Agarose Gel Electrophoresis

Agarose gel electrophoresis is used by molecular biologists to separate pieces of **nucleic acid** (usually **deoxyribonucleic acid**, DNA, but sometimes **ribonucleic acid**, RNA, as well). Agarose is an organic gel, derived from seaweed, that is nontoxic and easy to manipulate (unlike SDS/polyacrylamide). Since every piece of nucleic acid is highly negatively charged, nucleic acids can be separated effectively on the basis of size even without the charge masking provided by SDS. Agarose gels are stained with a compound called ethidium bromide, which binds to nucleic acids and is visualized by its fluorescence under ultraviolet light.

Agarose gel electrophoresis can also be used preparatively by cutting the desired band out of the gel and eluting out the nucleic acid.

B. Sds-Polyacrylamide Gel Electrophoresis

SDS-polyacrylamide gel electrophoresis separates proteins on the basis of mass, not charge. Polyacrylamide gel (PAGE) is the standard medium for electrophoresis. SDS is sodium dodecyl sulfate, which disrupts noncovalent interactions. It binds to proteins and creates large negative net charges, neutralizing the protein's original net charge. As proteins move through the gel, the only variable affecting their velocity is f, the frictional coefficient, which is dependent on mass. After separation, the gel is stained so that the protein bands can be visualized.

C. Isoelectric Focusing

A protein may be characterized by its **isoelectric point**, pI, which is the pH at which its net charge (the sum of the charges on all of its component amino acids) is zero. If a mixture of proteins is placed in an electric field in a gel with a pH gradient, the proteins will move until they reach the point at which the pH is equal to their pI. At this location, the protein will be uncharged and will no longer move in the field. Molecules differing by as little as one charge can be separated in this manner, which is called **isoelectric focusing**.

SUMMARY OF PURIFICATION METHODS

BRIDGE

Since amino acids and proteins are organic molecules, the fundamental principles of acid-base chemistry apply to them as well.

- At a low pH, [H+] is relatively high. Thus, at a pH < pI, proteins will tend to be protonated and, as a result, positively charged.
- At a relatively high (basic) pH, [H+] is fairly low and proteins will tend to be depronated—thus carrying a negative charge.

Method	Use
Extraction	Separates dissolved substances based on differential solubility in aqueous versus organic solvents.
Filtration	Separates solids from liquids.
Recrystallization	Separates solids based on differential solubility; temperature is important here.
Sublimation	Separates solids based on their ability to sublime.
Centrifugation	Separates large things (like cells, organelles, and macromolecules) based on mass and density.
Distillation	Separates liquids based on boiling point, which in turn depends on intermolecular forces.
Chromatography	Uses a stationary phase and a mobile phase to separate compounds based on how tightly they adhere (generally due to polarity but sometimes size as well).
Electrophoresis	Used to separate biological macromolecules (such as proteins or nucleic acids) based on size and sometimes charge.

13

Spectroscopy

Once an organic compound is isolated, it must be characterized and identified. If it is a known compound, identification can often be made from elemental analysis or determination of the melting point. With new or more complex compounds, other methods must be used. **Spectroscopy** is the process of measuring the energy differences between the possible states of a molecular system by determining the frequencies of electromagnetic radiation (light) absorbed by the molecules. The possible states are quantized energy levels associated with different types of molecular motion, including molecular rotation, vibration of bonds, and electron movement. Different types of spectroscopy measure these different types of molecular motion, identifying specific functional groups and how they are connected.

Spectroscopy is useful because only a very small quantity of sample is needed. In addition, the sample may be reused after an IR, NMR, or UV spectrum is obtained.

INFRARED

A. Basic Theory

Infrared (IR) spectroscopy measures molecular vibrations, which include bond **stretching, bending,** and **rotation.** The useful absorptions of infrared light occur in the 3,000–30,000 nm region, which corresponds to 3,500–300 cm^{-1} (called **wavenumbers**). When light of these wavelengths/wavenumbers is absorbed, the molecules enter higher (excited) vibrational states.

Bond stretching (which can be of two types: symmetric or asymmetric) involves the largest change in energy and is observed in the region 1,500–4,000 cm^{-1}. Bending vibrations are observed in the region 400–1500 cm^{-1}. Four types of vibration that can occur are shown in Figure 13.1.

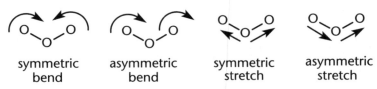

| symmetric | asymmetric | symmetric | asymmetric |
| bend | bend | stretch | stretch |

Figure 13.1

In addition to bending and stretching vibrations, more complex vibrations may occur. These can be combinations of bending, stretching, and rotation frequencies or complex frequency patterns caused by the motion of the whole molecule. Absorptions of these types are seen in the region 1,500–400 cm⁻¹. This region of the spectrum is known as the **fingerprint region** and is characteristic of a molecule; it is, therefore, frequently used to identify a substance.

For an absorption to be recorded, the motion must result in a change in a bond dipole moment. Molecules comprised of atoms with the same electronegativity, as well as symmetrical molecules, do not experience a changing dipole moment and, therefore, do not exhibit absorption. For example, O_2 and Br_2 do not absorb, but HCl and CO do.

A typical spectrum is obtained by passing infrared light (of frequencies from approximately 4,000–400 cm⁻¹) through a sample and recording the absorption pattern. Percent transmittance is plotted versus frequency, where percent transmittance = absorption⁻¹ ($\%T = A^{-1}$); absorptions appear as valleys on the spectrum.

KEY CONCEPT

Symmetric stretches do not show up in IR spectra since they involve no net change in dipole movement.

REMEMBER

Wavenumbers (cm⁻¹) are not the same as frequency.

$v = \dfrac{c}{\lambda}$ while wave number $= \dfrac{1}{\lambda}$.

B. Characteristic Absorptions

Particular functional groups absorb at localized frequencies. For example, alcohols absorb around 3,300 cm⁻¹, carbonyl groups around 1,700 cm⁻¹, and ethers around 1,100 cm⁻¹. Table 13.1 lists the specific absorptions of key functional groups and the vibrations with which they are associated.

C. Application

A great deal of information can be obtained from an IR spectrum. Most of the useful functional group information is found between 1,400 and 4,000 cm⁻¹. Figure 13.2 shows the IR spectrum of an aliphatic alcohol. The large peak at 3,300 cm⁻¹ is due to the presence of the hydroxyl group, while the peak at 3,000 cm⁻¹ can be attributed to the alkane portion of the molecule.

Table 3.1. Common Infrared Absorption Peaks

Functional Group	Frequency (cm⁻¹)	Vibration
Alkanes	2,800–3,000	C—H
	1,200	C—C
Alkenes	3,080–3,140	=C—H
	1,645	C=C
Alkynes	2,200	C≡C
	3,300	≡C—H
Aromatic	2,900–3,100	C—H
	1,475–1,625	C—C
Alcohols	3,100–3,500	O—H (broad)
Ethers	1,050–1,150	C—O
Aldehydes	2,700–2,900	(O)C—H
	1,725–1,750	C=O
Ketones	1,700–1,750	C=O
		C=O
Carboxylic Acids	1,700–1,750	C=O
	2,900–3,300	O—H (broad)
Amines	3,100–3,500	N—H (sharp)

KEY CONCEPT

IR spectroscopy is best used for identification of functional groups. The most important peaks to know are those for alcohols (don't forget this is a BROAD peak), acids (BROADEST peak), ketones, and amines (SHARP peak). If you know nothing else here, know these!

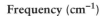

Frequency (cm⁻¹)

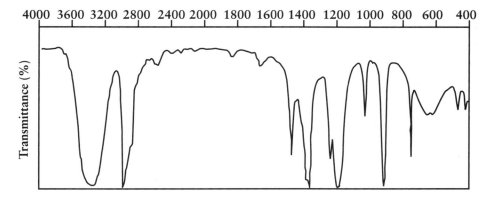

Figure 13.2

NUCLEAR MAGNETIC RESONANCE

A. Basic Theory

Nuclear magnetic resonance (NMR) spectroscopy is one of the most widely used spectroscopic tools in organic chemistry. NMR is based on the fact that certain nuclei have magnetic moments that are normally oriented at random. When such nuclei are placed in a magnetic field, their magnetic moments tend to align either with or against the direction of this applied field. Nuclei whose magnetic moments are aligned with the field are said to be in the α **state** (lower energy), while those whose moments are aligned against the field are said to be in the β **state** (higher energy). If the nuclei are then irradiated with electromagnetic radiation, some will be excited into the α state. The absorption corresponding to this excitation occurs at different frequencies depending on an atom's environment. The nuclear magnetic moments are affected by other nearby atoms that also possess magnetic moments. Hence, a compound may contain many nuclei that resonate at different frequencies, producing a very complex spectrum.

A typical NMR spectrum is a plot of frequency versus absorption of energy during resonance. Frequency *decreases* toward the right. Alternatively, varying magnetic field may be plotted on the x-axis, *increasing* towards the right. Because different NMR spectrometers operate at different magnetic field strengths, a standardized method of plotting the NMR spectrum has been adopted. An arbitrary variable, called **chemical shift** (represented by the symbol δ), with units of **parts per million (ppm)** of spectrometer frequency, is plotted on the x-axis.

NMR is most commonly used to study ^1H nuclei (protons) and ^{13}C nuclei, although any atom possessing a nuclear spin (any nucleus with an odd atomic number or odd mass number) can be studied, such as ^{19}F, ^{17}O, ^{14}N, ^{15}N, or ^{31}P.

B. ^1H-NMR

REMEMBER

TMS provides a reference peak. The signal for its H atoms is assigned a d = 0.

Most ^1H nuclei come into resonance between 0 and 10 δ downfield from tetramethylsilane (TMS). Each distinct set of nuclei gives rise to a separate peak. The compound dichloromethyl methyl ether has two distinct sets of ^1H nuclei. The single proton attached to the dichloromethyl group is in a different magnetic environment than are the three protons on the methyl group, and the two classes resonate at different frequencies. The three protons on the methyl group are magnetically equivalent due to rotation about the oxygen-carbon single bond and resonate at the same frequency. Thus, two separate peaks are expected, as shown in Figure 13.3.

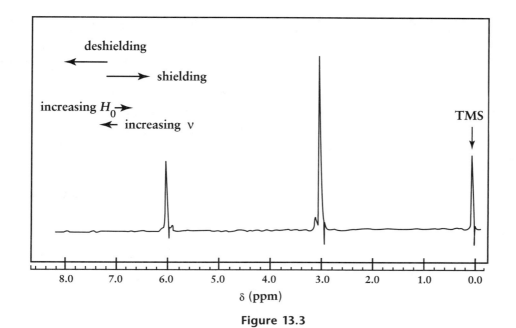

Figure 13.3

KEY CONCEPT

- Each peak represents a single proton or a group of equivalent protons. (The number of peaks represents the number of groups of nonequivalent protons.)
- The relative area of each peak reflects the ratio of the protons producing each peak.
- The position of the peak (upfield or downfield) due to shielding or deshielding effects reflects the chemical environment of the protons.

The left-hand peak corresponds to the single dichloromethyl proton and the middle peak to the three methyl protons (the one on the far right is the TMS reference peak). Notice that if the areas under the peaks are integrated, the ratio between them is 3:1, corresponding to the number of protons producing each peak.

The single proton comes into resonance downfield from the methyl protons. This phenomenon is due to the electron-withdrawing effect of the chlorine atoms. The electron cloud that surrounds the ^{1}H nucleus ordinarily screens the nucleus somewhat from the applied magnetic field. The chlorine atoms pull away the electron cloud and **deshield** the nucleus. Thus, the nucleus resonates in a lower field than it would otherwise. By the same rationale, electron-donating atoms, such as the silicon atoms in TMS, **shield** the ^{1}H nuclei, causing them to come into resonance at a higher field.

If two magnetically different protons are within three bonds of each other, a phenomenon known as **coupling,** or **splitting,** occurs. Consider two protons, H_a and H_b, on the molecule 1,1-dibromo-2,2-dichloroethane (Figure 13.4).

REMEMBER

Downfield is Deshielded.

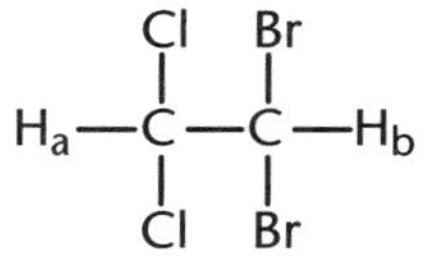

Figure 13.4

At any given time, H_a can experience two different magnetic environments, since H_b can be in either the α or the β state. These different states of H_b influence nucleus H_a (if the two H atoms are within three bonds of each other), causing slight upfield and downfield shifts. Since there is approximately a 50 percent chance that H_b will be in either state, this results in a **doublet**, two peaks of equal intensity equally spaced around the true chemical shift of H_a. H_b experiences the two different states of H_a and is likewise coupled. The magnitude of the splitting, usually denoted in Hz, is called the **coupling constant, J**.

KEY CONCEPT

The splitting of the peak represents the number of adjacent hydrogens. A peak will be split into $n + 1$ peaks, where n is the number of adjacent hydrogens.

In 1,1-dibromo-2-chloroethane (Figure 13.5), the H_a nucleus is affected by two nearby H_b nuclei, and can experience four different states: $\alpha\alpha$, $\alpha\beta$, $\beta\alpha$, or $\beta\beta$.

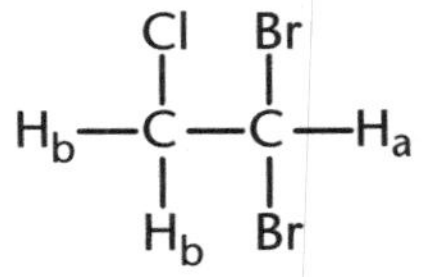

Figure 13.5

The $\alpha\beta$ and $\beta\alpha$ states have the same net effect on the H_a nucleus, and the resonances occur at the same frequency. The $\alpha\alpha$ and $\beta\beta$ states resonate at frequencies different from each other and from the $\alpha\beta/\beta\alpha$ frequency. The result is three peaks centered around the true chemical shift with an area ratio of 1:2:1. In general, n hydrogen atoms couple to give $n + 1$ peaks, whose area ratios are given by Pascal's triangle, shown in Table 13.2.

Table 13.2. Pascal's Triangle

Number of Adjacent Hydrogens	Total Number of Peaks	Area Ratios
0	1	1
1	2	1:1
2	3	1:2:1
3	4	1:3:3:1
4	5	1:4:6:4:1
5	6	1:5:10:10:5:1
6	7	1:6:15:20:15:6:1
7	8	1:7:21:35:35:21:7:1

Table 13.3 indicates the chemical shift ranges of several different types of protons:

Table 13.3. Chemical Shifts

Type of Proton	Approximate Chemical Shift δ (ppm) Downfield from TMS
RCH_3	0.9
RCH_2	1.25
R_3CH	1.5
$-CH=CH$	4.6–6.0
$-C\equiv CH$	2.0–3.0
Ar–H	6.0–8.5
–CHX	2.0–4.5
–CHOH/–CHOR	3.4–4.0
RCHO	9.0–10.0
RCHCO–	2.0–2.5
–CHCOOH/–CHCOOR	2.0–2.6
–CHOH–CH_2OH	1.0–5.5
ArOH	4.0–12.0
–COOH	10.5–12.0
–NH_2	1.0–5.0

> **KEY CONCEPT**
>
> Proton MR is good for
> 1. determining the relative number of protons and their relative chemical environments.
> 2. showing how many adjacent protons there are by splitting patterns.
> 3. showing certain functional groups.

C. ^{13}C-NMR

^{13}C-NMR is very similar to ^{1}H-NMR. Most ^{13}C-NMR signals, however, occur 0–200 δ downfield from the carbon peak of TMS. Another significant difference is that only 1.1 percent of carbon atoms are ^{13}C atoms. This has two effects: First, a much larger sample is needed to run a ^{13}C spectrum (about 50 mg compared with 1 mg for ^{1}H-NMR), and second, coupling between carbon atoms is generally not observed.

Coupling *is* observed, however, between carbon atoms and the protons directly attached to them. This one-bond coupling is analogous to the three-bond coupling in ^{1}H-NMR. For example, if a carbon atom is attached to two protons, it can experience four different states of those protons, and the carbon signal is split into a triplet with the area ratio 1:2:1.

An additional feature of ^{13}C-NMR is the ability to record a spectrum *without* the coupling of adjacent protons. This is called **spin decoupling**, and it produces a spectrum of **singlets**, each corresponding to a separate, magnetically equivalent carbon atom. For example, compare two spectra of 1,1,2-trichloropropane. One (Figure 13.6) is a typical **spin-decoupled spectrum**, and the other (Figure 13.7) is spin coupled.

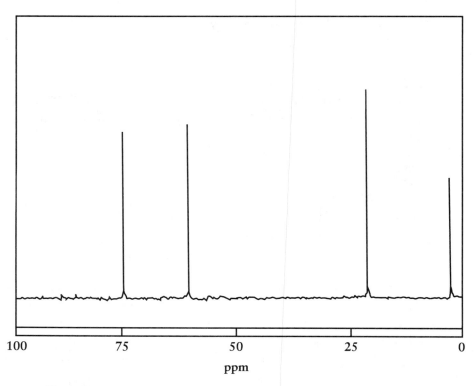

Figure 13.6. Spin-Decoupled Spectrum of 1,1,2-Trichloropropane

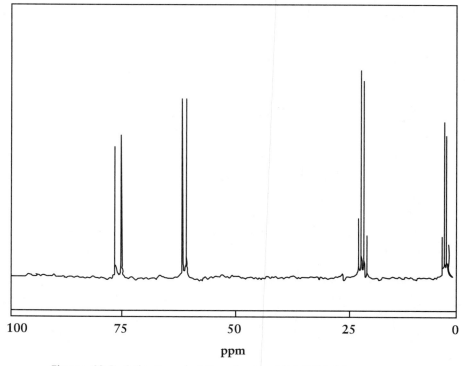

Figure 13.7. Spin-Coupled Spectrum of 1,1,2-Trichloropropane

In general, NMR spectroscopy provides information about the carbon skeleton of a compound, along with some suggestion of its functional groups. Specifically, NMR can provide the following types of information:

1. the number of nonequivalent nuclei, determined from the number of peaks
2. the magnetic environment of a nucleus, determined by the chemical shift
3. the relative numbers of nuclei, determined by integrating the peak areas
4. the number of neighboring nuclei, determined by the splitting pattern observed (except for ^{13}C in the spin-decoupled mode)

ULTRAVIOLET SPECTROSCOPY

A. Basic Theory

Ultraviolet spectra are obtained by passing ultraviolet light through a chemical sample (usually dissolved in an inert, nonabsorbing solvent) and plotting absorbance versus wavelength. The wavelength of maximum absorbance provides information on the extent of the conjugated system, as well as other structural and compositional information.

> **KEY CONCEPT**
>
> UV spectroscopy is most useful for studying compounds containing double bonds and/or hetero atoms with lone pairs.

MASS SPECTROMETRY

A. Basic Theory

Mass spectrometry differs from the methods thus far discussed in that it is not true spectroscopy (i.e., no absorption of electromagnetic radiation is involved) and in that it is a destructive technique—mass spectrometry, does not allow for reuse of the sample once the analysis is complete. Most commonly used mass spectrometers utilize a high-speed beam of electrons to ionize the sample to be analyzed, a particle accelerator to put the charged particles in flight, a magnetic field to deflect the accelerated cationic fragments, and a detector that records the number of particles of each mass exiting the deflector area. The initially formed ion is the molecular cation-radical (M^+) resulting from a single electron being removed from a molecule of the sample. This unstable species usually decomposes rapidly into a cationic fragment and a radical fragment. Since there are many molecules in the sample and (usually) more than one way for the initially formed cation-radical to decompose into fragments, a typical mass spectrum is composed of many lines, each corresponding to a specific mass/charge ratio (*m/e*). The spectrum itself plots mass/charge on the horizontal axis and relative abundance of the various cationic fragments on the vertical axis (see Figure 13.8).

B. Characteristics

The tallest peak, belonging to the most common ion, is called the **base peak**, and it is assigned the relative abundance value of 100 percent. The peak with the highest m/e ratio (see Figure 13.8) is generally the **molecular ion peak (parent ion peak)**, **M+**, from which the molecular weight, M, can be obtained. The charge value is usually 1; hence, the m/e ratio can usually be read as the mass of the fragment.

C. Application

Fragmentation patterns often provide information that helps identify or distinguish certain compounds. In particular, the fragmentation pattern provides clues to the compound's structure. For example, while IR spectroscopy would be of little use in distinguishing between propionaldehyde and butyraldehyde, a mass spectrum would allow unambiguous identification.

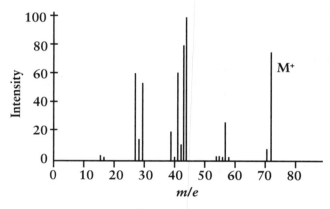

Figure 13.8

Figure 13.8 shows the mass spectrum of butyraldehyde. The peak at $m/e = 72$ corresponds to the molecular cation-radical, M^+, while the base peak at $m/e = 44$ corresponds to the cationic fragment resulting from the loss of a C_2H_4 neutral fragment ($M - 28 = 44$). Other peaks of note include those at $57(M - 15$, loss of CH_3 radical), $43(M - 29$, loss of C_2H_5 radical), and at 29 ($M - 43$, loss of C_3H_7 radical). The small peak at $m/e = 15$ can be attributed to the unstable (and therefore not abundant) methyl cation.

Carbohydrates

14

Carbohydrates are compounds containing carbon, hydrogen, and oxygen in the form of polyhydroxylated aldehydes or ketones. They have the general formula $C_n(H_2O)_n$ and serve many functions in biological systems, most notably as the chemical energy source for most organisms. A single carbohydrate unit is a **monosaccharide** (simple sugar), and a molecule with two sugars is a **disaccharide**. **Oligosaccharides** are short carbohydrate chains, while **polysaccharides** are long carbohydrate chains.

> **KEY CONCEPT**
>
> Carbohydrates are aldehydes or ketones with many hydroxyl groups.

MONOSACCHARIDES

Monosaccharides are single sugar subunits. Examples of monosaccharides include fructose, glucose, galactose, and mannose. Monosacchaides are classified according to the number of carbons they possess.

For example, **trioses**, **tetroses**, **pentoses**, and **hexoses** have 3, 4, 5, and 6 carbons, respectively. The basic structure of monosaccharides is exemplified by the simplest, glyceraldehyde.

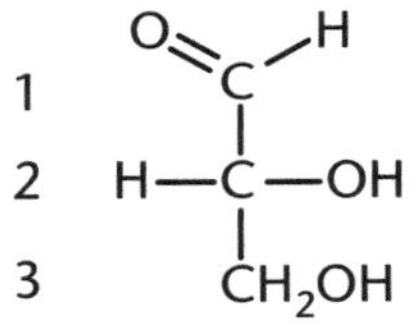

> **KEY CONCEPT**
>
> Monosaccharides are the simplest units and are classified by the number of carbons.

Figure 14.1. Glyceraldehyde

Glyceraldehyde is a polyhydroxylated aldehyde or **aldose** (aldehyde sugar). A polyhydroxylated ketone is called a **ketose** (ketone sugar). The numbering of the carbon atoms in a monosaccharide begins with the end closest to the carbonyl group.

> **REMEMBER**
>
> As usual, number the molecule from the end closest to the carbonyl.

A. Stereochemistry

The stereochemistry of monosaccharides can be understood by studying the enantiomeric configurations of glyceraldehyde (see Figure 14.2).

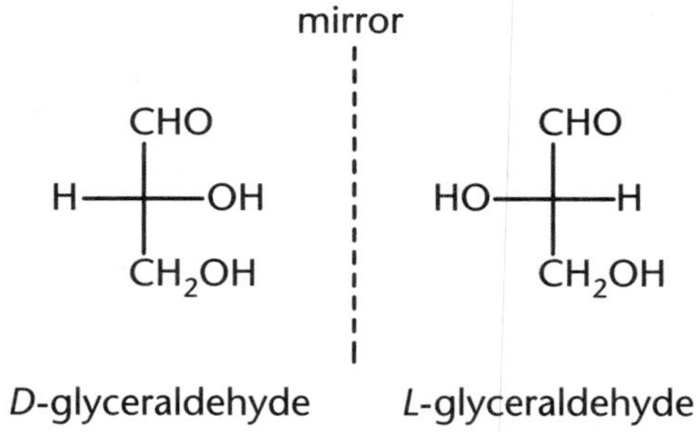

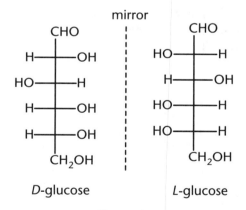

Figure 14.2

The *D* and *L* configurations of glyceraldehyde were assigned early in this century (before the *R* and *S* configurations were used) to designate the optical rotation of each enantiomer. *D*-glyceraldehyde was later determined to exhibit a positive rotation (designated as *D*-(+)-glyceraldehyde), and *L*-glyceraldehyde a negative rotation (designated as *L*-(–)-glyceraldehyde. However, other monosaccharides are assigned the *D* or *L* configuration depending on their relationship to glyceraldehyde: A molecule whose highest-numbered chiral center (the chiral center farthest from the carbonyl) has the same configuration as *D*-(+)-glyceraldehyde is classed as a *D*-sugar. A molecule that has its highest-numbered chiral center in the same configuration as *L*-(–)-glyceraldehyde is classed as an *L*-sugar. This is illustrated Figure 14.3.

Figure 14.3

Monosaccharide stereoisomers are divided into two optical families, *D* and *L*; the stereoisomers within one family are known as **diastereomers**. Aldose diastereomers that differ only about the configuration of one carbon are known as **epimers**. For instance, *D*-ribose and *D*-arabinose are pentose epimers. They differ in configuration only at C–2 (see Figure 14.4). Some important monosaccharides are shown in Figure 14.5.

KEY CONCEPT

The *D* and *L* designations are based on the sterochemistry of glyceraldehyde. Further, they are enantiomers.

REMEMBER

If Lowest –OH is on the Left, the molecule is L. If the –OH is on the Right, it's D (from the Latin root dextro, meaning "right").

KEY CONCEPT

Epimers differ in configuration at only one carbon.

REMEMBER

Fructose is a ketose while glucose, galactose, and mannose are all aldoses.

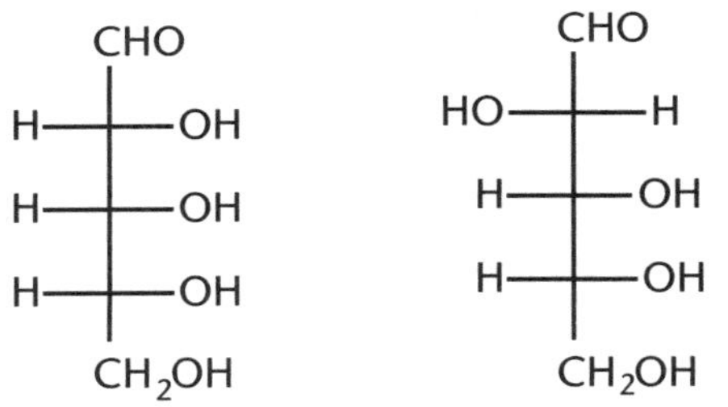

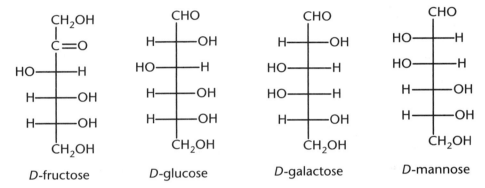

D-ribose *D*-arabinose

Figure 14.4

D-fructose *D*-glucose *D*-galactose *D*-mannose

Figure 14.5

B. Ring Properties

Because monosaccharides contain both a hydroxyl group and a carbonyl group, they can undergo intramolecular reactions to form cyclic hemiacetals (or hemiketals, in the case of ketoses). These cyclic molecules are stable in solution and may exist as six-membered **pyranose** rings (as in glucose) or five-membered **furanose** rings. Like cyclohexane, the pyranose rings adopt a chairlike configuration, and the substituents assume axial or equatorial positions so as to minimize steric hindrance. When converting the monosaccharide from its straight-chain Fischer projection to the Haworth projection (shown in Figure 14.6), it is important to remember that any group on the right of the Fischer projection will be pointing down, while any group on the left side of the Fischer projection will be pointing up. The following reaction scheme depicts the formation of a cyclic hemiacetal from *D*-glucose.

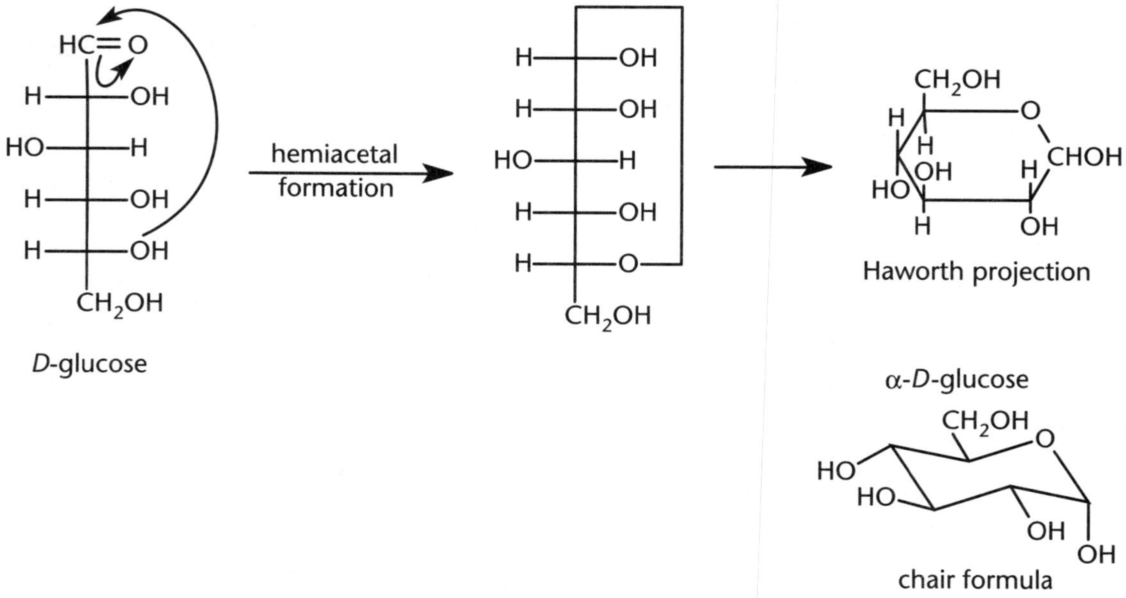

Figure 14.6

KEY CONCEPT

Anomers differ in configuration only at the newly formed chiral center.

α = down or axial. β = up.

When a straight-chain monosaccharide is converted to its cyclic form, the carbonyl carbon (C1 for glucose) becomes chiral. Cyclic stereoisomers differing about the new chiral carbon are known as **anomers**. In glucose, the alpha anomer has the –OH group of C1 *trans* (or *a*xial) to the CH_2OH substituent (down), while the beta anomer has the –OH group of C1 *cis* to the CH_2OH substituent (up).

When exposed to water, hemiacetal rings spontaneously open and then reform. Because of bond rotation between C1 and C2, either the alpha or beta anomer may be formed. The reaction is more rapid when catalyzed by an acid or a base. The spontaneous change of configuration about C1 is known as **mutarotation**, and it results in a mixture containing both anomers in their equilibrium concentrations (for glucose, 36 percent alpha:64 percent beta). The alpha configuration is less favored because the hydroxyl group of C1 is axial, making the molecule more sterically strained.

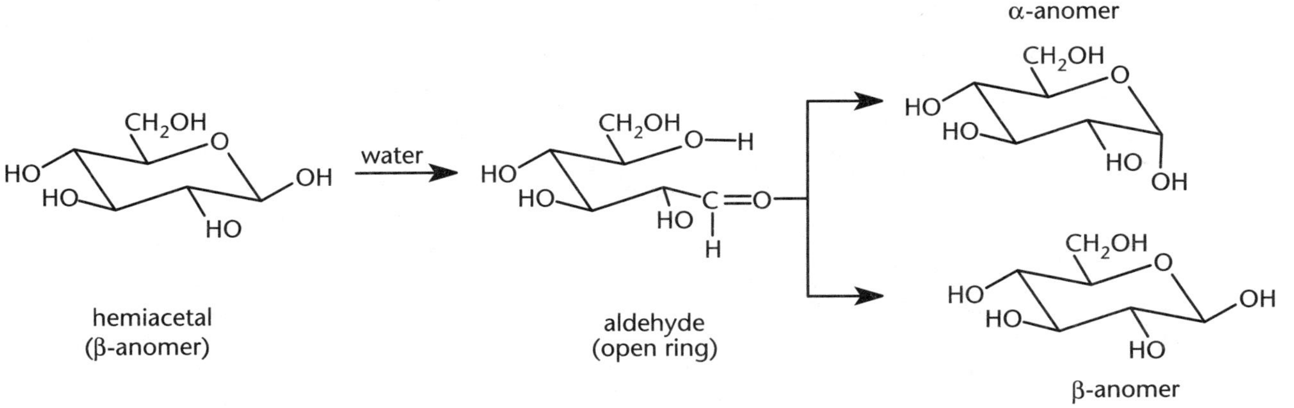

Figure 14.7

C. Monosaccharide Reactions

1. ESTER FORMATION

Monosaccharides contain hydroxyl groups and can undergo many of the same reactions as simple alcohols. Therefore, they may be converted to either esters or ethers. In the presence of acid anhydride and base, all of the hydroxyl groups will be esterified. The reaction shown in Figure 14.8 is an example of glucose esterification.

> **KEY CONCEPT**
>
> Reaction types are determined by the functional groups that are present. Think of alcohols and carbonyls.

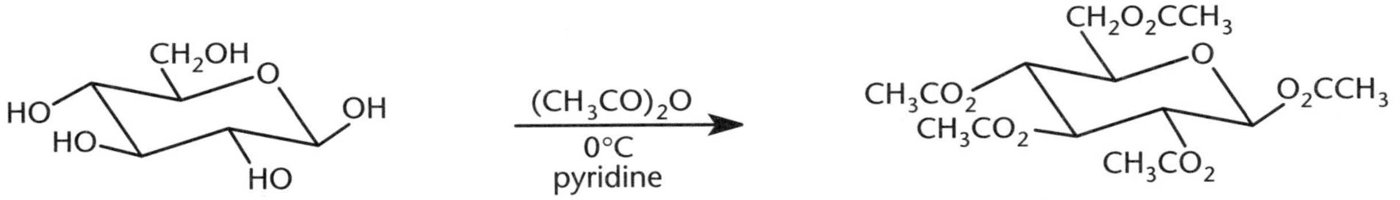

β-D-glucose   penta-O-acetyl- β-D-glucose

Figure 14.8

2. OXIDATION OF MONOSACCHARIDES

As they switch between anomeric configurations, the hemiacetal rings spend a short time in the open-chain aldehyde form. Like all aldehydes, these can be oxidized to carboxylic acids called **aldonic acids**. Thus, the aldoses are reducing agents. Any monosaccharide with a hemiacetal ring (–OH on C1) is considered a **reducing sugar** and can be oxidized. Both Tollens' reagent and Benedict's reagent can be used to detect the presence of reducing sugars. A positive Tollens' test involves the reduction of Ag^+ to form metallic silver. When Benedict's reagent is used, a red precipitate of Cu_2O indicates the presence of a reducing sugar. Ketose sugars are also reducing sugars and give positive Tollen's and Benedict's tests, because they can isomerize to aldoses via keto-enol shifts.

> **KEY CONCEPT**
>
> Key reactions of monosaccharides include:
> - ester formation
> - oxidation
> - glycosidic reactions

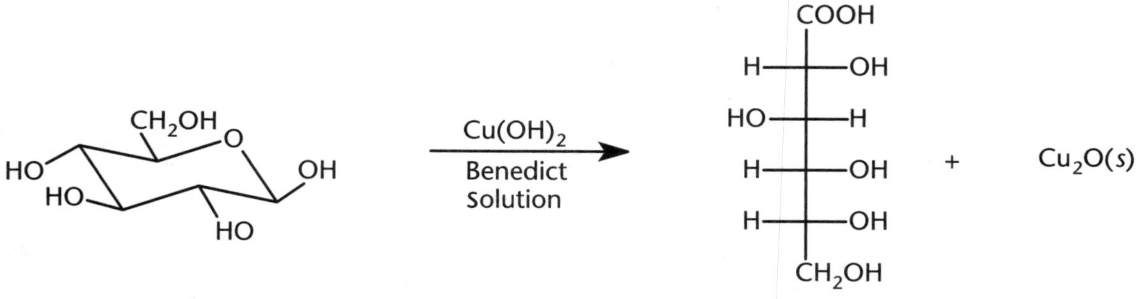

β-*D*-glucose → [Cu(OH)₂ / Benedict Solution] → *D*-gluconic acid (an aldonic acid) + Cu₂O(s) (red solid)

Figure 14.9

3. GLYCOSIDIC REACTIONS

Hemiacetal monosaccharides will react with alcohols under acidic conditions. The anomeric hydroxyl group is transformed into an alkoxy group, yielding a mixture of the alpha and beta acetals. The resulting bond is called a **glycosidic linkage**, and the acetal is known as a **glycoside**. An example is the reaction of glucose with ethanol (see Figure 14.1). Glycosides do not mutarotate and are stable in water.

β-*D*-glucose → [C_2H_5OH / HCl] → ethyl-α-*D*-glucoside (an acetal) + ethyl-β-*D*-glucoside (an acetal) + H_2O

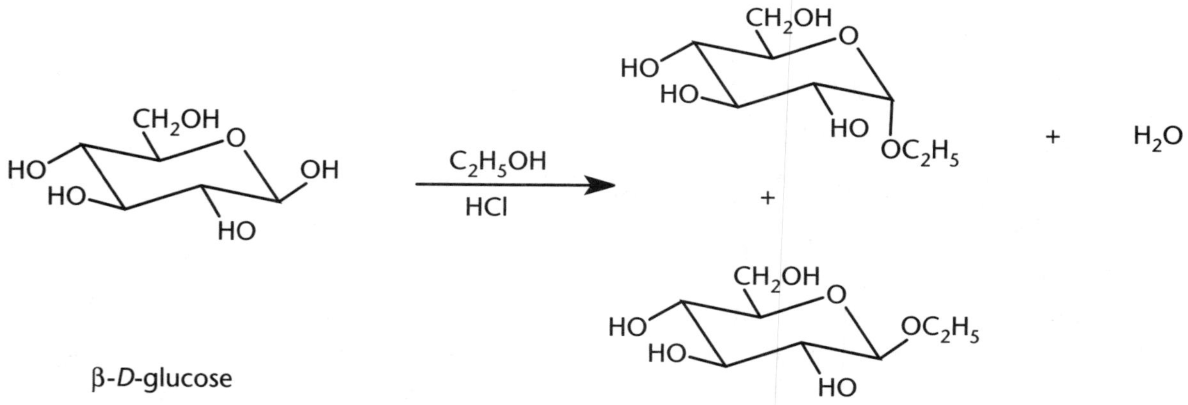

Figure 14.10

DISACCHARIDES

As discussed above, a monosaccharide may react with alcohols to give acetals. When that alcohol is another monosaccharide, the product is called a **disaccharide**. The formation of a disaccharide is shown in Figure 14.11.

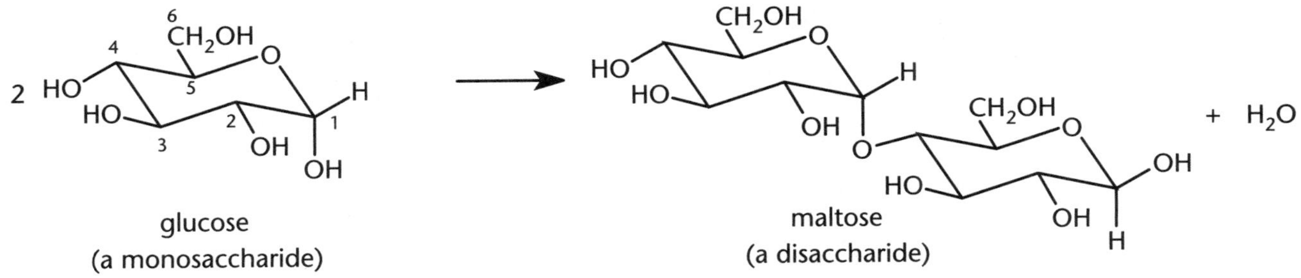

Figure 14.11

The most common glycosidic linkage occurs between C1 of the first sugar and C4 of the second, and it is designated as a 1,4' link; 1,6' and 1,2' bonds are also observed. The glycosidic bonds may be either alpha or beta, depending on the orientation of the hydroxyl group on the anomeric carbon.

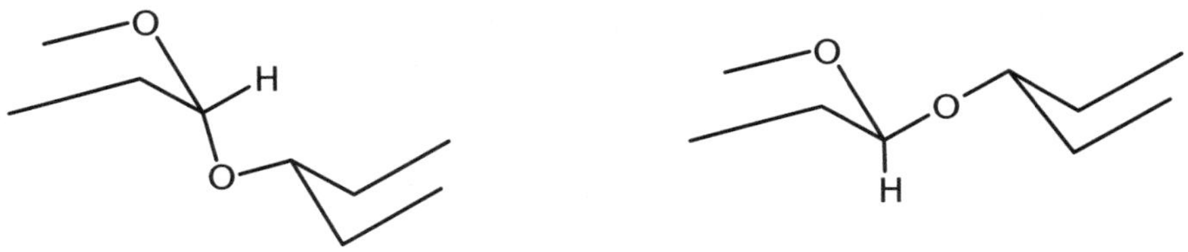

α-glycosidic linkage   β-glycosidic linkage

Figure 14.12

BRIDGE

In the body, enzymes are needed to ensure that the correct glycosidic linkages form. Without enzymes, the reactions are nonspecific and tend to keep going, never stopping at the disaccharide level.

These glycosidic linkages can often be cleaved in the presence of aqueous acid. For example, the glycosidic linkage of maltose, a disaccharide, can be cleaved to yield two molecules of glucose.

POLYSACCHARIDES

Polysaccharides are formed via linkage of monosaccharide units with glycosidic bonds. The three most important biological polysaccharides are **cellulose**, **starch**, and **glycogen**. Cellulose is comprised of D-glucose linked by 1,4'-beta-glycosidic bonds. Cellulose is the structural component of plants. Starch stores energy in plants, and glycogen stores energy in animals; both are formed by linking glucose units in 1,4'-alpha-glycosidic bonds, with occasional 1,6'-alpha-glycosidic bonds creating branches. While all three are composed of glucose subunits, the orientation about the anomeric carbon

BRIDGE

Key biological polysaccharides:
- Cellulose (1,4' beta)
- Starch and glycogen (mostly 1,4' alpha; some 1,6' alpha)

gives them biological differences. Cellulose cannot be digested by humans, while starch and glycogen can and are important energy sources for living organisms.

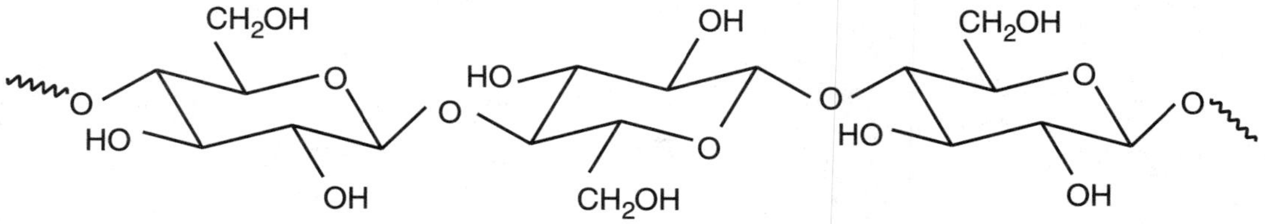

cellulose, a 1,4', -β-*D*-glucose polymer

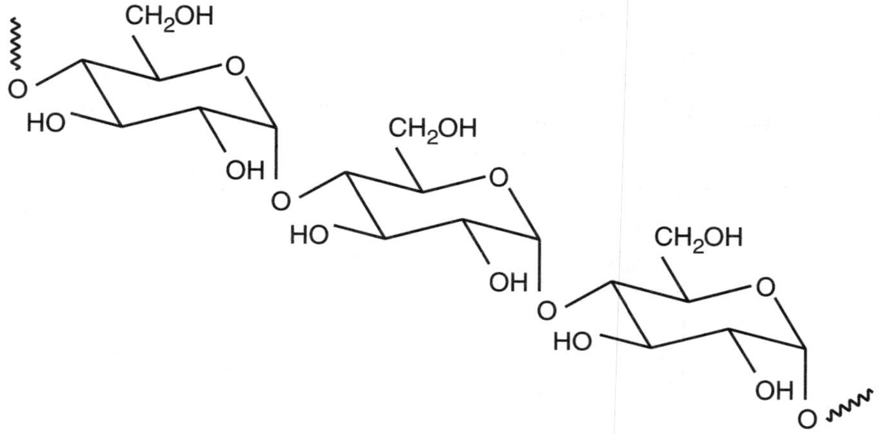

starch, a 1,4', -α-*D*-glucose polymer

Figure 14.13

15

Amino Acids, Peptides, and Proteins

Proteins are large polymers composed of many amino acid subunits. Proteins have diverse biological roles; for example, they provide structure (keratin, collagen), regulate body metabolism via hormonal control (insulin), and serve as catalysts (enzymes).

AMINO ACIDS

Amino acids contain an amine group and a carboxyl group attached to a single carbon atom (the alpha carbon atom). The other two substituents of the alpha carbon are usually a hydrogen atom and a variable side chain referred to as the **R-group**.

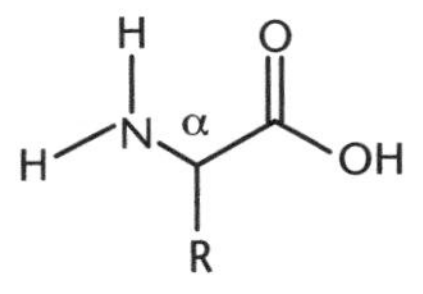

Figure 15.1

The alpha carbon is a chiral center (except in glycine, the simplest amino acid, where R=H), and thus all amino acids (except for glycine) are optically active. Naturally occurring amino acids (of which there are 20) are *L*-enantiomers.

By convention, the Fischer projection for an amino acid is drawn with the amino group on the left (see Figure 15.2).

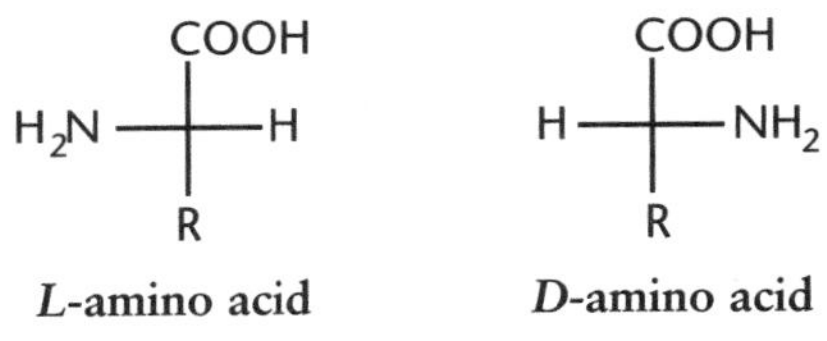

L-amino acid   *D*-amino acid

Figure 15.2

A. Acid-Base Characteristics

Amino acids have an acidic carboxyl group and a basic amino group on the same molecule. As a result, when they are in solution, amino acids sometimes take the form of dipolar ions, or **zwitterions** (from German *zwitter,* hybrid). The two halves of the molecules neutralize each other so that at neutral pH, they exist in the form of internal salts.

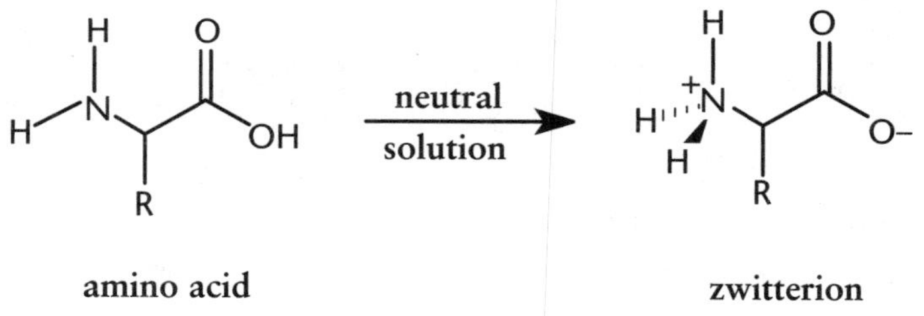

amino acid   zwitterion

Figure 15.3

Amino acids are **amphoteric** (i.e., they may act as either acids or bases, depending on their environment). Amino acids in acidic solution (see Figure 15.4) are fully protonated. Since they have two protons that can dissociate—one from the carboxyl group and one from the amino group—amino acids have at least two dissociation constants, K_{a1} and K_{a2}.

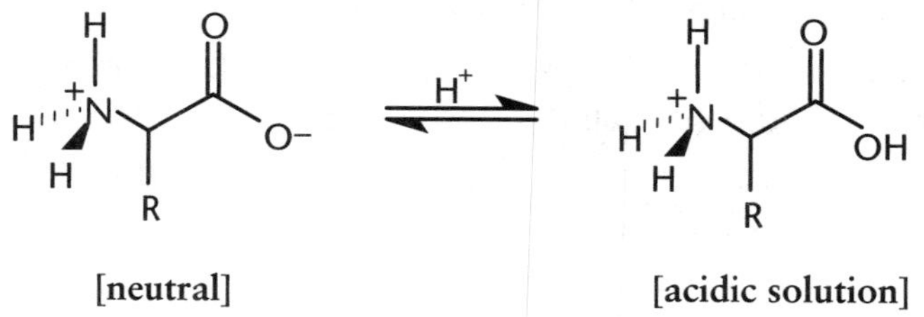

[neutral]   [acidic solution]

Figure 15.4

Amino acids in basic solution (see Figure 15.5) are deprotonated. They have two proton-accepting groups and, therefore, at least two dissociation constants, K_{b1} and K_{b2}.

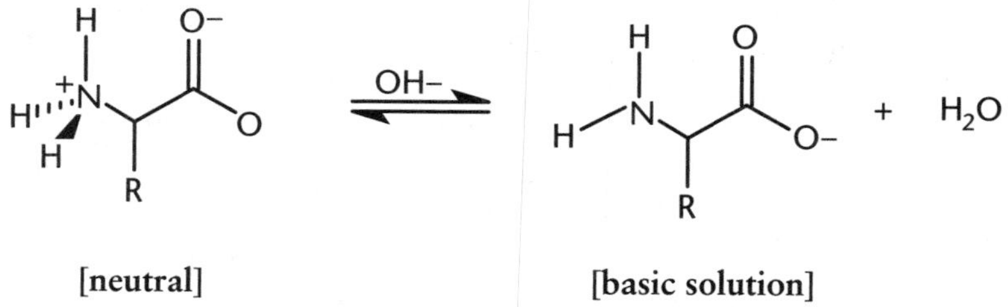

[neutral]   [basic solution]

Figure 15.5

At low pH, the amino acid carries an excess positive charge, and at high pH, the amino acid carries an excess negative charge. The intermediate pH, at which the amino acid is electrically neutral and exists as a zwitterion, is the **isoelectric point (pI)**, or **isoelectric pH**, of the amino acid.

The isoelectric pH lies between pK_{a1} and pK_{a2}.

B. Titration of Amino Acids

Because of their acidic and basic properties, amino acids can be titrated. The titration of each proton occurs as a distinct step resembling that of a simple monoprotic acid. The titration curve of glycine is shown in Figure 15.6.

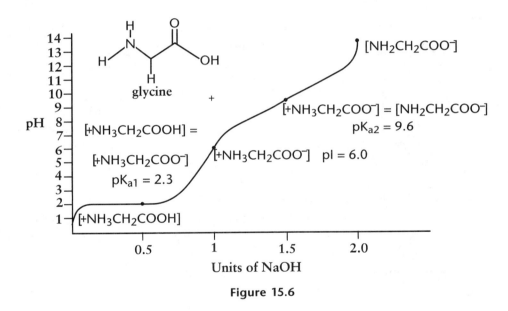

Figure 15.6

A 1M glycine solution is acidic; the glycine exists predominantly as $^+NH_3CH_2COOH$. The amino acid is fully protonated and carries a positive charge. As the solution is titrated with NaOH, carboxyl groups lose a proton. During this stage, the amino acid acts as a buffer, and the pH changes very slowly. When 0.5 mol of base has been added to the amino acid solution, the concentrations of $^+NH_3CH_2COOH$ and $^+NH_3CH_2COO^-$ (its zwitterion) are equimolar. At this point, the pH is equal to the pK_{a1}, and the solution is buffered against pH changes.

As more base is added, all of the carboxyl groups are deprotonated. The amino acid loses buffering capacity, and thus the pH rises more rapidly. When 1 mol of base has been added, glycine exists predominantly as $^+NH_3CH_2COO^-$. The amino acid is now electrically neutral; the pH is equal to glycine's pI.

Glycine passes through a second buffering stage during which pH change is slow because continued titration deprotonates amino groups. When 1.5 mol of base have been added, the concentrations of $^+NH_3CH_2COO^-$ and $NH_2CH_2COO^-$ are equimolar, and the pH is equal to pK_{a2}.

As another 0.5 mol of base is added, all of the amino groups are deprotonated to $NH_2CH_2COO^-$; glycine is now completely deprotonated.

Certain things should be noted about the titration of amino acids:

1. When adding base, the carboxyl group loses its proton first; after all of the carboxyl groups are fully deprotonated, the amino group loses its acidic proton.

2. Two moles of base must be added in order to deprotonate one mole of most amino acids. The first mole deprotonates the carboxyl group, while the second mole deprotonates the amino group.

3. The buffering capacity of the amino acid is greatest at or near the two dissociation constants, K_{a1} and K_{a2}. At the isoelectric point, its buffering capacity is minimal.

4. It is possible to perform the titration in reverse, from alkaline pH to acidic pH, with the addition of acid; the sequence of events is reversed.

C. Henderson-Hasselbalch Equation

The ratio of an amino acid's ions are dependent on pH. The **Henderson-Hasselbalch equation** defines the relationship between pH and the ratio of conjugate acid to conjugate base, and it provides a mathematical expression for the dissociation constants of amino acids.

$$pH = pK_a + \log \frac{[\text{conjugate base}]}{[\text{conjugate acid}]}$$

When the pK_{a1} of glycine is known, the ratio of conjugate acid to conjugate base for a particular pH can be determined. For example, at pH 3.3, glycine, which has a pK_a of 2.3, will have these ratios:

$$3.3 = 2.3 + \log \frac{[H_3N^+CH_2COO^-]}{[H_3N^+CH_2COOH]}$$

By subtraction: $\log \dfrac{[H_3N^+CH_2COO^-]}{[H_3N^+CH_2COOH]} = 1$

The antilog of 1 = 10. Thus: $\dfrac{[H_3N^+CH_2COO^-]}{[H_3N^+CH_2COOH]} = \dfrac{10}{1}$

So, in this example, there are ten times as many zwitterions as there are of the fully protonated form.

The Henderson-Hasselbalch equation can be used experimentally to prepare buffer solutions of amino acids. The best buffering regions of amino acids occur within one pH unit of the pK_a or pK_b. For example, the carboxyl group of glycine, which has a pK_a of 2.3, shows high buffering capacity between pH 1.3 and 3.3.

D. Amino Acid Side Chains

Amino acid side chains (R-groups) give chemical diversity to the backbone of the amino acid molecule. They also give proteins some distinguishing features. The 20 amino acids are classified according to whether their side chains are **nonpolar, polar** (but uncharged), **acidic,** or **basic**.

1. NONPOLAR AMINO ACIDS

Nonpolar amino acids (see Figure 15.7) have R-groups that are saturated hydrocarbons. The R-groups are hydrophobic and decrease the solubility of the amino acid in water. Amino acids with nonpolar side chains are usually found buried within protein molecules, away from the aqueous cellular environment.

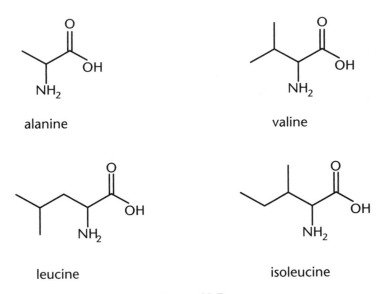

alanine

valine

leucine

isoleucine

Figure 15.7a

> **KEY CONCEPT**
>
> Nonpolar amino acids are often found at the core of globular proteins or in trans-membrane regions of proteins that are in contact with the hydrophobic portion of the phospholipid membrane.

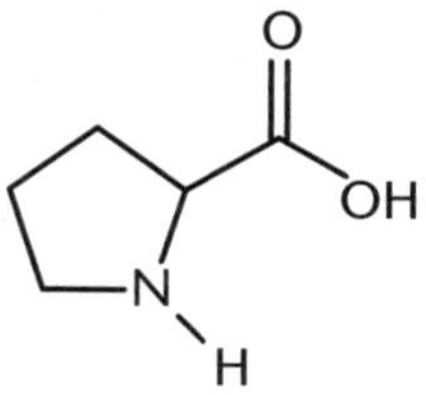

proline

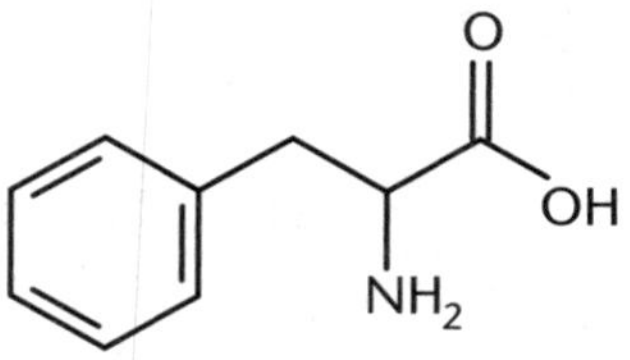

phenylalanine

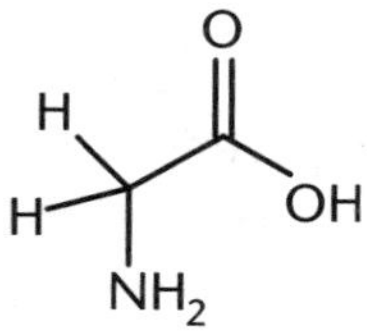

glycine

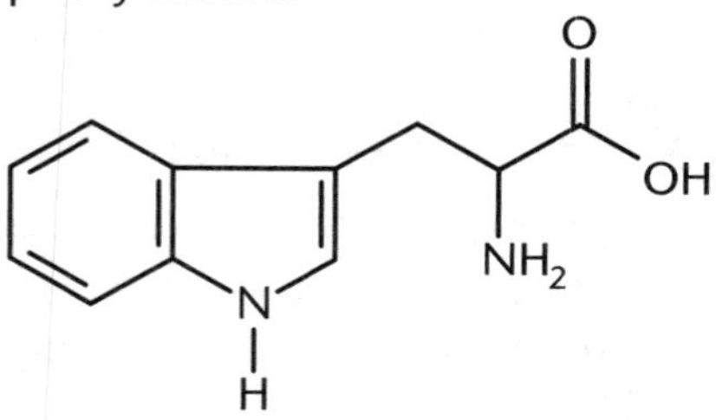

tryptophan

Figure 15.7b

KEY CONCEPT

The other types of amino acids (polar, acidic, and basic) are found in regions of proteins that are exposed to the aqueous, polar environment.

2. POLAR AMINO ACIDS

Polar amino acids (see Figure 15.8) have polar, uncharged R-groups that are hydrophilic, increasing the solubility of the amino acid in water. They are usually found on protein surfaces.

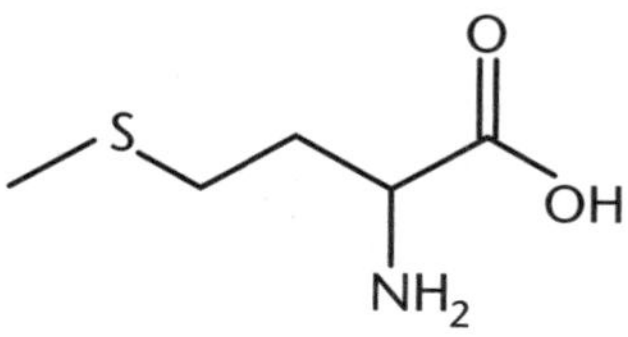

methionine

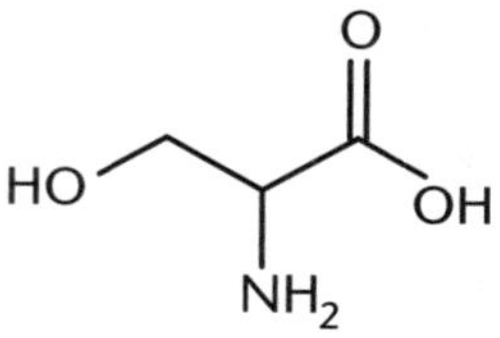

serine

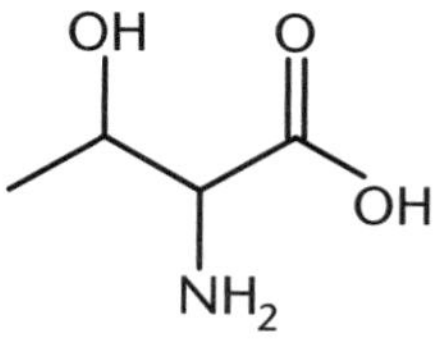

threonine

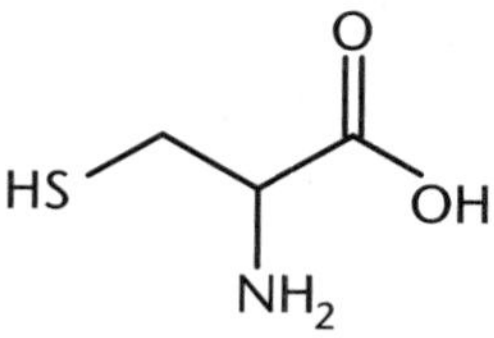

cysteine

Figure 15.8a

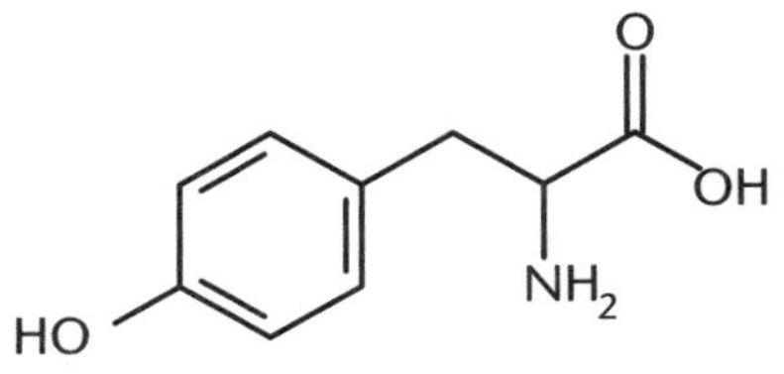

tyrosine

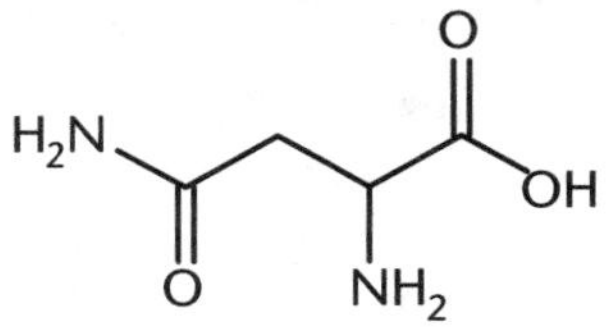

asparagine

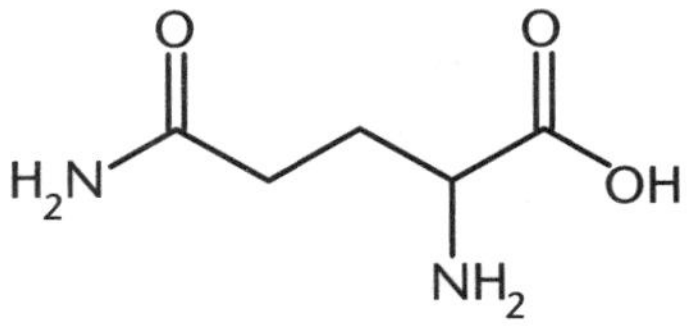

glutamine

Figure 15.8b

3. ACIDIC AMINO ACIDS

Amino acids whose R-group contains a carboxyl group are called acidic amino acids (see Figure 15.9). They have a net negative charge at physiological pH (pH 7.4) and exist in salt form in the body. They often play important roles in the substrate-binding sites of enzymes.

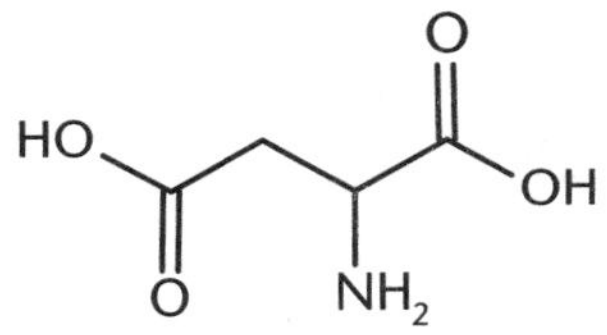

aspartic acid

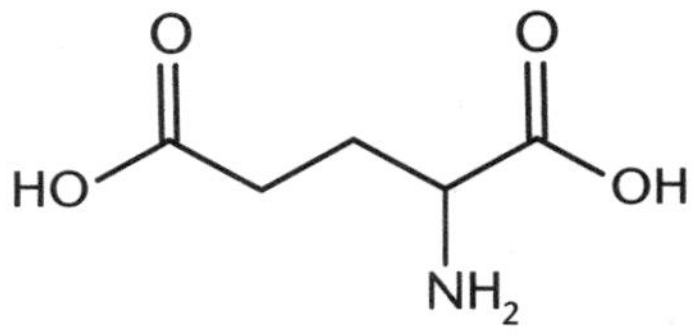

glutamic acid

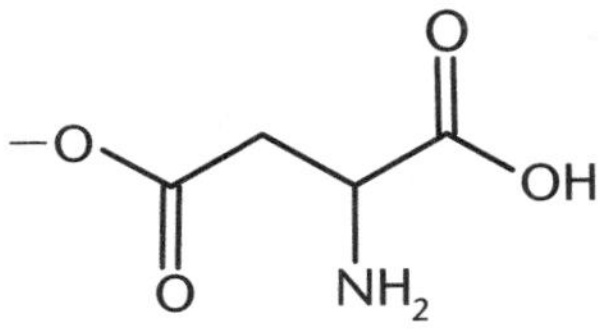

(salt is aspartate)

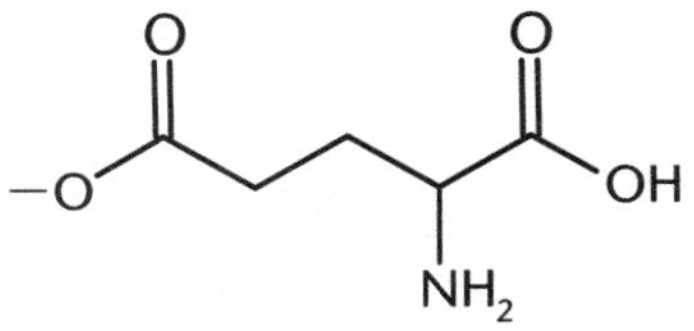

(salt is glutamate)

Figure 15.9

Aspartic acid and glutamic acid each have three groups that must be neutralized during titration (two –COOH and one –NH₃⁺). Therefore, their titration curve is different from the standard curve for amino acids (exemplified by glycine). The molecule has three distinct dissociation constants—pK_{a1}, pK_{a2}, and pK_{a3}—although the neutralization curves of the two carboxyl groups overlap to a certain extent. Because of the additional carboxyl group, the isoelectric point is shifted towards an acidic pH. Three moles of base are needed to deprotonate one mole of an acidic amino acid.

4. BASIC AMINO ACIDS

Amino acids whose R-group contains an amino group are called basic amino acids and carry a net positive charge at physiological pH (see Figure 15.10).

KEY CONCEPT

At physiological pH, basic amino acids have a net positive charge. They also have three dissociation constants.

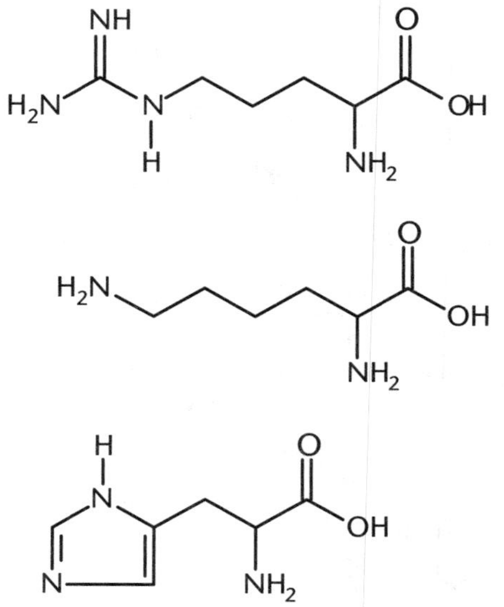

arginine

lysine

histidine

Figure 15.10

KEY CONCEPT

You can use pI to predict an amino acid's charge at a given pH.

- If pH < pI, think positive charge.
- If pH > pI, think negative charge.

The titration curve of amino acids with basic R-groups is modified by the additional amino group that must be neutralized. Although basic amino acids have three dissociation constants, the neutralization curves for the two amino groups overlap. The isoelectric point is shifted toward an alkaline pH. Three moles of acid are needed to neutralize one mole of a basic amino acid.

Understanding titration curves and isoelectric points helps predict the charge of particular amino acids at a given pH. For example, in a mixture of glycine, glutamic acid, and lysine at pH 6.0, glycine will be neutral, glutamic acid will be negatively charged, and lysine will be positively charged.

REMEMBER

Amino acids can undergo electrophonesis. This is based on the isoelectric point, which is the pH at which the amino acid has a net zero charge.

PEPTIDES

Peptides are composed of amino acid subunits, sometimes called **residues,** linked by **peptide bonds**. Peptides are small proteins (the distinction between a peptide and protein is vague). Two amino acids joined together form a **dipeptide**, three form a **tripeptide**, and many amino acids linked together form a **polypeptide**.

BRIDGE

A peptide bond is an amide bond.

A. Reactions

Amino acids are joined by **peptide bonds** (amide bonds) between the carboxyl group of one amino acid and the amino group of another. This bond is formed via a condensation reaction (a reaction in which water is lost). The reverse reaction, hydrolysis (cleavage with the addition of water) of the peptide bond, is catalyzed by an acid or base.

Certain enzymes digest the chain at specific peptide linkages. For example, **trypsin** cleaves at the carboxyl end of arginine and lysine; chymotrypsin cleaves at the carboxyl end of phenylalanine, tyrosine, and tryptophan.

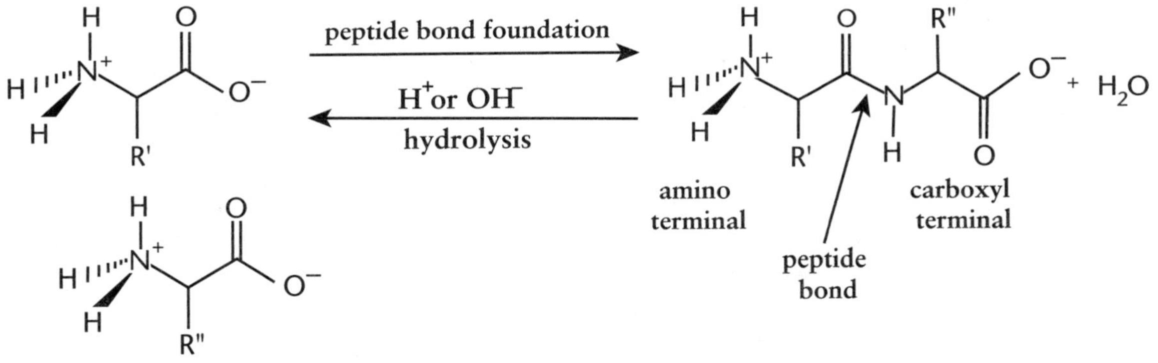

Figure 15.11

B. Properties

The terminal amino acid with a free alpha-amino group is known as the **amino-terminal** or **N-terminal** residue, while the terminal residue with a free carboxyl group is called the **carboxy-terminal** or **C-terminal** residue. By convention, peptides are drawn with the N-terminal end on the left and the C-terminal end on the right.

KEY CONCEPT

Rotation is limited around the peptide bond because resonance gives the C–N bond partial double-bond character.

Amides have two resonance structures, and the true structure is a hybrid with partial double-bond character. As a result, rotation about the C–N bond is restricted. The bonds on either side of the peptide unit, however, have a great deal of rotational freedom.

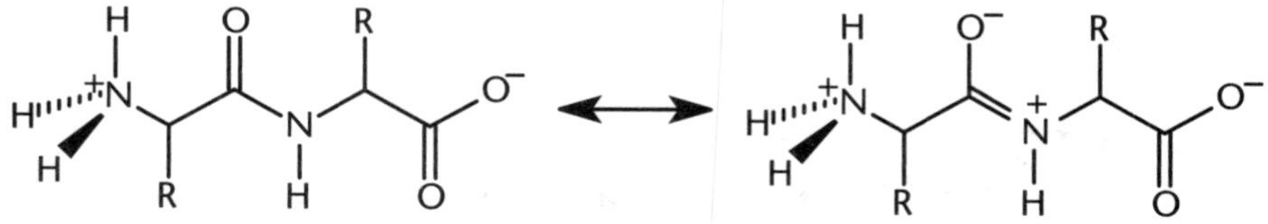

Figure 15.12

PROTEINS

Proteins are polypeptides that can range from only a few to more than a thousand amino acids in length. Proteins serve many diverse functions in biological systems, acting as enzymes, hormones, membrane pores, receptors, and elements of cell structure. Four structural levels of protein structure—**primary, secondary, tertiary,** and **quaternary**—are described below.

A. Primary Structure

The primary structure of the protein refers to the sequence of amino acids, listed from the N-terminus to the C-terminus, linked by covalent bonds between neighboring residues in the chain.

The higher-level structures of a protein are dependent on the primary sequence; in other words, a protein will assume whatever secondary, tertiary, and quaternary structures are most energetically favorable given its primary structure and environment. The primary structure of a protein can be determined using a laboratory procedure called **sequencing**.

B. Secondary Structure

The secondary structure of a protein refers to the local structure of neighboring amino acids, governed mostly by hydrogen bond interactions within and between peptide chains. The two most common types of secondary structures are the α-**helix** and the β-**pleated sheet**.

1. α-HELIX

The α-helix is a rod-like structure in which the peptide chain coils clockwise about a central axis. The helix is stabilized by intramolecular hydrogen bonds between carbonyl oxygen atoms and amine hydrogen atoms four residues away. The side chains point away from the structure's core and interact with the cellular environment. A typical protein with this structure is **keratin**, which is found in feathers and hair.

2. β-PLEATED SHEET

In β-pleated sheets, the peptide chains lie alongside each other in rows. The chains are held together by intramolecular hydrogen bonds between carbonyl oxygen atoms on one peptide chain and amine hydrogen atoms on another. To accommodate the maximum number of hydrogen bonds, the β-pleated sheet assumes a rippled, or pleated, shape (see Figure 15.14). The R-groups of the amino residues point above and below the plane of the β-pleated sheet. Silk fibers are composed of β-pleated sheets.

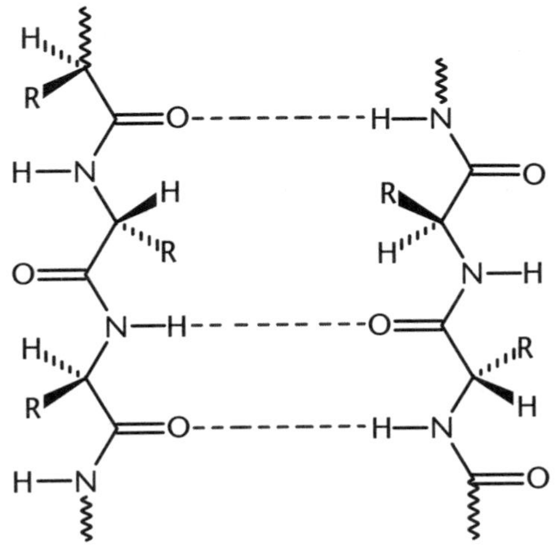

β-pleated sheet

Figure 15.13

C. Tertiary Structure

Tertiary structure refers to the three-dimensional shape of the protein, as determined by hydrophilic and hydrophobic interactions between the R-groups of amino acids that are far apart on the chain and by the distribution of disulfide bonds. In a disulfide bond, two **cysteine** molecules become oxidized to form **cystine**. Disulfide bonds create loops in the protein chain.

KEY CONCEPT

- Primary structure consists of the amino acid sequence.
- Secondary structure refers to the local structure of a protein, largely determined by hydrogen bond interactions within and between neighboring amino acids.
- Tertiary structure is the three- dimensional shape of the protein.
- Quaternary structure is the arrangement of polypeptide subunits.
- Conjugated proteins have prosthetic groups.

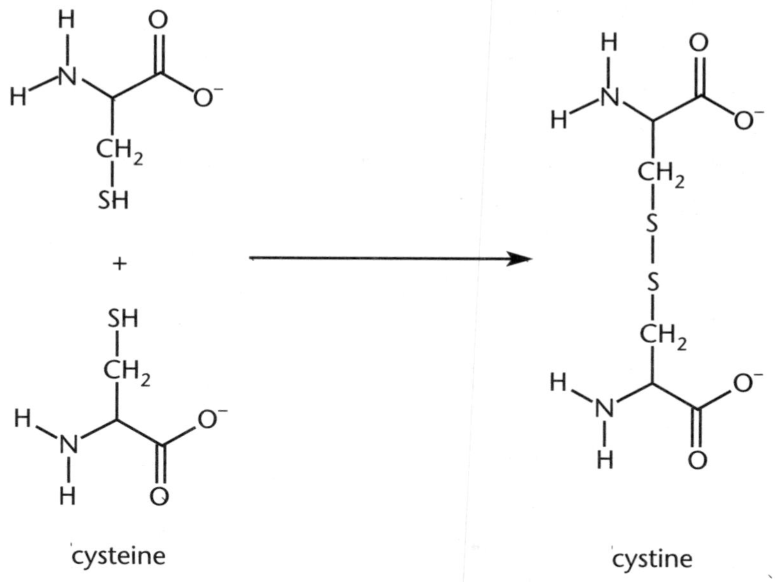
cysteine
cystine

Figure 15.14

REMEMBER

Think of:

- Primary structure as linear or one dimensional.
- Secondary structure as two dimensional.
- Tertiary structure as three dimensional.
- Quaternary structure as two chains bonding after each has attained tertiary structure.

Other amino acids have significant effects on tertiary structures as well. For instance, proline, because of its shape, cannot fit into an α-helix, thereby causing a kink in the chain.

Amino acids with hydrophilic (polar and charged) R-groups tend to arrange themselves toward the outside of the protein, where they interact with the aqueous cellular environment. Amino acids with hydrophobic R-groups tend to be found close together, protected from the aqueous environment by polar amino and carboxyl groups.

Proteins are divided into two major classifications on the basis of tertiary structure. **Fibrous proteins**, such as **collagen**, are found as sheets or long strands, while **globular proteins**, such as **myoglobin**, are spherical in shape.

D. Quaternary Structure

Some proteins contain more than one polypeptide subunit. The quaternary structure refers to the way in which these subunits arrange themselves to yield a functional protein molecule. **Hemoglobin**, which is composed of four polypeptide chains, possesses quaternary structure.

E. Conjugated Proteins

Certain proteins, known as **conjugated proteins**, derive part of their function from covalently attached molecules called **prosthetic groups**. Prosthetic groups may be organic molecules or metal ions. Many vitamins are prosthetic groups. Proteins with lipid, carbohydrate, and nucleic acid prosthetic groups are referred to as **lipoproteins**, **glycoproteins**, and **nucleoproteins**, respectively. Prosthetic groups play major roles in determining the function of the proteins with which they are associated. For example, the **heme group** carries oxygen in both myoglobin and hemoglobin. The heme is composed of an organic porphyrin ring with an iron atom bound in the center. Hemoglobin is inactive without the heme group.

F. Denaturation of Proteins

Denaturation, or **melting**, is a process in which proteins lose their three-dimensional structure and revert to a **random-coil** state. Denaturation can be caused by detergent or by changes in pH, temperature, or solute concentration. The weak intermolecular forces keeping the protein stable and functional are disrupted. When a protein denatures, the damage is usually permanent. However, certain gentle denaturing agents do not permanently disrupt the protein; removing the reagent might allow the protein to **renature** (regain its structure and function).

REAL-WORLD ANALOGY

Permanent denaturation occurs when cooking egg whites. They denature and form a solid, rubbery mass that cannot be transformed back to its clear liquid form.

VI

PHYSICS

Units and Kinematics

In this first chapter we will review some of the basic mathematics necessary for the study of OAT® physics, such as scientific notation, basic trigonometric functions, and vectors. In addition, the topic of units is presented with emphasis on the three systems of units that you need to be familiar with, i.e., MKS, CGS, and FPS. Finally, the topic of kinematics, which is the study of motion, is discussed. Here, a review is given of the basic quantities of displacement, speed, velocity, and acceleration. These basic quantities are then applied to the study of motion with constant acceleration. The case of one-dimensional motion is discussed, including an example of free-fall. The case of projectile motion, which is motion in two dimensions, is also covered in a detailed example.

UNITS

A. Fundamental Measurements and Dimensions

Physics is the most basic of all the sciences. Everything in the world around us is subject to the laws of physics. In order to describe nature, physicists use the language of mathematics, in the form of equations, to make their quantitative descriptions.

These descriptions, however, mean nothing if they are not expressed in some kind of units. While explaining how you were pulled over on the highway doing seventy might mean something amongst friends, a scientist would ask whether your speed was 70 miles per hour or 70 kilometers per hour or some other speed. Scientists have developed systems of units that give meaning to all the numbers in the formulas. The "British," or **FPS** system is commonly used in America but virtually nowhere else in the world (not even in Britain). Basic units for length, weight, and time are the foot (ft), the pound (lb), and the second (s), respectively. The most common system of units is the metric system where the basic units include length, mass (instead of weight like in FPS), and time. The metric system comes in two main variations. One

> **REMEMBER**
>
> Don't mix units! Your wrong answer may be one of the choices.

metric system uses meter (m), kilogram (kg), and second (s) as its base, and is referred to as **MKS** and also **SI** (SI being the initials of the French abbreviation for the International System of Units). The other metric system uses centimeter (cm), gram (g), and second (s), and is referred to as **CGS**. The **SI** system is becoming the standard.

The following chart lists some important units in the three different systems:

Some Important Units

Quantity	CGS	SI	FPS
Length	centimeter (cm)	meter (m)	foot (ft)
Mass	gram (g)	kilogram (kg)	slug (sl)
Force	dyne (dyn)	Newton (N)	pound (lb)
Time	second (s)	second (s)	second (s)
Work & Energy	erg	Joule (J)	foot-pound (ft•lb)
Power	erg/second	Watt (W)	foot-pound/sec

In atomic-sized systems, due to the extremely small scale of the interactions, some different scales are used that make the numbers a little easier to handle. Useful length units on the atomic scale include the angstrom (Å where 1 Å = 10^{-10} m) and the nanometer (nm), where 1 nm = 10^{-9} m. Also important at this level is the unit of energy called the electron–volt (eV), which is the energy acquired by an electron accelerating through a potential difference of 1 volt. Compared to the SI unit of energy, the Joule, the electron–volt is very small (1 eV = 1.6×10^{-19} J).

Metric system prefixes are often added to units to make numbers easier to handle. The chart below lists prefixes sometimes encountered.

Multiples

Factor	Prefix	Prefix abbreviation
10^9	giga	G (or B)
10^6	mega	M
10^3	kilo	k

REMEMBER

Most common prefixes:

m = 10^{-3}, k = 10^3, μ = 10^{-6}, M = 10^6, n = 10^{-9}

Submultiples

Factor	Prefix	Prefix abbreviation
10^{-2}	centi	c
10^{-3}	milli	m
10^{-6}	micro	µ
10^{-9}	nano	n
10^{-12}	pico	p

B. Scientific Notation

Scientific notation is a convention for expressing numbers which simplifies computation and standardizes results. To express a number in scientific notation, convert it into a number between 1 and 10, then multiply it by 10 raised to the appropriate power.

Example: $123 = 1.23 \times 10^2$

$\qquad$ 1.23 is the **mantissa** and 2 is the **exponent** (power of ten).

Example: $0.042 = 4.2 \times 10^{-2}$

One can easily obtain products and quotients of numbers expressed in scientific notation. When multiplying, one simply multiplies the mantissas and adds the exponents to find the new mantissa and exponent of the answer. Some additional conversion may be necessary so that the new mantissa is again between 1 and 10, as in the third example on this page.

Example: $(1.1 \times 10^6)(5.0 \times 10^{17}) = ?$

Solution: Multiply the mantissas 1.1 and 5.0, and add the exponents 6 and 17.

The answer is 5.5×10^{23}.

The quotient of two numbers expressed in scientific notation is obtained by dividing the mantissa in the numerator by the mantissa in the denominator, and subtracting the power of 10 in the denominator from the power of 10 in the numerator.

Example: $\dfrac{6.2 \times 10^5}{2.0 \times 10^{-7}}$

Solution: Divide 6.2 by 2.0 and subtract –7 from 5 (note that $5 - (-7)$ $= 5 + 7 = 12$).

The answer is 3.1×10^{12}.

> **KEY CONCEPT**
>
> Check the exponent before calculating. It is often possible to arrive at the correct solution based on its order alone.

When a number expressed in scientific notation is raised to a power, the mantissa is raised to that power and the exponent is multiplied by that number.

Example: $(6.0 \times 10^4)^2$

Solution: Square the 6.0 and multiply the exponent by 2.

$$(6.0)^2 \times 10^{4 \times 2} = 36.0 \times 10^8 = 3.6 \times 10^9$$

When adding or subtracting numbers expressed in scientific notation they must have the **same** power of 10; when they do not, the appropriate conversion must be made first.

Example: $3.7 \times 10^4 + 1.5 \times 10^3 = ?$

Solution: First convert 1.5×10^3 to 0.15×10^4 so both numbers have the same exponent. Then $3.7 \times 10^4 + 0.15 \times 10^4 = 3.85 \times 10^4$, rounded to 3.9×10^4.

C. Trigonometric Relations

For the right triangle, the trigonometric functions for angle θ are:

$$\sin \theta = \frac{y}{h} = \frac{\text{opposite side}}{\text{hypotenuse}}$$

$$\cos \theta = \frac{x}{h} = \frac{\text{adjacent side}}{\text{hypotenuse}}$$

$$\tan \theta = \frac{y}{x} = \frac{\text{opposite side}}{\text{adjacent side}}$$

Some important values of the trigonometric functions:

θ	$\sin \theta$	$\cos \theta$
0°	0	1
30°	$\frac{1}{2}$	$\frac{\sqrt{3}}{2}$
45°	$\frac{\sqrt{2}}{2}$	$\frac{\sqrt{2}}{2}$
60°	$\frac{\sqrt{3}}{2}$	$\frac{1}{2}$
90°	1	0
180°	0	−1

D. Vectors and Scalars

Scalars are those numerical quantities that have **magnitude** but no direction, such as distance, speed and mass. **Vector** quantities have **both magnitude and direction.** Some vector quantities are displacement, velocity, and force.

1. VECTOR REPRESENTATION

We can represent a vector by an arrow. The direction of the arrow corresponds to the direction of the vector. The length of the arrow **may or may not** be proportional to the magnitude of the vector. Common notations for a vector quantity are either an arrow or **boldface.** For example, vector A can be written as $\vec{A}$ or **A**. The magnitude of vector A can be represented as $|\vec{A}|$, $|A|$, or simply A (no arrow or boldface).

2. VECTOR ADDITION

The **sum** of two or more vectors is called the **resultant** of the vectors. The terms vector sum and resultant are interchangeable.

One method of finding the resultant **A + B** of the two vectors **A** and **B** is to place the tail of **B** at the tip of **A** (without changing the length or direction of either arrow). In this method of vector addition the lengths of the arrows **must** be proportional to the magnitudes of the vector. The vector sum **A + B** is the vector joining the tail of **A** to the tip of **B** and pointing toward the tip of **B**. For three or more vectors, proceed similarly (see Figure 1.1 below).

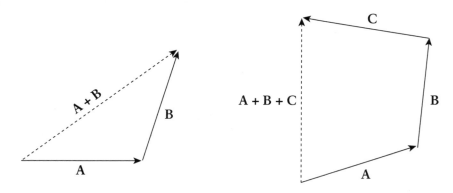

Figure 1.1

Another method more commonly used for finding the resultant of several vectors involves breaking each vector into perpendicular (X and Y) components. These components are often, but not always, horizontal and vertical.

Given any vector **V**, we can find the X component and the Y component by drawing a right triangle with **V** as the hypotenuse (see Figure 1.2 below). If θ is the angle between **V** and the x direction, then $\cos \theta = X/V$ and $\sin \theta = Y/V$. In other words:

$$X = V \cos \theta$$
$$Y = V \sin \theta$$

Example: V = 10 m/s
          $\theta = 30°$

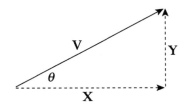

$$X = 10 \cos 30° = \frac{10\sqrt{3}}{2}$$
$$= 5\sqrt{3} \text{ m/s}$$
$$Y = 10 \sin 30° = \frac{10}{2} = 5 \text{ m/s}$$

Figure 1.2

Conversely, if we know X and Y we can find V by using the Pythagorean theorem: $X^2 + Y^2 = V^2$; or $V = \sqrt{X^2 + Y^2}$.

Example: X = 3 m/s
          Y = 4 m/s

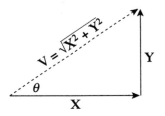

$$V = \sqrt{3^2 + 4^2} = \sqrt{25}$$
$$= 5 \text{ m/s}$$

(Also note that we can find θ from $\tan \theta = Y/X$. In this example $\tan \theta = 4/3$, so $\theta = 53°$.)

Figure 1.3

The X component of the resultant vector is the sum of the X components of the vectors being added. Similarly, the Y component of the resultant vector is the sum of the Y components of the vectors being added.

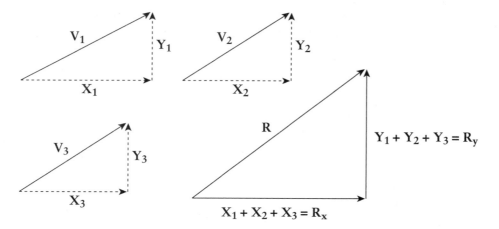

Figure 1.4

To find the resultant (**R**) using the components method:

1. Resolve the vectors to be summed into their X and Y components.

2. Add the X components to get the X component of the resultant (**R$_x$**). In the same way, add the Y components to get the Y component of the resultant (**R$_y$**).

3. Find the magnitude of the resultant by using the Pythagorean theorem. If **R$_x$** and **R$_y$** are the components of the resultant then:

$$R = \sqrt{R_x^2 + R_y^2}$$

4. Find the direction (θ) of the resultant by using the relation $\tan θ = \dfrac{R_y}{R_x}$ From the value of tan θ you can find θ, the angle **R** makes with the x direction.

> **REMEMBER**
>
> Magnitude of a vector V:
>
> $V = \sqrt{V_x^2 + V_y^2}$

Example: Find the horizontal and vertical components of **V.**

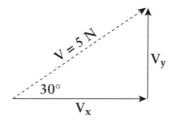

Figure 1.5

Solution: Let x be the horizontal direction and y be the vertical direction, then:

$$\mathbf{V_x} = \mathbf{V} \cos \theta = 5 \cos 30° = \frac{5\sqrt{3}}{2} = 2.5 \sqrt{3}\,\text{N} \approx 4.3 \text{ N}$$

$$\mathbf{V_y} = \mathbf{V} \sin \theta = 5 \sin 30° = \frac{5}{2} = 2.5 \text{ N}$$

Example: Find the resultant of **A**, **B**, **C**, and **D**.

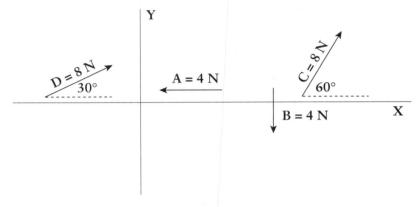

Figure 1.6

Solution: Resolve the vectors into their horizontal (x) and vertical (y) components. Note that we have x components going both left and right, and y components going both up and down. **In each case choose one direction as the positive direction. The other direction is then automatically the negative direction.** In this example we chose going to the right as the positive x direction (so to the left is negative), and up as the positive y direction (so down is negative). **A component in the positive direction is then positive and a component in the negative direction is then negative.**

a. $\mathbf{A_x} = -4$ N

$\mathbf{B_x} = 0$

$\mathbf{C_x} = 8 \cos 60° = \dfrac{8}{2} = 4$ N

$\mathbf{D_x} = 8 \cos 30° = \dfrac{8\sqrt{3}}{2} = 4\sqrt{3}$ N

b. $\mathbf{A_y} = 0$

$\mathbf{B_y} = -4$ N

$\mathbf{C_y} = 8 \sin 60° = \dfrac{8\sqrt{3}}{2} = 4\sqrt{3}$ N

$\mathbf{D_y} = 8 \sin 30° = \dfrac{8}{2} = 4$ N

Add the components of **A**, **B**, **C**, and **D** to get the components of the resultant R:

a. $R_x = (-4) + 0 + 4 + 4\sqrt{3} = 4\sqrt{3}$ N
b. $R_y = 0 + (-4) + 4\sqrt{3} + 4 = 4\sqrt{3}$ N

Find the magnitude of the resultant:

$$R = \sqrt{R_x{}^2 + R_y{}^2}$$

$$R = \sqrt{(4\sqrt{3})^2 + (4\sqrt{3})^2} = \sqrt{96} = 4\sqrt{6} \text{ N}$$

Find the angle the resultant makes with the horizontal:

$$\tan \theta = \frac{4\sqrt{3}}{4\sqrt{3}} = 1; \; \theta = 45°$$

Thus, we have found that **R** is a vector of magnitude of $4\sqrt{6}$ N, making an angle of 45° with the horizontal. (In general, $\tan \theta = |R_y/R_x|$ where θ is the smallest angle with the x-axis.)

3. VECTOR SUBTRACTION

Subtracting two vectors is exactly the same as adding the negative of the vector being subtracted. When expressed in a mathematical formula, the idea looks like this:

$$A - B = A + (-B)$$

By –**B** we mean a vector with the same magnitude as **B** but pointing in the opposite direction.

Example: What is the resultant of **A** – **B** as pictured below?

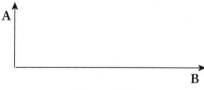

Figure 1.7

Solution: The first thing to do is make the vector –**B**. This is done by erasing the arrowhead at the tip of **B**, and redrawing it where the tail used to be (see Figure 1.8(a)). Now, add this to **A**. To do this move the tip of **A** to the tail of –**B**, and join the tail of **A** to the tip of –**B** (see Figure 1.8(b)).

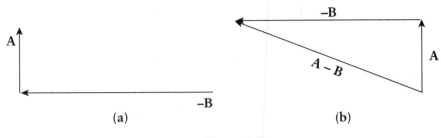

Figure 1.8

To find –**B** using the method whereby the vectors are broken up into their horizontal and vertical components, each vector component is multiplied by –1 before adding.

Example: If **A** has components $A_x = 3$ and $A_y = 4$ and **B** has components $B_x = 2$ and $B_y = 1$, then what is **A** – **B**?

Solution: First, remember **A** – **B** = **A** + (–**B**). Since **B** has components B_x and B_y, –**B** has components $-B_x$ and $-B_y$.

$$R_x = A_x - B_x = 3 - 2 = 1$$
$$R_y = A_y - B_y = 4 - 1 = 3$$

To get the magnitude of the final resultant vector **R**:

$$R = \sqrt{(1^2 + 3^2)}$$
$$= \sqrt{(1 + 9)} = \sqrt{10}$$

To get the direction:

$$\tan\theta = \frac{R_y}{R_x} = 3$$
$$\theta = 72°$$

4. MULTIPLYING A VECTOR BY A SCALAR

Now consider the case where a vector is multiplied by a scalar, **B** = n**A**. To find the magnitude of **B** simply multiply the magnitude of **A** by the absolute value of n, **B** = |n|**A**. If n is a positive number, then **B** and **A** are in the same direction. However, if n is a negative number, then **B** and **A** are in opposite directions. For example, if vector **A** is multiplied by +3, the resultant vector **B** will be three times as long as **A** and point in the same direction. However, if **A** is multiplied by –3, then **B** would again be three times as long as **A**, but it would point in the opposite direction.

KINEMATICS

Kinematics is the branch of mechanics dealing with the description of motion. In physics, the **position** of an object or particle is defined on a three-dimensional coordinate axis. Most questions you will have to deal with concerning motion will involve only one or two dimensions.

A. Displacement

The **displacement** ($\Delta \mathbf{x}$) of an object is a vector quantity that describes the change in position. It goes (in a straight line) from the initial position to the final position without regard to the actual path taken. Since this is a vector quantity, displacement has both direction and magnitude.

Example: A man walks 2 km east, 2 km north, 2 km west, and then 2 km south. His actual total distance traveled is 8 km, since distance is a scalar. But his displacement is a vector quantity that is the change in position. In this case his displacement is zero, since the man ends up in the same place he started (see Figure 1.9).

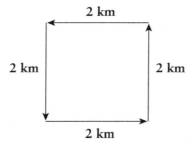

Figure 1.9

B. Velocity

1. AVERAGE VELOCITY

The **average velocity** of a particle is the ratio of the displacement vector over the change in time. It is a vector quantity.

$$\bar{\mathbf{v}} = \Delta \mathbf{x}/\Delta t$$

$\bar{\mathbf{v}}$ has the same direction as $\Delta \mathbf{x}$.

2. INSTANTANEOUS VELOCITY

The **instantaneous velocity** or **velocity** refers to a single instant of time. It is the average velocity as Δt approaches 0. This can be represented as:

$$v = \lim_{\Delta t \to 0} \frac{\Delta x}{\Delta t}$$

Graphically, this corresponds to the slope of the graph of the object's position with respect to time at the particular time, t.

3. SPEED

The **average speed** is given by:

$$\bar{s} = d/\Delta t$$

where d is the actual distance traveled. It is a scalar. Since actual distance traveled is not always the same as the magnitude of the displacement vector, average speed is not always the same as the magnitude of the average velocity.

The **instantaneous speed** or **speed** is the magnitude of the instantaneous velocity vector. It is also a scalar.

C. Acceleration

1. AVERAGE ACCELERATION

Acceleration is the rate of change of an object's velocity. It is a vector quantity. **Average acceleration** $\bar{a}$ is the change in instantaneous velocity over the time period Δt:

$$\bar{a} = \Delta v/\Delta t$$

2. INSTANTANEOUS ACCELERATION

The **instantaneous acceleration**—the acceleration at one point of a particle's path—is defined the same way as instantaneous velocity, i.e., it is the average acceleration as Δt approaches 0.

$$v = \lim_{\Delta t \to 0} \frac{\Delta x}{\Delta t}$$

Graphically, this corresponds to the slope of the graph of the object's velocity with respect to time at the particular time t. The direction of the acceleration vector is not always along the direction of the velocity vector. The direction of **a** is the same as the direction of Δv.

MOTION WITH CONSTANT ACCELERATION

The acceleration of a body is proportional to the force (see Chapter 2) applied to that body. When a body is under the influence of a constant force, the acceleration is also constant. In the following sections it is assumed that the acceleration is constant.

A. Linear Motion

In linear motion the acceleration and velocity vectors are along the line of motion. Note that the linear motion need not be in the horizontal direction. One-dimensional motion of this kind can be fully described by the following equations:

Notes:

$v = v_0 + at$

1. v_0, x_0 are v and x at t = 0.

$x - x_0 = v_0t + \dfrac{at^2}{2}$

2. When the motion is vertical, we use y instead of x.

$v^2 = v_0^2 + 2a(x - x_0)$

$\bar{v} = \dfrac{(v_0 + v)}{2}$

3. As illustrated below, in using these equations, we must remember that velocity and acceleration are vector quantities.

$x - x_0 = \bar{v}\, t = \dfrac{(v_0 + v)}{2}t$

By way of an example let's examine free-falling bodies. Free-fall means that the only force acting on a body is its own weight (gravity) and neglects, for example, any force of air resistance. All objects in free-fall have the same acceleration, called **the acceleration due to gravity (g),** which in SI units is 9.8 m/s². The following example demonstrates the use of the above equations in the analysis of free-falling bodies.

Example: A ball is thrown vertically up into the air with an initial velocity of 10 m/s.

   a. Find the position and velocity of the ball after 2 seconds.

   b. Find the distance and time at which the ball reaches its maximum height.

Solution: a. Remember that velocity and acceleration are vector quantities. Taking the initial position of the ball $y_0 = 0$, and taking "up" as positive, the initial velocity is $v_0 = +10$ m/s and the acceleration is g = –9.8 m/s². Notice g is negative because its direction is down, and we are taking "up" to be the positive direction. Velocity after 2 seconds can be found using the equation:

$$v = v_0 + at$$ (Minus sign for v means that
$$= (+10) + (-9.8)(2)$$ the ball is coming down.)
$$= -9.6 \text{ m/s}$$

After 2 seconds, the position of the ball is found using the equation:

$$y = v_0 t + \frac{at^2}{2} \quad (y_0 = 0)$$
$$= 10(2) + \frac{(-9.8)(2)^2}{2}$$
$$= 20 - 19.6$$
$$= +0.4 \text{ m}$$

b. When the ball is at its maximum height the velocity, v, which has been decreasing on the way up, is zero. Using the following equation and plugging in values, we can find the maximum height the ball reaches above the ground:

$$v^2 = v_0^2 + 2ay$$
$$0 = (10)^2 + 2(-9.8)y$$
$$y = 5.1 \text{ m}$$

The time at which the ball reaches its maximum height can be found from the equation:

$$v = v_0 + at$$
$$0 = 10 + (-9.8)t$$
$$t = 1.0 \text{ s}$$

B. Projectile Motion

Note again that we have been considering only linear motion in the above example. In the case of **projectile motion**, however, the object has velocity and position components in both the vertical and horizontal directions. The two components of the velocity vector v_x and v_y are independent, so the change in the vertical velocity v_y due to gravity does not affect and is not affected by the constant horizontal velocity v_x. The following example demonstrates how projectile motion is analyzed.

Example: A projectile is fired from ground level with an initial velocity of 50 m/s and an initial angle of elevation of 37°. Assuming $g = 10$ m/s^2, find:

a. the projectile's total time in flight.
b. the maximum height attained.
c. the total horizontal distance traveled.

d. the final horizontal and vertical velocities just before it hits the ground.

$$(\sin 37° = 0.6; \cos 37° = 0.8)$$

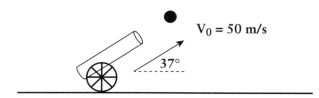

Figure 1.10

Solution: a. Let y equal the vertical height; let up be the positive direction.

$$a = -10 \text{ m/s}^2$$

$$y = v_{0_y}t + \frac{1}{2}at^2 \ (y_0 = 0)$$

$$v_{0_y} = v_0 \sin 37°$$

$$v_{0_y} = 50(0.6) = 30 \text{ m/s}$$

$$y = 30t - 5t^2$$

$y = 0$ both when the projectile is first fired and when it hits the ground later. Its time of flight will be the time from the launch ($y_0 = 0$) until landing ($y = 0$).

$$30t - 5t^2 = 0$$

$$5t(6 - t) = 0$$

$$t = 0 \text{ (first fired)}, t = 6 \text{ (hits the ground)}$$

Time in flight = 6 − 0 = 6 s

b. To find the maximum height attained:

$$v_y^2 = v_{0y}^2 + 2a(y - y_0)$$

$$0 = 30^2 + 2(-10)(y - 0)$$

$$y = \frac{900}{20}$$

$$y = 45 \text{ m}$$

c. To find the horizontal distance traveled:

$$x = v_x t \ (a_x = 0)$$

$$v_x = 50 \cos 37° = 40 \text{ m/s}$$

$$x = 40(6) = 240 \text{ m}$$

> **REMEMBER**
>
> Horizontal motion is the same as a particle moving with constant horizontal speed = V_{0_x}.

d. The horizontal velocity remains constant, so $v_x = 40$ m/s. To find the vertical velocity at impact:

$$v_y = v_{0y} + at$$
$$v_y = 30 - 10(6)$$
$$v_y = 30 - 60$$
$$v_y = -30 \text{ m/s}$$

Since we chose up as positive, the minus sign means the vertical component of the velocity is directed down.

2

Newtonian Mechanics

This chapter covers an important area of OAT® physics, namely Newton's laws of motion. Basic to the study of Newton's laws are the fundamental concepts of force and mass, which are discussed along with the distinction between mass and weight, and a detailed example of obtaining the resultant of two or more forces. The classic example of a block sliding down a frictionless incline is presented as an exercise for applying Newton's 2nd law in a situation where there are forces in two directions. Translational and rotational equilibrium are discussed as examples of cases where the net force or net torque respectively vanishes. The real-world problem of motion in the presence of friction is briefly discussed qualitatively, followed by a detailed numerical example. Lastly, the topic of circular motion is discussed along with the associated concepts of tangential and centripetal acceleration, and centripetal force.

NEWTON'S THREE LAWS

A. Force

Force is a vector quantity. Forces are observed as the push or pull on an object. Forces can either be exerted between bodies in contact (such as the force a person exerts to push a box across the floor), or between bodies not in contact (such as the force of gravity holding the earth in its orbit around the sun). The unit for force in SI units is the Newton (N), and is equivalent to kilogram•meter/second^2.

> **REMEMBER**
>
> Newtons can be broken down into fundamental units using $F = ma$.

B. Mass and Weight

The mass of an object should not be mistaken for the weight of an object. **Mass (m)** is a scalar quantity that measures a body's inertia, while **weight (W)** is a force vector that measures a body's gravitational attraction to the earth. The two are related by the equation:

$$\mathbf{W} = \mathbf{mg}$$

where **g** is the acceleration due to gravity. The unit for weight is the same as for any other force, the Newton (N).

When one of the forces acting on a body is its own weight, the entire force due to gravity can be thought of as applied at a single point, called the center of gravity. For a homogeneous body the center of gravity is at its geometric center.

C. Newton's Laws of Motion Stated

Mechanics is the study of bodies in motion and at rest. Newtonian mechanics is a way of describing the effect forces have on macroscopic bodies. In order to carry out such a description, it is first necessary to have an understanding of Newton's three laws of motion and how to apply them to various situations. Newton's three laws are:

REAL-WORLD ANALOGY

Why are collapsible guard rails actually safer than more rigid ones?

What's dangerous in a collision is the average impact force, which equals the mass of the colliding vehicle times the average acceleration experienced. The average acceleration equals the change in speed experienced by the vehicle divided by the time over which the change occurs or the collision time. Given equal changes in speed, a collapsible guard rail results in a longer collision time and thus a smaller average impact force.

1. A body either at rest or in motion with constant velocity will remain that way unless a net force acts upon it.

2. A net force applied to a body of mass m will result in that body undergoing an acceleration in the same direction as the net force. The magnitude of the body's acceleration is directly proportional to the magnitude of the net force and inversely proportional to the body's mass. This can be expressed in general terms as:

$$\mathbf{F}_{net} = \Sigma\mathbf{F} = m\mathbf{a}$$

or in components as:

$$\Sigma F_x = ma_x$$
$$\Sigma F_y = ma_y$$

Note that the acceleration in the x-direction depends only on the forces (or components of forces) in the x-direction (and the same is true for the y-direction).

REMEMBER

When you see $F_{net} = 0$, think a = 0 and vice versa.

3. If body A exerts a force **F** on body B, then B exerts a force –**F** back on A (equal in magnitude and opposite in direction). In Newton's words, "to every action there is always an opposed but equal reaction."

$$\mathbf{F}_{BA} = -\mathbf{F}_{AB}$$

D. Free-Body Diagram

Another concept useful in force problems is the **free-body diagram,** which helps to clarify what forces are applied and what their directions are. The examples below demonstrate the use of this technique.

Example: Three people are pulling on ropes tied to a tire with forces of 100 N, 150 N, and 200 N, as shown in Figure 2.1. Find the magnitude and direction of the resultant force.

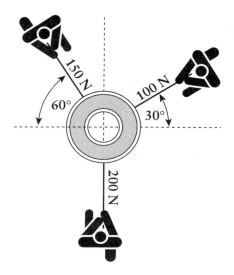

Figure 2.1

Solution: First we draw a free-body diagram that shows the forces acting on the tire. Its purpose is to identify and better visualize the acting forces.

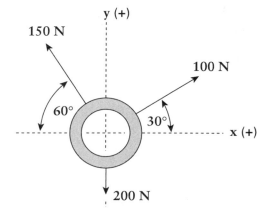

Figure 2.2

The resultant force is simply the sum of the forces. To find the resultant force vector, first we need the sum of the force components:

$$R_x = \Sigma F_x = 100 \cos 30° - 150 \cos 60°$$
$$= 86.6 - 75$$
$$= 11.6 \text{ N (positive x direction, to the right)}$$

$$R_y = \Sigma F_y = 100 \sin 30° + 150 \sin 60° - 200$$
$$= 50 + 129.9 - 200$$
$$= -20.1 \text{ N (negative y direction, down)}$$

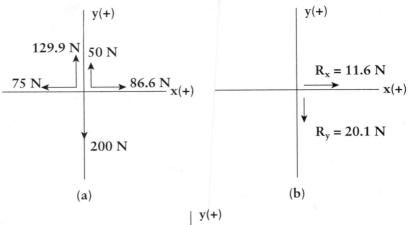

(a)

(b)

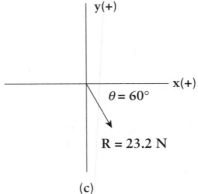

(c)

Figure 2.3

$$R = \sqrt{(11.6)^2 + (-20.1)^2}$$
$$= 23.2 \text{ N}$$

$$\tan \theta = \frac{-20.1}{11.6}$$
$$\theta = -60° \text{ (R is in the 4th quadrant)}$$

Example: Starting from rest, a 5 kg block takes 4 s to slide down a frictionless incline. Find the normal force, the acceleration of the block, and the vertical height h the block starts from, if the plane is at an angle of 30°.

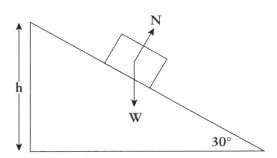

Figure 2.4

It is usually best to choose the x-and y-axes such that one of the axes is parallel to the surface, even when the surface is not horizontal. This is what we will do here. The force that the surface exerts on the block is broken up into two components, one perpendicular to the surface, called the **normal force (N)**, and the other parallel to the surface, called the **friction force (f)**. In this problem the incline is frictionless (i.e., no **f**), so we have only the normal force, **N**. The block's weight **W** is, of course, vertically down. We need to find the components of **W** parallel and perpendicular to the inclined surface (i.e., the components of **W** in the x and y directions, W_x and W_y).

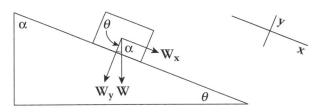

Figure 2.5

Note that in Figure 2.5 the angle **W** makes with the x-axis is α, and we would normally use this angle in expressing the components of **W**; $W_x = W \cos \alpha$ and $W_y = W \sin \alpha$. However, it is more useful to express the components of **W** in terms of the angle θ which the inclined surface makes with the horizontal. In terms of θ the components of **W** are:

$$W_x = W \sin \theta = mg \sin \theta \ (W = mg)$$
$$W_y = W \cos \theta = mg \cos \theta$$

So let the x-axis be parallel to the inclined surface, and let the y-axis be perpendicular to it. The motion is along the inclined surface, in other words, along the x-axis. Therefore, any acceleration is only in the x direction, and a_y is automatically zero.

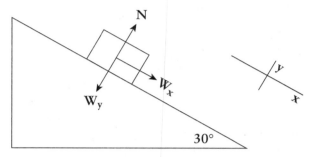

Figure 2.6

Only the forces in the x direction affect the motion of the block. Since there is no acceleration in the y direction, the sum of those forces equals zero.

$$\Sigma F_x = W_x = (5)(9.8) \sin 30° = 24.5 \text{ N} = ma_x$$
$$\Sigma F_y = ma_y = N - W_y = 0$$

From the second equation we can solve for N:

$$N = (5)(9.8) \cos 30° = 42.4 \text{ N}$$

From the first equation we can solve for a_x: (Note that $a_x = a$ since $a_y = 0$.)

$$a = \frac{F}{m}$$
$$= \frac{24.5}{5}$$
$$= 4.9 \text{ m/s}^2$$

The length d of the incline from where the block started can now be found using:

$$d = \frac{at^2}{2} \quad (V_0 = 0)$$
$$= \frac{(4.9)(4)^2}{2}$$
$$= 39.2 \text{ m}$$

From trigonometry, the vertical height h is readily available:

$$\sin 30° = \frac{h}{d}$$

$$h = 39.2 \sin 30°$$

$$= 19.6 \text{ m}$$

E. Gravity

Gravity is an attractive force that is felt by all forms of matter. The magnitude of the **gravitational force (F)** is given as:

$$F = \frac{Gm_1m_2}{r^2}$$

where G is the gravitational constant (6.67×10^{-11} N•m^2/kg^2), m_1 and m_2 are the masses of the two objects, and r is the distance between their centers.

Example: Find the gravitational attraction between an electron and a proton at a distance of 10^{-11} m. (Proton mass = 10^{-27} kg; electron mass = 10^{-30} kg)

Solution: Using Newton's law of gravitation:

$$F = \frac{Gm_1m_2}{r^2}$$

$$= \frac{(6.67 \times 10^{-11})(10^{-27})(10^{-30})}{(10^{-11})^2}$$

$$= 6.67 \times 10^{-46} \text{ N}$$

EQUILIBRIUM

If several forces act on an object simultaneously, their vector sum may cancel, leaving the motion of the body unchanged. This balancing phenomenon is called **equilibrium**.

A. Translational Equilibrium

An unbalanced force acting on an object accelerates the object in the direction of the force. For an object to be in **translational equilibrium**, the sum of the forces pushing the object through space in one direction must be counterbalanced by the sum of the forces acting in the opposite direction. This is called the first condition of equilibrium and can be written as:

$$\Sigma F = 0 \text{ (vector sum)}$$

or, if the vectors are resolved into their x and y components:

$$\Sigma F_x = 0 \quad \Sigma F_y = 0$$

Example: A block of mass 20 kg is supported as shown in the diagram. Find the tensions T_1 and T_2.

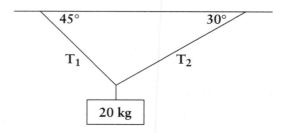

Figure 2.7

Solution: A free-body diagram at the point of intersection of the three cords will help solve this problem. Cords, strings, and the like can only exert pulling forces, and these are in the direction of each cord. Note also that the tension in the vertical cord is equal to the weight of the 20 kg mass, as shown in the other free-body diagram on the right.

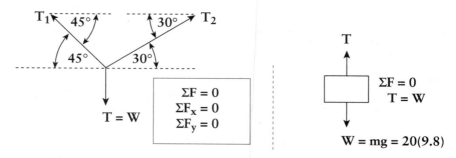

Figure 2.8

The force components are:

$$\Sigma F_x = 0 = T_2 \cos 30° - T_1 \cos 45°$$
$$\Sigma F_y = 0 = T_1 \sin 45° + T_2 \sin 30° - 20(9.8)$$

Solve the second equation for T_1:

$$T_1 = \frac{20(9.8) - T_2 \sin 30°}{\sin 45°}$$

$$= \frac{20(9.8) - T_2 / 2}{\sqrt{2} / 2}$$

$$= \frac{196 - T_2}{\sqrt{2}}$$

Substitute this into the first equation:

$$\frac{T_2\sqrt{3}}{2} - \frac{\sqrt{2}}{2}\left(\frac{196 - T_2}{\sqrt{2}}\right) = 0$$

$$T_2(\sqrt{3} + 1) = 196$$

$$T_2 = \frac{196}{\sqrt{3} + 1}$$

$$= 71.8 \text{ N}$$

And now T_1 follows from this:

$$T_1 = \frac{196 - 71.8}{\sqrt{2}}$$

$$= 87.8 \text{ N}$$

B. Rotational Equilibrium

Unlike translational motion, rotational motion depends not only on the magnitude and direction of the force, but also on the distance from the force to the axis of rotation. The greater the distance, the greater the change in rotational motion that will be produced by a given force. (As an example, try closing a door first by pushing on it a few inches from the hinge, then by pushing far from the hinge. You'll find it's much easier to close the door when you push farther from the hinge because the distance between the axis and the force is greater.)

The quantity that causes rotation is called the **moment of the force** or the **torque** τ, and is given by:

$$\tau = rF \sin \theta$$

where F is the magnitude of the force, r is the distance between the axis and the force (also called the lever arm), and θ is the angle between **F** and **r**.

Torque can act in two directions about a pivot point, clockwise and counterclockwise. Counterclockwise is the positive direction and clockwise the negative direction. For **rotational equilibrium** to occur, the sum of the torques in both these directions must be equal. Since torques causing a rotation in the clockwise direction are negative and torques causing counterclockwise rotations are positive, we can also say that the sum of all the torques must be zero:

$$\Sigma\tau = 0$$

This is called the second condition of equilibrium.

KEY CONCEPT

Maximum torque when $\theta = 90°$ ($\tau_{max} = rF$), minimum torque when $\theta = 0°$ ($\tau_{min} = 0$).

REMEMBER

Clockwise torques are negative, counterclockwise torques are positive.

Example: A seesaw with a mass of 5 kg has one block of mass 10 kg 2 meters to the left of the fulcrum and another block 0.5 m to the right of the fulcrum. If the seesaw is in equilibrium,

a.   find the mass of the second block.

b.   find the force exerted by the fulcrum.

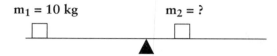

Figure 2.9

Solution: a.   To find τ, take the point of the fulcrum as the pivot point. This way both the normal force and the weight of the seesaw will be eliminated from the equation ($r = 0$). Let's call the 10 kg mass object 1 and the block whose mass we are trying to find object 2.

$$\Sigma \tau = 0 = m_1 g r_1 - m_2 g r_2$$

$$m_2 = \frac{m_1 r_1}{r_2}$$

$$= \frac{10(2)}{0.5}$$

$$= 40 \text{ kg}$$

b.   To find the normal force, N, exerted by the fulcrum, $\Sigma F_y = 0$. There is the upward force exerted by the fulcrum and the downward weights of the seesaw and the two masses. Don't forget that $W = mg$. Taking up as positive:

$$N - 5(9.8) - 10(9.8) - 40(9.8) = 0$$

$$N = 49 + 98 + 392 = 539 \text{ N}$$

MOTION

A.   Translational Motion

Translational motion is defined as motion in which there is no rotation. An example of translational motion is a block sliding on an inclined plane. With Newton's three laws and enough initial conditions, any translational motion problem can be solved.

B. Friction

Whenever two objects are in contact, their surfaces rub together creating a friction force. **Static friction, f_s,** is the force which must be overcome to set an object in motion. Its equation is:

$$0 \le f_s \le \mu_s N$$

where μ_s is the **coefficient of static friction** and **N** is the normal force. Note that static friction can have any value up to some maximum $\mu_s N$. For example, to send a book that is at rest sliding across a table, a force greater than the maximum static friction force is required. Once the book starts to slide, though, the friction force is not quite as strong. This new friction force is called **kinetic friction, f_k,** and its equation is:

$$f_k = \mu_k N$$

where μ_k is the **coefficient of kinetic friction** and **N** is the normal force. Remember that friction always acts to oppose motion.

Example: Two blocks are in static equilibrium as shown in Figure 2.10.

    a. If block A has a mass of 15 kg and the coefficient of static friction μ_s equals 0.20, then find the maximum mass of block B.

    b. If an extra 5 kg are added to B, find the acceleration of A and the tension T in the rope. (μ_k equals 0.14)

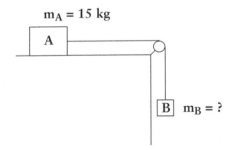

$$m_A = 15 \text{ kg}$$

A

B $m_B = ?$

Figure 2.10

Solution: a.

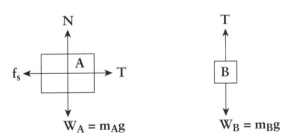

N   T

f_s A   T   B

$W_A = m_A g$ $W_B = m_B g$

Figure 2.11

KEY CONCEPT

An object at rest on a real surface requires a force greater than $\mu_s N$ to start moving.

For block B:

$$\Sigma F_y = 0 = T - W_B$$
$$T = W_B = m_B g$$

For block A:

Asking for the maximum mass of block B means that the coefficient of static friction holding block A is at its maximum, $f_s = \mu_s N$.

$$\Sigma F_y = 0 = N - W_A$$
$$N = W_A = m_A g$$
$$\Sigma F_x = 0 = T - \mu_s N$$
$$T = \mu_s m_A g$$
$$T = (0.2)(15)(9.8)$$
$$T = 29.4 \text{ N}$$

Since block B is in static equilibrium, the tension in the rope must equal the weight of the block, so we have:

$$m_B g = 29.4$$
$$m_B = 3 \text{ kg}$$

b.

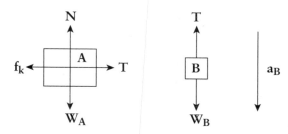

Figure 2.12

We found the maximum mass of B for the system to be in static equilibrium. Adding an extra 5 kg to B means that the system is now in motion.

For block B:

$$\Sigma F_y = m_B g - T = m_B a_B$$

For block A:

$$\Sigma F_x = T - \mu_k N$$
$$= T - \mu_k m_A g$$
$$= m_A a_A$$

Since the blocks are connected by the string, the magnitude of the acceleration for both of them is the same:

$$a_A = a_B = a$$

and

$$m_B g - T = m_B a$$
$$T - \mu_k m_A g = m_A a$$

Adding the two equations gives:

$$m_B g - T + T - \mu_k m_A g = (m_A + m_B)a$$

Solving for a:

$$a = \frac{(m_B - \mu_k m_A)g}{(m_A + m_B)}$$

$$= \frac{(8 - (0.14)(15))9.8}{(15 + 8)}$$

$$= 2.5 \text{ m/s}^2$$

Substituting this value into the equation $m_A a = T - \mu_k m_A g$ and solving for the tension gives:

$$T = m_A(\mu_k g + a)$$
$$= 15(0.14(9.8) + 2.5)$$
$$= 58.1 \text{ N}$$

CIRCULAR MOTION

The velocity vector is always tangent to the circular path. In general, the acceleration vector can be broken into radial and tangential components as shown in Figure 2.13.

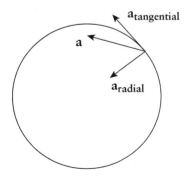

Figure 2.13

In uniform circular motion, the speed of the object remains constant. When uniform circular motion is assumed, there is no tangential acceleration. The radial component of the acceleration is always directed toward the center of the circle and is called **centripetal acceleration.** Its magnitude is given by:

$$a = \frac{v^2}{r}$$

The centripetal acceleration toward the center of the circle must be the result of some force also directed toward the center. Whatever the particular force happens to be, it is called the **centripetal force.** Using the relationship a = v²/r for the centripetal acceleration, the magnitude of the centripetal force on a particle in circular motion is given by:

$$F = ma = \frac{mv^2}{r}$$

In nonuniform circular motion, the speed of the object changes. In this case there is a tangential component of acceleration, and therefore the resultant acceleration is not directed toward the center of the circle. Instead its direction is given by the resultant of the radial component of the acceleration and the tangential component of the acceleration.

Consider a mass tied to a string, moving with circular motion. To keep the mass moving in a circular path, the string must constantly pull the object toward the center. In this particular case, the force exerted by the string is the centripetal force. If at some point the string breaks, the inward force no longer acts and the mass flies off along a path tangential to the circle.

There is always some force that causes circular motion. As another example, consider a planet in orbit around the sun. In this case, the centripetal force is the force of gravity.

3

Work, Energy, and Momentum

In this chapter we will review the fundamental concepts of energy and momentum and the associated concepts of work and impulse. Essentially, you can think of work as responsible for changing the energy of an object, and impulse as responsible for changing the momentum of an object. Regarding energy and momentum, the great laws of conservation of energy and conservation of momentum are discussed along with concrete examples of problems that make use of these laws for their solution. The topic of collisions is discussed in detail as the most common example on the OAT® of the application of conservation of momentum. The concept of work is applied to the problem of pulley systems resulting in the definition of the efficiency of a simple machine. The chapter closes with a review of the equivalent concepts of center of mass and center of gravity.

WORK

A. Work Defined

As was shown in Chapter 2, solving mechanics problems using Newtonian methods involves analyzing the forces acting on a system. In this chapter, energy and momentum considerations, rather than forces, will be used to solve problems. Before we undertake a discussion of energy, though, it is important that we first talk about work. For a constant force **F** acting on an object which moves through a distance d, the **work W** is:

$$W = Fd \cos \theta$$

where θ is the angle between **F** and **d**. Units for work (and energy) are the Joule (J) in SI (1 Joule = 1 Newton•meter) and the foot•pound in FPS. Only the component of the force parallel to the path, $F \cos \theta$, is relevant. For a force perpendicular to the motion, $W = 0$ ($\theta = 90°$, thus $\cos 90° = 0$). Note that for a force opposite to the motion ($\theta > 90°$), the work will be negative ($\cos \theta < 0$).

KEY CONCEPT

When force and displacement are perpendicular, the work done is zero, therefore the centripetal force does no work.

Example: A block weighing 100 N is pushed up a frictionless incline over a distance of 20 m to a height of 10 m. Find:

a. the minimum force required to push the block;

b. the work done by the force;

c. the force required and the work done by the force if the block were simply lifted vertically 10 m.

Solution:

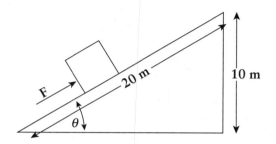

Figure 3.1

a. A free-body diagram of the forces acting on the block:

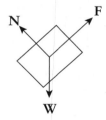

Figure 3.2

The minimum force needed is a force parallel to the plane which will push the block with no acceleration. Since $a = 0$, $\Sigma F = 0$:

$$\Sigma F = 0 = F - mg \sin \theta$$
$$F = mg \sin \theta$$
$$mg = 100 \text{ N}; \sin \theta = \frac{10}{20}. \text{ Therefore:}$$
$$F = 100\frac{10}{20}$$
$$= 50 \text{ N}$$

b. The work done by F is:

$$W = Fd \cos \theta$$

In this case θ is the angle between the force vector and the displacement vector. Since they are parallel, $\theta = 0$, therefore cos θ = 1. Substituting the numbers into the equation:

$$W = 50(20)(1)$$
$$= 1,000 \text{ J}$$

c. To raise the block vertically, the force should also be vertical and equal to the object's weight.

$$F = mg$$
$$= 100 \text{ N}$$

The work done by the lifting force is:

$$W = Fd \cos \theta$$
$$= 100(10)(1)$$
$$= 1,000 \text{ J}$$

The same amount of work is required in both cases, but twice the force is needed to raise the block vertically compared with pushing it up the incline.

B. Power

Often, the amount of work required to perform an operation is less important than the amount of time required to do the work. The rate at which work is done is called **power** (P), and is given as:

$$P = \frac{W}{t}$$

Units of power are the Watt (W) in SI (1 Watt = 1 Joule/sec) and foot•pound/sec in FPS.

Example: Find the power required to raise the block (of the previous example) in 4 seconds in each case.

Solution: When lifted up the incline, power is:

$$P = \frac{W}{t}$$
$$= \frac{1,000}{4}$$
$$= 250 \text{ W}$$

When lifted straight up, the power equals:

$$P = \frac{1,000}{4}$$

$$= 250 \text{ W}$$

ENERGY

A. Kinetic Energy

A body in motion possesses energy. This energy of motion is called **kinetic energy,** and is defined for a body of mass m and velocity v as:

$$K = \frac{mv^2}{2}$$

Units for kinetic energy are Joules (J) in SI.

Example: A 15 kg block, initially at rest, slides down a frictionless incline and comes to the bottom with a velocity of 7 m/s. What is the kinetic energy at the top and at the bottom?

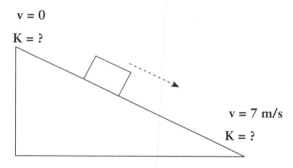

$v = 0$

$K = ?$

$v = 7$ m/s

$K = ?$

Figure 3.3

Solution: At the top v = 0, so kinetic energy is:

$$K = \frac{mv^2}{2}$$

$$= \frac{15(0)}{2}$$

$$= 0$$

At the bottom:

$$K = \frac{15(7)^2}{2}$$

$$= 367.5 \text{ J}$$

B. Potential Energy

Another form of energy a body can possess is **potential energy.** Unlike kinetic energy, which depends upon a body's motion, potential energy depends upon a body's **position.** One example of potential energy is the gravitational potential energy an object has when it is raised to a height h. Objects on the earth possess greater potential energy the higher they are from the surface. Gravitational potential energy (U) is given as:

$$U = mgh$$

where m is the mass of the body, g is the acceleration due to gravity, and h is the height of the body. Just as for work and kinetic energy, potential energy's units are Joules (J).

Example: An 80 kg diver leaps from a 10 m cliff into the sea. Find the diver's potential energy at the top of the cliff and just as he hits the water (set height equal to zero at sea level).

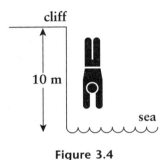

Figure 3.4

Solution: At the top of the cliff:

$$U = mgh$$
$$= 80(9.8)(10)$$
$$= 7,840 \text{ J}$$

At the water's surface:

$$U = 80(9.8)(0)$$
$$= 0$$

C. Total Mechanical Energy

Kinetic and potential energy are both forms of mechanical energy. The total mechanical energy (E) is the sum of the kinetic and potential E = K + U, where K is the kinetic energy of a system and U is the potential energy. Mechanical energy is conserved when the sum of the potential and kinetic energies remains constant. Mechanical energy is not always conserved, though. For example, when friction is present, mechanical energy is drained away in the form of heat.

CONSERVATION OF ENERGY

A. Work-Energy Theorem

The work-energy theorem relates the work performed by **all** the forces acting on a body in a certain time interval to the change in kinetic energy during that time. In equation form, the theorem is:

$$W = \Delta K$$

Example: A baseball of mass 0.25 kg is thrown straight up in the air with an initial velocity of 30 m/s. Assuming no air resistance, find the work done by the force of gravity when the ball is at its maximum height.

Solution: Neglecting air resistance, the only force acting on the ball is gravity. Since the ball's speed is 0 at its maximum height, using the work-energy theorem:

$$W = \Delta K$$
$$= 0 - \frac{mv^2}{2}$$
$$= \frac{-(0.25)(30)^2}{2}$$
$$= -112.5 \text{ J}$$

B. Conservative and Nonconservative Forces

Conservative forces have associated potential energies (e.g., gravity). There are two equivalent tests that are used to determine whether a force is conservative or not:

1. If the work done to move a particle in any round-trip path is zero, the force is conservative.

2. If the work needed to move a particle between two points is the same regardless of the path taken, then the force is conservative.

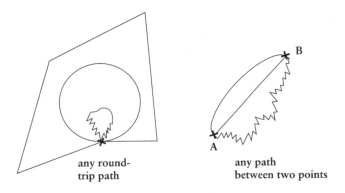

any round-
trip path

any path
between two points

Figure 3.5

For our purposes we will simply use the following rule of thumb: A force which has an associated potential energy (e.g., gravity) is conservative. Since an object's weight is just another name for the gravitational force on the object, an object's weight is a conservative force.

C. Conservation of Energy

When the work done by the nonconservative forces is 0 (or when there are no nonconservative forces, for example an object falling without air resistance), the total mechanical energy remains constant, and we have **conservation of energy:**

$$E = K + U = \text{constant}$$

or equivalently:

$$\Delta E = \Delta K + \Delta U = 0$$

However, when nonconservative forces such as friction or air resistance are present, mechanical energy is **not** conserved. The equation for a nonconservative system is:

$$W' = \Delta E = \Delta K + \Delta U$$

where **W′ is the work done by the nonconservative forces only.** Note that if the work done by the nonconservative forces is zero (which is automatically true if there aren't any such forces), $W' = 0 = \Delta E = \Delta K + \Delta U$ and we have conservation of energy.

Example: A baseball of mass 0.25 kg is thrown in the air with an initial speed of 30 m/s, but because of air resistance the ball returns to the ground with a speed of 27 m/s. Find the work done by air resistance.

KEY CONCEPT

In the presence of friction: $E_{initial} > E_{final}$, and the lost energy goes into heat.

Solution: Air resistance is a nonconservative force. To solve this problem, the energy equation for a nonconservative system is needed. The work done by air resistance is W'.

$$W' = \Delta E = \Delta K + \Delta U$$

Since $\Delta U = 0$ (final height = initial height):

$$W' = \Delta K$$
$$= \frac{mv_f^2}{2} - \frac{mv_i^2}{2}$$
$$= \frac{1}{2}(0.25)[(27)^2 - (30)^2]$$
$$= -21.4 \text{ J}$$

REMEMBER

$W < 0$ means the object slows down; the force opposes motion.

PULLEYS

Pulley systems allow heavy weights to be lifted using a much smaller force. Consider first the heavy block in Figure 3.6, suspended from two ropes. The force that the block exerts downward is equaled by the sum of the tensions in the two ropes. For a symmetrical system, the tensions in the two ropes are the same and are equal to half the weight of the block.

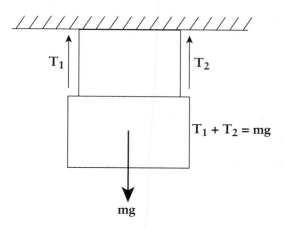

Figure 3.6

Now consider the pulley setup in Figure 3.7, with the block being held stationary. The tension in both vertical ropes will be equal; if they were different, then the pulleys would turn until the tensions on both sides were equal. Since the tensions are equal, each rope supports half the total weight of the block. This means that the force required to raise the block is now only half the total weight of the block. Though only half the force is now required to lift the block, the length of rope that must be pulled through is twice the distance that the block moves upward. This can be visualized more clearly in considering a case when a block is raised 5 meters. For this to happen, both sides of the supporting rope have to shorten 5 meters, and the only way to accomplish this is by pulling through 10 meters of rope.

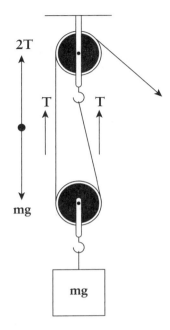

Figure 3.7

In a frictionless pulley system where the pulleys themselves have no mass, the work expended pulling the rope and the potential energy gained by the mass would be equal. However, no pulley system has these properties, since the pulleys do have mass and are not frictionless. This implies that no real pulley system is 100 percent efficient. At this point it is worth defining some terms. The weight of the object being lifted is the **load**, and the distance it rises is the **load distance.** The force exerted on the rope when lifting the load is known as the **effort**, and the distance through which the effort is exerted is the **effort distance.** It has been mentioned previously that work is force multiplied by the distance that the force moves an object through. Work input is, therefore, the product of the effort and the effort distance, and work output is the product of the load and the distance the load moves through. A measure of the **efficiency** of the system is given by the ratio of the work output to the work input, and is given by

$$\text{Efficiency} = \frac{W_{out}}{W_{in}}$$

$$= \frac{\text{Load} \times \text{Load distance}}{\text{Effort} \times \text{Effort distance}}$$

Efficiencies are often spoken of as percentages (multiply decimal by 100 to get percent), but in doing calculations efficiencies have to be decimals or fractions (divide percent by 100 to get a decimal). The efficiency gives a measure of the amount of work a person puts into a machine that comes out as useful work.

Consider the pulley system in Figure 3.8. By increasing the number of pulleys, it is possible to reduce the effort still further. In this case, the load has been divided among six strands of the rope, so the effort required is now only one-sixth the load. However, it is important to note that, generally speaking, as the number of pulleys increases, the efficiency decreases. This decrease in efficiency is caused by the added weight of each pulley as well as the increase in frictional forces.

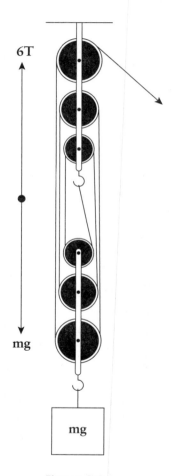

Figure 3.8

Example: The pulley system of Figure 3.8 has an efficiency of 80% and a person is required to lift 200 kg. Find:

a. the distance through which the effort must move to raise the load a distance of 4 m.

b. the effort required to lift the load.

    c.   the work done by the person lifting the load through a height of 4 m.

Solution: a.   For the load to move through a vertical distance of 4 m, all six of the supporting ropes must shorten 4 m also. This may only be accomplished by pulling $6 \times 4 = 24$ m of rope through. So the effort must move through a distance of 24 m.

    b.   To calculate the effort required, the equation for efficiency must be used. The load is the weight of the object being lifted and is equal to the mass times the acceleration due to gravity g. Since g is approximately 10 m/s^2 and all the other parameters except the effort are known, it is possible to substitute into this equation to calculate the effort:

$$\text{Efficiency} = \frac{\text{Load} \times \text{Load distance}}{\text{Effort} \times \text{Effort distance}}$$

$$0.80 = \frac{(200)(10)(4)}{(\text{Effort})(24)}$$

$$\text{Effort} = \frac{(2,000)(4)}{(0.80)(24)}$$

$$= 417 \text{ N}$$

    c.   The work done is given by:

$$\text{Work done} = \text{Effort} \times \text{Effort distance}$$

$$= 417 \times 24$$

$$= 10,000 \text{ J}$$

CONSERVATION OF MOMENTUM

A. Momentum

In nonrelativistic physics, **momentum p** means the product of mass and velocity. Momentum, like velocity, is a vector quantity. In equation form it is given as:

$$\mathbf{p} = m\mathbf{v}$$

For two or more objects, the total momentum is the vector sum of the individual momentums.

B. Impulse

Applying a force to an object over time will cause that object's momentum to change. The product of the force applied **F** and the time it was

---

KEY CONCEPT

$F = ma = m\Delta v/\Delta t$, so $F\Delta t = m\Delta v = \Delta p$, i.e., we just derived impulse $J = \Delta p = F\Delta t$.

applied for t is a vector quantity, and is given the name **impulse J**. For constant forces, impulse and momentum are related by the equation:

$$J = Ft = mv - mv_0 = \Delta p$$

In one-dimensional problems the forces and velocities are either in the positive or negative direction, and the equation becomes a single scalar equation:

$$J = Ft = mv - mv_0$$

(In this equation, J, F, v, and v_0 are positive or negative depending on whether the corresponding vectors are in the positive or negative direction.)

Example: A 7 kg bowling ball initially at rest is acted on by a 110 N force for 3.5 s. Find the final speed of the ball.

Solution: From the equation for impulse:

$$Ft = mv - mv_0$$

$$v = v_0 + \frac{Ft}{m}$$

$$= 0 + \frac{110(3.5)}{7}$$

$$= 55 \text{ m/s}$$

C. Conservation of Momentum

Those forces that one part of a system exerts on another part are called **internal forces**. Those forces that are exerted on any part of a system from outside the system are called **external forces**. The principle of **conservation of momentum** states that when the net impulse of the external forces acting on a system is zero, the total momentum of the system remains constant. This condition is automatically satisfied when there are no external forces, or when their vector sum is zero.

D. Collisions

One of the most common applications of conservation of momentum occurs when two objects collide in an idealized collision: one that occurs instantaneously at a specific location. Because there are no external forces, conservation of momentum applies. Conservation of momentum means that the total momentum before the collision equals the total momentum after the collision. For a collision between two objects a, and b, this is given by:

$$p_{ai} + p_{bi} = p_{af} + p_{bf}$$

REAL-WORLD CONCEPT

Many cars are now equipped with airbags as a safety feature. From the viewpoint of basic physics, why do airbags make cars safer? The answer has to do with the concept of impact force, which is the average force exerted on a passenger during a collision. The definition of impulse says that the average force exerted on an object, times the time over which the force is applied, equals the change in momentum of the object. The impact force then equals the change in momentum divided by the time over which the force is applied. The change in momentum of a passenger in a collision is fixed by the mass of the passenger and the initial speed of the vehicle. Airbags, however, can increase the time over which the passenger's momentum changes, thereby reducing the impact force. Since impact force is what's dangerous, airbags are useful as safety devices.

KEY CONCEPT

Conservation of momentum means $p_{initial} = p_{final}$ (p's are total initial and final momentum).

---

where $\mathbf{p}_{ai}$, $\mathbf{p}_{bi}$ are the momenta before the collision, and $\mathbf{p}_{af}$, $\mathbf{p}_{bf}$ are the momenta after the collision. Since momentum has been defined previously as $\mathbf{p} = mv$, the conservation of momentum equation may be written as:

$$m_a\mathbf{v}_{ai} + m_b\mathbf{v}_{bi} = m_a\mathbf{v}_{af} + m_b\mathbf{v}_{bf}$$

where $\mathbf{v}_{ai}$, $\mathbf{v}_{bi}$ are the velocities before the collision, and $\mathbf{v}_{af}$, $\mathbf{v}_{bf}$ are the velocities after the collision.

In one-dimensional problems, velocities are either in the positive direction or in the negative direction, and the conservation of momentum equation becomes a simple scalar equation:

$$m_av_{ai} + m_bv_{bi} = m_av_{af} + m_bv_{bf}$$

v_{ai}, v_{bi}, v_{af}, and v_{bf} are the magnitudes of the respective velocity vectors. They have positive signs if the velocities are in the positive direction, and negative signs if the velocities are in the negative direction. The positive direction is chosen arbitrarily.

Example: Figure 3.9 shows two bodies moving toward each other on a frictionless air track. Body A has a mass of 2 kg and a speed of 4 m/s; body B has a mass of 3 kg and has a speed of 1 m/s. After the bodies collide, body A moves away with a velocity of 2 m/s to the left. What is the final velocity of body B?

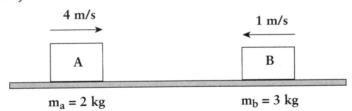

4 m/s   1 m/s

A   B

$m_a = 2$ kg $m_b = 3$ kg

Figure 3.9

Solution: This problem may be solved by equating the total momentum before the collision with the total momentum after the collision. Let the final velocity of body B be v_{bf}. Taking the right as positive (and therefore the left as negative):

$$m_av_{ai} + m_bv_{bi} = m_av_{af} + m_bv_{bf}$$

$$2(4) + 3(-1) = 2(-2) + 3(v_{bf})$$

$$v_{bf} = \frac{8 - 3 + 4}{3}$$

$$v_{bf} = 3 \text{ m/s}$$

The fact that the solution is positive means that body B is moving to the right after the collision.

In many typical one-dimensional problems the velocities before the collision are known, and **both** velocities after the collision are unknown. The two most common types of such problems are **completely inelastic collisions** and **completely elastic collisions**.

1. COMPLETELY INELASTIC COLLISIONS

A completely inelastic collision is one in which the colliding bodies stick together after the collision. This means that the final velocities of the two bodies are equal, and hence:

$$v_{af} = v_{bf} = v_f$$

Thus, there is only one unknown final velocity. This can be combined with the principle of the conservation of momentum to give:

$$m_a v_{ai} + m_b v_{bi} = (m_a + m_b) v_f$$

Example: Two rail freight cars are being hitched together. The first car has a mass of 15,750 kg and is moving at a speed of 4 m/s toward the second car, which is stationary and which has a mass of 19,250 kg. Calculate the final velocity of the two cars.

Solution: Using the modified equation above for the conservation of momentum:

$$m_a v_{ai} + m_b v_{bi} = (m_a + m_b) v_f$$

$$v_f = \frac{m_a v_{ai} + m_b v_{bi}}{m_a + m_b}$$

Taking the direction of the initial velocity of the car as the positive direction:

$$v_f = \frac{15,750(4) + 19,250(0)}{(15,750 + 19,250)}$$

$$v_f = 1.8 \text{ m/s}$$

The fact that v_f is positive means that after the collision, the two cars together are moving in the direction that the first car was moving initially.

2. COMPLETELY ELASTIC COLLISIONS

A completely elastic collision is one in which kinetic energy is conserved. The final velocities are not necessarily equal. If neither is given, then from the conservation of momentum equation there is one equation and two unknowns. However, in a completely elastic collision, the kinetic energy is conserved. That is to say, the sum of the kinetic energies just after the collision equals the sum of the kinetic energies just before the collision. This provides the needed second equation.

Conservation of momentum:

$$m_a v_{ai} + m_b v_{bi} = m_a v_{af} + m_b v_{bf}$$

Conservation of kinetic energy:

$$\frac{1}{2} m_a v_{ai}^2 + \frac{1}{2} m_b v_{bi}^2 = \frac{1}{2} m_a v_{af}^2 + \frac{1}{2} m_b v_{bf}^2$$

> **REMEMBER**
>
> Use conservation of energy and conservation of momentum in elastic collisions.

Example: Using the results obtained from the example on pages 629-630, establish whether the collision was completely elastic.

Solution: For the collision to be completely elastic, both the kinetic energy and the momentum must be conserved. The second condition has already been satisfied. Now the kinetic energy before the collision and the kinetic energy after the collision must be calculated, and only if these values are equal can it be said that the collision was completely elastic.

The kinetic energy before the collision is:

$$\frac{1}{2} m_a v_{ai}^2 + \frac{1}{2} m_b v_{bi}^2$$
$$= \frac{1}{2}(2)(4)^2 + \frac{1}{2}(3)(-1)^2$$
$$= 17.5 \text{ J}$$

The kinetic energy after the collision is:

$$\frac{1}{2} m_a v_{af}^2 + \frac{1}{2} m_b v_{bf}^2$$
$$= \frac{1}{2}(2)(-2)^2 + \frac{1}{2}(3)(3)^2$$
$$= 17.5 \text{ J}$$

> **KEY CONCEPT**
>
> In elastic collisions: (total kinetic energy before collision) = (total kinetic energy after collision).

Since the kinetic energy is not changed by the collision, it can be said that the collision was completely elastic.

CENTER OF MASS

Every object has a special point known as the **center of mass.** Consider a tennis racket being thrown into the air. Each part of the racket moves in its own way, so it's not possible to represent the motion of the racket as a single particle. However, there will be one point along the axis of the racket that moves in a simple parabolic path, very similar to the flight of a tennis ball. It is this point that is known as the center of mass. This is shown more clearly in Figure 3.10.

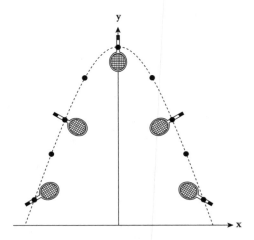

Figure 3.10

For a system of two masses m_1, m_2 lying along the x-axis at points x_1 and x_2 respectively, the center of mass is:

$$X = \frac{m_1 x_1 + m_2 x_2}{m_1 + m_2}$$

For a system with several masses strung out along the x-axis the center of mass is given by

$$X = \frac{m_1 x_1 + m_2 x_2 + m_3 x_3 + \ldots}{m_1 + m_2 + m_3 + \ldots}$$

For a system in which the particles are distributed in all three dimensions, the center of mass is defined by the three coordinates:

$$X = \frac{m_1 x_1 + m_2 x_2 + m_3 x_3 + \ldots}{m_1 + m_2 + m_3 + \ldots}$$

$$Y = \frac{m_1 y_1 + m_2 y_2 + m_3 y_3 + \ldots}{m_1 + m_2 + m_3 + \ldots}$$

$$Z = \frac{m_1 z_1 + m_2 z_2 + m_3 z_3 + \ldots}{m_1 + m_2 + m_3 + \ldots}$$

The **center of gravity** is the point at which the entire force due to gravity can be thought of as acting. It is found from similar formulas:

$$X = \frac{W_1 x_1 + W_2 x_2 + W_3 x_3 + \ldots}{W_1 + W_2 + W_3 + \ldots}$$

$$Y = \frac{W_1 y_1 + W_2 y_2 + W_3 y_3 + \ldots}{W_1 + W_2 + W_3 + \ldots}$$

$$Z = \frac{W_1 z_1 + W_2 z_2 + W_3 z_3 + \ldots}{W_1 + W_2 + W_3 + \ldots}$$

Since $W = mg$, the center of gravity and the center of mass will be the same point as long as g is constant.

REMEMBER

When you see the words "center of gravity," think center of mass, and vice versa.

Example: Find the center of mass with respect to the x- and y-axes of two uniform metal cubes that are attached to each other as shown in the figure below. One cube has a mass of 2 kg and is 0.4 m on its side, the other has a mass of 0.5 kg and is 0.2 m on its side.

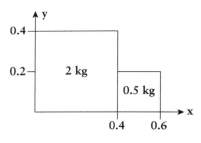

Figure 3.11

KEY CONCEPT

The force of gravity on an object acts through the center of gravity.

Solution: The fact that the cubes are uniform implies that the center of mass for each cube is located at the center of that cube. Therefore, the problem becomes finding the center of mass of two point masses; one is a 2 kg mass located at 0.2 m along the x-axis and 0.2 m along the y-axis, and the other is a 0.5 kg mass located at 0.5 m along the x-axis and 0.1 m along the y-axis.

Let's consider the x-coordinate first. The x component of the center of mass can be determined by the following formula:

$$X = \frac{m_1 x_1 + m_2 x_2 + m_3 x_3 + \ldots}{m_1 + m_2 + m_3 + \ldots}$$

Taking m_1 as 2 kg, x_1 as 0.2 m, m_2 as 0.5 kg, and x_2 as 0.5 m:

$$X = \frac{m_1 x_1 + m_2 x_2}{m_1 + m_2}$$

REMEMBER

The center of mass of a uniform object is in the center of the object, i.e., the center of mass of a uniform bar is in the center of the bar.

$$= \frac{2(0.2) + 0.5(0.5)}{2 + .05}$$

$$= \frac{0.65}{2.5}$$

$$= 0.26 \text{ m}$$

The y component of the center of mass can be determined by the following formula:

$$Y = \frac{m_1y_1 + m_2y_2 + m_3y_3 + \ldots}{m_1 + m_2 + m_3 + \ldots}$$

Taking m_1 as 2 kg, y_1 as 0.2 m, m_2 as 0.5 kg, and y_2 as 0.1 m:

$$Y = \frac{m_1y_1 + m_2y_2}{m_1 + m_2}$$

$$= \frac{2(0.2) + 0.5(0.1)}{2 + 0.5}$$

$$= \frac{0.45}{2.5}$$

$$= 0.18 \text{ m}$$

4

Thermodynamics

Thermodynamics is the study of heat and its effects. Primary to this study are the concepts of temperature, heat, pressure, volume, work, internal energy, and entropy. As applications of these concepts, we will review thermal expansion, heat transfer processes, the notion of specific heat, heat of transformation (latent heat), and p-v diagrams, including the relationship between work, pressure, and volume. The 1st law of thermodynamics, or conservation of energy in the presence of heat transfer, is reviewed, as is the 2nd law of thermodynamics along with the associated concept of entropy.

TEMPERATURE

A. Temperature

All bodies possess a property called **temperature**. In common usage, temperature is the relative measure of how hot or cold something is. In the study of thermodynamics, however, temperature must be measured quantitatively on a defined scale. There are three scales used to make these measurements of temperature on a thermometer: the **Fahrenheit** (°F), the **Celsius** (°C), and the **Kelvin** (K) scales. Absolute zero and the boiling and freezing points of water for the three scales are listed in the table below.

> **KEY CONCEPT**
>
> Temperature is a measure of the random kinetic energy of the molecules of a substance.

Temperature Scales

Situation	K	°C	°F
Absolute zero	0	−273	−460
Freezing point of water	273	0	32
Boiling point of water	373	100	212

The Kelvin scale is most commonly used for scientific measurements and is a base unit in SI. The Celsius scale is convenient for everyday usage because of its phase change points for water. The Kelvin degree and Celsius degree are the same size. The following formulas are used to convert from one scale to another:

$$T_C = T_K - 273$$

$$T_F = \frac{9}{5}T_C + 32$$

where T_C stands for degrees Celsius, T_K stands for degrees Kelvin, and T_F stands for degrees Fahrenheit.

Example: If the weatherperson says that the temperature will reach a high of 303 K today, what will be the temperature in °C and in °F?

KEY CONCEPT

A change of 1 K = a change of 1°C. 0°C = 273 K.

Solution: To convert from Kelvin to Celsius, use:

$$T_C = T_K - 273$$
$$= 303 - 273$$
$$= 30°C$$

Now to convert from Celsius to Fahrenheit use:

$$T_F = \frac{9}{5}T_C + 32$$

$$= \frac{9}{5}(30) + 32$$

$$= 86°F$$

B. Thermal Expansion

KEY CONCEPT

When you see the symbol Δ in front of a quantity, think final minus initial value.

Rising temperatures cause most solids to increase in length. The amount of expansion, known as **thermal expansion**, is proportional to the length of the solid and the increase in temperature:

$$\Delta L = \alpha L \Delta T$$

where ΔL is the change in length, L is the original length, and ΔT is the change in temperature. The **coefficient of linear expansion** α is a constant that characterizes how a specific material's length changes as the temperature changes. This usually has units of K^{-1}, though it may sometimes be quoted as $°C^{-1}$. Note that since a change of 1 K is the same as a change of 1°C, α quoted in units of K^{-1} is absolutely equal to α quoted in units of $°C^{-1}$.

Example: A metal rod of length 2 m and a coefficient of expansion of 11×10^{-6} K^{-1} is heated from 30°C to 1,080°C. By what amount does the rod expand?

Solution: By using the information given in the problem, we can substitute directly into the thermal expansion formula:

$$\Delta L = \alpha L \Delta T$$
$$= (11 \times 10^{-6})(2)(1,080 - 30)$$
$$= 0.023 \text{ m}$$

Liquids also expand when heated, but in their case the only meaningful parameter of expansion is **volume expansion.** The formula that governs this expansion for both solids and liquids is:

$$\Delta V = \beta V \, \Delta T$$

where $\beta = 3\alpha$.

Example: Assume that a thermometer with 1 ml of mercury is taken from a freezer with a temperature of –25°C and placed near an oven at 225°C. If the coefficient of volume expansion of mercury is 1.8×10^{-4} K^{-1}, by how much will the liquid expand?

Solution: Using the information given:

$$\Delta V = \beta V \, \Delta T$$
$$= (1.8 \times 10^{-4})(1)(225 - (-25))$$
$$= 0.045 \text{ ml}$$

HEAT

As was stated in the earlier section, all macroscopic objects have a property called temperature. What exactly does a body's temperature say about that body? The answer is that a body's temperature is related to the internal energy of that body. At constant volume, an increase in temperature indicates an increase in internal energy, and a decrease in temperature indicates a decrease in internal energy.

When two objects that are at different temperatures are brought into contact, the object with a higher temperature will give off **heat** energy to the cooler body until both objects have the same temperature. Heat can be defined as the energy transferred between two objects as a result of a difference in temperature. Note that heat can never be transferred from a cooler body to a warmer body without doing work on the system.

A. Heat Transfer

Heat energy can be transferred by conduction, convection, or radiation (or any combination of these processes). **Conduction** is the direct transfer of energy from molecule to molecule through molecular collisions.

Metals are the best heat conductors, since mobile electrons play a role in the transfer of heat from one molecule to the next. Gases tend to be the poorest heat conductors. An example of heat transfer through conduction is the heat that is rapidly conducted to your finger when you touch a hot stove.

Convection is the transfer of heat by the physical motion of the heated material. Since convection involves a flow of material, it can take place only in fluids (liquids and gases). During convection, heated portions of fluid rise from the source of heat, while colder portions sink. Thus, convection involves the transfer of heat through a flow of material.

Radiation is the transfer of energy by electromagnetic waves, which can travel through a vacuum. An example of this form of heat transfer is the warming effect the sun has on the earth.

B. Units

Units of heat are either the **calorie** (cal) for SI, or the **British thermal unit** (Btu) for English units. Note that the calorie defined here (lower-case c) and the term **Calorie** used in nutrition (uppercase C) are not the same. One food Calorie is equal to one thousand calories.

Since heat is equivalent to energy, the **Joule** is also suitable.

The conversion factors among the heat units are as follows:

$$1 \text{ Cal} = 10^3 \text{ cal} = 3.97 \text{ Btu} = 4{,}184 \text{ J}$$

C. Specific Heat

The heat Q gained or lost by an object and the change in temperature of that object ΔT are related by the equation:

$$Q = mc\ \Delta T = mc(T_f - T_i)$$

where m is the mass of the object and c is a proportionality constant called the **specific heat**. The specific heat can be defined as the amount of heat required to raise 1 kg of a substance 1 K or 1°C, and depends solely on the material of the object. This formula applies provided that the phase of the object — solid, liquid, or gas — does not change.

D. Heat of Transformation

The formula discussed above, $Q = mc\ \Delta T$, applies only when there is no change of phase. During a phase change the temperature remains constant and the heat gained or lost is related to the amount of material which changes phase. The amount of heat needed to change the phase of 1 kg of a substance is the **heat of transformation** L. The total amount of heat gained or lost by a substance during a phase change is given by:

$$Q = mL$$

where Q is the heat gained or lost, m is the mass of the substance, and L is the heat of transformation of the substance.

The phase change from liquid to solid, or solid to liquid, occurs at the melting point temperature. The corresponding heat of transformation is often referred to as the **heat of fusion**. On the other hand, the phase change from liquid to gas, or gas to liquid, occurs at the boiling point temperature. Here the heat of transformation is often referred to as the **heat of vaporization.**

Example: Silver has a melting point of roughly 1,000°C and a heat of fusion of 1×10^5 J/kg. The specific heat of silver is roughly 250 J/kg•°C. Approximately how much heat is required to completely melt a 1 kg silver chain, whose initial temperature is 20°C?

Solution: Before melting the chain, we must first get the temperature of the chain to the melting point. To figure out how much heat is required we use the formula:

$$Q = mc(T_f - T_i)$$
$$= 1(250)(1,000 - 20)$$
$$= 245,000 \text{ J}$$
$$= 245 \text{ kJ}$$

This tells us we have to add 245 kJ of heat to the chain just to get the chain's temperature to the melting point. The chain is still in the solid phase. To melt it (change its phase to liquid) we must continue to add heat in accordance with the formula:

$$Q = mL$$
$$= 1(1 \times 10^5)$$
$$= 100,000 \text{ J}$$
$$= 100 \text{ kJ}$$

The total heat needed to melt the solid silver chain is 245 kJ + 100 kJ = 345 kJ.

BRIDGE

Temperature is constant during a phase transition, i.e., when melting ice at 0°C, all of the ice must melt before the temperature increases. For more on phase transitions, see Chapter 8 of the General Chemistry Notes.

FIRST LAW OF THERMODYNAMICS

A. Pressure

Consider a gas contained in a box. The gas particles move in random directions and some of them hit the wall of the box. As the gas particles hit the wall of the box, they impart a force to the wall. If many particles hit the wall, the net force on the wall increases. The force per unit area is the **pressure** of the gas:

$$P = \frac{F}{A}$$

The SI unit of pressure is the Pascal (Pa). The Pascal is equivalent to a Newton/meter^2. Since this unit is a relatively low pressure, often you will see the pressure quoted in kilopascals (kPa) where 1 kPa = 10^3 Pa. The pressure at sea level can also be used as a unit. This is called an atmosphere (atm), and one atm is equal to 1.013×10^5 Pa.

B. Work

When dealing with the various problems of thermodynamics, the concept of a system is used. To describe a physical process there are two things to take into account: the system whose behavior is being observed and everything else (the environment).

A good example of a system is a gas contained in a cylinder with a piston that is able to move up when the gas expands and down when the gas is compressed. When the piston moves up, a force is exerted by the gas inside the cylinder to physically expand the system. Since the volume of the system has increased because of a pressure applied by it, work is said to have been done **by** the system. When the piston is compressed, causing the system's volume to decrease, work is done **on** the system by the environment. This implies that work, in thermo-dynamics problems, depends on pressure and volume.

During any thermodynamic process, a system goes from some initial state with an initial pressure and volume to some other state with a different pressure or volume. These thermodynamic processes are often represented in graphical form with volume on the x-axis and pressure on the y-axis [see Figure 4.1(a)–4.1(d)]. There are an infinite number of paths between an initial and final state. Different paths require different amounts of work. You can calculate the work done on or by a system by finding the area under the pressure-volume curve. Note that if volume doesn't change, then there can be no work done because there is no area to calculate. On the other hand, if pressure remains constant, the area under the curve is a rectangle of length P and width ($V_f - V_i$) or ΔV. Thus, for processes in which the pressure remains constant, $W = P \, \Delta V$.

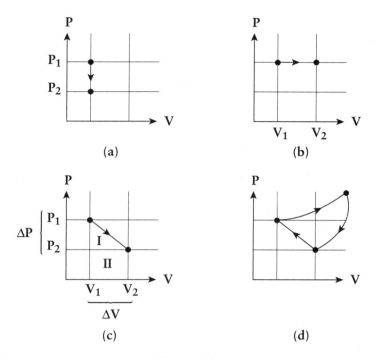

Figure 4.1

KEY CONCEPT

Net work done by a gas = (work done by gas) – (work done on gas). Work = (area under p-v curve) and = 0 if volume is constant.

Figure 4.1(a) shows that the system undergoes a decrease in pressure from P_1 to P_2. The work done in this process is zero, because volume is constant. In Figure 4.1(b) the system expands from V_1 to V_2 at constant pressure. When the pressure remains constant, the process is called **isobaric**. Here the work done is found using the formula shown above. The work in this case is positive. Figure 4.1(c) shows a case in which neither pressure nor volume is held constant. The total area under the graph (Regions I and II) gives the work done. Region I is a triangle whose base is ΔV and whose height is ΔP so the area is:

$$A_I = \frac{1}{2} \Delta V \Delta P$$

Region II is a rectangle with base ΔV and height P_2 so its area is:

$$A_{II} = P_2 \Delta V$$

Work now is the sum of Regions I and II:

$$W = A_I + A_{II}$$

Figure 4.1(d) shows a closed cycle in which, after certain interchanges of work and heat, the system returns to its initial state. Here, the work done is the area enclosed by the curve.

C. First Law of Thermodynamics

Internal energy (U) is the measure of all the energy, potential and kinetic, possessed by molecules in a system. The internal energy of a system can be increased by doing work on it or by adding heat to it. This change in internal energy ΔU is calculated from the **First Law of Thermodynamics:**

$$\Delta U = Q - W$$

where Q is the heat energy transferred to the body and W is the work done by the system. Note, we have chosen to use the more common letter U to represent internal energy; however, you may see it also represented by E. Also, note the following **sign convention:** Work done by the system is positive, but work done on the system is negative; heat flow into the system is positive, but heat flow out of the system is negative. The table below gives some special cases of the First Law:

Some Special Cases of the First Law of Thermodynamics

Process	First Law Becomes
Adiabatic ($Q = 0$)	$\Delta U = -W$
Constant Volume ($W = 0$)	$\Delta U = Q$
Closed Cycle ($\Delta U = 0$)	$Q = W$

Example: A gas in a cylinder is kept at a constant pressure of 3.5×10^5 Pa while 300 kJ of heat are added to it, causing the gas to expand from 0.9 m^3 to 1.5 m^3 Find:

  a. the work done by the gas.

  b. the change in internal energy of the gas.

Solution: a. The pressure is held constant through the entire process so the work can be found using the equation:

$$W = P\Delta V$$
$$= (3.5 \times 10^5)(1.5 - 0.9)$$
$$= 2.1 \times 10^5 \text{ J}$$

  b. The change in internal energy can be found from the First Law of Thermodynamics:

$$\Delta U = Q - W$$
$$= 3 \times 10^5 - 2.1 \times 10^5$$
$$= 0.9 \times 10^5$$
$$= 9 \times 10^4 \text{ J}$$

ENTROPY AND THE SECOND LAW OF THERMODYNAMICS

Entropy can be defined as the measure of disorder of a system. One way to picture entropy is to imagine a pool divided in two by an impermeable barrier; one side is filled with water, and the other with ink. This system is highly ordered because the ink molecules and water molecules are physically separated. The position of a particular ink molecule is limited to one half of the pool; therefore, there is some degree of certainty as to where a given ink molecule can be found. If someone were to remove the barrier, however, the water and ink would mix until there was no discernible difference between them. The position of a particular ink molecule is less certain now because it has access to the entire pool, as opposed to half of it. Therefore, the order of the system has decreased and its entropy has increased.

The Second Law of Thermodynamics states that in any thermodynamic process that moves from one equilibrium state to another, the entropy of the system and environment together will either increase or remain unchanged. The entropy of the system and environment together will not change during a totally reversible process, but the entropy will increase in an irreversible process. (For a complete discussion of reversible and irreversible processes see Chapter 5 of the General Chemistry Home Study Notes.) Reexamination of the pool described above shows that it is perfectly acceptable for the ink and water to diffuse and mix together, but it is a violation of the Second Law for the mixture to spontaneously separate into two distinct sections of water and ink.

Isothermal processes are processes in which the temperature remains constant throughout. For reversible isothermal processes, the change in entropy of the system or of the environment can be found from:

$$\Delta S = \frac{Q}{T}$$

where T is the constant temperature of the system or environment in Kelvins.

Example: If, in a reversible process, 6.66×10^4 J of heat is used to change a 200 g block of ice to water at a temperature of 273 K, what is the change in the entropy of the system? (The heat of fusion of ice = 333 kJ/kg.)

KEY CONCEPT

The entropy of an isolated system increases for all real (irreversible) processes. The entropy of a system (not isolated) can decrease as long as the entropy of its surroundings increases by at least as much (refrigerators are examples of such a system).

Solution: We know that during a change of phase the temperature is constant, in this case 273 K. From the information given,

$$\Delta S = \frac{Q}{T}$$

$$= \frac{6.66 \times 10^4}{273}$$

$$= 244 \text{ J/K}$$

Note that we did not need to know the mass.

Fluids and Solids

In this chapter we review the physics of both fluids and solids. The basic concepts of density and pressure are covered as well as the applied concept of the pressure as a function of depth in a fluid. Hydrostatics, or the study of fluids at rest, is presented from the point of view of the two dominant concepts of hydrostatics: Pascal's principle, and Archimedes' principle. Hydro-dynamics, or the study of fluids in motion, takes us into a discussion of the continuity equation and Bernoulli's equation, as well as a brief discussion of the viscosity and behavior of real fluids. Finally, the elastic properties of solids are discussed along with the associated concepts of stress, strain, Young's modulus, shear modulus, and the bulk modulus.

FLUIDS AND SOLIDS

Both liquids and gases are classified as fluids; solids are not. Fluids are char-acterized by their ability to flow and to conform to the boundaries of any container they are put in. Solids, however, are characterized by their rigidity. While both fluids and solids can exert forces perpendicular to their surfaces, only solids can withstand shear (tangential) forces.

DENSITY AND PRESSURE

Density ρ is a scalar quantity that is defined as mass m per unit volume V. In equation form:

$$\rho = \frac{m}{V}$$

The units of density are kg/m^3 (SI). From the definition of density, the weight of an object can be expressed as the product of its density, volume, and the acceleration due to gravity:

$$W = mg$$
$$m = \rho V$$
$$W = \rho V g$$

The density of water is 10^3 kg/m^3 (= 1 gm/cm^3). The ratio of the density of a substance to the density of water is called **specific gravity**. Since it is a ratio, specific gravity has no units.

Example: Find the specific gravity of benzene, given that the density of benzene is 879 kg/m^3.

Solution: The ratio of the density of benzene to the density of water is the specific gravity.

$$\text{specific gravity} = \frac{\rho_{\text{benzene}}}{\rho_{\text{water}}}$$

$$= \frac{879}{1,000}$$

$$= 0.879$$

Pressure P is also a scalar quantity. It is defined as the magnitude of the normal force F per unit area A. As an equation it reads:

$$P = \frac{F}{A}$$

The SI unit of pressure is the Newton per square meter, also called the Pascal (1 Pa = 1 N/m^2). Another commonly used unit of pressure is the atmosphere, which is the average atmospheric pressure at sea level. It is related to the SI unit of pressure by:

$$1 \text{ atm} = 1.013 \times 10^5 \text{ Pa}$$

Example: The window of a skyscraper measures 2.0 m by 3.5 m. If a storm passes by and lowers the pressure outside the window to 0.997 atm while the pressure inside the building remains at 1 atm, what net force is pushing the window out?

Solution: The forces acting inside and outside the building are needed. However, before the forces may be calculated, the values of the pressure both inside and outside the building must be converted from atmospheres to Pascals.

$$1 \text{ atm} = 1.013 \times 10^5 \text{ Pa}$$
$$0.997 \text{ atm} = (0.997)(1.013 \times 10^5)$$
$$= 1.010 \times 10^5 \text{ Pa}$$

Using the equation for pressure, the force inside pushing out is,

$$F_i = P_i A$$
$$F_i = (1.013 \times 10^5)(7.0)$$
$$= 7.091 \times 10^5 \text{ N}$$

and the force outside pushing in is:

$$F_o = P_oA$$
$$F_o = (1.010 \times 10^5)(7.0)$$
$$= 7.070 \times 10^5 \text{ N}$$

The net force is the difference of these two:

$$F_{net} = 7.091 \times 10^5 - 7.070 \times 10^5$$
$$= 2,100 \text{ N}$$

To find the **absolute pressure P** in a fluid due to gravity somewhere below the surface, use the equation:

$$P = P_0 + \rho gh$$

where P_0 is the pressure at the surface, ρ is the density of the fluid, g is the acceleration due to gravity, and h is the depth. In many applications the pressure at the surface is atmospheric pressure, $P_0 = P_{atm} = 1.013 \times 10^5$ Pa. More common in everyday usage than the absolute pressure is what is called the **gauge pressure**. Automobile tire pressure is reported as gauge pressure. Gauge pressure P_g, is simply the difference between the absolute and atmospheric pressure. The equation for gauge pressure is:

$$P_g = P - P_{atm}$$

Note that if $P_0 = P_{atm}$, then $P_g = \rho gh$ at a depth h.

Example: A diver in the ocean is 20 m below the surface.

   a.   What is the absolute pressure he experiences? (density of sea water = 1,025 kg/m^3)

   b.   What is the gauge pressure?

Solution: a.   Using the equation for absolute pressure in a liquid:

$$P = P_{atm} + \rho gh$$
$$= 1.013 \times 10^5 + (1,025)(9.8)(20)$$
$$= 3.02 \times 10^5 \text{ Pa}$$

   b.   Using the equation for gauge pressure:

$$P_g = P - P_{atm}$$
$$= (3.02 - 1.013) \times 10^5$$
$$= 2.01 \times 10^5 \text{ Pa}$$

KEY CONCEPT

Pressure increases linearly with depth below the surface of a liquid, and depends on the density of the liquid but not on the density of the object in the liquid.

HYDROSTATICS

A. Pascal's Principle

Pascal's principle deals with the transmission of pressures in enclosed fluids. The principle states:

A change in the pressure applied to an enclosed fluid is transmitted undiminished to every portion of the fluid and to the walls of the containing vessel.

For example, a fluid in a tube exerts pressure on an object at any depth below the surface of the fluid. When the pressure on the fluid is increased, pressure will be increased throughout the fluid and on any submerged object in the fluid.

Pascal's principle is the basis of the hydraulic lever (see Figure 5.1). Consider the case when an external force of magnitude F_1 is applied to the left-hand piston of area A_1. To keep the system in equilibrium, a force of magnitude F_2 must be applied to the right-hand piston of area A_2.

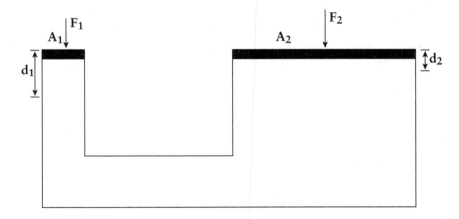

Figure 5.1

Pascal's principle states that a change in pressure is transmitted to every portion of the fluid. Since the system remains in equilibrium as the pressure changes, the change in pressure in both pistons must be equal and is given by:

$$\Delta P = \frac{F_1}{A_1} = \frac{F_2}{A_2}$$

$$F_2 = F_1 \frac{A_2}{A_1}$$

This equation shows that F_2 can be made larger if $A_2 > A_1$.

When piston 1 is moved down a distance d_1, piston 2 moves up a distance d_2. If the fluid is incompressible, then the volume in the system must remain constant. This implies that:

$$V = A_1d_1 = A_2d_2$$

$$d_2 = d_1 \frac{A_1}{A_2}$$

By combining the above two equations the expression below is obtained:

$$F_1d_1 = F_2d_2 = W$$

where work W is the product of force and distance. This shows that no additional work is being done by the greater force; the greater force is moving through a smaller distance.

Example: A hydraulic press has a piston of radius 5 cm, which pushes down on an enclosed fluid. A 45 kg weight rests on this piston. The other piston has a radius of 20 cm. Taking g = 10 m/s², what force is needed on the larger piston to keep the press in equilibrium?

Solution: Using Pascal's principle:

$$\frac{F_2}{A_2} = \frac{F_1}{A_1}$$

$$F_2 = \frac{F_1A_2}{A_1}$$

Since $F_1 = mg$, and $A = \pi r^2$, it is possible to solve for F_2:

$$F_2 = \frac{45(10)\pi(0.2)^2}{\pi(0.05)^2}$$

$$= 7{,}200 \text{ N}$$

B. Archimedes' Principle

Archimedes' principle deals with the buoyancy of objects when placed in a fluid. It explains why ships float and why objects seem lighter when underwater. The principle states:

A body wholly or partially immersed in a fluid will be buoyed up by a force equal to the weight of the fluid that it displaces.

In other words, when any object is placed in a fluid, it displaces some of that fluid, and the weight of the displaced fluid equals the magnitude of the upward buoyant force which the fluid exerts on the object. If the volume of fluid displaced by the object has a weight greater than the object's weight, then the object will float. If the weight of fluid displaced is less than the object's weight, then the object will sink deeper until the weight of the displaced fluid exceeds its own weight. If the weight of the displaced fluid is less than the object's weight even when fully submerged, then the object will sink. In terms of density, if the average density of the object is less than that of the surrounding fluid, then the object will float. However, if the average density of the object is greater than that of the surrounding fluid, then the object will sink.

Example: A wooden block floats in the ocean with half its volume submerged. Find the density of the wood ρ_b. (The density of seawater is 1,024 kg/m³.)

Solution: The weight of the block of total volume V_b is:

$$W_b = m_b g = \rho_b V_b g$$

The weight of the displaced seawater is the buoyant force and is given by:

$$W_w = F_{buoy} = m_w g = \rho_w V_w g$$

where ρ_w is the density of seawater (1,024 kg/m³) and V_w is the volume of displaced water, which is also the volume of that part of the block which is submerged. Since the block is floating, the buoyant force equals the block's weight:

$$W_b = F_{buoy}$$
$$\rho_b V_b g = \rho_w V_w g$$

We are given that half the block is submerged, so $V_w = V_b/2$.

$$\rho_b V_b g = \frac{1}{2} \rho_w V_b g$$

$$\rho_b = \frac{1}{2} \rho_w$$

$$\rho_b = \frac{1}{2} (1,024)$$

$$= 512 \text{ kg/m}^3$$

C. Surface Tension

There are two types of forces that the molecules of a liquid experience. The first type is **adhesion**, which is the attractive force that a molecule of the liquid feels toward the molecules of some other substance. For example, the adhesive force causes water droplets to stick to the windshield of a car even though gravity is pulling them downward.

The second type of force experienced by the molecules in a liquid is **cohesion**. Cohesion is the attractive force that a molecule of the liquid feels toward the other molecules of the liquid. Below the surface of the liquid, the cohesive forces cancel out since any one molecule is surrounded on all sides by the other molecules of the liquid. However, on the surface, the molecules feel an unbalanced force pulling them back toward the liquid. This causes the surface to behave like a skin and results in what is known as the **surface tension**. An example of the force of the surface tension is the fact that an insect can float on water even though its density is greater than that of water.

HYDRODYNAMICS

A. Streamlines

When talking about flowing fluids it is helpful to use streamlines. Streamlines are the paths followed by tiny fluid elements (sometimes called fluid particles) as they move. The velocity of a fluid particle will always be tangent to the streamline at that point. It is important to note that streamlines may never cross.

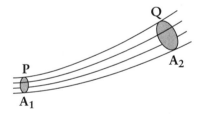

Figure 5.2

Figure 5.2 shows a tube of flow defined by streamlines that form its boundary. Mass flows from cross sectional area A_1 to A_2. The mass of fluid flowing per second through cross sectional area A is given by $Av\rho$, where v is the velocity and ρ is the density. Since matter is conserved, the mass flow rate of fluid must remain constant from one cross-section to another. It is also assumed that the fluid is incompressible, which implies that the densities are equal. Therefore, canceling the density, we find that the volume flow rate is given by:

$$v_1A_1 = v_2A_2 = \text{constant}$$

which is known as the **continuity equation**. This equation states that in narrow passages the flow is faster than in wider passages.

B. Bernoulli's Equation

The continuity equation, stated previously, results from the conservation of the mass of the fluid. This equation is a statement of the fluid's incompressibility as it flows from one point to another. Energy is also conserved as the fluid flows, and Bernoulli formulated this fact into the following equation that bears his name:

$$P_1 + \frac{\rho v_1^2}{2} + \rho g y_1 = P_2 + \frac{\rho v_2^2}{2} + \rho g y_2 = \text{a constant}$$

where P is the absolute pressure of the fluid, ρ is the density of the fluid, v is the velocity of the fluid, g is the acceleration due to gravity, and y is the height of the fluid relative to some reference height. Like the continuity equation, the Bernoulli equation also refers to two distinct points along the fluid flow labeled by subscripts 1 and 2 respectively. An important relation is derived for the case in which the height of the fluid doesn't change from point 1 to point 2 ($y_1 = y_2$). The pressure of the fluid then decreases as the velocity of the fluid increases and vice versa.

Example: An office building with a bathroom 40 m above ground has its water enter the building through a pipe at ground level with an inner diameter of 4 cm. If the flow velocity when entering is 3 m/s and at the top is 8 m/s, find the cross-sectional area of the pipe at the top and the pressure needed at the bottom so that pressure in the bathroom is 3×10^5 Pa.

Solution: The cross-sectional area of the pipe in the bathroom is calculated using the continuity equation, where point 1 is the ground level and point 2 is the bathroom:

$$A_2 = A_1 \frac{v_1}{v_2}$$

$$= \pi(0.02)^2 \frac{3}{8}$$

$$= \pi(1.5 \times 10^{-4})$$

$$= 4.71 \times 10^{-4} \text{ m}^2$$

The pressure can be found from Bernoulli's equation:

$$P_1 + \frac{1}{2}\rho v_1{}^2 + \rho g y_1 = P_2 + \frac{1}{2}\rho v_2{}^2 + \rho g y_2$$

$$P_1 = P_2 + \frac{1}{2}\rho(v_2{}^2 - v_1{}^2) + \rho g(y_2 - y_1)$$

$$= 3 \times 10^5 + \frac{1}{2}(1 \times 10^3)((8)^2 - (3)^2) + (1 \times 10^3)(9.8)(40)$$

$$= 7.2 \times 10^5 \text{ Pa}$$

C. Viscosity

Viscosity η is a measure of the internal friction of a fluid. Because of viscosity, a force must be exerted to cause one layer of fluid to slide past another. Both liquids and gases have viscosity, though the viscosity of gases is much lower than that of liquids since a gas has a much lower density. Consider a person moving a hand through air. Little effort is required to move the air out of the way, hence the viscosity of air is very low. However, for the same person to move the same hand through a tub of water is much more difficult. This is because water has a much higher viscosity than air, and so a greater force is required to move the water out of the way.

The SI unit of viscosity is the Newton•second/meter^2 (N•s/m^2). The CGS unit is the dyne•second/centimeter^2 (dyn•s/cm^2), also called the poise. 1 N•s/m^2 = 10 poise.

> **REMEMBER**
>
> Viscosity is a measure of the frictional force in a fluid. Don't forget, frictional forces always oppose the motion of an object.

D. Laminar and Turbulent Flow

The simplest type of flow in a tube is **laminar flow**: thin layers of liquid sliding over one another. However, when the velocity of a fluid flowing in a tube exceeds a certain critical velocity v_c (dependent on the properties of the fluid and the diameter of the tube), the nature of the flow becomes very complex. In this case laminar flow occurs only in a very thin layer adjacent to the walls, called the boundary layer. The flow velocity is zero at the tube walls and increases uniformly throughout the layer. Beyond the boundary layer, the motion is highly irregular. Here, random local circular currents called vortices develop within the fluid, and this results in a large increase in resistance to flow. This type of flow is known as **turbulence**.

For a fluid flowing through a tube of diameter D, a critical velocity v_c exists below which the flow is laminar and above which it is turbulent. This critical velocity can be calculated from the properties of the fluid flow and is given by:

$$v_c = \frac{N_R \eta}{\rho D}$$

where N_R is a dimensionless constant called the Reynolds number, η is the viscosity of the fluid, ρ is the density of the fluid, and D is the diameter of the tube.

ELASTIC PROPERTIES OF SOLIDS

A. Young's Modulus

The elasticity of a solid is characterized by a number of different quantities called **moduli.** When subjected to a stretching or tensile force F, a material will stretch a length ΔL. Defining a modulus in terms of F and ΔL is difficult because two bodies made of the same substance might require differing forces to yield the same ΔL. This ambiguity is eliminated by defining the tensile stress as the force per unit area, where the force is perpendicular to the area. Similarly, the change in length ΔL may vary for identical materials of different starting lengths L. This ambiguity is also eliminated by defining a quantity called the **strain,** which is the elongation per unit length $\Delta L / L$. It is assumed that upon termination of the stress, the material returns to its original length. Young's modulus Y is then defined as the quotient of stress over strain and is given by:

$$Y = \frac{(F/A)}{(\Delta L /L)} = \frac{\text{stress}}{\text{strain}}$$

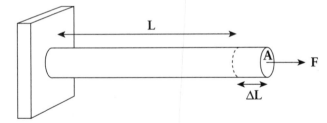

Figure 5.3

Yield strength is the point beyond which a material will not return to its original dimensions once the force is removed. If more stress is applied, eventually the ultimate strength is reached. Beyond that point, rupture occurs.

B. Shear Modulus

Another type of deforming stress is **shearing,** which is measured in units of force per unit area. However, in this case the force vector lies parallel to the area as shown in Figure 5.4. The corresponding deformation or strain is x, the movement in the direction of the force, divided by h.

The **shear modulus** is defined as the ratio of the stress to the strain and is given by:

$$S = \frac{(F/A)}{(x/h)}$$

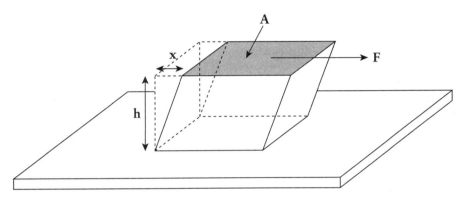

Figure 5.4

C. Bulk Modulus

The **bulk modulus** relates the change in pressure acting on the surfaces of a solid or fluid to the change in volume that is produced. The stress is the change in pressure ΔP and the strain is $\Delta V/V$, where V is the original volume and ΔV is the decrease in volume. This leads to the following equation for the bulk modulus:

$$B = \frac{\Delta P}{\Delta V / V}$$

REMEMBER

Bulk modulus describes the change in volume of a material, whereas Young's modulus describes the change in length of a material.

6

Electrostatics

Electrostatics is the study of stationary or static charges and the forces between them. In this chapter we will review Coulomb's law, which gives the electrostatic force between two charges and then discuss the concept of the electric field, which gives the electrostatic force per unit charge. The topic of electric potential energy is discussed along with the related topic of the electric potential, which is electric potential energy per unit charge. One can think of the electric potential being related to the electric potential energy in the same way as the electric field is related to the electric force. Associated with the electric field and electric potential are the concepts of field lines and equipotential lines which are reviewed separately.

CHARGES

Charge may be either positive or negative. A positive charge and a negative charge attract one another; positive repels positive; and negative repels negative. To summarize: **unlike charges attract, like charges repel.** The force that exists between stationary charges is known as the **electrostatic** force.

Net charge can appear on a macroscopic object due to friction. If a glass rod is rubbed on a piece of silk, electrons, which are negatively charged, flow from the glass rod to the silk cloth. This results in the glass rod being positively charged and the silk cloth being negatively charged. The rod and cloth then attract each other; this is known as static cling.

The SI unit of charge is the **Coulomb** and the **fundamental unit of charge** is:

$$e = 1.60 \times 10^{-19} \text{ C}$$

Both protons and electrons have this amount of charge, though protons are positively charged ($q = +e$), and electrons are negatively charged ($q = -e$).

COULOMB'S LAW

Coulomb's law gives the magnitude of the electrostatic force F between two charges, q_1 and q_2 whose centers are separated by a distance r:

$$F = k\frac{q_1 q_2}{r^2}$$

where k is called **Coulomb's constant** or the **electrostatic constant**, and is a number that depends on the units used in the equation. In SI units $k = 1/4\pi\varepsilon_0 = 8.99 \times 10^9$ N•m²/C², where $\varepsilon_0 = 8.85 \times 10^{-12}$ C²/N•m² and is called the **permittivity of free space**.

Coulomb's law in SI units is therefore:

$$F = k\frac{q_1 q_2}{r^2} = \frac{1}{4\pi\varepsilon_0}\frac{q_1 q_2}{r^2} = 8.99 \times 10^9 \frac{q_1 q_2}{r^2}$$

where the force F is in Newtons, the charges q_1 and q_2 are in Coulombs, and the distance r is in meters. The direction of the force may be obtained by remembering that unlike charges attract and like charges repel. The force always points along the line connecting the centers of the two charges.

Example: A positive charge is attracted to a negative charge a certain distance away. The charges are then moved so that they are separated by twice the distance. How has the force of attraction changed between them?

Solution: Coulomb's law states that the force between two charges varies as the inverse of the square of the distance between them. Therefore, if the distance is doubled, the square of the distance is quadrupled and the force is reduced to 1/4 of what it was originally. Note that it was not necessary to know the distance or the units being used, but only the fact that the distance was doubled and that the relation was an inverse square law.

Example: Negatively charged electrons are electrostatically attracted to positively charged protons (together they form hydrogen atoms). Because electrons and protons have mass, they will be gravitationally attracted to each other as well. Compare the two forces using Coulomb's law and Newton's law of gravitation.

(Use $m_p = 1.67 \times 10^{-27}$ kg, $m_e = 9.11 \times 10^{-31}$ kg, and a Bohr radius separation between the electron and proton so that $r = 5.29 \times 10^{-11}$ m.)

Solution: Both Coulomb's law and Newton's law state that the attractive forces between the electron and proton vary as the inverse of the square of the distance between them. As calculated in Chapter 2, the gravitational attractive force is:

$$F_N = \frac{Gm_pm_e}{r^2}$$

$$= \frac{(6.67 \times 10^{-11})(1.67 \times 10^{-27})(9.11 \times 10^{-31})}{(5.29 \times 10^{-11})^2}$$

$$= 3.63 \times 10^{-47} \text{ N} \approx 10^{-47} \text{ N}$$

On the other hand, the magnitude of the electrostatic attractive force is:

$$F_c = \frac{1}{4\pi\varepsilon_0} \frac{q_pq_e}{r^2}$$

$$= \frac{(8.99 \times 10^9)(1.60 \times 10^{-19})(1.60 \times 10^{-19})}{(5.29 \times 10^{-11})^2}$$

$$= 8.22 \times 10^{-8} \text{ N} \approx 10^{-7} \text{ N}$$

Note that the electrostatic attraction between the electron and proton is stronger than the gravitational attraction by a factor of approximately 10^{40}.

ELECTRIC FIELD

Every electric charge sets up a surrounding **electric field**. The electric field can be detected by the force it exerts on other electric charges. It is defined as the force on a stationary positive test charge q_0 divided by the charge. It is therefore a vector quantity given by:

$$E = \frac{F}{q_0}$$

The electric field **E** points in the direction of the force **F** on the positive test charge q_0. In SI units, **E** is measured in Newtons/Coulomb, which equals Volts/meter. The Volt will be defined in the next section where the electric potential is discussed.

Given an electric field **E** in some region of space, any charge q placed in the field experiences a force **F** given by:

$$F = qE$$

REMEMBER

The electric field is a vector with units given by $E = \frac{F}{q_0} =$ Newtons/Coulomb.

REMEMBER

A positive charge in an electric field feels a force in the direction of the field. A negative charge in an electric field feels a force in the direction opposite the field.

In this vector equation we keep the sign of the charge, so that the force **F** is in the direction of q**E**: that is, in the same direction as **E** itself if q is positive, but in the opposite direction to **E** if q is negative.

The force on a positive test charge q_0 placed a distance r from a charge q is given by Coulomb's Law:

$$F = k\frac{qq_0}{r^2}$$

Using this equation and the fact that the electric field $E = F/q_0$, we get an equation for the electric field at any distance r from a charge q:

$$E = k\frac{q}{r^2}$$

REMEMBER

The electric field of a positive charge points radially outward from the charge. The electric field of a negative charge points radially inward toward the charge.

The **direction** of the electric field vector is such that it points away from q if q is a positive charge, but it points toward q if q is a negative charge.

In order to visualize the direction and magnitude of the electric field vector over a wide number of points, it is helpful to think of **field lines.** Field lines, or **lines of force**, as they are sometimes called, are imaginary lines that represent how a positive test charge would be accelerated in the electric field. For example, the field lines for a negatively charged particle such as an electron would point radially toward the charge, since the positive test charge would be attracted toward a negative charge. Similarly, the field lines point radially away from a positive charge, such as a proton, since the positive test charge would be repelled away from another positive charge.

REMEMBER

The electric field strength is stronger where the field lines are closer together and weaker where the field lines are farther apart.

The direction of the electric field, at a given point, is always tangent to the field line at that point and in the same direction. Field lines also indicate the relative strength of the electric field. Where the field lines are closer together the electric field is stronger; where the field lines are farther apart the electric field is weaker.

For a collection of charges, the total electric field at a point in space is the **vector sum** of the electric field due to each charge:

$$E_{total} = E_{q_1} + E_{q_2} + E_{q_3} + ... \text{ (vector sum)}$$

REMEMBER

Electric fields of separate charges add as vectors.

The vector sum must be carried out using the rules of vector addition, as shown in the following example.

Example: A positive charge of $+1 \times 10^{-5}$ C is located one meter away from another positive charge of $+2 \times 10^{-5}$ C. At what point along the line between the two charges is the electric field equal to zero?

Solution: In order for the sum of two vectors to be zero, they must be equal in magnitude and opposite in direction. Because both of the charges are positive, the electric field vector of each charge points away from the charge. Along the line between the two charges the two electric field vectors point in opposite directions. If the charges were equal in magnitude, the point at which the two fields have the same magnitude (and therefore where the resultant field is zero) would be exactly halfway between them. However, the charges are not equal, since one charge is half the charge of the other. Let x be the distance from the $+1 \times 10^{-5}$ C charge. The distance from the other charge is the total distance of one meter minus x, or $(1 - x)$.

Setting the magnitudes of the two fields equal to each other to find the distance x that will make them equal, we have:

$$k\frac{(1 \times 10^{-5})}{x^2} = k\frac{(2 \times 10^{-5})}{(1-x)^2}$$

$$\frac{1}{x^2} = \frac{2}{(1-x)^2}$$

$$2x^2 = (1-x)^2$$

$$\sqrt{2}\,x = 1 - x$$

$$x(1 + \sqrt{2}) = 1$$

$$x = \frac{1}{\sqrt{2}+1}$$

$$x = 0.41 \text{ m}$$

As might be expected, this point is closer to the smaller charge since the field of the larger charge is stronger.

ELECTRIC POTENTIAL

Just as work is required to lift an object against the Earth's gravitational field, work must be done to move an electric charge in an electric field. The **electric potential** at a point is defined as the amount of work needed to move a positive test charge q_0 from infinity to that point divided by the test charge q_0:

$$V = \frac{W}{q_0}$$

In SI units electric potential is measured in **Volts** (V) where 1 Volt = 1 Joule/ Coulomb. The electric potential at a distance r from a point charge q is:

$$V = k\frac{q}{r}$$

REMEMBER

The electric potential, V, has units of Volts and is electric potential energy per unit charge, so Volt = Joule/ Coulomb.

REMEMBER

The electric potential of a positive/negative charge is a positive/negative number.

V is a scalar quantity whose sign is determined by the sign of the charge q. For a positive charge V is positive, but for a negative charge V is negative. For a collection of charges, the total electric potential at a point in space is the **scalar sum** of the electric potential due to each charge:

$$V_{total} = V_{q_1} + V_{q_2} + V_{q_3} + \text{... (scalar sum)}$$

Potential difference (voltage) is the difference in potential between two points. If V_a and V_b are the electric potentials at points a and b, then the potential difference between a and b is $V_b - V_a$. From the definition of electric potential, it follows that the potential difference between a and b can be expressed as:

$$V_b - V_a = \frac{W_{ab}}{q_0}$$

where W_{ab} is the work needed to move a test charge q_0 through an electric field from a to b. The work depends only on the potentials at the two points a and b, and is independent of the path. This means that like the gravitational force in Chapter 3, the electrostatic force is a conservative force.

EQUIPOTENTIAL LINES

An **equipotential line** is one for which the potential at every point is the same. The potential difference between any two points on an equipotential line is zero. From the above equation it follows that no work is done when moving a test charge q_0 from one point to another on an equipotential line. Work will be done in going from one line to another, but the **work depends only on the potential difference of the two lines and not on the path.**

Example: In Figure 6.1 an electron goes from point a to point b in the vicinity of a very large positive charge. The electron could be made to follow any of the paths shown. Which path requires the least work to get the electron charge from a to b?

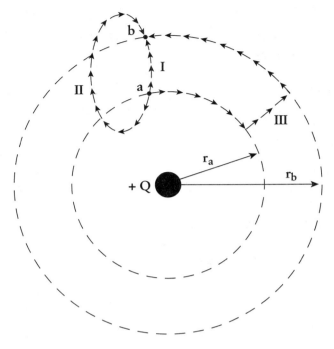

Figure 6.1

Solution: As stated, the **work depends only on the potential difference and not on the path,** so any of the paths shown would require the same amount of work in moving the electron from a to b, namely:

$$W_{ab} = q_e(V_b - V_a)$$

$$= q_e(k\frac{Q}{r_b} - k\frac{Q}{r_a})$$

So paths I, II, and III all require the same amount of work to move the electron. (Note that W_{ab} is positive in this example since $r_a < r_b$ and $q_e = -e$.)

ELECTRIC POTENTIAL ENERGY

We have already defined the electric potential V at a point in space as the amount of work W required to move a positive test charge q_0 from infinity to that point divided by q_0. We now define the electric potential energy U of an arbitrary charge q at that point in space to be the amount of work needed to move it from infinity to the point. Using the definition of the electric potential we get:

$$U = W = qV$$

where V is the electric potential due to the other charges. Note that the sign of U depends on the signs of q and V. Since U = qV, it may be said that V = U/q; electric potential can also be thought of as electric potential energy per unit charge. When V is due to just one other charge Q, V is given by kQ/r, and U may be rewritten as:

$$U = k\frac{qQ}{r}$$

$$= \left(\frac{1}{4\pi\varepsilon_0}\right)\frac{qQ}{r}$$

If the charges are both positive or both negative (in other words, like charges), U will be positive, but if one charge is positive and the other negative (that is, unlike charges), U will be negative.

Example: If a charge of +2e and a charge of –3e are separated by a distance of 3 nm, what is the potential energy of the system? (e is the fundamental unit of charge equal to 1.6×10^{-19} C.)

Solution: $U = k\dfrac{qQ}{r}$

From the question stem we know that q = +2e, Q = –3e, and r = 3nm = 3×10^{-9}m. So, putting these numbers into the equation, and approximating k as 9.0×10^9:

$$U = (9 \times 10^9)\frac{(2)(1.6 \times 10^{-19})(-3)(1.6 \times 10^{-19})}{3 \times 10^{-9}}$$

$$= -4.6 \times 10^{-19}\text{ J}$$

THE ELECTRIC DIPOLE

Two equal and opposite charges a small distance d away from each other form what is called an **electric dipole**. Suppose there is a dipole with charges +q and –q, as shown in Figure 6.2.

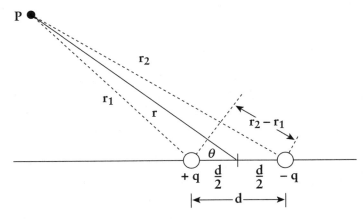

Figure 6.2

The potential at any point P is given by the sum of the two potentials:

$$V = k\frac{q}{r_1} - k\frac{q}{r_2}$$

$$= kq\left(\frac{r_2 - r_1}{r_1 r_2}\right)$$

For points relatively far from the dipole (compared to d), $r_1 r_2 \cong r^2$ and $r_2 - r_1 \cong d\cos\theta$. With these approximations the potential becomes:

$$V = k\frac{qd}{r^2}\cos\theta$$

The product of qd is defined as the **dipole moment p** with SI units of C•m. This is a vector quantity. Its magnitude is equal to the product qd, and its direction lies along the line connecting the charges (dipole axis) and points from the negative charge toward the positive charge. (Beware! Chemists often reverse this convention, having **p** point from the positive toward the negative charge.) In terms of dipole moment, one can rewrite the dipole potential as:

$$V = k\frac{p}{r^2}\cos\theta$$

Note that the potential is zero for $\theta = 90°$ and that this is the plane that lies halfway between +q and –q (called the perpendicular bisector of the dipole).

The electric field produced by the dipole at any point is the vector sum of each of the individual fields due to each of the two charges. Along the perpendicular bisector of the dipole the magnitude of the electric field can be approximated as:

$$E = \frac{1}{4\pi\varepsilon_0} \frac{p}{r^3}$$

The field will point in the opposite direction to **p**.

Example: The H_2O molecule has a dipole moment of 1.85 D, where D = Debye unit = 3.34×10^{-30} C•m. Calculate the electric potential due to an H_2O molecule at a point 89 nm away along the axis of the dipole. (Use $k = 9 \times 10^9$ N•m^2/C^2.)

Solution: Since the question asks for the potential along the axis of the dipole, the angle θ is given by 0°. Substituting the values into the equation for the dipole potential and multiplying 1.85 D by 3.34×10^{-30} to convert it to C•m:

$$V = k\frac{p}{r^2} \cos\theta$$

$$= 9 \times 10^9 \frac{(1.85)(3.34 \times 10^{-30})(\cos 0°)}{(89 \times 10^{-9})^2}$$

$$= 7 \times 10^{-6} \text{ V}$$

Now consider the case when an electric dipole is placed in a uniform external electric field. If there is no field present, the dipole moment will assume any random orientation. With a uniform external electric field present, however, each of the equal but opposite charges that make up the dipole will feel a force exerted on it by the external electric field. The net force will be zero, since the force on each charge is equal in magnitude but opposite in direction. The dipole therefore feels no translational force. However, there will be a nonzero torque about the center:

$$\tau = F\frac{d}{2}\sin\theta + F\frac{d}{2}\sin\theta$$

$$= Fd\sin\theta$$

$$= qEd\sin\theta$$

$$= (qd)E\sin\theta$$

$$= pE\sin\theta$$

where p is the magnitude of the dipole moment (p = qd), E is the magnitude of the uniform external electric field, and θ is the angle the dipole moment makes with the electric field. This torque will cause the dipole to reorient itself by rotating, so that its dipole moment, **p**, aligns with the electric field **E**. This is shown in Figure 6.3.

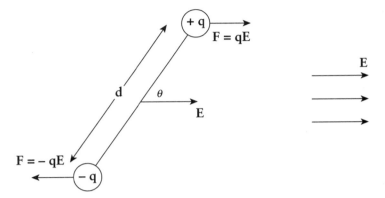

Figure 6.3

For more information on dipole moments, see Chapter 3 of the General Chemistry Notes.

7

Magnetism

In this chapter we will review the subject of magnetism. Unlike electrostatics where electric charges create electric fields which exert forces on other electric charges, magnetism has no fundamental magnetic charges. Instead, magnetic fields are created by moving charges, currents in wires, and permanent magnets. These magnetic fields, in turn, exert magnetic forces on the very things that create them, i.e., moving charges, currents in wires, and permanent magnets.

The first half of the chapter is concerned with the determination of the magnetic force due to a given magnetic field. Since force is a vector, both the magnitude and direction of the magnetic force are considered. The second half of the chapter then examines sources of magnetic fields, including a brief review of magnetic materials, and also a discussion of the two most common current configurations, the straight wire and the loop of wire.

KEY CONCEPT

Magnetic fields are created by moving charges and permanent magnets, and in turn exert forces on moving charges and permanent magnets.

THE MAGNETIC FIELD

In discussing the magnetic force on moving charges and on current carrying wires, we will assume the presence of a fixed and uniform magnetic field **B**. Of course, this field must be produced by some external source such as a magnet or arrangement of current-carrying wires, but for our purposes we are only concerned with the strength and direction of this field.

Like all physical quantities, magnetic fields have units. The SI unit of the magnetic field is the Tesla (T) where $1 \text{ T} = 1 \dfrac{N \bullet s}{m \bullet C}$. Small magnetic fields are sometimes measured in Gauss where 1 Tesla = 10^4 Gauss.

A. Force on a Moving Charge

When a charge moves in a magnetic field, a magnetic force is exerted on it. This force, like all forces, is a vector. The **magnitude** of F is given by:

$$F = qvB \sin \theta$$

In using this formula, θ is the smallest angle between the vectors q**v** and **B** (more on q**v** below), q is the charge of the moving particle, v is the particle's speed, and B = |**B**| is the magnitude of the magnetic field vector.

Right-hand rule for the direction of the magnetic force on a moving charge. Turning our attention to the **direction** of the magnetic force, we should first note that qv is a vector that depends on the velocity vector **v** and the sign of the charge q. If q is nonzero and positive (positive charge), then qv points in the same direction as **v**. If q is nonzero and negative (negative charge), then qv points in the opposite direction as **v**. (If q or v is zero, then the magnetic force will be zero.) The direction of the magnetic force will be **perpendicular** to the plane defined by qv and **B**, but this could be either of two directions. To find the correct direction let the thumb of the **right hand** (left-handed people must be careful to use the correct hand) point in the direction of the vector qv (that is, parallel to **v** if q is positive and antiparallel to **v** if q is negative). Let the remaining fingers of the **right hand** point in the direction of **B**. Your **palm** now points in the direction of **F**, the magnetic force on q.

REMEMBER

To find the direction of the magnetic force, use whichever (valid) right-hand rule you prefer.

(Note: The right-hand rule as stated above may differ from what you have previously learned. A different version would have the right index finger in the direction of qv and right middle finger in the direction of **B** and, holding the thumb perpendicular to these two fingers, the right thumb points in the direction of **F**. It is important only to get the direction correct no matter which rule you use. **If you have committed to memory another version of the rule, and it works, then feel free to use it.**)

KEY CONCEPT

The symbol "x" means the magnetic field direction is into the page, and the symbol "." means the magnetic field direction is out of the page.

Because of the three-dimensional nature of problems involving magnetic fields, scientists have chosen the following conventions to denote magnetic fields going into the page, or coming out of the page. The symbol x represents a field going into the page. The x represents the tail end of an arrow travelling into the page. The symbol • represents a field coming out of the page. The • represents the tip of an arrow coming out of the page.

Example: Suppose a proton, whose charge is +1.6 × 10⁻¹⁹ C, is moving with a speed of 15 m/s in a direction parallel to a uniform magnetic field of 3.0 T. What is the magnitude and direction of the magnetic force on the proton?

Solution: Because the proton is positively charged, the vector qv is in the same direction as **v**, which is the same direction as **B** as stated in the problem. Since qv and **B** are pointing in the same direction, the angle between the vectors is zero. Since sin 0° = 0 and F = qvB sin θ, the magnetic force on the proton is zero, too. Note that if the charge had been negative (an electron, for example), the angle between qv and **B** would have been 180° and since sin 180° = 0, the magnetic force on a negative charge moving parallel to a uniform magnetic field would be zero as well. In general, the magnetic force on a moving charge will be zero if the charge is moving parallel or antiparallel to the magnetic field.

Example: Suppose a proton whose charge equals $+1.6 \times 10^{-19}$ C is moving with a speed of 15 m/s toward the top of the page and through a uniform magnetic field of 3.0 T directed into the page (see Figure 7.1(a)). What is the magnitude and direction of the magnetic force on the proton?

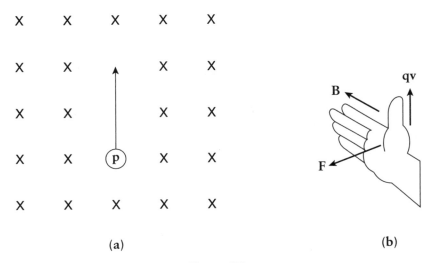

(a)   (b)

Figure 7.1

Solution: Because the proton is positively charged, the vector qv is in the same direction as **v**, which is perpendicular to **B** as stated in the problem. (**B** is perpendicular to the plane of the page.) Because qv and **B** are perpendicular, the angle between the vectors is θ = 90°, and since sin 90° = 1, the magnetic force on the proton is:

$$F = qvB \sin \theta$$
$$= qvB$$
$$= (1.6 \times 10^{-19})(15)(3.0)$$
$$= 7.2 \times 10^{-18} \text{ N}$$

By holding the thumb of the **right hand** so that it is directed toward the top of the page, then holding the remaining fingers of the **right hand** so that they point toward (into) the page, one's **right hand** palm points to the left (see

Figure 7.1(b)). Hence, the proton is deflected to the left on its upward journey. As the velocity of the proton changes, so does the magnetic force that it experiences. Note that if the charge had been negative (an electron, for example), the angle between qv and **B** still would have been 90°, but the right-hand rule would have required that qv point toward the bottom of the page, meaning one's right-hand palm would point to the right. Hence an electron is deflected to the right on its upward journey. One can readily see that the direction of the magnetic force on a negative charge moving through a magnetic field is opposite to the direction of the magnetic force acting on a positive charge moving in the same direction.

When a charged particle moves **perpendicular** to a **constant, uniform magnetic field**, the resulting motion is circular motion with constant speed in the plane perpendicular to the magnetic field. A centripetal force is always associated with circular motion. In this case the centripetal force is the magnetic force (F = qvB). Since the centripetal acceleration equals v^2/r, we get:

$$F = qvB = \frac{mv^2}{r}$$

From this equation one can solve for the orbit radius, the magnetic field, and so on:

$$r = \frac{mv}{qB} \qquad B = \frac{mv}{qr}$$

Example: Suppose the proton of the previous example is allowed to circle (counterclockwise) in the same perpendicular magnetic field of 3.0 T with the same speed of 15 m/s (as in Figure 7.2(a)). What is the orbit radius r? (The mass of a proton is 1.67×10^{-27} kg.)

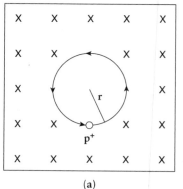

(a)

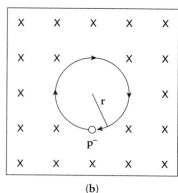

(b)

Figure 7.2

Solution: By equating the centripetal acceleration to the magnetic force and solving for the orbit radius as shown above:

$$r = \frac{mv}{qB}$$

$$= \frac{(1.67 \times 10^{-27})(15)}{(1.6 \times 10^{-19})(3)}$$

$$= 5.2 \times 10^{-8} \text{ m}$$

Note that the direction of the magnetic force on a negative charge moving through a uniform magnetic field is opposite to the direction of the magnetic force acting on a positive charge moving in the same direction. Therefore, if the charge had been negative (an antiproton, for example, which has the mass of the proton but is negatively charged), it would have circled in the **clockwise** direction with the same orbit radius. (See Figure 7.2 (b).)

REMEMBER

For a given field direction, if positive charges circle clockwise, then negative charges circle counterclockwise.

B. Current

Electric current will be discussed more completely in Chapter 8. However, it is important to realize that when two points at different electric potentials are connected with a conductor (such as a metal wire), charge flows between the two points. The flow of charge is called an **electric current**. The magnitude of the current i is the amount of charge Δq passing through the conductor per unit time Δt, or in the form of an equation:

$$i = \frac{\Delta q}{\Delta t}$$

KEY CONCEPT

Current is in the direction that positive charges would flow.

The SI unit of current is the Ampere (1 A = 1 Coulomb/second).

Charge is transmitted by a flow of electrons in a conductor. Since electrons are negatively charged, they go from lower potentials to higher potentials. But, **by convention**, the direction of **current** is the direction in which **positive charge** would flow, or from high to low potential. **Thus the direction of current is opposite to the direction of electron flow.**

C. Force on a Current-Carrying Wire

Since moving charge is subject to magnetic forces and electric current is a flow of charge, it should come as no surprise that magnetic forces can act on a current-carrying wire. For a straight wire of length L carrying a current i in a direction that makes an angle θ with a uniform magnetic field **B**, the magnitude of the magnetic force on the current-carrying wire is:

KEY CONCEPT

A current in a magnetic field behaves similarly to a positive charge moving in a magnetic field since current is a collection of moving positive charges.

$$F = iLB \sin \theta$$

The direction of the force is given by a simple right-hand rule, the **right-hand rule for the magnetic force on currents.** The force will be **perpendicular** to the plane defined by **B** and the direction of the current flow, but this could be either of two directions. To find the correct direction let the thumb of the **right hand** (left-handed people must be careful to use the correct hand) point in the direction of the current i. Now let the remaining fingers of the **right hand** point in the direction of **B**. The palm of the **right hand** now points in the direction of **F,** the magnetic force on the current-carrying wire. (Note: This rule is virtually the same as the rule given above for moving charges. Again, you should feel free to use any right-hand rule that you have committed to memory and that gives the correct direction.)

Example: Suppose a wire of length 2.0 m is conducting a current of 5.0 A toward the top of the page and through a 30 Gauss uniform magnetic field directed into the page (see Figure 7.3(a)). What is the magnitude and direction of the magnetic force on the wire?

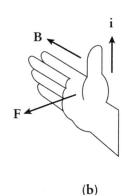

(a)　　　　　　　　　　　　　　　　　　(b)

Figure 7.3

Solution: Since 1 T = 10^4 Gauss, 1 Gauss = 10^{-4} T, 30 Gauss = 30 × 10^{-4} T = 3×10^{-3} T. The wire is conducting current toward the top of the page and the magnetic field points into the page; therefore, the current is perpendicular to **B**. The angle between them is $\theta = 90°$, and since $\sin 90° = 1$, the magnetic force on the wire is:

$$F = iLB \sin \theta = iLB$$
$$= 5.0(2.0)(3.0 \times 10^{-3})$$
$$= 3.0 \times 10^{-2} \text{ N} = 0.03 \text{ N}$$

By holding the thumb of the **right hand** so that it is directed toward the top of the page, then holding the remaining fingers toward (into) the page, the palm of the **right hand** points to the left. Hence the force on the wire is to the left.

SOURCES OF MAGNETIC FIELD

The previous section dealt with the magnetic force on a moving charge and a current-carrying wire, but did not discuss how the field was generated. Any moving charge creates a magnetic field. Magnetic fields may be set up by the "flow" of charge in permanent magnets, or electric currents, or simply by individual moving charges (e.g., an electron moving through space). This section deals only with permanent magnets and current-carrying wires, but it is important to realize that each of these sources of magnetic field has, in one sense or another, a flow of charge or a current—it is the movement of charge that gives rise to the magnetic field.

As with electric fields, magnetic **field lines** can be used to visualize the magnetic field. At any point along a field line the magnetic field itself is in the tangential direction.

A. Magnetic Materials

Materials are classified as diamagnetic, paramagnetic, and ferromagnetic. In a **diamagnetic material** the individual atoms have no net magnetic field. Diamagnetic materials will be repelled from the pole of a strong bar magnet, so they are sometimes called weakly antimagnetic. In **para-magnetic** and **ferromagnetic** materials the individual atoms do have a net magnetic field, but normally these individual atomic fields are randomly oriented so the material itself exhibits no net magnetic field. In a paramagnetic material under certain conditions, some degree of alignment of the individual atomic magnetic fields can occur. Paramagnetic materials will be attracted toward the pole of a strong bar magnet, so they are sometimes called weakly magnetic. In a ferromagnetic material a special effect takes place when the temperature drops below a critical value that allows a high degree of alignment of the magnetic fields of the individual atoms to occur. Above this critical temperature, called the Curie temperature, the material is paramagnetic. Ferromagnetic materials are sometimes called strongly magnetic and include iron, nickel, and cobalt. When the Curie temperature is above room temperature, ferromagnetic materials are permanently magnetized at room temperature (for example, the familiar bar magnet).

When a paper with iron filings is placed on top of a permanent bar magnet, the iron filings tend to form lines connecting the top of the magnet to the bottom of the magnet. The iron filings are showing the

FLASHBACK

Magnetic field lines are analogous to electric field lines, i.e., the magnetic field is tangent to the magnetic field line at any point.

REAL-WORLD ANALOGY

A compass is simply a small permanent magnet designed so that it can rotate to whatever direction it naturally seeks. In particular, the compass needle will align itself with the local magnetic field direction in such a way that the north pole of the compass magnet points in the field direction. The earth also acts like a permanent magnet, having north and south magnetic poles and field lines that go from the north to the south magnetic pole. So when the north pole of a compass magnet points along the local field line of earth's magnetic field it is actually pointing toward a magnetic south pole. Thus, what we call the northern direction is actually in the direction of a magnetic south pole.

magnetic field lines. All bar magnets have a **north** and **south** pole. The north pole is the place where the magnetic field lines emerge; the south pole is where they enter. Given two bar magnets, opposite poles attract each other; like poles repel.

B. Current-Carrying Wires

A current-carrying wire will produce a magnetic field in its vicinity. The magnetic field of a current-carrying wire is the vector sum of the magnetic fields due to the individual moving charges that comprise the current. The final result depends on the shape of the wire. Special cases include a long straight wire and the center of a circular loop of wire.

At a perpendicular distance r from an infinitely long and straight current-carrying wire the magnitude of the magnetic field produced by the current i in the wire is given by:

$$B = \frac{\mu_0 i}{2\pi r}$$

where μ_0 is the **permeability of free space** $= 4\pi \times 10^{-7}$ Tesla • meter/ Ampere $= 1.26 \times 10^{-6}$ T•m/A. The above equation shows that for a long straight wire, the field strength drops off with distance.

The magnetic field lines are concentric perpendicular circles about the wire. You can use a **right-hand rule to find the direction of the magnetic field produced by a long straight wire.** This rule differs from the previous ones. In this rule your **right thumb** points in the direction of the current. Your remaining **right fingers** mimic the circular magnetic field lines and curl around the wire. Your fingers now show you the direction of the magnetic field lines and the direction of B itself at any point. Note that this rule differs from the previous two in that it gives the direction of the field lines produced by the current instead of starting with a given direction of **B** to find the direction of a force. Also note that, as shown in a later example, this rule may be applied to current loops as well as straight wires.

Example: A straight wire carries a current of 5 A toward the top of the page (see Figure 7.4(a)). What is the magnitude and direction of the magnetic field at point P, which is 10 cm to the left of the wire? What is the magnitude and direction of the magnetic field at point Q, which is 2 cm to the right of the wire?

KEY CONCEPT

Magnetic field lines come out of north poles and go into south poles. Opposite magnetic poles attract and like poles repel.

REMEMBER

Magnetic field lines encircle currents. Use the right-hand rule (different than the rule for magnetic force on a moving charge) to find the field direction.

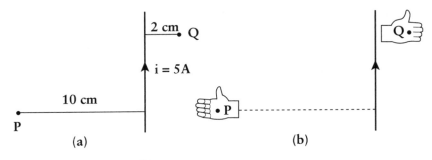

Figure 7.4

Solution: To find the magnitude at point P:

$$B = \frac{\mu_0 i}{2\pi r}$$

$$= \frac{(4\pi \times 10^{-7})(5)}{2\pi(0.1)}$$

$$= 10^{-5} \text{ T} = 0.1 \text{ Gauss}$$

To find the magnitude at point Q:

$$B = \frac{(4\pi \times 10^{-7})(5)}{2\pi(0.02)}$$

$$= 5 \times 10^{-5} \text{ T} = 0.5 \text{ Gauss}$$

Now to get the direction of the field for each of these points, we use the right-hand rule. Hold your **right thumb** toward the top of the page. Now curl your fingers around the wire. At Q your fingers should point into the page. Keep curling around and you notice that at point P your fingers come out of the page. (See Figure 7.4 (b).) So your answer should be: **B** (at P) = 0.1 Gauss, pointing out of the page, and **B** (at Q) = 0.5 Gauss, pointing into the page. Note that as we move farther from the wire the magnitude of magnetic field decreases.

The magnitude of the magnetic field at the center of a circular loop of current-carrying wire of radius r is:

$$B = \frac{\mu_0 i}{2r}$$

Notice that these two laws for magnetic fields look similar. For the long straight wire, r refers to the perpendicular distance from the wire and gives B for any point away from the wire. However, r in the second case is the radius of the loop and the expression gives the magnetic field at the loop's center point only. The following example illustrates how to find directions.

Example: Suppose a wire is formed into a loop that carries current clockwise (that is, electrons flow counterclockwise) as in Figure 7.5(a). Find the direction of the magnetic field produced by this loop:

a. within the loop.

b. outside of the loop.

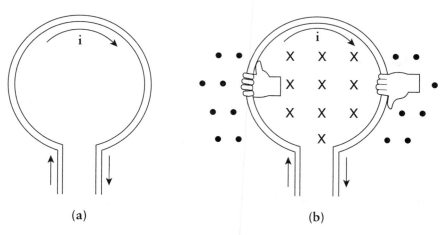

(a)   (b)

Figure 7.5

Solution: Look at Figure 7.5(b). By holding your **right thumb** anywhere around the loop in the direction of current flow (clockwise) and encircling the wire with the remaining fingers of the **right hand,** your **right fingers** should point:

a. into the page. Thus the magnetic field within the loop points into the page.

b. out of the page. Thus the magnetic field outside the loop points out of the page.

8

DC and AC Circuits

Electric circuits pervade our everyday world, existing in myriad forms in the various necessities of modern day living, most notably, TVs and stereos. In this chapter we will review the essentials of DC circuits, touching only briefly and qualitatively on the subject of AC circuits. Included are the usual topics of DC circuit theory: emf, resistance, power dissipated by resistors, Kirchhoff's laws, parallel and series resistor circuits, capacitors, parallel and series capacitor circuits, and a brief discussion of dielectrics. Although the topic of DC circuits can be a place to encounter a substantial amount of algebra when solving complicated circuits, the emphasis on the OAT® and in this chapter is on the essential concepts involved and on applying those concepts in simple situations. Let's begin with a short review of conductors and insulators, the essential materials of the wires of any circuit.

Some materials allow electric charge to move freely within the material. These materials are called electrical **conductors.** Metal atoms can easily lose one or more of their outer electrons, which are then free to move around in the metal. This makes most metals good electrical conductors. In most conductors, the positive ions remain fixed and the liberated electrons are free to move.

In other materials electric charge is bound to the constituent atoms and is not free to move. These materials severely retard the flow of electricity and are called **insulators.** Most nonmetals are good insulators.

The wires to most appliances have a conducting core of copper wire perhaps, with an insulating sheath of some plastic. The copper wire conducts the electricity to the appliance from the wall socket. The insulating sheath protects you from touching the wire and getting an electric shock.

DIRECT CURRENT

A. Current and Circuit Voltage

The flow of charge is called an **electric current**. The magnitude of the current, i, is the amount of charge, Δq, passing a given point per unit time Δt, and is given by:

$$i = \frac{\Delta q}{\Delta t}$$

The SI unit of current is the **Ampere** (1 A = 1 Coulomb/second). The two basic types of current flow are **direct current** (DC), where the charge flows in one direction only, and **alternating current** (AC), where the flow changes direction periodically. AC will be discussed later.

When two points at different electric potentials are connected by a conductor (such as a metal wire), charge flows between the two points. In a conductor, only negatively charged electrons are free to move. These act as the charge carriers, and move from low to high potentials. By convention, however, the direction of the **current** is taken as the direction in which **positive charge** would flow, from high to low potential. **Thus the direction of current is opposite to the direction of electron flow.**

A voltage (potential difference) can be produced by an electric generator, a voltaic cell, or by a group of cells wired into a battery. **Electromotive force** (emf or ε) is the name given to the voltage across the terminals of a cell when no current is flowing. Electromotive force should not be confused with a force or an electric field; it is a potential difference and is measured in Volts.

Because cells typically have a small internal resistance r_{int} of their own, the voltage they actually furnish to a circuit is reduced by ir_{int}, where i is the current supplied by the cell. The voltage V across the terminals of the cell when current is flowing out, is given in terms of the cell's emf and internal resistance by:

$$V = \varepsilon - ir_{int}$$

Note that if the cell is supplying no current (i = 0), or if the cell has no internal resistance (r_{int} = 0), then V = ε. For cases in which the current supplied is greater than zero and the internal resistance is not negligible, then V < ε. When a cell is supplying current (discharging), the current flows out of the positive terminal and into the negative terminal. When a cell is being recharged, current from another source is sent into the positive terminal.

B. Resistance

1. RESISTANCE AND OHM'S LAW

Resistance R can be thought of as the opposition within a conductor to the flow of an electric current. This opposition takes the form of an energy loss or drop in potential. **Ohm's law** states that the voltage drop across a resistor is proportional to the current it carries, with R being the proportionality constant:

$$V = iR$$

This equation applies to a single resistor within a circuit, to any part of a circuit, or to an entire circuit (provided one knows how to add resistances in series and parallel). Note that the current is unchanged as it passes through the resistor. This is because no charge is lost inside the resistor. Therefore, the current that is supplied to several resistors wired in series must all flow through each resistor. The SI derived unit of electrical resistance is the **Ohm** (Ω).

2. RESISTANCE OF A CONDUCTOR

The resistance of an object depends on its size, the type of material from which it is made, and its temperature. Specifically the resistance depends on:

a. Length (L)

Resistance is directly proportional to length. A longer conductor means greater resistance, because there is a longer path that current-carrying electrons must travel. For example, two wires, identical in every respect except that one is twice as long as the other, will have different resistances. The longer one will have twice the resistance of the shorter one.

b. Cross-sectional area (A)

The resistance of a conductor is inversely proportional to its cross-sectional area. An increase in cross-sectional area causes a decrease in resistance. This is because there is an increase in the number of conduction paths electrons can follow. For example, two wires, identical in every respect except that one has twice the cross-sectional area of the other, will have different resistances. The thinner wire will have twice the resistance of the thicker wire.

c. Resistivity of the conductor (ρ)

Some materials are intrinsically better conductors of electricity than others. For example, copper conducts electricity much better than does glass. The number that characterizes the intrinsic resistance to current flow in a material is called the **resistivity** (ρ),

> **REMEMBER**
>
> - The resistance of a wire increases with increased length.
> - The resistance of a wire decreases with increased cross-sectional area.

> **REMEMBER**
>
> Resistivity, ρ, is a measure of the intrinsic resistance of a type of material, independent of length and cross-sectional area.

where the SI unit of resistivity is the Ohm•meter. The resistivity is therefore defined as the proportionality constant relating a conductor's resistance to the ratio of its length over its cross-sectional area:

$$R = \rho \frac{L}{A}$$

d. Temperature

Most conductors have greater resistance at higher temperatures. This is due to increased thermal oscillations of atoms in the conductor which produce a greater resistance to electron flow. The resistivity can then be thought of as a function of temperature. A few materials, such as glass, pure silicon, and most semiconductors are exceptions to this general rule.

3. POWER DISSIPATED BY A RESISTOR

Electric potential is electric potential energy per unit positive charge. Since current is a flow of charge, it should come as no surprise that through a current-carrying resistor there is a **flow of energy.** In a resistor, this electric energy is converted into heat. The **rate** at which the energy loss occurs is equal to the power dissipated by the resistor and is given by:

$$P = iV$$

where i is the current flowing through the resistor and V is the potential drop across the resistor. Using Ohm's law this expression can be rewritten as:

$$P = i^2R = V^2/R$$

C. Circuit Laws

An electric circuit is a conducting path that usually has one or more voltage sources (such as a cell) connected to one or more **passive circuit elements** (such as resistors). This subsection deals primarily with voltages, resistances, and currents in DC circuits.

1. KIRCHHOFF'S LAWS

a. **At any point or junction in a circuit the sum of currents directed into that point equals the sum of currents directed away from that point.** This is a consequence of the **conservation of electric charge.**

Example: Three wires (a, b, and c) meet at a junction point P as in Figure 8.1. A current of 5 A flows into P along wire a, and a current of 3 A flows away from P along wire b. What is the magnitude and direction of the current along wire c?

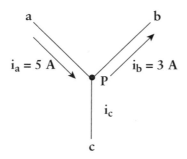

Figure 8.1

Solution: The sum of the currents entering P must equal the sum of the currents leaving P. Assume for now that i_c flows out of P. If we find that it is negative, then we know that it flows into P.

$$i_a = i_b + i_c$$
$$i_c = 5 - 3$$
$$i_c = 2 \text{ A}$$

Thus a current of 2 A flows **out** of P along wire c. Note that the total current into and out of P is then zero.

b. **The sum of voltage sources is equal to the sum of voltage (potential) drops around a closed circuit loop.** This is a consequence of the conservation of energy: All the electrical energy supplied by a source gets fully used up by the rest of the circuit. No excess energy appears or disappears. (But remember that voltage is energy per unit charge, not just energy.)

2. RESISTORS IN SERIES

It has already been mentioned that the same current flows through all the resistors in series and from the above laws we can deduce that voltage drops add in series. Therefore, using Ohm's law we find that resistances add in series (see Figure 8.2). That is:

$$R_s = R_1 + R_2 + R_3 + \dots + R_n$$

> **KEY CONCEPT**
>
> Energy is conserved in one complete loop of a circuit. Energy lost in the resistors is gained back in the battery.

> **KEY CONCEPT**
>
> Each additional resistor in a series of resistors increases the total resistance and thus decreases the total current.

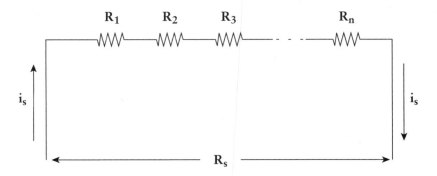

Figure 8.2

Example: A circuit is wired with one cell supplying 5 V (neglect the internal resistance of the cell) in series together with three resistors of 3 Ω, 5 Ω, and 7 Ω also wired in series as shown in Figure 8.3. What is the resulting voltage across, and current through, each resistor of this circuit, as well as the entire circuit?

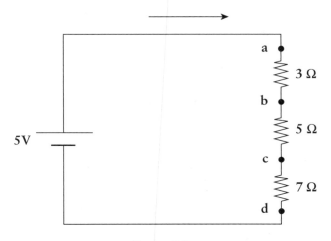

Figure 8.3

REMEMBER

Ohm's law can be applied to the entire circuit at once, using total resistance.

Solution: The total resistance of the resistors is:

$$R_s = R_1 + R_2 + R_3$$
$$= 3 + 5 + 7$$
$$= 15 \ \Omega$$

Now use Ohm's law to get the current through the entire circuit (since everything is in series this is also the current through each element):

$$i_s = \frac{V_s}{R_s} = \frac{5}{15} = \frac{1}{3}A$$

Now use Ohm's law for each of the resistors in turn. From a to b the voltage drop across R_1 is:

$$iR_1 = (1/3)(3)$$
$$= 1.0 \text{ V}$$

From b to c the voltage drop across R_2 is:

$$iR_2 = (1/3)(5)$$
$$= 1.67 \text{ V}$$

From c to d the voltage drop across R_3 is:

$$iR_3 = (1/3)(7)$$
$$= 2.33 \text{ V}$$

REMEMBER

Ohm's law can be applied to each resistor separately.

3. RESISTORS IN PARALLEL

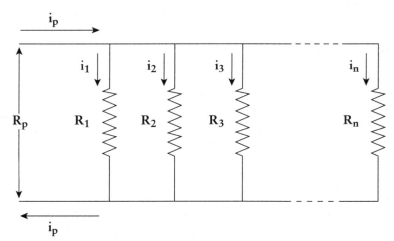

Figure 8.4

When resistors are wired in parallel, they are all wired with a common high-potential terminal and a common low-potential terminal (see Figure 8.4). The effect of **adding resistors in parallel** is the same as that of increasing the cross-sectional area of a conductor. It increases the paths by which current can flow and thereby **decreases resistance** (there is also the analogy to viscous blood flow through capillaries—flow resistance is reduced when several capillaries are arranged in parallel). The rule for combining resistances in parallel is a bit more complicated than the previous rules. It states that the reciprocal of the equivalent resistance equals the sum of the reciprocals of their individual resistances. In equation form this may be written as:

$$\frac{1}{R_p} = \frac{1}{R_1} + \frac{1}{R_2} + \frac{1}{R_3} + \ldots + \frac{1}{R_n}$$

KEY CONCEPT

Each additional resistor added in parallel acts to decrease the total resistance and thus increase the current.

When resistors are in parallel, the voltage drop across each is the same and is equal to the voltage drop across the entire combination:

$$V_p = V_1 = V_2 = V_3 = \ldots = V_n$$

Example: Consider two equal resistors wired in parallel. What is the equivalent resistance of the two?

Solution: The equation for summing resistors in parallel is:

$$\frac{1}{R_p} = \frac{1}{R_1} + \frac{1}{R_2}$$

Find the common denominator of the right-hand side and take the inverse to find:

$$R_p = \frac{R_1 R_2}{(R_1 + R_2)}$$

Since $R_1 = R_2$ in this special case, let $R = R_1 = R_2$:

$$R_p = \frac{R^2}{2R} = \frac{R}{2}$$

REMEMBER

Parallel resistors experience the same voltage drop.

In the above example, it is seen that the total resistance is **halved** by wiring two identical resistors in parallel. More generally, when n identical resistors are wired in parallel, the total resistance is given by R/n. Note that the voltage across each of the parallel resistors is equal, and that for equal resistances the current flowing through each of the resistors is also equal.

Example: Consider two resistors wired in parallel with $R_1 = 5\ \Omega$ and $R_2 = 10\ \Omega$. If the voltage across them is 10 V, what is the current through each of the two resistors?

Solution: First the current flowing through the whole circuit must be found. To do this, the combined resistance must be determined:

$$\frac{1}{R_p} = \frac{1}{R_1} + \frac{1}{R_2} \qquad \textbf{OR} \qquad R_p = \frac{R_1 R_2}{(R_1 + R_2)}$$

$$= \frac{1}{10} + \frac{1}{5} \qquad\qquad R_p = \frac{(5)(10)}{(5 + 10)}$$

$$= \frac{3}{10} \qquad\qquad\qquad R_p = \frac{50}{15}\Omega = \frac{10}{3}\Omega$$

$$R_p = \frac{10}{3}\Omega$$

Using Ohm's law to calculate the current flowing through the circuit gives:

$$i_p = \frac{V_p}{R_p}$$
$$= \frac{10}{(10/3)}$$
$$= 3 \text{ A}$$

Three Amps flow through the combination R_1 and R_2. Since the resistors are in parallel $V_p = V_1 = V_2 = 10$ V. Apply Ohm's law to each resistor individually:

$$i_1 = \frac{V_p}{R_1} = \frac{10}{5} = 2A$$

$$i_2 = \frac{V_p}{R_2} = \frac{10}{10} = 1A$$

As a check, note that $i_p = 3$ A $= i_1 + i_2 = 2 + 1 = 3$ A. More current flows through the smaller resistance. In particular note that R_1 with half the resistance of R_2 has twice the current. Once i_p was found to be 3 A, the problem could have been solved by noting that because R_1 is half of R_2, $i_1 = 2i_2$, and $i_1 + i_2 = 3$ A.

D. Capacitors and Dielectrics

1. CAPACITORS AND CAPACITANCE

When two electrically neutral plates of metal are connected to a voltage source, positive charge builds up on the plate connected to the positive terminal and an equal amount of negative charge builds up on the plate connected to the negative terminal. The two-plate system stores charge and is called a **capacitor**. It is important to remember that charge collects on a capacitor any time there is a potential difference between the plates. The **capacitance** C of a capacitor is defined as the ratio of charge stored (meaning the absolute value of the charge on one plate) to the total potential difference across the capacitor. So, if a voltage difference V is applied across the plates of the capacitor and a charge Q collects on it (with +Q on the positive plate and –Q on the negative plate), then the capacitance is given by:

$$C = \frac{Q}{V}$$

The SI unit of capacitance is the **Farad** (where 1 F = 1 Coulomb/Volt). Because one Coulomb is such a large amount of charge, one Farad is a very large capacitance. Capacitances are therefore quoted in submultiples of the Farad such as microfarads (1 $\mu F = 10^{-6}$ F), or nanofarads (1 $nF = 10^{-9}$ F), or picofarads (1 $pF = 10^{-12}$ F). Note also that the Farad should not be confused with the Faraday, the unit of charge equal to the charge on a mole of elementary charges (= 9.65×10^4 Coulombs).

The capacitance of a capacitor is dependent on the geometry of the two conducting surfaces. For the simple case of the parallel plate capacitor, the capacitance is given by:

$$C = \varepsilon_0 \frac{A}{d}$$

where ε_0 is the **permittivity of free space** ($\varepsilon_0 = 8.85 \times 10^{-12}$ F/m), A is the area of overlap of the two plates, and d is the separation of the two plates. The separation of charges sets up an electric field between the plates of the capacitor. The electric field between the plates of a parallel plate capacitor is a uniform field whose magnitude at any point is given by:

$$E = \frac{V}{d}$$

The direction of the electric field at any point between the plates is toward the negative plate and away from the positive plate.

2. DIELECTRIC MATERIALS

When an insulating material (such as glass, plastic, or certain metal oxides) is placed between the plates of a charged-up capacitor, the voltage across the capacitor decreases. Such insulating materials are called **dielectrics**. By lowering the voltage across the charged-up capacitor the dielectric has "made room for" even more charge, hence, the capacitance of the capacitor is increased. Dielectric materials are characterized by a dimensionless number called the **dielectric constant K**, which tells by what factor the capacitance of a capacitor is increased:

$$C' = KC$$

where C' is the new capacitance with the dielectric, and C is the original capacitance.

Example: The voltage across the terminals of an isolated 3 μF capacitor is 4 V. If a piece of ceramic having dielectric constant K = 2 is placed between the plates, find:

   a.   the new charge on the capacitor.

   b.   the new capacitance of the capacitor.

   c.   the new voltage across the capacitor.

Solution: a.   The introduction of a dielectric by itself has no effect on the charge stored on the isolated capacitor. There is no new charge, so the charge is the same as before. The charge stored is therefore given by:

$$Q' = Q$$
$$= CV$$
$$= (3 \times 10^{-6})(4)$$
$$= 12 \times 10^{-6} \text{ C}$$
$$= 12 \text{ } \mu C$$

   b.   By introducing a dielectric with a value of 2, the capacitance of the capacitor is doubled (C' = KC). Hence the new capacitance is 6 μF.

   c.   Using the relationship V' = Q'/C', the new voltage across the capacitor may be determined. Putting numbers into the equation gives:

$$V' = \frac{12 \times 10^{-6}}{6 \times 10^{-6}}$$
$$= 2 \text{ V}$$

Example: The voltage across the terminals of a 3 μF capacitor is 4 V. Now suppose a piece of ceramic having dielectric constant K = 2 is placed between the plates **and the voltage is held constant** (e.g., by a battery). What is the new charge on the capacitor?

Solution: By introducing the dielectric ceramic, the capacitance of the capacitor has been altered. But because the voltage was held constant, the charge on the capacitor plates must have been altered. From the definition of dielectric constant and from the above example it is clear that the new capacitance is:

$$C' = KC$$
$$= 6 \text{ μF}$$

But the new voltage is still 4 V, so the new charge must be:

$$Q' = C'V'$$
$$= (6 \times 10^{-6})(4)$$
$$= 24 \times 10^{-6} \text{ C}$$
$$= 24 \ \mu C$$

Since the original charge was $Q = CV = (3 \times 10^{-6})(4) = 12 \ \mu C$, by keeping the voltage constant the battery had to supply an additional $+12 \ \mu C$ of charge to the positive plate and $-12 \ \mu C$ to the negative plate.

3. CAPACITORS IN PARALLEL

When wired in parallel, capacitors can be added directly. The capacitors wired in parallel can be thought of as combining to form a single capacitor with increased capacitance. Since the wire from one capacitor to the next is a conductor and an equipotential surface, the potential of all the plates on one side are the same (see Figure 8.5).

$$C_p = C_1 + C_2 + C_3 + \dots + C_n$$

The voltage across each parallel capacitor is the same, and is equal to the voltage across the entire combination:

$$V_p = V_1 = V_2 = V_3 = \dots = V_n$$

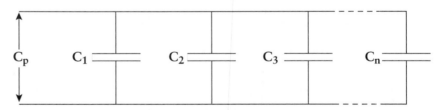

Figure 8.5

4. CAPACITORS IN SERIES

Each additional capacitor added in series decreases the total capacitance of the circuit, so just as for resistors in parallel, the reciprocal of the total capacitance in series is equal to the sum of the reciprocals of the individual capacitances (see Figure 8.6).

$$\frac{1}{C_s} = \frac{1}{C_1} + \frac{1}{C_2} + \frac{1}{C_3} + \dots + \frac{1}{C_n}$$

For capacitors in series, the total voltage is the sum of the individual voltages:

$$V_s = V_1 + V_2 + V_3 + ... + V_n$$

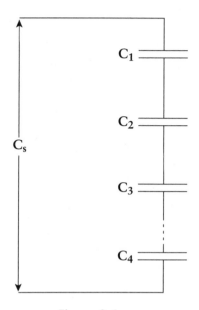

Figure 8.6

E. A Summary of Circuit Element Addition

SERIES

$$R_s = R_1 + R_2 + R_3 + ... + R_n$$

$$\frac{1}{C_s} = \frac{1}{C_1} + \frac{1}{C_2} + \frac{1}{C_3} + ... + \frac{1}{C_n}$$

PARALLEL

$$\frac{1}{R_p} = \frac{1}{R_1} + \frac{1}{R_2} + \frac{1}{R_3} + ... + \frac{1}{R_n}$$

$$C_p = C_1 + C_2 + C_3 + ... + C_n$$

ALTERNATING CURRENT

A. Alternating Current

Alternating current (AC) changes its direction of flow periodically. The most common form of AC current oscillates in a sinusoidal way as shown in Figure 8.7. Note that for half of the cycle the current flows in one direction, and for the other half of the cycle the current flows in the opposite direction. Such a current can be described by the equation

$$i = I_{max} \sin (2\pi ft)$$
$$= I_{max} \sin \omega t$$

where i is the instantaneous current at the time t, I_{max} is the maximum current, f is the frequency, and $\omega = 2\pi f$ is the angular frequency.

The most common sinusoidal current is the ordinary AC house current that oscillates with a frequency f of 60 Hz. In some countries, such as England, the frequency is 50 Hz.

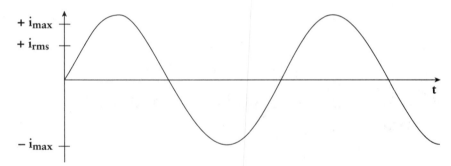

Figure 8.7

B. RMS Current

In AC circuits the magnitude of the current varies from a maximum positive value to a minimum negative value. A problem arises when one tries to calculate the average current for sinusoidal AC currents: for one cycle, the sum of the positive current flowing in one direction is exactly canceled by the sum of the negative current that flows in the other direction. Yet there is AC current; it delivers power. Consider the power dissipated in a resistor R that carries an AC current i. It is given by the equation $P = i^2R$. Therefore, in order to find the average power dissipated we must find the average of i^2 over one period. This is equal to I_{rms}^2, where I_{rms} is the root-mean-square (rms) current given by:

$$I_{rms} = \frac{I_{max}}{\sqrt{2}}$$

Example: What is the rms current of an AC signal that will produce a maximum current of 1.00 A?

Solution:
$$I_{rms} = \frac{I_{max}}{\sqrt{2}}$$

$$= \frac{1.00}{\sqrt{2}}$$

$$= \frac{1.00}{1.41}$$

$$= 0.71 \text{ A}$$

C. RMS Voltage

Voltage in AC circuits, like current, is sinusoidal and changes sign back and forth over time. It can be described by an equation similar to the equation for sinusoidal current. So just as for current, one can calculate an **rms voltage**:

$$V_{rms} = \frac{V_{max}}{\sqrt{2}}$$

Example: The AC current used in a home is frequently called "120 V AC." Assuming that this refers to the rms voltage, what is the maximum voltage?

Solution: Using the above equation gives:

$$V_{max} = \sqrt{2}\,V_{rms}$$

$$= \sqrt{2}\,(120)$$

$$= 170 \text{ V}$$

9

Periodic Motion, Waves, and Sound

OSCILLATIONS

Oscillating systems are those that continuously show repetitive movement of some kind. There are many different examples of oscillatory motion in the natural world, from the waves in the ocean to the waves of light that illuminate our world to the waves of sound that literally bring music to our ears. In this chapter, we will first lay the foundation for understanding wave phenomena by reviewing the subject of simple harmonic motion. General properties of waves are then introduced including the concepts of amplitude, wavelength, frequency, wave speed, and resonance. The superposition of two waves is discussed along with the related concepts of constructive vs. destructive interference and the production of standing waves, both in strings and open and closed pipes. The subject of sound is reviewed as a subject which is rich in wave related phenomena such as beats and the Doppler effect. A brief summary is also given of sound production by musical instruments.

A. Simple Harmonic Motion

A very important type of oscillation, or periodic motion, is **simple harmonic motion** (SHM). In SHM, a particle or mass oscillates about an equilibrium point subject to a linear restoring force. A linear restoring force has two characteristics: (i) it is always directed back toward the equilibrium position, and (ii) its magnitude is directly proportional to the displacement from the equilibrium position. By Newton's second law, the particle's acceleration is also proportional to the displacement from equilibrium:

$$\mathbf{F} = -k\mathbf{x}$$
$$a = -\omega^2 x$$

where the angular frequency ω is given by:

$$\omega = \sqrt{k/m}$$

> **KEY CONCEPT**
>
> The equilibrium point is the point where the net force is zero.

> **REMEMBER**
>
> The minus sign in F = –kx means that the restoring force is in the opposite direction to the displacement.

A mass attached to a spring, and a simple pendulum (provided the angle of swing is not too large) are two examples of simple harmonic oscillators. A stretched or compressed spring exerts a linear restoring force, where the constant k is called the **spring constant** (or force constant), and the equation F = –kx is called **Hooke's Law.** k is a measure of the stiffness of the spring. Figure 9.1(a) shows a spring-mass system with the mass at the equilibrium position. Figure 9.1(b) shows the same system with the mass displaced a distance x from the equilibrium position.

For other systems that execute SHM, k may be related to other properties of the system. In the case of a simple pendulum, k = mg/L where m is the mass, and L is the length of the pendulum. Figure 9.1(c) shows a simple pendulum displaced at an angle θ with the vertical.

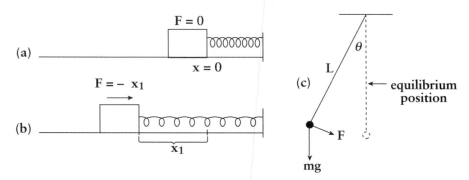

Figure 9.1

Let X be the particle's amplitude (maximum displacement x from the equilibrium position). Then assuming the particle has a maximum displacement at t = 0, the equation that describes the particle's displacement x is:

$$x = X \cos (\omega t)$$

where t is the time and ω is the angular frequency. ($\omega = 2\pi f = 2\pi/T$, where f is the frequency and T is the period.)

One final consideration in SHM is energy. If the forces are conservative and the system is frictionless, by the conservation of energy:

$$E = K + U = constant$$

where K is the kinetic energy and U is the potential energy. Kinetic energy for both the mass attached to the spring and the pendulum mass is given by:

$$K = \frac{1}{2}mv^2$$

For the pendulum, the potential energy is the gravitational potential energy (mgh) as it swings up. For the spring, the potential energy is given by:

$$U(\text{spring}) = \frac{1}{2}kx^2$$

When the mass is at the equilibrium position the potential energy is zero and the kinetic energy is a maximum given by $E = K_{max}$. However, when the oscillation reaches its maximum displacement the mass has zero speed. At this point the kinetic energy is zero and the potential energy is a maximum given by $E = U_{max}$.

The chart below gives important information on both the mass-spring system and the simple pendulum and shows the similarities between them. Note that when talking about a simple pendulum we commonly refer to the angle θ which it makes with the vertical.

NOTE: Period (T) is the time to complete 1 cycle, frequency (f) is the number of cycles completed in 1 second, and angular frequency $\omega = 2\pi f = 2\pi/T$. In SHM the frequency and period are independent of the amplitude.

	Mass-spring	**Simple pendulum**
force constant k	spring constant k	mg/L
period T	$2\pi\sqrt{m/k}$	$2\pi\sqrt{L/g}$
ang. freq. ω	$\sqrt{k/m}$	$\sqrt{g/L}$
frequency f	1/T or $\omega/2\pi$	1/T or $\omega/2\pi$
kinetic energy K	$\frac{1}{2}mv^2$	$\frac{1}{2}mv^2$
Kmax occurs at	x = 0	$\theta = 0$ (vertical position)
potential energy U	$\frac{1}{2}kx^2$	mgh
Umax occurs at	x = ±X	max value of θ
max acceleration at	x = ±X	max value of θ

Example: What is the length of a pendulum that has a period of 1 second?

Solution: Using our equation for the period of a simple pendulum we can find the length:

$$T = 2\pi \sqrt{L/g}$$
$$L = T^2 g/4\pi^2$$
$$= g/4\pi^2$$
$$= 0.25 \text{ m}$$

B. Uniform Circular Motion and SHM

Consider a particle moving around a circular path at constant angular frequency ω. If the path were projected onto a line adjacent to the circle (Figure 9.2), it is obvious that the particle is oscillating back and forth between +X and −X and obeying the laws of SHM. This fact helps give some insight as to where the idea of angular frequency comes from.

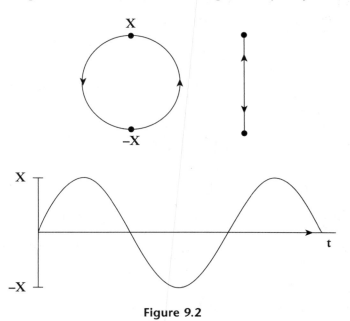

Figure 9.2

GENERAL WAVE CHARACTERISTICS

A. Transverse and Longitudinal Waves

This chapter will be primarily concerned with sinusoidal waves. In such waves the individual particles oscillate back and forth with simple harmonic motion. In the case of **transverse waves** the particles oscillate perpendicular to the direction of the wave motion as shown in Figure 9.3(a). The oscillating string elements are moving at right angles to the direction of travel of the wave. In the case of **longitudinal waves** the particles oscillate along the direction of the wave motion, and this is illustrated in Figure 9.3(b). In this case, the longitudinal wave created by the person moving the piston back and forth consists of oscillating air molecules that move parallel to the direction of motion of the wave.

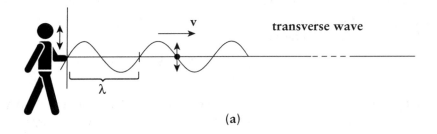

(a)

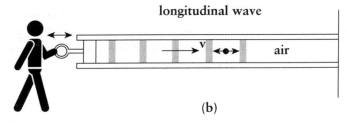

(b)

Figure 9.3

B. Describing Waves

The displacement y of a particle may be plotted at each point x along the direction of the wave's motion. It is given mathematically by:

$$y = Y \sin(kx - \omega t)$$

where Y is the amplitude (maximum displacement), k is the wave number (not to be mistaken with the *k* of Hooke's law), ω is the angular frequency, and t is the time.

The distance from one maximum (crest) of the wave to the next is the wavelength, λ. The frequency f is the number of wavelengths passing a fixed point per second (cycles per second (cps) or Hertz (Hz)). The speed of the wave v is related to the frequency and wavelength by the very important equation:

$$v = f\lambda$$

REMEMBER

The maximum displacement or amplitude is Y, since the maximum of the sin function is 1.

REMEMBER

The speed of a wave is also the speed at which a crest or trough propagates through space.

The following relations define k and ω:

$$k = \frac{2\pi}{\lambda}$$

$$\omega = 2\pi f = \frac{2\pi}{T}$$

where the period T is the time for the wave to move one wavelength (f = 1/T). The following relationships for the velocity of the wave follow from the above definitions:

$$\upsilon = f\lambda = \frac{\omega}{k} = \frac{\lambda}{T}$$

Example: If a wave on a string were described by the equation y = (0.01) sin (2x − 10t), find the frequency, wavelength, and speed of the wave. (Assume units of meters and seconds.)

Solution: Everything that is needed to find the frequency, wavelength, and speed is given in the wave's equation, y = Y sin (kx − ωt) = (0.01) sin (2x − 10t). Remembering that frequency is given by f = 1/T and that T = 2π/ω:

$$f = \omega/2\pi$$
$$= 5/\pi$$
$$= 1.59 \text{ Hz}$$

The wavelength is given by:

$$\lambda = 2\pi/k$$
$$= 2\pi/2$$
$$= \pi$$
$$= 3.14 \text{ m}$$

and the speed by:

$$v = f\lambda$$
$$= (5/\pi)\pi$$
$$= 5 \text{ m/s}$$

C. Phase

REMEMBER

A phase difference between two waves means that the crests (or troughs) don't occur at the same points in space.

When comparing two waves we often speak about a **phase difference.** This phase difference describes how "in step" two waves are with each other. Let's take two separate waves that have the same frequency, amplitude, and wavelength. If the waves are perfectly in phase, the maxima and minima of each wave coincide, i.e., they occur at the same point. In this case the phase difference is zero. However, if the two waves are out of phase, then one wave is shifted with respect to the other by some definite fraction of a cycle. This phase difference is usually expressed as an angle. In Figure 9.4(a), waves y_1 and y_2 are nearly in phase; their phase difference is approximately 0°. In Figure 9.4(b), wave y_2 is shifted nearly one-half wavelength with respect to y_1. The phase difference in this case is almost 180°.

D. Principle of Superposition

The principle of superposition states simply that when waves interact with each other the result is a sum of the waves. When the waves are in phase, the amplitudes add together (**constructive interference**) but when waves are 180° out of phase, the resultant amplitude is the difference between interacting amplitudes (**destructive interference**). Figures 9.4(a) and (b) show the interference between two waves when they are nearly in phase and when they are nearly 180° out of phase.

> **REMEMBER**
>
> When two waves are in phase and interfere, the resultant amplitude is the sum of the two separate amplitudes.

> **REMEMBER**
>
> When two waves are out of phase by 180°, the resultant amplitude is the difference between the two separate amplitudes.

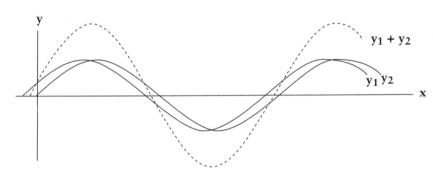

Figure 9.4(a)

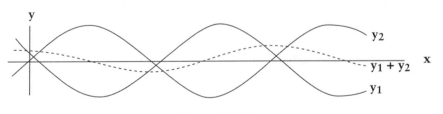

Figure 9.4(b)

E. Traveling and Standing Waves

If a string fixed at one end is moved from side to side, it is seen that a wave travels or propagates down the string. Such a wave is known as a **traveling wave**. When the wave reaches the fixed boundary it is reflected and inverted (see Figure 9.5). If the free end of the string is continuously moved from side to side there will then be two waves: the original wave moving down the string and the reflected wave moving the other way. These waves will then interfere with each other.

> **KEY CONCEPT**
>
> Standing waves occur because of the interference of two or more waves.

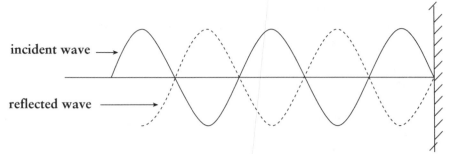

incident wave →

reflected wave →

Figure 9.5

Consider now the case when both ends of the string are fixed and traveling waves are excited in the string. Certain wave frequencies can result in a waveform remaining in a stationary position, while the amplitude fluctuates. These waves are known as **standing waves**. Points in the wave that remain at rest are known as **nodes**, and points that are midway between these nodes are known as **antinodes**. Antinodes are points that fluctuate with maximum amplitude.

It is also possible to set up standing waves in pipes in much the same way as in a string. Standing waves in strings and pipes are discussed in more detail in Section E of "Sound."

F. Resonance

In any oscillatory system there will be one or more **natural frequencies** (normal modes) of vibration; that is to say that the system will oscillate at one of these natural frequencies if there are no external forces involved (in the case of the free-swinging pendulum there is only one natural frequency, whereas a stretched string will have an infinite number of natural frequencies).

If a periodically varying force is applied to the system, the system will then be driven at a frequency equal to the frequency of the force. This is known as a **forced oscillation**. The amplitude of this motion will generally be small. However, if the frequency of the applied force is close to that of the natural frequency of the system, then the amplitude becomes much larger.

If the frequency of the periodically varying force is equal to a natural frequency of the system, then the system is said to be **resonating**, and the amplitude of the oscillation is a maximum. If the oscillating system were frictionless, then the periodically varying force would continually add energy to the system, and the amplitude would increase indefinitely. However, since no system is completely frictionless there is always some damping that results in a finite amplitude of oscillation.

SOUND

Sound is transmitted by oscillation of particles along the direction of motion of the sound wave. It is therefore a longitudinal wave. More generally, sound is a mechanical disturbance propagated through a deformable medium, and so can be transmitted through solids, liquids, and gases, but NOT through a vacuum. Sound travels faster in a solid than in a liquid, and faster in a liquid than in a gas.

This section will be primarily concerned with waves that, when they strike the ear, produce the sensation we call sound. For humans, such waves are called **audible waves** and have frequencies ranging from 20 Hz to 20,000 Hz. Waves whose frequencies are below 20 Hz are called **infrasonic waves**, and those whose frequencies are above 20,000 Hz are called **ultrasonic waves**. For sound waves in air at 0°C, the speed of sound is 331 m/s.

A. Characteristics of Sound

Intensity is defined as the average rate per unit area at which energy is transported across a perpendicular surface by the wave. In other words, the intensity is the power transported per unit area. In SI it has units of W/m^2. The amplitude of the sound wave is a measure of its energy. The total power P carried across a surface area (such as an eardrum) equals the product of the intensity I and the surface area A when the intensity is uniformly distributed. Mathematically, one can write:

$$P = IA$$

The **sound level,** β, is measured in decibels and is defined as:

$$\beta = 10 \log \frac{I}{I_0}$$

where I_0 is a reference intensity of 10^{-12} W/m^2, corresponding to the faintest sound that can be heard by humans.

Example: A detector with a surface area of 1 square meter is placed 1 meter from an operating jackhammer. It measures the power of the jackhammer's sound to be 10^{-3} W. Find:

   a. the intensity and the sound level of the jackhammer.

   b. the ratio of the intensities of the jackhammer and a jet engine (Assume β_{jet} = 130 dB).

Solution: a. Intensity is equal to power divided by area.

$$I = \frac{P}{A}$$

$$= \frac{10^{-3}}{1}$$

$$= 10^{-3} \text{ W/m}^2$$

The sound level is given by:

$$\beta = 10 \log \frac{I}{I_0}$$

$$= 10 \log \left(\frac{10^{-3}}{10^{-12}} \right)$$

$$= 10 \log 10^9$$

$$= 90 \text{ dB}$$

b. The ratio of two intensities of sound can be found from the difference of their sound levels:

$$\beta_{jet} - \beta_{jack} = 10 \log \left(\frac{I_{jet}}{I_{jack}} \right)$$

$$130 - 90 = 10 \log \left(\frac{I_{jet}}{I_{jack}} \right)$$

$$4 = \log \left(\frac{I_{jet}}{I_{jack}} \right)$$

$$10,000 = \left(\frac{I_{jet}}{I_{jack}} \right)$$

Thus the jet engine's sound is 10,000 times more intense than the jackhammer's.

Another characteristic of sound is **pitch**. This refers to the sensation of sound that enables one to classify the frequency of a note.

B. Production of Sound

For sound to be produced, there must be a longitudinal oscillation of air molecules. This oscillation can be produced by the vibration of a solid object that sets adjacent air molecules into motion, or by means of an acoustic vibration in an enclosed space.

Sound produced by the vibration of a solid object includes sound that is created by string and percussion instruments such as the guitar, violin, and piano. In this case, a string or several strings are set into motion and vibrate at their normal mode frequencies. Since the strings are very thin, it makes them ineffective in transmitting their vibration to the surrounding air. For this reason, a solid body is employed to provide a better coupling to the air. In the case of a guitar, the vibration is transmitted through the bridge to the body of the instrument, which vibrates at the same frequency as the string.

Sound created by acoustic vibration includes sound from instruments such as organ pipes, the flute, and the recorder. There are no moving parts, and sound is produced by a vibrating motion of air within the instrument. In the case of an organ pipe, the pitch is determined by the length of the pipe. However, instruments such as the recorder and the flute are able to generate more than one pitch by the opening and closing of holes.

In the case of the human voice, sound is created by passing air between the vocal cords. The pitch is controlled by varying the tension of the cords. This is very similar to the production of sound in wind instruments such as the oboe and the clarinet, but these use a reed instead of vocal cords. Pitch in this case is controlled both by the opening and closing of holes and by varying the tension across the reed.

C. Beats

Beats are heard when two waves that have nearly equal frequencies are superimposed. By the principle of superposition, the two waves add together, and what results is a periodic variation in loudness called beats. The beat frequency is:

$$f_{beat} = |f_1 - f_2|$$

Example: Two tuning forks are sounded. One has a frequency of 250 Hz while the other has a frequency of 245 Hz. What is the frequency of the beats?

Solution: The frequency of the beats is the difference of the frequencies of the interacting waves:

$$f_{beat} = f_1 - f_2$$
$$= 250 - 245$$
$$= 5 \text{ Hz}$$

REAL-WORLD ANALOGY

The frequency of sound produced by a guitar string, violin string, or piano string is the frequency of vibration of the string.

REAL-WORLD ANALOGY

Musicians who play woodwind instruments such as saxophones, clarinets, or flutes have all experienced the effect of air temperature on the pitch of the notes they are trying to play. If the air temperature drops significantly below the temperature they are used to playing at, they find that the pitch of all notes also drops. Remembering that pitch is just frequency, this is equivalent to saying that the frequency of the notes drops with decreasing air temperature. Given that $v = \lambda f$, we see that $f = v/\lambda$ so that a decreased frequency means either a decreased wave velocity or an increased wavelength. The wavelength, however, is fixed, being simply the wavelength of the standing wave corresponding to a particular note. Since the length of the instrument is essentially independent of temperature for the temperatures that musicians play at, the wavelengths of the standing waves are also independent of temperature. The velocity of sound, however, is proportional to the square root of the absolute temperature. Thus as the temperature drops the wave velocity also does, causing the frequency or pitch to drop.

D. Doppler Effect

A qualitative description of the **Doppler effect** is that when a source emitting sound and the detector of that sound are moving relative to each other along the line joining them, the perceived frequency of the sound received, f', differs from the actual frequency emitted, f. If the source and detector are moving toward each other the observed frequency increases, and if the source and detector are moving away from each other the observed frequency decreases. This can be seen from the following equation:

$$f' = f\frac{(v \pm V_D)}{(v \mp V_S)}$$

where v is the speed of sound in the medium, V_D is the speed of the detector relative to the medium, and V_S is the speed of the source relative to the medium. The upper sign on V_D (V_S) is used when the detector (source) moves toward the source (detector), while the lower sign is used when it moves away.

Example: The siren of a police car cruising at 144 km/hr is going while the car is in pursuit of a speeding motorist. Assume that the speed of sound is 330 m/s. The siren emits sound at a frequency of 1450 Hz. What is the frequency heard by a stationary observer when:

a. the police car is moving toward the observer?

b. the police car has passed the observer?

Solution: a. To solve this problem the speed of the police car must first be converted to m/s.

$$\frac{144\ km}{hr} \bullet \frac{10^3 m}{km} \bullet \frac{hr}{3,600\ s} = 40\ m/s$$

Since the police car is moving toward the stationary observer, the denominator is $v - V_S$, and the numerator is simply v (since $V_D = 0$). This gives:

$$f' = f\frac{v}{v - V_S}$$

$$= \frac{1,450(330)}{330 - 40}$$

$$= 1,650\ Hz$$

b. In this part of the question the police car is now moving away from the observer, so the denominator is $v + V_s$. The numerator remains unchanged since the observer is still stationary.

$$f' = f\frac{v}{v + V_s}$$

$$= \frac{1{,}450(330)}{330 + 40}$$

$$= 1{,}293 \text{ Hz}$$

This example shows precisely why the pitch of a siren changes when an ambulance or police car passes you on the street. In this case, when the police car is moving toward the observer the perceived frequency is 1,650 Hz, whereas when the car has passed the observer the perceived frequency has decreased to 1,293 Hz.

E. Standing Waves

1. STRINGS

Consider a string fixed rigidly at both ends. Since the string is fixed at both ends, each end must be a node (a point in a wave that remains at rest). This implies that if the string is to support a standing wave, the string's length L must be equal to some integer multiple of half a wavelength (e.g., $\lambda/2$, $2\lambda/2$, $3\lambda/2$, and so on). This string will be able to support standing waves with wavelengths:

$$\lambda = 2L, \frac{2L}{2}, \frac{2L}{3}, \ldots \frac{2L}{n} \qquad (n = 1,2,3,\ldots)$$

From the relationship that $f = v/\lambda$, where v is the speed of the wave, the possible frequencies are:

$$f = \frac{v}{2L}, \frac{2v}{2L}, \frac{3v}{2L} \ldots, \frac{nv}{2L} \qquad (n = 1,2,3,\ldots)$$

The lowest frequency that the string can support is given by v/2L and is known as the **fundamental frequency (first harmonic)**. The frequency given by n = 2 is known as the first overtone (second harmonic) and so on. All the possible frequencies that the string can support are said to form a **harmonic series**. The waveforms of the first three harmonics are shown in Figure 9.6 below. (Note: N stands for node and A for antinode.)

REMEMBER

The 1st harmonic or fundamental is n = 1. The mth harmonic is n = m.

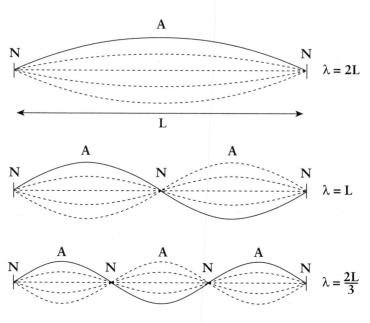

Figure 9.6

2. PIPES

Whereas strings are typically fixed at both ends, pipes may be open or closed at each end. In pipes the standing waves (if they occur) are sound waves originating in the air column. A closed end of a pipe corresponds to a fixed end of a string, and if standing waves occur a node will be at a closed end. On the other hand, at an open end of a pipe there will be an antinode. One end of the pipe will typically be open to allow air to enter. The pipe is then called open or closed depending on whether the other end is open or closed. The rules for the wavelengths and frequencies of the possible standing waves in a pipe of length L depend on whether the pipe is open (both ends are open) or closed (one end is open and the other end is closed).

Open pipes

An open pipe supports standing waves with antinodes at both ends. It is more difficult to illustrate the standing wave patterns in a pipe, since a sound wave is longitudinal. However, Figure 9.7 gives a symbolic representation, and it can be seen that this produces the same rule as for the string:

$$\lambda = \frac{2L}{n} \qquad (n = 1, 2, 3, \ldots)$$

$$f = \frac{nv}{2L} \qquad (n = 1, 2, 3, \ldots)$$

where v is the speed of the waves.

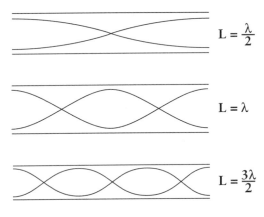

$$L = \frac{\lambda}{2}$$

$$L = \lambda$$

$$L = \frac{3\lambda}{2}$$

Figure 9.7

Closed pipes

In the case of a pipe open at one end but closed at the other, there is a node at the closed end. As in the case of the open pipe, the open end has an antinode. A symbolic representation of the standing wave patterns for a closed pipe is shown in Figure 9.8.

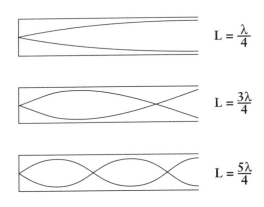

$$L = \frac{\lambda}{4}$$

$$L = \frac{3\lambda}{4}$$

$$L = \frac{5\lambda}{4}$$

Figure 9.8

It can be seen that in this case, because the wave goes from a node to an antinode, the length of the pipe needed to produce the fundamental frequency must be a quarter-wavelength long. The first overtone occurs when the pipe is $3/4\lambda$; the next at $5/4\lambda$; etc. This can be represented by the general expression:

$$\lambda = \frac{4L}{n} \qquad (n = 1, 3, 5, \ldots \text{odd integers only})$$

$$f = \frac{nv}{4L} \qquad (n = 1, 3, 5, \ldots \text{odd integers only})$$

10

Light and Optics

In this chapter we will review the basics of optics, which is the study of the reflection and transmission of light through material media and through constrictions such as apertures and slits. Our review will cover the two main areas of optics. The first is termed geometrical optics because we treat light as moving in a straight line path and can apply simple geometry to determine its behavior. Geometrical optics pertains to the study of mirrors and lenses along with the concepts of reflection and refraction. The second topic is concerned with the wave nature of light and particularly the way in which light does not travel in straight-line paths when it is passed through apertures and slits. The concepts of superposition and interference are explained in order to understand this behavior. A brief review is also provided of the physical nature of light itself, i.e., the electromagnetic wave.

ELECTROMAGNETIC SPECTRUM

A. Electromagnetic Waves

A changing magnetic field can cause a change in the electric field, and a changing electric field can cause a change in the magnetic field. Since changing electric fields affect changing magnetic fields that affect changing electric fields (and so on and so on), we can begin to see how **electromagnetic waves** occur in nature. One field affects the other, totally independent of matter, and electromagnetic waves can travel through a vacuum.

Electromagnetic waves are transverse waves because the oscillating electric and magnetic field vectors are perpendicular to the direction of propagation. Furthermore, the electric field and the magnetic field are perpendicular to each other. This is illustrated in Figure 10.1.

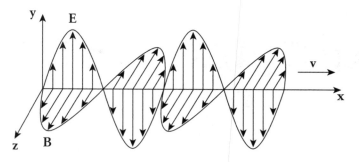

Figure 10.1

The **electromagnetic spectrum** is a term used to describe the full range in frequency and wavelength of electromagnetic waves. The following prefixes are often used when quoting wavelength: 1 mm = 10^{-3} m, 1 μm = 10^{-6} m, 1 nm = 10^{-9} m, and 1 Å = 10^{-10}m. The full spectrum is broken up into many regions which, in descending order of wavelength, are: radio (10^9 m to 1 mm), infrared (1 mm to 700 nm), visible light (700 nm to 400 nm), ultraviolet (400 nm to 50 nm), X ray (50 nm to 10^{-2} nm), and gamma ray (smaller than 10^{-2} nm). These regions have arbitrary boundaries, and some authors quote slightly different values: For example, one person will call 50 nm "short wavelength ultraviolet," while another may call it "long wavelength X ray."

Electromagnetic waves can vary in frequency or wavelength, but in a vacuum all electromagnetic waves travel at the same speed called the **speed of light**. This constant is represented by the letter c and is equal to: 3.00×10^8 m/s. To a first approximation, electromagnetic waves also travel in air with this velocity. Now the familiar equation $v = f\lambda$ becomes:

$$c = f\lambda$$

for all electromagnetic waves in a vacuum and, to a first approximation, in air.

B. Color and the Visible Spectrum

We just mentioned that the electromagnetic spectrum is broken up into many regions. The visible part of the spectrum is the only part that is perceived as light by the human eye. Within this region different wavelengths induce sensations of different colors, with violet at one end of the visible spectrum (400 nm) and red at the other end of the visible spectrum (700 nm).

Light that contains all of the colors in equal intensity is seen as white. The color of an object that does not emit its own light is dependent on the color of light that it reflects. So, an object that appears red is one that absorbs all light except red. This implies that a red object receiving green light will appear black, since it absorbs the green light and has no light to reflect.

GEOMETRICAL OPTICS

When light travels through a single homogeneous medium it travels in a straight line. This is known as rectilinear propagation. The behavior of light at the boundary of a medium or interface between two media is described by the theory of geometrical optics.

A. Reflection

Reflection is the rebounding of incident light waves at the boundary of a medium.

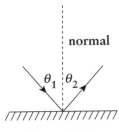

Figure 10.2

The law of reflection is:

$$\theta_1 = \theta_2$$

Important note: In optics, angles are always measured from a line drawn perpendicular to the boundary of a medium, often referred to as the **normal.**

1. PLANE MIRRORS

Parallel incident rays remain parallel after reflection from a plane mirror. In general, images created by a mirror can be either real or virtual. An image is said to be **real** if the light actually converges at the position of the image. An image is **virtual** if the light only *appears* to be coming from the position of the image but does not converge there.

Plane mirrors always create virtual images. In a plane mirror the image appears to be the same distance behind the mirror as the object's distance in front of it. Because the reflected light remains in front of the mirror but the image is behind the mirror, the image is virtual.

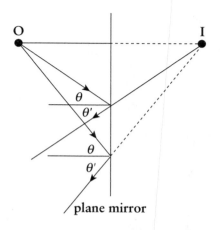

Figure 10.3

2. SPHERICAL MIRRORS

Spherical mirrors come in two varieties, **concave** and **convex**. The word "spherical" implies that the surface of the mirror has the shape of a sphere. In other words, if you had a sphere made out of a mirrorlike material, a spherical mirror would be a small portion cut out of that sphere. Therefore, spherical mirrors have a **center of curvature** C and a **radius of curvature** r associated with them.

If you were to look from the inside of a sphere to its surface, you would see a concave surface. However, if you were to look from outside the sphere you would see a convex surface. The **focal length** f is the distance between the focal point and the mirror. For all spherical mirrors f = r/2. For a convex surface the center of curvature and the focal point are behind the mirror. Concave mirrors are called **converging mirrors** and convex mirrors are called **diverging mirrors**.

There are several important distances associated with mirrors. The focal length f is the distance between the focal point F and the mirror; the radius of curvature r is the distance between C and the mirror (remember that r = 2f); the distance of the object from the mirror is o; the distance of the image from the mirror is i. There is a simple relation satisfied by these distances:

$$\frac{1}{o} + \frac{1}{i} = \frac{1}{f} = \frac{2}{r}$$

While it is not important which units of distance are used in this equation, it is important that all values used have the same units, be they centimeters, meters, or whatever.

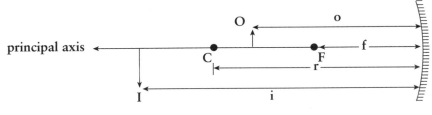

Figure 10.4

Often you will use this equation to calculate the image distance. If the image has a positive distance it is a real image, which implies that the image is in front of the mirror. If the image has a negative distance, it is virtual and thus located behind the mirror. Note also that for a plane mirror $r = f = \infty$ and the equation becomes $1/o + 1/i = 0$ or $i = -o$ (virtual image).

The **magnification** (m) is a dimensionless value that is the ratio of the image's height to the object's height. Following the sign convention given below, the orientation of the image compared with the object can also be determined. A negative magnification signifies an inverted image, while a positive value means the image is upright.

$$m = -\frac{i}{o}$$

If $|m| < 1$ the image is reduced, if $|m| > 1$ the image is enlarged, and if $|m| = 1$ the image is the same size as the object.

Figure 10.5 shows ray diagrams for a concave spherical mirror with the object at three different points. A ray diagram is useful for getting an approximation of where the image is. In general, there are three important rays to draw. For a concave mirror, a ray that strikes the mirror parallel to the horizontal is reflected back through the focal point. A ray that passes through the focal point before reaching the mirror is reflected back parallel to the horizontal. A ray which strikes the mirror right where the normal intersects it gets reflected back with the same angle (measured from the normal).

A single diverging mirror forms only a virtual erect image, regardless of the position of the object. The image formed by a single converging mirror depends on the position of the object as is demonstrated by Figure 10.5. When the object is farther away from the mirror than the focal point, the image is real and inverted. By moving the object to the focal point, the image disappears as the light rays reflect off the mirror parallel to each other and never converge. Moving the object closer to the mirror than the focal length makes an image that is virtual and erect.

A wineglass offers an easy opportunity to simultaneously view the image of the same object reflected off of both a convex and concave mirror. Looking straight on at the glass, the surface closest to you is convex, and the surface on the other side of the glass is concave. Since some of the light that hits the surface is reflected, the surfaces of the glass act as convex or concave mirrors. If you're careful, you can see two images, one from the convex side closest to you, and the other from the concave side. The image from the convex side is upright as images from convex mirrors always are. The image from the concave side will be inverted. This is because you, the object, are outside of the focal length of the mirror.

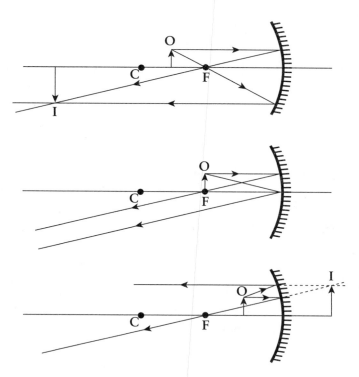

Figure 10.5

3. SIGN CONVENTION

The following chart gives the proper signs for various instances when dealing with single mirrors. Note that R side is used to denote Real side, which for mirrors is in front of the mirror. Similarly, V side stands for Virtual side, which is behind the mirror.

Sign Chart for Single Mirrors

Symbol	Positive	Negative
o	object is in front of mirror (R side)	object is behind mirror (V side)
i	image is in front of mirror (R side)	image is behind mirror (V side)
r	concave mirrors	convex mirrors
f	concave mirrors	convex mirrors
m	image is upright (erect)	image is inverted

Note that in almost all problems the object will be in front of the mirror, and thus the object distance o will be positive.

Example: An object is placed 7 cm in front of a concave mirror that has a 10 cm radius of curvature. Determine the image distance, the magnification, whether the image is real or virtual, and whether it is inverted or upright.

Solution: Using the mirror equation:

$$\frac{1}{i} + \frac{1}{o} = \frac{2}{r}$$

$$\frac{1}{i} = \frac{2}{r} - \frac{1}{o}$$

$$\frac{1}{i} = \frac{2}{10} - \frac{1}{7}$$

$$i = +17.5 \text{ cm}$$

The magnification m is:

$$m = -\frac{i}{o}$$

$$= -\frac{17.5}{7}$$

$$= -2.5$$

The image is in front of the mirror (i is positive) and therefore real. The image is inverted (m is negative) and 2.5 times larger ($|m| = 2.5$).

B. Refraction

1. SNELL'S LAW

When light is not in a vacuum, its speed is less than c. (As previously noted, when light is in air $v \cong c$.) For a given medium:

$$n = \frac{c}{v}$$

where c is the speed of light in a vacuum, v is the speed of light in the medium, and n is a dimensionless quantity called the **index of refraction** of the medium. Because $v < c$, $n > 1$. For air, to a first approximation, $v = c$ and $n = 1$.

Refracted rays of light obey **Snell's law** as they pass from one medium to another:

$$n_1 \sin \theta_1 = n_2 \sin \theta_2$$

REMEMBER

Light travels more slowly in material media (like glass) than in a vacuum. The wavelength changes accordingly while the frequency remains constant.

n_1 and θ_1 are for the medium the light is coming from, and n_2 and θ_2 are for the medium the light is going into. Note that θ is measured with respect to the perpendicular (normal) to the boundary.

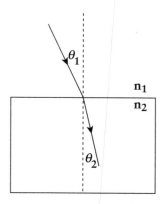

Figure 10.6

In general, when light enters a medium with a higher index of refraction ($n_2 > n_1$) it bends toward the normal so that $\theta_2 < \theta_1$. Conversely, if the light travels into a medium where the index of refraction is smaller ($n_2 < n_1$) the light will bend away from the normal so that $\theta_2 > \theta_1$.

Example: A penny sits at the bottom of a pool of water ($n = 1.33$) at a depth of 3.0 m. If an observer 1.8 m tall stands 30 cm away from the ledge, how close to the side can the penny be and still be visible?

Solution: First draw a picture of the situation, as in Figure 10.7. Note that the light is coming from the water ($n_1 = 1.33$) and going into the air ($n_2 = 1$), so the light is bent away from the normal ($\theta_2 > \theta_1$).

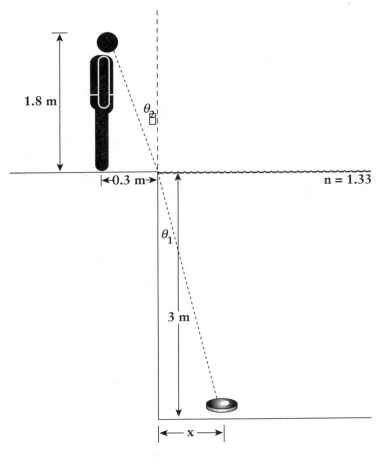

Figure 10.7

We need to find the angles that the light rays make with the normal to the water's surface:

$$\tan \theta_2 = \frac{0.3}{1.8}$$

$$\theta_2 = 9.51°$$

Using Snell's law we can solve for θ_1:

$$\sin \theta_1 = \frac{n_2}{n_1} \sin \theta_2$$

$$= \frac{0.165}{1.33}$$

$$\theta_1 = 7.1°$$

We can find x using trigonometry:

$$x = 3 \tan \theta_1$$
$$= 0.37 \text{ m}$$
$$= 37 \text{ cm}$$

2. TOTAL INTERNAL REFLECTION

When light travels from a medium with a higher index of refraction to a medium with a lower index of refraction, the refracted angle is larger than the angle of incidence ($\theta_2 > \theta_1$). As the angle of incidence is increased, a special angle is reached, called the **critical angle** (θ_c), where for this value of θ_1 the refracted angle θ_2 equals 90°. The critical angle can be found from Snell's Law:

$$n_1 \sin \theta_1 = n_2 \sin \theta_2$$
$$n_1 \sin \theta_c = n_2 \sin 90° = n_2$$
$$\sin \theta_c = \frac{n_2}{n_1}$$

KEY CONCEPT

Total internal reflection can only occur when going from a medium of greater index of refraction to one of lesser index of refraction.

Total **internal reflection**, a condition where all the light incident on a boundary is reflected back into the original material, results for any angle of incidence greater than θ_c.

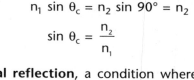

Figure 10.8

Example: From the previous example, suppose another penny is 10 times farther out than the first one. Will a light ray going from this penny to the top edge of the pool emerge from the water?

Solution: First find the critical angle:

$$\sin \theta_c = \frac{n_2}{n_1}$$

$$= \frac{1}{1.33}$$

$$\theta_c = 48.8°$$

The angle made by the second penny's light ray is:

$$\tan \theta_1 = \frac{0.37 \times 10}{3} = 1.23$$

$$\theta_1 = 51°$$

$\theta_1 > \theta_c$, therefore the light ray will be totally internally reflected and will not emerge.

3. THIN SPHERICAL LENSES

There is an important difference between lenses and mirrors aside from the obvious fact that lenses refract light while mirrors reflect it. When working with lenses, you are dealing with *two* surfaces that affect the light path. For example, a person wearing glasses sees light that travels from an object through the air into the glass lens (first surface). Then the light travels through the glass until it reaches the other side, where again it travels out of the glass into the air (second surface).

A thin lens is a lens whose thickness can be neglected. Since light can be coming from either side of a lens, a lens has two focal points (one on each side of the lens) and two focal lengths (see Figure 10.9). For thin spherical lenses the focal lengths are equal, and so we speak of the focal length.

Figure 10.9(a) also illustrates that a **converging lens** is always thicker at the center, while Figure 10.9(b) illustrates that a **diverging lens** is always thinner at the center.

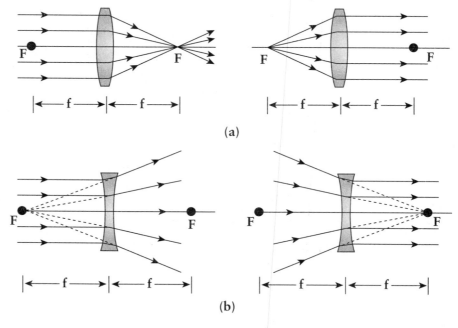

(a)

(b)

Figure 10.9

The basic formulas for finding image distance and magnification for spherical mirrors (except r = 2f,) also apply to lenses. The object distance o, image distance i, focal length f, and magnification m are related by:

$$\frac{1}{o} + \frac{1}{i} = \frac{1}{f}$$

$$m = -\frac{i}{o}$$

For lenses where the thickness cannot be neglected, the focal length is related to the curvature of the lens surfaces and the index of refraction of the lens by the **lensmaker's equation:**

$$\frac{1}{f} = (n - 1)\left(\frac{1}{r_1} - \frac{1}{r_2}\right)$$

where r_1 is the radius of curvature of the first lens surface and r_2 is the radius of curvature of the second lens surface.

Note that sign conventions change slightly for lenses. (Sign conventions are the trickiest part to optics.) For both lenses and mirrors, positive magnification means upright images and negative magnification means inverted images. Also, for both lenses and mirrors a positive image distance means that the image is real and is located on the R side, whereas a negative image distance means that the image is virtual and located on the V side.

However, where to place the R side and V side confuses most people because it is different for mirrors and lenses. To place the R side, remember that the R side is where the light really goes after interacting with the mirror or lens. For mirrors, light is reflected and therefore stays in front of the mirror. The image may either appear in front of or behind the mirror, but the light rays always remain in front of the mirror. Since the R side is in front of the mirror, the V side is behind the mirror. For lenses, it is different: Light travels through the lens and comes out on the other side. The light really travels to the other side of the lens, and therefore, for lenses, the R side is on the opposite side of the lens from where the light came from. Thus, the V side must be the side of the lens that the light came from. Although the object of a single lens is on the V side, this does not make the object virtual. Objects are real, with a positive object distance, unless they are in certain multiple lens systems.

Focal lengths have a simple sign convention. For both mirrors and lenses, converging lenses and mirrors have positive focal lengths and diverging mirrors and lenses have negative focal lengths. For radii of curvature you have to remember that a lens has two surfaces each with its own radius of curvature (r_1 and r_2, where the surfaces are numbered in the order that they are encountered by the traveling light). For both mirrors and lenses, a radius of curvature is positive if the center of curvature is on the R side and negative if the center of curvature is on the V side.

Sign Chart for Single Lenses

Symbol	Positive	Negative
o	object on side of lens light is coming from	object on side of lens light is going to
i	image on side of lens light is going to (R side)	image on side of lens light is coming from (V side)
f	converging lens	diverging lens
m	image erect	image inverted
r	when on R side (convex surface as seen from side the light is coming from)	when on V side (concave surface as seen from side the light is coming from)

Optometrists often describe a lens in terms of its **power** (P). This is measured in **diopters** when f is in meters, and is given by the equation:

$$P = \frac{1}{f}$$

P has the same sign as f and is therefore positive for a converging lens and negative for a diverging lens.

4. MULTIPLE LENS SYSTEMS

Lenses in contact are a series of lenses with neglible distances between them. These systems behave as a single lens with equivalent focal length given by:

$$\frac{1}{f} = \frac{1}{f_1} + \frac{1}{f_2} + \dots$$
$$(P = P_1 + P_2 + \dots)$$

A good example is the eye.

For **lenses not in contact** the image of one lens is used to make the object of another lens. The image from the last lens is the image of the system. Microscopes and telescopes are good examples. The magnification for the system is $M = m_1 \times m_2 \times m_3 \times \dots$

Example: An object is 15 cm to the left of a thin diverging lens with a 45 cm focal length as shown below. Find:

a. where the image is formed, if it is upright or inverted, and if it is real or virtual.

b. the radii of curvature assuming the lens is symmetrical and made of glass (n = 1.50).

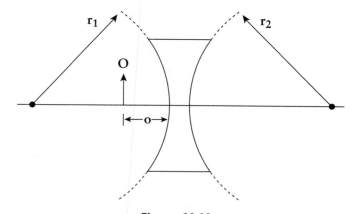

Figure 10.10

Solution: a.   The image distance (i) is found using the equation:

$$\frac{1}{i} + \frac{i}{o} = \frac{1}{f}$$

$$\frac{1}{i} = \frac{1}{f} - \frac{i}{o}$$

Since the lens is diverging the focal length takes a negative sign, $f = -45$ cm. The object (like all objects in a single lens system) has a positive sign, $o = 15$ cm. Solving for i:

$$\frac{1}{i} = \frac{-1}{45} - \frac{1}{15}$$

$$= \frac{-1}{45} - \frac{3}{45}$$

$$= \frac{-4}{45}$$

$$i = -11.25 \text{ cm}$$

The negative sign indicates that the image is on the left side of the lens and therefore virtual (the light went through the lens and is on the right side). To find out whether the image is upright or inverted we need to calculate the magnification:

$$m = -\frac{i}{o}$$

$$= -\frac{-11.25}{15}$$

$$= \frac{11.25}{15}$$

$$= 0.75$$

Since the magnification is positive, the image is upright. Furthermore, since $|m| < 1$, the image is smaller than the object.

b. Since the lens is symmetrical, the radii are equal but opposite in sign. They can be found from the lensmaker's equation:

$$\frac{1}{f} = (n - 1)\left(\frac{1}{r_1} - \frac{1}{r_2}\right)$$

As the light progresses from left to right, the first surface of the lens is concave (r_1 negative) and the second surface of the lens is convex (r positive). So:

$$\frac{1}{f} = (n - 1)\left(\frac{1}{-r} - \frac{1}{r}\right)$$

$$= (n - 1)\left(-\frac{2}{r}\right)$$

We know that f = −45 cm (diverging lens). Therefore:

$$-\frac{1}{45} = (1.5 - 1)\left(-\frac{2}{r}\right)$$

$$= \frac{-1}{r}$$

$$r = 45 \text{ cm}$$

C. Dispersion

As noted earlier, the speed of light for all wavelengths in a vacuum is the same. However, when light travels through a medium, different wavelengths travel at different velocities. This fact also implies that the index of refraction of a medium is a function of the wavelength, since the index of refraction is related to the velocity of the wave by n = c/v. When the speed of the wave varies with wavelength a material exhibits **dispersion**. The most common example of dispersion is the splitting of white light into its component colors using a prism.

If a source of white light is incident on one of the faces of a prism, the light emerging from the prism is spread out into a fan-shaped beam, as shown in Figure 10.11. The light has been dispersed into a spectrum. This occurs because violet light "sees" a greater index of refraction than red does and so is bent to a greater extent.

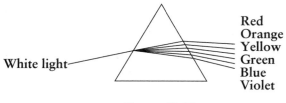

Figure 10.11

DIFFRACTION

When we first began discussing geometrical optics, we asserted that light travels in straight lines. But there are situations where this is not strictly true. For example, when light passes through a narrow opening (an opening whose size is on the order of wavelengths), the light waves seem to spread out as is seen in Figure 10.12. As the slit narrows, the light is spread out more. This spreading out of light as it passes through a narrow opening is called **diffraction**.

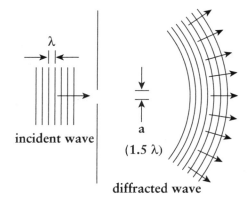

incident wave

Figure 10.12

> **REMEMBER**
>
> Diffraction is really the interference of an infinite number of waves, where each point along the slit acts as a wave source.

If a lens is placed between a narrow slit and a screen, a pattern is observed consisting of a bright central fringe with alternating dark and bright fringes on each side (see Figure 10.13). The central bright fringe is twice as wide as the bright fringes on the sides, and as the slit becomes narrower the central maximum becomes wider. The location of the dark fringes is given by the following formula:

$$a \sin \theta = n\lambda \ (n = 1, 2, 3, \ldots)$$

where a is the width of the slit, λ is the wavelength of the incident wave, and θ is the angle made by the line drawn from the center of the lens to the dark fringe and the line perpendicular to the screen. Note that bright fringes are halfway between dark fringes.

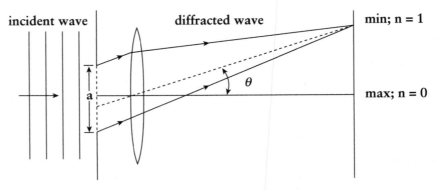

Figure 10.13

INTERFERENCE

By the superposition principle, when waves interact with each other the amplitudes of the waves add together in a process called **interference** (see Chapter 9). Young's experiment showed that two light waves can interfere with one another, and this contributed to the wave theory of light. Figure 10.14(a) shows the typical setup for Young's double-slit experiment. When monochromatic light illuminates the slits, an interference pattern is observed on a screen placed behind the slits. Monochromatic light is light that consists of just one wavelength, and coherent light consists of light waves whose phase difference does not change with time. Regions of constructive interference between the two light waves appear as regions of maximum light intensity on the screen. Conversely, in regions where the light waves interfere destructively, the light is at a minimum intensity and the screen is dark. An interference pattern produced by a double-slit setup is shown in Figure 10.14(b).

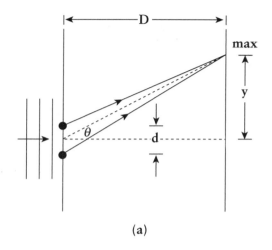

(a)

Zeroth fringe

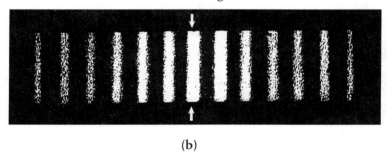

(b)

Figure 10.14

The position of maxima and minima on the screen can be found from the following equations:

(maxima) $\quad d \sin \theta = m\lambda \quad\quad\quad m = 0, 1, 2, \ldots$

(minima) $\quad d \sin \theta = (m + \frac{1}{2})\lambda \quad\quad m = 0, 1, 2, \ldots$

where d is the distance between the slits, θ is the angle between the dashed lines shown in Figure 10.14a, λ is the wavelength of the light, and m is an integer representing the order.

Example: What is the linear distance y between the sixth and eighth maxima on the screen? The wavelength λ is 550 nm, the slits are separated by 0.14 mm, and the screen is 70 cm from the slits.

KEY CONCEPT

When one refers to the 2nd order maximum or 4th order minimum, one simply substitutes m = 2 or m = 4 into the appropriate equation.

Solution: Using the small angle approximation $\sin\theta \approx \tan\theta \approx \theta$, the equation for the distance between maxima is derived as follows:

$$\sin\theta = \frac{m\lambda}{d}$$

$$\tan\theta = \frac{y}{D} \approx \frac{m\lambda}{d}$$

$$\Delta y \approx \frac{\Delta m\lambda D}{d}$$

where Δm is the difference between fringe numbers. Substituting the numbers gives:

$$y = \frac{2(550\times10^{-9})(0.70)}{0.14\times10^{-3}}$$

$$= 5.5 \text{ mm}$$

POLARIZATION

Plane-polarized light is light in which the electric fields of all the waves are oriented in the same direction, i.e., their electric field vectors are parallel. It is true that their magnetic field vectors are also parallel, but convention dictates that the plane of the electric field identifies the plane of polarization.

Unpolarized light corresponds to a random orientation of the electric field vectors. Sunlight is a prime example. However, there are filters called polarizers, often used in cameras and sunglasses, which allow only light whose electric field is pointing in a particular direction to pass. If you hold one polarizer out the window, it will let through only that portion of the daylight that has a given E vector orientation. If you now hold up another polarizer and slowly turn it, you will see the light transmitted through the two polarizers vary from total darkness to the level of the original polarizer alone. When both the first and second polarizer are polarizing in the same direction, all the light that passed through the first also passes through the second. When the second polarizer is turned so that it polarizes in a direction perpendicular to the first, no light gets through at all.

11

Atomic Phenomena

Toward the end of the nineteenth century and throughout the twentieth, research has shown that different sets of laws take effect at short distances, due to the wave nature of the discrete bits of matter. The theory that was developed to explain such phenomena is known as quantum mechanics. This chapter will primarily cover particular applications of quantum mechanical ideas to atomic phenomena but will not cover the formal theory of quantum mechanics. The first two topics covered here, blackbody radiation and the photoelectric effect, provided a first look at the quantum or discrete aspects of nature at the atomic level, particularly the discrete or particle nature of light. The quantum theory was later applied to the structure of the hydrogen atom, thus uncovering the discrete nature of the electron energies in hydrogen. This theory of the hydrogen atom, Bohr's theory, is reviewed along with a discussion (also due to physicist Niels Bohr) of the interaction of electromagnetic quanta (photons) with atoms. The application of quantum mechanics to nuclear phenomena is discussed in Chapter 12 of General Chemistry.

THERMAL BLACKBODY RADIATION

At any temperature above absolute zero, matter will emit electromagnetic radiation. The amount of radiant energy emitted at a given wavelength depends on the temperature of the emitter. In addition, different materials may emit different amounts of radiant energy at a particular wavelength due to the differences in their atomic structure. Because of these complications, physicists at the turn of the century turned their attention to an **ideal radiator** known as a **blackbody** (because of the fact that any ideal radiator is also an ideal absorber and would appear totally black if it were at a lower temperature than its surroundings). In practice, a blackbody radiator can be approximated rather closely by radiation produced in a cavity within a hot object. Hence blackbody radiation is approximated by what is called **cavity radiation**.

Physicist Max Planck developed the theoretical derivation of the blackbody spectrum. His radiant spectrum for two blackbodies at different temperatures is shown in Figure 11.1. In the derivation Planck had to use a number called **Planck's constant** (h) whose value is given by:

$$h = 6.63 \times 10^{-34} \text{ J} \cdot \text{s} = 4.14 \times 10^{-15} \text{ eV} \cdot \text{s}$$

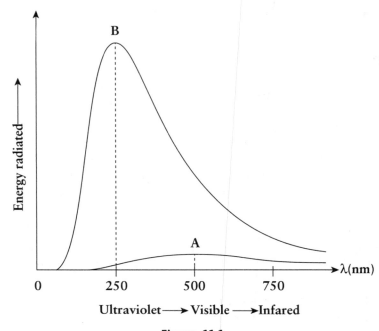

Figure 11.1

An analysis of Planck's formula for the blackbody spectrum shows that for a blackbody there is one wavelength at which the maximum amount of energy is emitted (λ_{peak}). This wavelength depends on the absolute temperature of the blackbody in a relation known as **Wien's displacement law,** which is expressed mathematically as:

$$\lambda_{peak} T = \text{constant}$$

The value of the constant is 2.90×10^{-3} m·K. Note that λ_{peak} is the wavelength at which more energy is emitted than any other wavelength. λ_{peak} **does not** refer to the maximum wavelength emitted.

Also, according to the **Stefan-Boltzmann law,** the total energy being emitted per unit area per second is proportional to the fourth power of the absolute temperature:

$$E_T = \sigma T^4$$

where σ is the Stefan-Boltzmann constant (5.67×10^{-8} J/s·m²·K⁴).

Example: In Figure 11.1 the radiant spectrum for two blackbodies is plotted. The first body is at temperature T_a, and the second body is at temperature T_b. How do the temperatures of the two blackbodies compare?

Solution: From the plots in Figure 11.1 we find that $\lambda_{peak-a} = 2\lambda_{peak-b}$, and from Wien's law we know that $T_b = 2T_a$. (By the Stefan-Boltzmann law the emitted energy per unit area per second of blackbody b is $2^4 = 16$ times greater than that of blackbody a.)

PHOTOELECTRIC EFFECT

When light of a sufficiently high frequency (typically, blue or ultraviolet light) is incident on a metal in a vacuum, the metal emits electrons. This phenomenon, first discovered by physicist Heinrich Hertz in 1887, is called the **photoelectric effect**. The minimum frequency of light that accomplishes this ejection of electrons is known as the **threshold frequency** f_T. The threshold frequency depends on the type of metal being exposed to the light. Einstein's explanation of these results was that the light beam consists of an integral number of light quanta, called photons, with the energy of each photon proportional to the frequency f of the light:

$$E = hf$$

The constant of proportionality h is Planck's constant.

It should also be noted that by knowing the frequency of the light you can easily find the wavelength λ via the relation:

$$\lambda = \frac{c}{f}$$

where c is the speed of light (3.00×10^8 m/s). These relations predict that shorter wavelength means higher frequency and therefore higher energy photons (toward the blue and ultraviolet end of the spectrum). Longer wavelength means lower frequency and therefore lower energy photons (toward the red and infrared end of the spectrum). Common units used for wavelength include nanometers (1 nm = 10^{-9} m) and Angstroms (1 Å = 10^{-10} m).

In the photoelectric effect, if the frequency of a photon incident on a metal is at the threshold frequency for the metal, the electron barely escapes from the metal. However, if the frequency of an incident photon is above the threshold frequency of the metal, the photon will have more than enough energy to eject a single electron, and the excess energy will be converted to kinetic energy of the ejected electron. The maximum kinetic energy can be calculated from the formula:

$$K = hf - W$$

KEY CONCEPT

Wavelength and frequency of light in a vacuum are related to speed of light by $c = \lambda f$, just as wavelength, frequency, and velocity of any wave are related by $v = \lambda f$.

KEY CONCEPT

$E = hf = hc/\lambda$, which says that higher frequency or shorter wavelength light has higher energy and lower frequency or longer wavelength light has lower energy.

where W is the **work function** of the metal in question (the minimum energy required to eject an electron), which is related to the threshold frequency of that metal by:

$$W = hf_T$$

So for $f > f_T$ the photon will eject electrons with the excess energy appearing as kinetic energy (K). For $f < f_T$ the photon does not carry enough energy to eject an electron from the metal.

We can think of all of the electrons liberated from the metal by the photo-electric effect as producing a net charge flow per unit time, or a current. Provided that a light beam's frequency is above the threshold frequency of the metal, light beams of greater intensity produce greater current. This is because the higher the intensity of the beam, the greater the number of photons per unit time that fall on an electrode, producing a greater number of electrons per unit time liberated from the metal. When the light's frequency is above threshold frequency, the current is directly proportional to the intensity of the light beam.

Example: If the work function of a metal is 2.00 eV and blue light of frequency 6.00×10^{14} Hz is incident on the metal, will there be photo-ejection of electrons? If so, how much kinetic energy will an electron carry away?

Solution: If the photons have a frequency of 6.00×10^{14} Hz, each photon has an energy given by:

$$E = hf$$
$$= (4.14 \times 10^{-15})(6.00 \times 10^{14})$$
$$= 2.48 \text{ eV}$$

Clearly then, any given photon has more than enough energy to get an electron in the metal to overcome the 2.00 eV barrier. In fact, the excess kinetic energy carried away by the electron turns out to be:

$$K = hf - W$$
$$= 2.48 - 2.00$$
$$= 0.48 \text{ eV}$$

KEY CONCEPT

A photon can liberate an electron from a metal surface (photoelectric effect) only if the energy of the photon, $E = hf$, is greater than or equal to the work function, W, of the metal.

THE BOHR MODEL OF THE HYDROGEN ATOM

A. Energy Levels

The hydrogen atom consists of an electron "in orbit" about a single, more massive, proton. As such, it is the simplest atom to describe and is a proving ground for any atomic theory. Before a more complete quantum mechanical description was developed, Niels Bohr proposed a model of the hydrogen atom consisting of the single electron in discrete circular orbits about the proton. It was necessary for Bohr to resort to new quantum ideas, since a classical model of hydrogen would require the electron to continuously radiate electromagnetic waves, thereby losing energy and spiraling into the proton. Bohr postulated that there were **specific stable, or allowed, orbits** of quantized (discrete) energy in which electrons did not radiate energy. This led him to deduce an **energy level formula.**

The Bohr energy corresponding to the closest allowed orbit to the nucleus or the **ground state** (n = 1) is –13.6 eV. The energies corresponding to orbits farther away from the nucleus (n = 2,3,4,...) are less negative and therefore greater, until the electron is given so much energy that it is free from the electrostatic (Coulomb) pull of the nucleus and can have any positive energy (**ionization**). An electron occupying one of these higher energy orbits or energy levels, but still bound to the proton, is said to be in an **excited state.** The quantum energy levels in the Bohr model of the hydrogen atom can be arranged from lowest to highest, each with an associated **principal quantum number** (n) that is a positive integer from n = 1 to n = ∞. The energy levels for hydrogen are given in electron-volts by the formula:

$$E_n = \frac{-13.6}{n^2} \text{ (hydrogen)}$$

> **REMEMBER**
>
> The lowest energy (ground state) of an electron in hydrogen is negative. Higher energy bound states are also negative but progressively smaller in magnitude.

Electron Energy Levels in Hydrogen

Principal quantum number	Energy level
n	E_n
1	$\dfrac{-13.6}{1}$ eV = -13.6 eV
2	$\dfrac{-13.6}{4}$ eV = -3.40 eV
3	$\dfrac{-13.6}{9}$ eV = -1.51 eV
4	$\dfrac{-13.6}{16}$ eV = -0.85 eV
•	• •
•	• •
•	• •
∞	$\dfrac{-13.6}{\infty}$ eV = 0 eV

Positive energy states have no principal quantum number, since the electron is not bound to the proton. It is in a free electron state and can have any positive energy.

B. Emission and Absorption of Light

It was found from experiments that hydrogen atoms radiate light only at particular frequencies. Bohr put forward a set of postulates that form the basis of his model. The postulates are:

1. Energy levels of the electron are stable and discrete. They correspond to specific orbits.

2. An electron emits or absorbs radiation **only** when making a transition from one energy level to another (from one allowed orbit to another).

3. To jump from a lower energy (inner orbit) to a higher energy (outer orbit), an electron must **absorb** a photon of precisely the right frequency such that the photon's energy (hf) equals the energy difference between the two orbits.

4. When jumping from a higher energy (outer orbit) to a lower energy (inner orbit) an electron **emits** a photon of a frequency such that the photon's energy (hf) is exactly the energy difference between the two orbits.

Bohr's initial ideas were replaced with the advent of full quantum mechanical theories of atomic structure. In contemporary theories, the electron is not envisioned as following a circular or elliptical path like the planets do in orbiting the sun. However, the Bohr model is still useful for certain calculations.

An electron in the lowest allowed energy level (n = 1 or ground state) cannot emit any more energy (though it could absorb radiation and jump up to a higher energy level). An electron occupying an **excited state** can either emit radiation when it jumps down to a lower energy level or absorb radiation when it jumps up to a higher energy level.

Bohr's 3rd and 4th postulates can be used to find the frequency of radiation emitted or absorbed by an electron in going from energy level E_i to energy level E_f. The change in the electron's energy is $\Delta E = E_f - E_i$. Since bound state energy levels are negative, if ΔE is negative then the electron has jumped from a higher, less negative energy state (less tightly bound state) to a lower, more negative energy state (more tightly bound state). There is then an **emission** of a photon of frequency f where:

$$\Delta E < 0$$

$$hf = -\Delta E \text{ (emission)}$$

On the other hand, if ΔE is positive, then the electron has **absorbed** a photon and jumped from a lower, more negative energy state to a higher, less negative energy state. The absorbed photon has a frequency f where:

$$\Delta E > 0$$

$$hf = \Delta E \text{ (absorption)}$$

Example: What wavelength of light is emitted by a hydrogen electron going from the n = 5 to the n = 2 energy levels?

Solution: For hydrogen, the energy for a given principal quantum number n is given in electron-volts by

$$E = \frac{-13.6}{n^2}$$

Since the electron goes **from** n = 5 **to** n = 2, the initial energy level is:

$$E_i = E_5 = \frac{-13.6}{25} = -0.544 \text{ eV}$$

The final energy level is:

$$E_f = E_2 = \frac{-13.6}{4} = -3.40 \text{ eV}$$

Therefore:

$$\Delta E = E_f - E_i$$
$$= -3.40 + 0.544$$
$$= -2.856 \text{ eV}$$

The negative value of ΔE confirms that the light is emitted. The frequency is found by:

$$f = \frac{|\Delta E|}{h}$$
$$= \frac{2.856}{4.14 \times 10^{-15}}$$
$$= 6.90 \times 10^{14} \text{ Hz}$$

REMEMBER

Use $E = hf$ to find frequency of photon given energy of photon.

Now we can easily find the wavelength (and convert to different units for comparison):

$$\lambda = \frac{c}{f}$$
$$= \frac{3.00 \times 10^8}{6.90 \times 10^{14}}$$
$$= 4.35 \times 10^{-7} \text{ m}$$
$$= 435 \text{ nm}$$
$$= 4350 \text{ Å}$$

REMEMBER

Use $c = \lambda f$ to find wavelength of photon from frequency of photon or vice versa.

Example: What wavelength of light is needed to free an electron from the ground state of hydrogen?

Solution: As previously mentioned, the electron in the ground state ($n = 1$) of hydrogen has an energy of -13.6 eV. Negative energies mean a bound state; positive energies mean a free state. It would take a photon of at least $+13.6$ eV to free the electron. Find the frequency:

$$f = \frac{E}{h}$$
$$= \frac{13.6}{4.14 \times 10^{-15}}$$
$$= 3.29 \times 10^{15} \text{ Hz}$$

KEY CONCEPT

The lowest energy an electron can have and be considered free is 0 eV. The energy necessary to free an electron equals the energy required to make the electron energy 0 eV.

Now the wavelength is given by:

$$\lambda = \frac{c}{f}$$

$$= \frac{3.00 \times 10^8}{3.29 \times 10^{15}}$$

$$= 9.12 \times 10^{-8} \text{ m}$$

$$= 91.2 \text{ nm}$$

$$= 912 \text{ Å}$$

FLUORESCENCE

Fluorescence refers to the process in which certain substances emit visible light when excited by other radiation, usually ultraviolet radiation. Photons corresponding to ultraviolet radiation have relatively high frequencies (short wavelengths). After being excited to a higher energy state by the ultraviolet radiation, the electron returns to its original state in two or more steps. By returning in two or more steps, each step involves less energy. In each step a lower frequency (longer wavelength) photon is emitted, whose wavelength may fall in the visible portion of the spectrum. This is the principle of the fluorescent light.

KEY CONCEPT

An excited electron may make one large jump back to the ground state, or a number of smaller jumps, i.e. an electron in n = 4 may jump from 4 to 1 or from 4 to 2 to 1, etc.

VII

FULL-LENGTH PRACTICE TEST

INSTRUCTIONS FOR
TAKING THE PRACTICE TEST

Before taking the practice test, find a quiet place where you can work uninterrupted. Make sure you have a comfortable desk and several No. 2 pencils.

Use the answer grid provided to record your answers. You'll find the answer key and score conversion chart following the test.

The test consists of four sections: Survey of the Natural Sciences (90 minutes), Reading Comprehension (50 minutes), Physics (50 minutes), and Quantitative Reasoning (45 minutes). Remember, if you finish a section early, you may review any questions within that section, but you may not go back or forward a section.

Good luck.

ANSWER SHEET

Mark one and only one answer to each question. Be sure to fill in completely the space for your intended answer choice. If you erase, do so completely. Make no stray marks.

RIGHT MARK: ●   WRONG MARKS: ⊘ ⊗ ⊙

Survey of the Natural Sciences

1. Ⓐ Ⓑ Ⓒ Ⓓ Ⓔ	11. Ⓐ Ⓑ Ⓒ Ⓓ Ⓔ	21. Ⓐ Ⓑ Ⓒ Ⓓ Ⓔ	31. Ⓐ Ⓑ Ⓒ Ⓓ Ⓔ	41. Ⓐ Ⓑ Ⓒ Ⓓ Ⓔ
2. Ⓐ Ⓑ Ⓒ Ⓓ Ⓔ	12. Ⓐ Ⓑ Ⓒ Ⓓ Ⓔ	22. Ⓐ Ⓑ Ⓒ Ⓓ Ⓔ	32. Ⓐ Ⓑ Ⓒ Ⓓ Ⓔ	42. Ⓐ Ⓑ Ⓒ Ⓓ Ⓔ
3. Ⓐ Ⓑ Ⓒ Ⓓ Ⓔ	13. Ⓐ Ⓑ Ⓒ Ⓓ Ⓔ	23. Ⓐ Ⓑ Ⓒ Ⓓ Ⓔ	33. Ⓐ Ⓑ Ⓒ Ⓓ Ⓔ	43. Ⓐ Ⓑ Ⓒ Ⓓ Ⓔ
4. Ⓐ Ⓑ Ⓒ Ⓓ Ⓔ	14. Ⓐ Ⓑ Ⓒ Ⓓ Ⓔ	24. Ⓐ Ⓑ Ⓒ Ⓓ Ⓔ	34. Ⓐ Ⓑ Ⓒ Ⓓ Ⓔ	44. Ⓐ Ⓑ Ⓒ Ⓓ Ⓔ
5. Ⓐ Ⓑ Ⓒ Ⓓ Ⓔ	15. Ⓐ Ⓑ Ⓒ Ⓓ Ⓔ	25. Ⓐ Ⓑ Ⓒ Ⓓ Ⓔ	35. Ⓐ Ⓑ Ⓒ Ⓓ Ⓔ	45. Ⓐ Ⓑ Ⓒ Ⓓ Ⓔ
6. Ⓐ Ⓑ Ⓒ Ⓓ Ⓔ	16. Ⓐ Ⓑ Ⓒ Ⓓ Ⓔ	26. Ⓐ Ⓑ Ⓒ Ⓓ Ⓔ	36. Ⓐ Ⓑ Ⓒ Ⓓ Ⓔ	46. Ⓐ Ⓑ Ⓒ Ⓓ Ⓔ
7. Ⓐ Ⓑ Ⓒ Ⓓ Ⓔ	17. Ⓐ Ⓑ Ⓒ Ⓓ Ⓔ	27. Ⓐ Ⓑ Ⓒ Ⓓ Ⓔ	37. Ⓐ Ⓑ Ⓒ Ⓓ Ⓔ	47. Ⓐ Ⓑ Ⓒ Ⓓ Ⓔ
8. Ⓐ Ⓑ Ⓒ Ⓓ Ⓔ	18. Ⓐ Ⓑ Ⓒ Ⓓ Ⓔ	28. Ⓐ Ⓑ Ⓒ Ⓓ Ⓔ	38. Ⓐ Ⓑ Ⓒ Ⓓ Ⓔ	48. Ⓐ Ⓑ Ⓒ Ⓓ Ⓔ
9. Ⓐ Ⓑ Ⓒ Ⓓ Ⓔ	19. Ⓐ Ⓑ Ⓒ Ⓓ Ⓔ	29. Ⓐ Ⓑ Ⓒ Ⓓ Ⓔ	39. Ⓐ Ⓑ Ⓒ Ⓓ Ⓔ	49. Ⓐ Ⓑ Ⓒ Ⓓ Ⓔ
10. Ⓐ Ⓑ Ⓒ Ⓓ Ⓔ	20. Ⓐ Ⓑ Ⓒ Ⓓ Ⓔ	30. Ⓐ Ⓑ Ⓒ Ⓓ Ⓔ	40. Ⓐ Ⓑ Ⓒ Ⓓ Ⓔ	50. Ⓐ Ⓑ Ⓒ Ⓓ Ⓔ

51. Ⓐ Ⓑ Ⓒ Ⓓ Ⓔ	61. Ⓐ Ⓑ Ⓒ Ⓓ Ⓔ	71. Ⓐ Ⓑ Ⓒ Ⓓ Ⓔ	81. Ⓐ Ⓑ Ⓒ Ⓓ Ⓔ	91. Ⓐ Ⓑ Ⓒ Ⓓ Ⓔ
52. Ⓐ Ⓑ Ⓒ Ⓓ Ⓔ	62. Ⓐ Ⓑ Ⓒ Ⓓ Ⓔ	72. Ⓐ Ⓑ Ⓒ Ⓓ Ⓔ	82. Ⓐ Ⓑ Ⓒ Ⓓ Ⓔ	92. Ⓐ Ⓑ Ⓒ Ⓓ Ⓔ
53. Ⓐ Ⓑ Ⓒ Ⓓ Ⓔ	63. Ⓐ Ⓑ Ⓒ Ⓓ Ⓔ	73. Ⓐ Ⓑ Ⓒ Ⓓ Ⓔ	83. Ⓐ Ⓑ Ⓒ Ⓓ Ⓔ	93. Ⓐ Ⓑ Ⓒ Ⓓ Ⓔ
54. Ⓐ Ⓑ Ⓒ Ⓓ Ⓔ	64. Ⓐ Ⓑ Ⓒ Ⓓ Ⓔ	74. Ⓐ Ⓑ Ⓒ Ⓓ Ⓔ	84. Ⓐ Ⓑ Ⓒ Ⓓ Ⓔ	94. Ⓐ Ⓑ Ⓒ Ⓓ Ⓔ
55. Ⓐ Ⓑ Ⓒ Ⓓ Ⓔ	65. Ⓐ Ⓑ Ⓒ Ⓓ Ⓔ	75. Ⓐ Ⓑ Ⓒ Ⓓ Ⓔ	85. Ⓐ Ⓑ Ⓒ Ⓓ Ⓔ	95. Ⓐ Ⓑ Ⓒ Ⓓ Ⓔ
56. Ⓐ Ⓑ Ⓒ Ⓓ Ⓔ	66. Ⓐ Ⓑ Ⓒ Ⓓ Ⓔ	76. Ⓐ Ⓑ Ⓒ Ⓓ Ⓔ	86. Ⓐ Ⓑ Ⓒ Ⓓ Ⓔ	96. Ⓐ Ⓑ Ⓒ Ⓓ Ⓔ
57. Ⓐ Ⓑ Ⓒ Ⓓ Ⓔ	67. Ⓐ Ⓑ Ⓒ Ⓓ Ⓔ	77. Ⓐ Ⓑ Ⓒ Ⓓ Ⓔ	87. Ⓐ Ⓑ Ⓒ Ⓓ Ⓔ	97. Ⓐ Ⓑ Ⓒ Ⓓ Ⓔ
58. Ⓐ Ⓑ Ⓒ Ⓓ Ⓔ	68. Ⓐ Ⓑ Ⓒ Ⓓ Ⓔ	78. Ⓐ Ⓑ Ⓒ Ⓓ Ⓔ	88. Ⓐ Ⓑ Ⓒ Ⓓ Ⓔ	98. Ⓐ Ⓑ Ⓒ Ⓓ Ⓔ
59. Ⓐ Ⓑ Ⓒ Ⓓ Ⓔ	69. Ⓐ Ⓑ Ⓒ Ⓓ Ⓔ	79. Ⓐ Ⓑ Ⓒ Ⓓ Ⓔ	89. Ⓐ Ⓑ Ⓒ Ⓓ Ⓔ	99. Ⓐ Ⓑ Ⓒ Ⓓ Ⓔ
60. Ⓐ Ⓑ Ⓒ Ⓓ Ⓔ	70. Ⓐ Ⓑ Ⓒ Ⓓ Ⓔ	80. Ⓐ Ⓑ Ⓒ Ⓓ Ⓔ	90. Ⓐ Ⓑ Ⓒ Ⓓ Ⓔ	100. Ⓐ Ⓑ Ⓒ Ⓓ Ⓔ

Reading Comprehension

1. Ⓐ Ⓑ Ⓒ Ⓓ Ⓔ	11. Ⓐ Ⓑ Ⓒ Ⓓ Ⓔ	21. Ⓐ Ⓑ Ⓒ Ⓓ Ⓔ	31. Ⓐ Ⓑ Ⓒ Ⓓ Ⓔ
2. Ⓐ Ⓑ Ⓒ Ⓓ Ⓔ	12. Ⓐ Ⓑ Ⓒ Ⓓ Ⓔ	22. Ⓐ Ⓑ Ⓒ Ⓓ Ⓔ	32. Ⓐ Ⓑ Ⓒ Ⓓ Ⓔ
3. Ⓐ Ⓑ Ⓒ Ⓓ Ⓔ	13. Ⓐ Ⓑ Ⓒ Ⓓ Ⓔ	23. Ⓐ Ⓑ Ⓒ Ⓓ Ⓔ	33. Ⓐ Ⓑ Ⓒ Ⓓ Ⓔ
4. Ⓐ Ⓑ Ⓒ Ⓓ Ⓔ	14. Ⓐ Ⓑ Ⓒ Ⓓ Ⓔ	24. Ⓐ Ⓑ Ⓒ Ⓓ Ⓔ	34. Ⓐ Ⓑ Ⓒ Ⓓ Ⓔ
5. Ⓐ Ⓑ Ⓒ Ⓓ Ⓔ	15. Ⓐ Ⓑ Ⓒ Ⓓ Ⓔ	25. Ⓐ Ⓑ Ⓒ Ⓓ Ⓔ	35. Ⓐ Ⓑ Ⓒ Ⓓ Ⓔ
6. Ⓐ Ⓑ Ⓒ Ⓓ Ⓔ	16. Ⓐ Ⓑ Ⓒ Ⓓ Ⓔ	26. Ⓐ Ⓑ Ⓒ Ⓓ Ⓔ	36. Ⓐ Ⓑ Ⓒ Ⓓ Ⓔ
7. Ⓐ Ⓑ Ⓒ Ⓓ Ⓔ	17. Ⓐ Ⓑ Ⓒ Ⓓ Ⓔ	27. Ⓐ Ⓑ Ⓒ Ⓓ Ⓔ	37. Ⓐ Ⓑ Ⓒ Ⓓ Ⓔ
8. Ⓐ Ⓑ Ⓒ Ⓓ Ⓔ	18. Ⓐ Ⓑ Ⓒ Ⓓ Ⓔ	28. Ⓐ Ⓑ Ⓒ Ⓓ Ⓔ	38. Ⓐ Ⓑ Ⓒ Ⓓ Ⓔ
9. Ⓐ Ⓑ Ⓒ Ⓓ Ⓔ	19. Ⓐ Ⓑ Ⓒ Ⓓ Ⓔ	29. Ⓐ Ⓑ Ⓒ Ⓓ Ⓔ	39. Ⓐ Ⓑ Ⓒ Ⓓ Ⓔ
10. Ⓐ Ⓑ Ⓒ Ⓓ Ⓔ	20. Ⓐ Ⓑ Ⓒ Ⓓ Ⓔ	30. Ⓐ Ⓑ Ⓒ Ⓓ Ⓔ	40. Ⓐ Ⓑ Ⓒ Ⓓ Ⓔ

ANSWER SHEET

Mark one and only one answer to each question. Be sure to fill in completely the space for your intended answer choice. If you erase, do so completely. Make no stray marks.

RIGHT MARK: ●   WRONG MARKS: ⊘ ⊗ ◉

Physics

1. Ⓐ Ⓑ Ⓒ Ⓓ Ⓔ	11. Ⓐ Ⓑ Ⓒ Ⓓ Ⓔ	21. Ⓐ Ⓑ Ⓒ Ⓓ Ⓔ	31. Ⓐ Ⓑ Ⓒ Ⓓ Ⓔ
2. Ⓐ Ⓑ Ⓒ Ⓓ Ⓔ	12. Ⓐ Ⓑ Ⓒ Ⓓ Ⓔ	22. Ⓐ Ⓑ Ⓒ Ⓓ Ⓔ	32. Ⓐ Ⓑ Ⓒ Ⓓ Ⓔ
3. Ⓐ Ⓑ Ⓒ Ⓓ Ⓔ	13. Ⓐ Ⓑ Ⓒ Ⓓ Ⓔ	23. Ⓐ Ⓑ Ⓒ Ⓓ Ⓔ	33. Ⓐ Ⓑ Ⓒ Ⓓ Ⓔ
4. Ⓐ Ⓑ Ⓒ Ⓓ Ⓔ	14. Ⓐ Ⓑ Ⓒ Ⓓ Ⓔ	24. Ⓐ Ⓑ Ⓒ Ⓓ Ⓔ	34. Ⓐ Ⓑ Ⓒ Ⓓ Ⓔ
5. Ⓐ Ⓑ Ⓒ Ⓓ Ⓔ	15. Ⓐ Ⓑ Ⓒ Ⓓ Ⓔ	25. Ⓐ Ⓑ Ⓒ Ⓓ Ⓔ	35. Ⓐ Ⓑ Ⓒ Ⓓ Ⓔ
6. Ⓐ Ⓑ Ⓒ Ⓓ Ⓔ	16. Ⓐ Ⓑ Ⓒ Ⓓ Ⓔ	26. Ⓐ Ⓑ Ⓒ Ⓓ Ⓔ	36. Ⓐ Ⓑ Ⓒ Ⓓ Ⓔ
7. Ⓐ Ⓑ Ⓒ Ⓓ Ⓔ	17. Ⓐ Ⓑ Ⓒ Ⓓ Ⓔ	27. Ⓐ Ⓑ Ⓒ Ⓓ Ⓔ	37. Ⓐ Ⓑ Ⓒ Ⓓ Ⓔ
8. Ⓐ Ⓑ Ⓒ Ⓓ Ⓔ	18. Ⓐ Ⓑ Ⓒ Ⓓ Ⓔ	28. Ⓐ Ⓑ Ⓒ Ⓓ Ⓔ	38. Ⓐ Ⓑ Ⓒ Ⓓ Ⓔ
9. Ⓐ Ⓑ Ⓒ Ⓓ Ⓔ	19. Ⓐ Ⓑ Ⓒ Ⓓ Ⓔ	29. Ⓐ Ⓑ Ⓒ Ⓓ Ⓔ	39. Ⓐ Ⓑ Ⓒ Ⓓ Ⓔ
10. Ⓐ Ⓑ Ⓒ Ⓓ Ⓔ	20. Ⓐ Ⓑ Ⓒ Ⓓ Ⓔ	30. Ⓐ Ⓑ Ⓒ Ⓓ Ⓔ	40. Ⓐ Ⓑ Ⓒ Ⓓ Ⓔ

Quantitative Reasoning

1. Ⓐ Ⓑ Ⓒ Ⓓ Ⓔ	11. Ⓐ Ⓑ Ⓒ Ⓓ Ⓔ	21. Ⓐ Ⓑ Ⓒ Ⓓ Ⓔ	31. Ⓐ Ⓑ Ⓒ Ⓓ Ⓔ	41. Ⓐ Ⓑ Ⓒ Ⓓ Ⓔ
2. Ⓐ Ⓑ Ⓒ Ⓓ Ⓔ	12. Ⓐ Ⓑ Ⓒ Ⓓ Ⓔ	22. Ⓐ Ⓑ Ⓒ Ⓓ Ⓔ	32. Ⓐ Ⓑ Ⓒ Ⓓ Ⓔ	42. Ⓐ Ⓑ Ⓒ Ⓓ Ⓔ
3. Ⓐ Ⓑ Ⓒ Ⓓ Ⓔ	13. Ⓐ Ⓑ Ⓒ Ⓓ Ⓔ	23. Ⓐ Ⓑ Ⓒ Ⓓ Ⓔ	33. Ⓐ Ⓑ Ⓒ Ⓓ Ⓔ	43. Ⓐ Ⓑ Ⓒ Ⓓ Ⓔ
4. Ⓐ Ⓑ Ⓒ Ⓓ Ⓔ	14. Ⓐ Ⓑ Ⓒ Ⓓ Ⓔ	24. Ⓐ Ⓑ Ⓒ Ⓓ Ⓔ	34. Ⓐ Ⓑ Ⓒ Ⓓ Ⓔ	44. Ⓐ Ⓑ Ⓒ Ⓓ Ⓔ
5. Ⓐ Ⓑ Ⓒ Ⓓ Ⓔ	15. Ⓐ Ⓑ Ⓒ Ⓓ Ⓔ	25. Ⓐ Ⓑ Ⓒ Ⓓ Ⓔ	35. Ⓐ Ⓑ Ⓒ Ⓓ Ⓔ	45. Ⓐ Ⓑ Ⓒ Ⓓ Ⓔ
6. Ⓐ Ⓑ Ⓒ Ⓓ Ⓔ	16. Ⓐ Ⓑ Ⓒ Ⓓ Ⓔ	26. Ⓐ Ⓑ Ⓒ Ⓓ Ⓔ	36. Ⓐ Ⓑ Ⓒ Ⓓ Ⓔ	46. Ⓐ Ⓑ Ⓒ Ⓓ Ⓔ
7. Ⓐ Ⓑ Ⓒ Ⓓ Ⓔ	17. Ⓐ Ⓑ Ⓒ Ⓓ Ⓔ	27. Ⓐ Ⓑ Ⓒ Ⓓ Ⓔ	37. Ⓐ Ⓑ Ⓒ Ⓓ Ⓔ	47. Ⓐ Ⓑ Ⓒ Ⓓ Ⓔ
8. Ⓐ Ⓑ Ⓒ Ⓓ Ⓔ	18. Ⓐ Ⓑ Ⓒ Ⓓ Ⓔ	28. Ⓐ Ⓑ Ⓒ Ⓓ Ⓔ	38. Ⓐ Ⓑ Ⓒ Ⓓ Ⓔ	48. Ⓐ Ⓑ Ⓒ Ⓓ Ⓔ
9. Ⓐ Ⓑ Ⓒ Ⓓ Ⓔ	19. Ⓐ Ⓑ Ⓒ Ⓓ Ⓔ	29. Ⓐ Ⓑ Ⓒ Ⓓ Ⓔ	39. Ⓐ Ⓑ Ⓒ Ⓓ Ⓔ	49. Ⓐ Ⓑ Ⓒ Ⓓ Ⓔ
10. Ⓐ Ⓑ Ⓒ Ⓓ Ⓔ	20. Ⓐ Ⓑ Ⓒ Ⓓ Ⓔ	30. Ⓐ Ⓑ Ⓒ Ⓓ Ⓔ	40. Ⓐ Ⓑ Ⓒ Ⓓ Ⓔ	50. Ⓐ Ⓑ Ⓒ Ⓓ Ⓔ

Survey of the Natural Sciences

100 questions–90 minutes

Directions: This examination is composed of 100 items: Biology (1–40), General Chemistry (41–70), and Organic Chemistry (71–100). Choose the best answer for each question from the five choices provided.

1 H 1.0																	2 He 4.0
3 Li 6.9	4 Be 9.0											5 B 10.8	6 C 12.0	7 N 14.0	8 O 16.0	9 F 19.0	10 Ne 20.2
11 Na 23.0	12 Mg 24.3											13 Al 27.0	14 Si 28.1	15 P 31.0	16 S 32.1	17 Cl 35.5	18 Ar 39.9
19 K 39.1	20 Ca 40.1	21 Sc 45.0	22 Ti 47.9	23 V 50.9	24 Cr 52.0	25 Mn 54.9	26 Fe 55.8	27 Co 58.9	28 Ni 58.7	29 Cu 63.5	30 Zn 65.4	31 Ga 69.7	32 Ge 72.6	33 As 74.9	34 Se 79.0	35 Br 79.9	36 Kr 83.8
37 Rb 85.5	38 Sr 87.6	39 Y 88.9	40 Zr 91.2	41 Nb 92.9	42 Mo 95.9	43 Tc (98)	44 Ru 101.1	45 Rh 102.9	46 Pd 106.4	47 Ag 107.9	48 Cd 112.4	49 In 114.8	50 Sn 118.7	51 Sb 121.8	52 Te 127.6	53 I 126.9	54 Xe 131.3
55 Cs 132.9	56 Ba 137.3	57 La* 138.9	72 Hf 178.5	73 Ta 180.9	74 W 183.9	75 Re 186.2	76 Os 190.2	77 Ir 192.2	78 Pt 195.1	79 Au 197.0	80 Hg 200.6	81 Tl 204.4	82 Pb 207.2	83 Bi 209.0	84 Po (209)	85 At (210)	86 Rn (222)
87 Fr (223)	88 Ra 226.0	89 Ac† 227.0	104 Unq (261)	105 Unp (262)	106 Unh (263)	107 Uns (262)	108 Uno (265)	109 Une (267)									

	58 Ce 140.1	59 Pr 140.9	60 Nd 144.2	61 Pm (145)	62 Sm 150.4	63 Eu 152.0	64 Gd 157.3	65 Tb 158.9	66 Dy 162.5	67 Ho 164.9	68 Er 167.3	69 Tm 168.9	70 Yb 173.0	71 Lu 175.0
*														
†	90 Th 232.0	91 Pa (231)	92 U 238.0	93 Np (237)	94 Pu (244)	95 Am (243)	96 Cm (247)	97 Bk (247)	98 Cf (251)	99 Es (252)	100 Fm (257)	101 Md (258)	102 No (259)	103 Lr (260)

GO TO THE NEXT PAGE

1. Which of the following might appear in an F_2 generation but could not appear in an F_1 generation if one parent is homozygous dominant and the other is homozygous recessive?

    A. Heterozygous genotype
    B. Dominant phenotype
    C. Recessive phenotype
    D. All of the above
    E. None of the above

2. Which of the following is NOT a distinction between plants and animals?

    A. Plants contain cell walls made of cellulose.
    B. Plants have intermediate larval stages.
    C. Plants are extensively branched.
    D. Animals are generally heterotrophic and motile.
    E. All of the above

3. Ectoderm : endoderm:

    A. Heart : stomach
    B. Retina : lungs
    C. Skeletal muscles : liver
    D. Skin : stomach muscle
    E. Taste buds : uterus

4. An organism is heterozygous with respect to three pairs of genes, namely Aa, Bb, and Cc. How many different types of gametes can be formed?

    A. 2
    B. 4
    C. 6
    D. 8
    E. 9

5. Breeding animals of close genotypes or phenotypes is known as

    A. inbreeding.
    B. hybridization.
    C. cross-breeding.
    D. selective breeding.
    E. test breeding.

6. $CO_2 + H_2O \rightarrow C_6H_{12}O_6 + O_2$

    The above reaction is catalyzed by
    A. light.
    B. ADP.
    C. CO_2.
    D. chlorophyll.
    E. None of the above

GO TO THE NEXT PAGE

7. The membrane that functions in respiration in the embryo is the

   A. amnion.
   B. allantois.
   C. chorion.
   D. umbilical cord.
   E. yolk sac.

8. A process that CANNOT take place in haploid cells is

   A. mitosis.
   B. meiosis.
   C. cell division.
   D. growth.
   E. digestion.

9. The Krebs cycle involves

   A. formation of NAD.
   B. regeneration of oxaloacetic acid.
   C. transamination.
   D. breaking of peptide bonds.
   E. glycogen formation.

10. Which is CORRECTLY associated?

    A. RNA : thymine
    B. DNA : uracil
    C. RNA : replication
    D. mRNA : picks up amino acids
    E. RNA : ribose sugar

11. Enzymes

    A. are carbohydrates.
    B. work best at pH greater than 8.
    C. always require a coenzyme.
    D. are necessary in respiration.
    E. are changed during a reaction.

12. A_____B C_____D

    If the diagram above represents genes on a chromosome, which genes would have the highest frequency of crossover?

    A. A and B
    B. A and D
    C. B and C
    D. B and D
    E. The frequencies are the same for all crossovers.

13. What is the BEST evidence that genes control synthesis of proteins?

    A. Proteins are macromolecules.
    B. RNA directs amino acid synthesis.
    C. Amino acid sequence of polypeptides is changed by gene mutation.
    D. DNA serves as a template for RNA.
    E. mRNA is found in the ribosome.

14. The different appearance of the rough endoplasmic reticulum compared to the smooth endoplasmic reticulum is due to the presence of

    A. lysosomes.
    B. ribosomes.
    C. mitochondria.
    D. Golgi apparati.
    E. histones.

15. In humans, the site of fertilization is the

    A. ovary.
    B. fallopian tube.
    C. uterus.
    D. cervix.
    E. vagina.

GO TO THE NEXT PAGE

16. Which of the following is found in eukaryotes but not prokaryotes?

    A. Ribosomal RNA
    B. Plasma membrane
    C. Nuclear membrane
    D. Ribosomes
    E. None of the above

17. A totipotent cell

    A. has 100% of its developmental potential.
    B. has limited developmental potential.
    C. has reached complete development.
    D. can develop into any organism.
    E. always forms a unicellular organism.

18. The hypothesis that chloroplasts and mitochondria were originally prokaryotic organisms living within eukaryotic hosts is supported by the fact that mitochondria and chloroplasts

    A. possess protein synthetic capability.
    B. possess genetic material.
    C. possess plasma membrane.
    D. possess characteristic ribosomes.
    E. All of the above

19. The site of storage and maturation of sperm is the

    A. seminiferous tubule.
    B. seminal vesicle.
    C. vas deferens.
    D. epididymis.
    E. prostate.

20. During the process of oxidative phosphorylation, oxygen serves as

    A. the initial acceptor of H electrons.
    B. the final acceptor of H electrons.
    C. a high-energy intermediate.
    D. a phosphorylating agent.
    E. a reducing agent.

21. From which germ layer do the kidneys form?

    A. Ectoderm
    B. Mesoderm
    C. Endoderm
    D. Ectoderm and mesoderm
    E. Mesoderm and endoderm

22. As a consequence of gastrulation, the embryo possesses

    A. an archenteron.
    B. a blastopore.
    C. a blastocoel.
    D. Two of the above
    E. All of the above

23. Neurulation is induced by cells of the

    A. archenteron.
    B. notochord.
    C. endodermal layer.
    D. neural ectoderm.
    E. neural crest.

GO TO THE NEXT PAGE

24. Which of the following statements regarding photosynthesis is NOT true?

    A. The light cycle occurs only during exposure to light.
    B. The dark cycle occurs only in the absence of light.
    C. During the light cycle, ATP is produced.
    D. During the dark cycle, sugars are produced.
    E. Red and blue light are optimal for photosynthetic function.

25. Which statement about the blastula stage of embryonic development is FALSE?

    A. It consists of a solid ball of cells.
    B. It contains a fluid-filled center called the blastocoel.
    C. It is the stage of development that precedes the gastrula.
    D. It is a more advanced stage than a morula.
    E. It is a less advanced stage than a neurula.

26. Which of the following foods contains the greatest amount of energy/gram?

    A. Sugar
    B. Starch
    C. Fat
    D. Protein
    E. Vitamins

27. The tRNA code for the amino acid valine is AAC. What is the mRNA code for valine?

    A. TTG
    B. GGU
    C. CCA
    D. CCG
    E. UUG

28. The source of oxygen given off in photosynthesis is

    A. water.
    B. carbon dioxide.
    C. glucose.
    D. starch.
    E. chlorophyll.

29. Laboratory mice are to be classified based on genes A, B, and C. How many genetically distinct offspring can be produced from a cross of an AaBbCc individual with an AaBBCc individual?

    A. 12
    B. 16
    C. 32
    D. 48
    E. 64

30. The BEST description of identical twins is

    A. twins of the same gender.
    B. twins from a single egg.
    C. twins from two eggs that have been fertilized by the same sperm.
    D. twins from two eggs fertilized by two separate sperm.
    E. twins from a single egg fertilized by two separate sperm.

31. The first major part of the photosynthetic process involves

    A. the conversion of water and carbon dioxide into starch and oxygen.
    B. the conversion of sugar into water and CO_2.
    C. the splitting of water into oxygen, hydrogen, and electrons.
    D. the changing of CO_2 into a bicarbonate ion.
    E. the splitting of CO_2 into carbon, oxygen, and an electron.

GO TO THE NEXT PAGE

32. The ABO human blood groups are inherited through a system of

    A. multiple alleles.

    B. dihybrid crosses.

    C. recessive alleles.

    D. independent assortments.

    E. spontaneous mutations.

33. Which of the following occurs in the cell nucleus?

    A. RNA synthesis

    B. Protein synthesis

    C. DNA synthesis

    D. A and C

    E. A, B, and C

34. The gene for red-green color blindness is recessive and located on the X chromosome. If a man suffering from red-green color blindness had children with an unaffected woman, how would their children be affected?

    A. 50% of the females would be carriers, 100% of the males would be affected.

    B. 100% of the females would be normal, 50% of the males would be affected.

    C. 100% of the females would be carriers, 100% of the males would be normal.

    D. 50% of the females would be affected, 100% of the males would be affected.

    E. 100% of the females would be normal, 50% of the males would be carriers.

35. A mutation in a gene in a somatic cell is deleterious because

    A. it will affect gamete formation.

    B. it will be dominant.

    C. it may be passed on to subsequent generations.

    D. it may lead to a tumor in that tissue.

    E. None of the above

36. A single nondisjunction may cause all of the following EXCEPT

    A. spontaneous miscarriage of the fetus.

    B. 47 chromosomes.

    C. 45 chromosomes.

    D. congenital diseases such as Down syndrome.

    E. breakage near the centromere.

37. Which of the following is FALSE regarding DNA replication?

    A. DNA replication is semiconservative.

    B. DNA replication occurs during prophase.

    C. Okasaki fragments are formed.

    D. Purines bind to pyrimidines.

    E. None of the above

38. Red is dominant over white in a certain flower. To test whether a red offspring is homozygous or heterozygous in this flower

    A. cross it with a red plant that had a white parent.

    B. cross it with a red plant that had two red parents.

    C. cross it with a white plant.

    D. Two of the above will work.

    E. None of the above will work.

39. Blood types A and B are dominant over type O. If a male with genotype AO marries a female with genotype AB, which of the following types is impossible for a first-generation child?

    A. Type B

    B. Type A

    C. Type O

    D. Type AB

    E. All blood types are possible.

GO TO THE NEXT PAGE

40. If one-twelfth of the males in a population are red-green color blind, what fraction of the females from that population are red-green color blind?

    A. $\frac{1}{6}$

    B. $\frac{1}{12}$

    C. $\frac{1}{48}$

    D. $\frac{1}{144}$

    E. No females will have color blindness because it is sex-linked.

41. A gaseous compound consists of element X (atomic weight = 12) and element Y (atomic weight = 1). Its empirical formula is XY_2, and its density is 1.25 g/L at STP. Its molecular formula is

    A. XY.

    B. XY_2.

    C. X_2Y_2.

    D. X_2Y_4.

    E. X_4Y_8.

42. How many grams of O_2 are necessary to oxidize 88 g of C_3H_8 to CO_2 and H_2O? (Atomic weights: C = 12, H = 1, O = 16)

    A. 32 g

    B. 64 g

    C. 120 g

    D. 160 g

    E. 320 g

43. What is the approximate mass of 1.204×10^{24} bromine atoms?

    A. 79.9 g

    B. 159.8 g

    C. 160.2 g

    D. 239.7 g

    E. 340.4 g

44. Element X has atomic number 16 and atomic weight 32. How many electrons are present in the ion X^{2-}?

    A. 2

    B. 14

    C. 16

    D. 18

    E. 32

45. Chlorophyll, the green pigment involved in photosynthesis, consists of 2.4312% Mg by mass. If you are given a 100-g sample of chlorophyll, how many Mg atoms will it contain?
    (Atomic weight of Mg: 24.312 g/mol)

    A. 6.02×10^{22}

    B. 6.02×10^{23}

    C. 6.02×10^{24}

    D. 6.02×10^{25}

    E. None of the above

46. If 88 g of C_3H_8 and 160 g of O_2 are allowed to react maximally to form CO_2 and H_2O, how many grams of CO_2 will be formed?
    (Atomic weights: C = 12, H = 1, O = 16)

    A. 33 g

    B. 66 g

    C. 132 g

    D. 264 g

    E. None of the above

47. The MOST important factor in determining the chemical properties of an element is

    A. the number of electrons in s orbitals.

    B. the number of protons.

    C. the number of valence electrons.

    D. the total number of electrons.

    E. the atomic mass.

GO TO THE NEXT PAGE

48. Which of the following is generally true of atomic radii?

   A. They increase from left to right across a period of the periodic table, and increase down a group.
   B. They decrease across a period from left to right and decrease down a group.
   C. They increase from left to right across a period and decrease down a group.
   D. They decrease from left to right across a period and increase down a group.
   E. Atomic radii do not vary in any regular pattern.

49. According to VSEPR theory, the molecular geometry of NF_3 is

   A. planar.
   B. tetrahedral.
   C. pyramidal.
   D. octahedral.
   E. linear.

50. Which of the following lists the atoms/ions in decreasing order by size?

   A. Te^{2-}, Cs^+, Xe, La^{3+}, I^-, Ba^{2+}
   B. Cs^+, Ba^{2+}, La^{3+}, Te^{2-}, I^-, Xe
   C. La^{3+}, Ba^{2+}, Cs^+, Xe, I^-, Te^{2-}
   D. Te^{2-}, I^-, Xe, Cs^+, Ba^{2+}, La^{3+}
   E. None of the above

51. If an electron on an atom has a principal quantum number of $n = 4$, what possible values of l can it have?

   A. 0
   B. 0, 1
   C. 0, 1, 2
   D. 0, 1, 2, 3
   E. 0, 1, 2, 3, 4

52. $Mg_3N_2 + 6H_2O \rightarrow 3Mg(OH)_2 + 2NH_3$

   How many moles of ammonia are liberated when 2 moles of Mg_3N_2 is reacted with 9 moles of H_2O?

   A. 1
   B. 2
   C. 3
   D. 4
   E. 5

53. Which of the following compounds is (are) held together by ionic bonds?

   $$NaH, MgH_2, NH_3$$

   A. NaH only
   B. MgH_2 only
   C. NaH and MgH_2
   D. All of the three
   E. None of the three

54. Calculate the heat released when 8.0 g of hydrogen react according to the following reaction:

   $$2H_2(g) + O_2(g) \rightarrow 2H_2O(g); \Delta H = -115.60 \text{ kcal}$$

   A. 57.80 kcal
   B. 115.60 kcal
   C. 173.4 kcal
   D. 231.2 kcal
   E. 462.4 kcal

55. The electron configuration $1s^2 2s^2 2p^6 3s^2 3p^6 3d^2$ represents

   A. an excited, neutral Ca atom.
   B. a ground state, neutral Ca atom.
   C. an excited, neutral Sc atom.
   D. an excited, neutral K atom.
   E. a ground state K^+ ion.

GO TO THE NEXT PAGE

56. If ΔH°_f of $CO_2(g)$ is –94.05 kcal/mol and ΔH°_f of $CO(g)$ is –26.41 kcal/mol, calculate ΔH for the following reaction:

$$CO(g) + \frac{1}{2}O_2(g) \rightarrow CO_2(g)$$

   A. –120.46 kcal
   B. –67.64 kcal
   C. 67.64 kcal
   D. 120.46 kcal
   E. None of the above

57. One mole of gas A exerts a pressure of 25 mmHg. How many molecules of gas B are required to exert a pressure of 125 mmHg in an identical container at the same temperature?

   A. 5.00
   B. 6.02×10^{23}
   C. 3.00×10^{23}
   D. 3.00×10^{24}
   E. Cannot be determined

58. If 0.15 mL of oxygen is obtained from analysis of a 1.0 mL sample of whole blood at STP, how many millimoles of oxygen would be obtained from 100.0 mL of the same blood at STP?

   A. $\dfrac{0.015}{22.4}$
   B. $\dfrac{15}{16}$
   C. $\dfrac{1.5}{32}$
   D. $\dfrac{15}{22.4}$
   E. $\dfrac{0.15}{32}$

59. The equilibrium

   $$4HI(g) + O_2(g) \leftrightarrow 2H_2O(g) + 2I_2(g) + \text{heat}$$

   has reached equilibrium at 350°C and 1.0 atm. To increase the yield of I_2, one could

   A. raise the temperature to 500°C.
   B. introduce a catalyst.
   C. add more oxygen.
   D. introduce H_2O into the reaction vessel.
   E. decrease the pressure.

60. Which of the following atoms has the largest electron affinity?

   A. He
   B. Li
   C. Na
   D. Br
   E. Cl

61. In an exothermic reaction, it is always TRUE that

   A. ΔG is positive.
   B. ΔH is positive.
   C. ΔH is negative.
   D. ΔG is negative.
   E. ΔS is positive.

62. When the following equation is balanced, what is the difference between the sum of the coefficients of the products and the sum of the coefficients of the reactants?

   $$KMnO_4 + NH_3 \rightarrow KNO_3 + MnO_2 + KOH + H_2O$$

   A. 3
   B. 4
   C. 5
   D. 6
   E. 7

GO TO THE NEXT PAGE

63. What could be the empirical formula of a compound that contains 6 g of C for each gram of H?
(Atomic weights: C = 12.011, H = 1.008)

   A. CH_3OH

   B. CH_4

   C. C_2H_4

   D. $C_6H_{12}O_6$

   E. CH_2O

64. ΔH°_f of $H_2O(g)$ is –57.798 kcal/mol, and ΔH°_f of $WO_3(s)$ is –200.84 kcal/mol. Calculate ΔH for the reaction

$$3H_2(g) + WO_3(s) \rightarrow W(s) + 3H_2O(g)$$

   A. –258.638 kcal

   B. –143.042 kcal

   C.   27.45 kcal

   D. 143.042 kcal

   E. 258.638 kcal

65. If an electron has a secondary quantum number of $l = 3$, what possible values of m_l can it have?

   A. –3, –2, –1, 0, 1, 2, 3

   B. 1, 2, 3, 4

   C. 0, 1, 2

   D. $-\frac{1}{2}, +\frac{1}{2}$

   E. None of the above

66. Which of the following ions has the smallest ionic radius?

$$Mg^{2+}, Ca^{2+}, Sr^{2+}, Be^{2+}$$

   A. Mg^{2+}

   B. Ca^{2+}

   C. Sr^{2+}

   D. Be^{2+}

   E. They all have the same ionic radius.

67. Which of the following will change the numerical value of an equilibrium constant?

   A. An increase in pressure

   B. A decrease in temperature

   C. An increase in the concentration of a reactant

   D. Addition of a catalyst

   E. An increase in the volume of the reaction vessel

68. If the temperature of an endothermic reaction is increased by 10°C, as a rule of thumb, which of the following is approximately doubled?

   A. Rate of reaction

   B. Velocity of molecules

   C. Concentration

   D. Pressure (of gases)

   E. Heat evolved

69. Approximately how many molecules are contained in 16.2 g of quinine, $C_{20}H_{24}N_2O_2$? (Atomic weights: C = 12.011, H = 1, N = 14.0, O = 15.999)

   A. 2.5×10^{21} molecules

   B. 3.0×10^{21} molecules

   C. 2.5×10^{22} molecules

   D. 3.0×10^{22} molecules

   E. 3.0×10^{23} molecules

70. Arrange the following elements in order of increasing metallic character.

$$Ge, Sn, Pb, Si$$

   A. Pb, Sn, Ge, Si

   B. Ge, Sn, Pb, Si

   C. Si, Ge, Sn, Pb

   D. Si, Sn, Ge, Pb

   E. All four are equally metallic.

GO TO THE NEXT PAGE

71. Acetylene is completely saturated through hydrogenation. The carbon-carbon bond distance in acetylene is 1.20 Å. After saturation, the carbon-carbon bond distance is

    A. 1.07 Å.
    B. 0.60 Å.
    C. 0.40 Å.
    D. 1.20 Å.
    E. 1.54 Å.

72. Which molecule is most likely to react via an S_N1 mechanism?

    A. $CH_3CH_2CH_2Br$
    B. $CH_3CH_2CHBrCH_3$
    C. $CH_3CH_2CBr(CH_3)_2$
    D.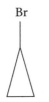
    E.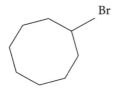

73. The isomerization of 2-butane from configuration A to configuration B requires

    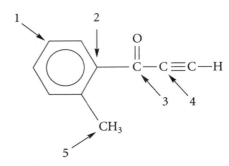

    A   B

    A. the breakage of one σ bond.
    B. the breakage of both a σ and a π bond.
    C. the breakage of one π bond and rotation about the σ bond.
    D. the breakage of one σ bond and rotation about the π bond.
    E. no breakage of bonds but simple rotation about the carbon-carbon bond.

74. Which of the following carbon atoms is *sp* hybridized?

    A. 1
    B. 2
    C. 3
    D. 4
    E. 5

GO TO THE NEXT PAGE

75. Which of the following structures has the largest number of stereoisomers?

(A)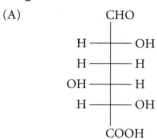

(B)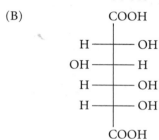

(C)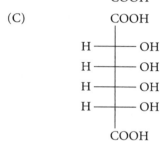

(D)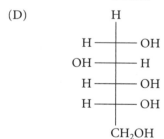

(E)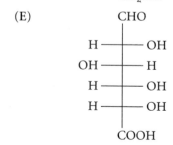

76. Which of the following is methyl acetate?

A. CH_3COOH

B. $CH_3COO^-Na^+$

C. CH_3OCH_3

D. $CH_3COOCH_2CH_3$

E. CH_3COOCH_3

77. Which of the following condition(s) favor(s) S_N2 reactions over S_N1 reactions?

A. Nonpolar solvent

B. Low temperature

C. Weak nucleophile

D. High concentration of nucleophile

E. All of the above

78. When an atom goes from its ground state to an excited state

A. the number of core electrons must decrease.

B. the number of valence electrons must decrease.

C. the total energy of the electrons must increase.

D. the total energy of the electrons must decrease.

E. the nucleus must always obtain a greater positive charge.

79. Dimethylpropylamine (*N,N*-dimethyl-1-propanamine) will be LEAST soluble in which of the following?

A. Dilute KOH(*aq*)

B. Dilute HCl(*aq*)

C. Dimethyl ether

D. Benzene

E. Concentrated H_2SO_4

GO TO THE NEXT PAGE

80. Benzene and cyclohexane are similar in which of the following ways?

    A. Both contain six carbon atoms.
    B. Both exist primarily in the chair conformation.
    C. Both are equally stable.
    D. A and C
    E. A, B, and C

81. The IUPAC name of the following structure is

$$CH_3 - \overset{\overset{\displaystyle CH_3}{|}}{\underset{\underset{\displaystyle CH_3}{|}}{C}} - CH_3$$

    A. *sec*-butyl methane.
    B. *tert*-butyl methane.
    C. 1,1-dimethyl isopropane.
    D. 2,2-dimethyl propane.
    E. None of the above

82. Which of the following Fischer projections are enantiomers of each other?

    I: Br—C(CH₃)(H)—Cl
    II: Cl—C(H)(CH₃)—Br
    III: Cl—C(CH₃)(H)—Br

    A. I and II only
    B. I and III only
    C. II and III only
    D. All are enantiomeric to each other.
    E. I and III and II and III are enantiomers, but I and II are not.

83. Which of the following is TRUE of benzene?

    A. Each pair of consecutive carbon atoms is connected only by a single bond.
    B. Each pair of consecutive carbon atoms is connected only by a double bond.
    C. All of the carbon-carbon bonds in benzene are the same length.
    D. Benzene exists as an equilibrium mixture of two energetically equivalent structures.
    E. Two of the above

84. What is wrong with the following Lewis structure?

    A. The carbon atom double bonded to oxygen should have a formal positive charge.
    B. The oxygen atom should have a formal positive charge.
    C. Six-membered rings containing carbon-oxygen double bonds never exist.
    D. Both B and C are correct.
    E. This structure is perfectly acceptable as shown.

GO TO THE NEXT PAGE

85. The name of the following alkane is

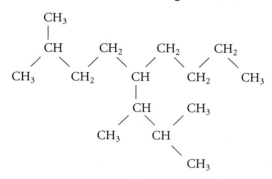

A. 5-(1,2-dimethylpropyl)-8-methylnonane.
B. 4-(3-methylbutyl)-2,3-methyloctane.
C. 5-(1,2-dimethylpropyl)-2-methylnonane.
D. 5-(1,2-dimethylpropyl)-2-methyldecane.
E. None of the above

86. Which of the following is/are aromatic?

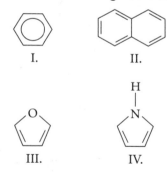

A. I only
B. I and II only
C. II and IV only
D. I, II, and IV only
E. All of the above

87. Arrange the following molecules in order of increasing boiling point.

   I. $CH_3(CH_2)_4CO_2H$
   II. $CH_3(CH_2)_5CH_3$
   III. $CH_3(CH_2)_5CO_2H$
   IV. $CH_3(CH_2)_4CH_2OH$
   V. $CH_3(CH_2)_4CH_2Br$

A. II, V, IV, I, III
B. II, V, IV, III, I
C. II, IV, V, III, I
D. V, II, IV, I, III
E. III, I, IV, II, V

88. Which of the following compounds is an amide?

A. $CH_3(CH_2)_5OCH_2NH_2$
B. $CH_3CH_2NHCH_3$
C.

$$CH_3\overset{\overset{\displaystyle O}{\|}}{C}-CH_2-N\begin{smallmatrix}CH_3\\ \\CH_3\end{smallmatrix}$$

D.

E. Two of the above

GO TO THE NEXT PAGE

89. How many different stereoisomers of the following molecule exist?

$$CH_3 - CH - CH - CH_3$$
$$\qquad\quad | \qquad |$$
$$\qquad\quad Cl \qquad I$$

   A. 1
   B. 2
   C. 4
   D. 8
   E. 16

90. The diagram below indicates a pair of *p* orbitals. What kind of bond is formed by overlapping *p* orbitals within a molecule?

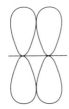

   A. σ bonds found in single bonds
   B. σ bonds found in single, double, and triple bonds
   C. π bonds found in triple but not in double bonds
   D. π bonds found in double but not in triple bonds
   E. π bonds found in double and triple bonds

91. The following compound is called

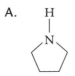

   A. neopentyl chloride.
   B. 1-chloro-2,2-dimethylpropane.
   C. 3-chloro-2,2-dimethylpropane.
   D. Two of the above
   E. All of the above

92. Which of the following is a secondary amine?

   A.

   B. $(CH_3)_3N$
   C. $(CH_3)_3CNH_2$
   D. $[(CH_3)_3CCH_2]_4N^+$
   E. NH_3

93. Rank the following alkenes in order of increasing stability:

   I. $CH_3CH = CHCH_3$
   II. $(CH_3)_2C = CHCH_3$
   III. $CH_2 = CH_2$
   IV. $(CH_3)_2C = C(CH_3)_2$
   V. $CH_3CH = CH_2$

   A. IV, II, I, V, III
   B. III, V, I, II, IV
   C. V, III, I, II, IV
   D. III, V, I, IV, II
   E. II, IV, I, V, III

GO TO THE NEXT PAGE

94. C_nH_{2n+2} + excess $O_2 \rightarrow$ products

    The above reaction

    A. is endothermic.
    B. is the oxidation of an alkene.
    C. yields CO_2 and H_2O as products.
    D. yields a mixture of alcohols as products.
    E. yields an alkene and H_2O as products.

95. Which of the following is NOT true of acetylene?

    A. It does not have a permanent dipole moment.
    B. The carbon atoms are sp^2 hybridized.
    C. Its formula is C_2H_2.
    D. It has two π bonds.
    E. It is a linear molecule.

96. Resonance structures do NOT contribute to the stability of which of the following?

    A. Benzene
    B.

    $\langle \text{O} \rangle$

    C. $CH_3 - C = O$
           $|$
           $O^{\ominus}$

    D. NH_2

    E. $CH_2 = C - CH_2^{\oplus}$

97. Which is the MOST stable carbocation?

    (A) $CH_3 - CH = CH - \overset{\oplus}{C}H_2$

    (B) $CH_3 - CH = CH - CH_2 - \overset{\oplus}{C}H_2$

    (C) $\langle \bigcirc \rangle - CH = CH - CH_2 - \overset{\oplus}{C}H_2$

    (D) $\langle \bigcirc \rangle - CH_2 - \overset{\oplus}{C}H_2$

    (E) $CH_2 = \overset{\oplus}{C}H$

98. Among molecules of similar formula weight, which of the following compound classes will exhibit the highest boiling point?

    A. Alcohol
    B. Ether
    C. Ketone
    D. Cyclic ether
    E. Alkane

GO TO THE NEXT PAGE

99. Which is the MOST stable isomer of di-bromo-di-phenyl ethene?

   A.

   B.

   C.

   D. Choices A and C
   E. Choices B and C

100. $C_2H_5ONa + CH_3I \rightarrow$ products

   The products of this synthesis are

   A. ethyl methyl ether and sodium iodide.
   B. ethyl iodide and sodium methoxide.
   C. propane, sodium iodide, and nascent oxygen.
   D. propyl alkoxide and sodium iodide.
   E. No reaction occurs.

STOP. IF YOU FINISH BEFORE TIME IS CALLED, YOU MAY CHECK YOUR WORK ON THIS SECTION ONLY. DO NOT TURN TO ANY OTHER SECTION IN THE TEST.

Reading Comprehension

40 questions—50 minutes

Directions: The following test consists of several reading passages and questions that test your comprehension of the passages. Choose the best answer for each question from the five choices provided.

Therapy for speech disorders is the joint concern of orthodontists and speech therapists. However, these two groups of specialists should by no means be thought of as working in an identical manner on identical problems. The contrast between the aims of speech therapy and orthodontics is analogous to the difference between treatment of functional and structural disorders.

The speech pathologist is concerned with a patient's functional disorders, employing therapy aimed simply at correcting the speech difficulty. Cases involving children with problems in sibilant articulation are generally important to the speech therapist, because of the fact that s sounds: 1) belong to the most difficult speech groups with regard to articulation, 2) generally appear last in the course of language development, and 3) are most easily disturbed by behavioral and/or pathological factors. Therefore, an examination of the methods employed by speech therapists for treating children with open bite or lisps is instructive.

A cardinal rule of speech therapy is that the patient must learn an entirely new sound to compensate for the one he or she is incapable of articulating. The therapist does not attempt to "improve" the faulty sound or require the child to imitate correct articulation. Either "passive" or "active" methods are used by therapists for correcting the sibilant problem.

Passive methods have as their purpose the direction of the child's articulatory organs into the proper position for making a correct sound. This is accomplished through the use of objects such as mirrors, probes, plates, or tubes, all of which enable the therapist to show the child what he or she is doing, and, where necessary, to manipulate the articulatory organs themselves. For example, illustration of correct tongue position is as follows: the therapist shows the child how to approximate the position of the front teeth, to touch or steady the tongue tip lightly against the lower front teeth, and then blow against the biting edge of the four inner incisor teeth.

Active methods of speech therapy are deductive in nature, beginning with sounds the child can already make and working toward the sound which is to be learned. In the case of sibilants, it is frequently observed that while one or more sounds are affected by lisping, many others in the sibilant series can be properly articulated by the child. In these cases, it is best to develop the desired new sound from the one which is already present. For example: children who are unable to pronounce the s may be able to articulate the Greek θ or th sound. The th corresponds to interdental protrusion of the tongue and is a rather common form of lisping. The therapist induces the child to pull the tongue tip back slightly while articulating a prolonged th. A correct s will occur spontaneously as soon as the tongue tip disappears behind the teeth. The most important action to avoid here is demonstration by the therapist of perfect pronunciation. Such demonstrations are generally of no use to the patient and may only create tension and nervousness, thus hindering progress.

As a form of preventive dentistry, orthodontics is usually concerned with the correction of dental anomalies for the purpose of heading off future difficulties. With regard to speech disorders, it has been demonstrated that misaligned teeth and tooth loss can cause or contribute to defects

GO TO THE NEXT PAGE

in articulation. Therefore, orthodontists are frequently called on to assist in the correction of speech disorders through the realignment or other adjustment of the patient's teeth.

In dealing with malocclusion—a faulty meshing of teeth in the upper and lower jaws when biting—the orthodontist generally places the child into one of three basic categories. The first, class I, includes patients who have irregularities in the front teeth, despite fairly normal relationships between the jaws and proper meshing of the back teeth (though other teeth may also be irregular). This condition can be treated with fixed or removable appliances that help turn or straighten irregular teeth. Fixed appliances work all the time, delivering even and consistent forces to the teeth. Removable appliances may be taken off on occasion, although neglect can bring progress to a halt.

Class II malocclusion involves an underdevelopment of the lower jaw, with upper molars falling in front of the lower ones. Frequently, this is accompanied by protrusion of the upper front teeth, a condition commonly referred to as "buck teeth." An appliance such as an elastic band and night brace may be worn for at least 13 hours each day and serves to push the molars back. If the other teeth do not then follow, they are moved individually into the proper alignment.

Class III children have prominent lower jaws and protruding lower front teeth. They are treated in much the same way as those in class II, through the use of the elastic band and night brace. The child's profile remains the same, with jaw structure correctable only through surgery.

Clearly, the speech pathologist and the orthodontist deal with the problems of improper speech in different contexts, one functional and the other structural. In many cases, the two are permitted to work together, as in the elimination of lisping by removing speech patterns with simultaneous speech correction. However, it has been shown that the problems of sibilant articulations, as well as other speech difficulties, can be treated with considerable success by speech therapy alone.

Also, there is abundant evidence that the correction by the orthodontist of dental anomalies such as malocclusion or missing teeth will spontaneously result in formal speech patterns. The conclusion drawn by many parents is that one or another of these types of therapy should suffice or that their effects are interchangeable.

This is a very dangerous assumption to make, however. It has often been the case that a child is taken to a speech pathologist for therapy when very young and achieves some success in overcoming his or her speech disorder. Then, he or she is taken to an orthodontist, who subjects the child to treatments for the correction of structural problems. The result is that the child must return to the speech therapist to begin a new sequence of treatment in order to acquire normal abilities in articulation.

The reason for this is simple. The speech therapist works with the child's existing articulatory organs and, with the help of artificial devices, helps the child to pronounce a particular sound in a particular way. By altering the structural context through orthodontics, the orthodontist has made the child's acquired techniques less effective, and a return to the therapist is necessary. This frequently results in emotional trauma for the child and, in most cases, inflicts a senseless and unnecessary burden.

The recommended attitude is one of isolating the very different approaches to speech improvement practiced by the speech therapist and the orthodontist. Our example of sibilant articulation in children leads to the conclusion that both specialists are able to employ methods and achieve significant results. If they worked together, the results would most probably be faster and more positive. Once the orthodontist has completed the correction of any dental problems, the speech therapist can reeducate the child's tongue and lips to function within the new structural context, thus assisting in maintaining the orthodontic results.

GO TO THE NEXT PAGE

1. According to the passage, the major difference between orthodontics and speech therapy is that orthodontics

   A. corrects structural anomalies rather than functional disorders.

   B. requires much more rigorous medical training than speech pathology.

   C. is contraindicated in cases of lisping.

   D. works best on adolescents, while speech therapy can begin much earlier.

   E. corrects functional disorders rather than structural anomalies.

2. A distinguishing feature of passive methods of speech therapy is that they

   A. begin with sounds the child can already articulate and develop gradually toward the correct sound.

   B. attempt to induce the child's speech organs to form the proper position for correct articulation.

   C. involve less personal contact between therapist and child than do active methods.

   D. tend to be effective even in cases of severe malocclusion.

   E. involve little manipulation of the articulatory organs.

3. Many of the children treated by speech therapists

   A. never achieve their desired results.

   B. are better served by orthodontic intervention.

   C. do not receive sufficient emotional support from their parents.

   D. must also contend with learning disabilities.

   E. do not require surgery.

4. Speech therapists in general believe that it is necessary to

   A. instruct the child by setting a correct example.

   B. treat children before any orthodontic treatment is attempted.

   C. employ active methods whenever possible.

   D. teach the child an entirely new sound.

   E. use passive methods over active methods.

GO TO THE NEXT PAGE

5. The essential characteristic of active methods of speech therapy is that they

   A. retrain the child's articulatory organs following orthodontic treatment.

   B. use related sounds that the child can already correctly articulate.

   C. avoid using mirrors or other external objects to cure speech disorders.

   D. eliminate the need for passive therapeutic methods.

   E. work with the physical manipulation of the mouth.

6. Problems with the articulation of sibilants

   A. can easily be corrected through speech therapy.

   B. are difficult to eliminate without surgery.

   C. are usually structural or anatomical in origin.

   D. often appear late in the child's language development.

   E. originate from early Greek alphabets.

7. One error speech therapists must avoid is

   A. treating children who have class III malocclusions.

   B. demonstrating to the child correct articulation.

   C. associating articulative mechanisms with particular sounds.

   D. attempting to correct lisps without the help of an orthodontist.

   E. teaching the child new sounds.

8. The author probably believes that, as a general rule, children with speech disorders

   A. benefit from speech therapy only if orthodontic work is not required.

   B. should never receive orthodontic treatment after completing speech therapy.

   C. could benefit from recent advances in dental surgery.

   D. respond best to a coordinated effort of speech therapist and orthodontist.

   E. should avoid any professional intervention.

GO TO THE NEXT PAGE

9. The night brace is used for treating

   A. open bite.

   B. tongue protrusion.

   C. problems in sibilant articulation.

   D. class I malocclusion.

   E. class II malocclusion.

10. According to the passage, orthodontics is considered a form of

    A. functional therapy.

    B. speech pathology.

    C. preventive dentistry.

    D. sibilant modification.

    E. active therapy.

11. Active methods of speech therapy are especially effective in cases of lisping where the child

    A. has already completed orthodontic treatment.

    B. has not yet begun orthodontic treatment.

    C. is able to articulate some sibilants correctly.

    D. is not suffering from severe malocclusion.

    E. suffers from class III malocclusion.

12. The passage indicates that a speech therapist employing passive methods might have the child begin by

    A. listening to recordings of the sound, articulated first incorrectly and then correctly.

    B. doing exercises to increase tongue flexibility.

    C. learning proper alignment of the front teeth.

    D. recognizing that changing one's speech habits is an emotional process as well as a physical one.

    E. wearing a night brace.

13. Patients receiving removable orthodontic appliances

    A. sometimes experience irritation of the gums.

    B. rarely correct their problems with the positioning of their teeth.

    C. are considered too young for fixed appliances.

    D. suffer from the condition commonly known as "buck teeth."

    E. may fail to make progress if they neglect to wear them.

GO TO THE NEXT PAGE

The population of the United States is growing older and will continue to do so until well into the next century. As the 1900s began, the median age of the U.S. population had risen from around 28, in the 1950s, to 33. It will be 36 by the beginning of the 21st century and 42 by the year 2050. The elderly—those people 65 and older—now outnumber teenagers for the first time in American history; the population of elders has doubled in just forty years. The U.S. Census Bureau projects that 39 million Americans will be 65 or older by the year 2010, 51 million by 2020, and 65 million by 2030. This demographic trend is due mainly to two factors: increased life expectancy and the occurrence of a "baby boom" in the generation born immediately after World War II.

To begin with, more people than ever before are surviving into old age. In 1900, the average life expectancy for a U.S. citizen was 47.3 years; only about one out of every ten Americans lived to the age of 65. Today, eight out of ten will see their 65th birthday, and the average life expectancy has increased to approximately 75 years. People are living well beyond the average life expectancy in greater numbers than ever before, too. In fact, the number of U.S. citizens 85 years old and older is growing six times as fast as the rest of the population.

Numerous subsidiary factors contribute to Americans' increased life expectancy, including improved methods of food production and public sanitation, the ever growing popularity of physical fitness, and federal and state aid for the poor and the elderly. Another important factor, of course, has been the explosive advancement of medicine in this century, which has helped sustain lives of all ages. Better prenatal and neonatal care, for example, have helped reduce infant mortality. Vaccines, new drugs and surgical techniques, and other technological innovations have vastly increased physicians' ability not only to save lives but also to extend them.

The "graying" of the United States is also due in large measure to the aging of the generation born after World War II, the "baby boomers." With the advent of peace, in an economic climate of unparalleled prosperity, the birth rate of post–World War II America increased dramatically. The baby boom peaked in 1957 with over 4.3 million births that year. More than 75 million Americans were born between 1946 and 1964, the largest generation in U.S. history. Today, millions of "boomers" are already moving into middle age; in less than two decades, they will join the ranks of America's elderly. Those ranks, it must be noted, will be predominantly female. In the United States, as in the rest of the world, the gender ratio at birth is 105 males for every 100 females. By the age of 65, however, there are only 81 men left for every 100 women, and at age 85 and above, only 41 men for every 100 women.

What will be the social, economic, and political consequences of the aging of America? One likely development will involve a gradual restructuring of the family unit, moving away from the traditional nuclear family and toward an extended, multi-generational family dominated by elders, not by their adult children. This restructuring has already begun to occur. With one out of every two U.S. marriages currently ending in divorce, a significant number of today's grandparents are suddenly faced with the task of raising or helping to raise their grandchildren, even as they continue to provide financial assistance to their adult children. Indeed, far from being a financial burden to their children, today's elders often find themselves acting as family bankers. Roughly 75 percent of today's elders already own their own homes, something their offspring are finding increasingly difficult to accomplish without parental assistance.

The aging of the U.S. population is also likely to have far-reaching effects on the nation's workforce. In 1989, there were approximately 3.5 workers for every person 65 and older; by the year 2030, there'll only be 2 workers for every person 65 and

GO TO THE NEXT PAGE

older. As the number of available younger workers shrinks, elderly people will become more attractive as prospective employees. Many will simply retain their existing jobs beyond the now-mandatory retirement age of 65. In fact, the phenomenon of early retirement, which has transformed the U.S. workforce over the past four decades, will probably become a thing of the past. In 1950, about 50 percent of all 65-year-old men still worked; today, only 15 percent of them do. The median retirement age is currently 61. Yet recent surveys show that almost half of today's retirees would prefer to be working, and in decades to come, their counterparts will be doing just that.

The housing needs of an aging population will generate further social and economic changes. Over the past 30 years, hundreds of thousands of senior citizens migrated south to Sunbelt states such as Arizona, California, and Florida, where they pioneered retirement communities and other congregate living arrangements that foreshadow some of the possible housing options for future retirees. But many demographic experts and social scientists predict that this southward migration will diminish in the future, since surveys have found that the great majority of people age 55 and older would prefer not to relocate. Tomorrow's elders may well decide to adapt the Sunbelt's retirement village format to the areas in which they have lived for the majority of their adult lives.

Finally, the great proportional increase in older Americans will have significant effects on the nation's economy in the areas of Social Security and health care. A recent government survey showed that 77 percent of elderly Americans have annual incomes of less than $20,000; only 3 percent earn more than $50,000. As their earning power declines and their need for health care increases, most elderly Americans come to depend heavily on federal and state subsidies. With the advent of Social Security in 1935 and Medicaid/Medicare in 1965, the size of those subsidies has grown steadily until by 1990,

spending on the elderly accounted for 30 percent of the annual federal budget.

Considering these figures, and the fact that the elderly population will double within the next forty years, it's clear that major government policy decisions lie ahead. In the first 50 years of its existence, for example, the Social Security fund has received $55 billion more in employee/employer contributions than it has paid out in benefits to the elderly. Yet time and again, the federal government has "borrowed" from this surplus—without repaying it—in order to pay interest on the national debt.

Similarly, the Medicaid/Medicare system is threatened by the continuous upward spiral of medical costs. The cost of caring for disabled elderly Americans is expected to double in the next decade alone. Millions of Americans of all ages are currently unable to afford private health insurance. In fact, the United States is practically unique among developed nations in lacking a national health care system. Its advocates say such a system would be far less expensive than the present state of affairs, but the medical establishment and various special interest groups have so far blocked legislation aimed at creating it. Nonetheless, within the next few decades, an aging U.S. population may well demand that such a program be implemented.

GO TO THE NEXT PAGE

14. According to the passage, the segment of the U.S. population currently aged 85 years and older

    A. is predominantly male.
    B. is located primarily in the Sunbelt states.
    C. is growing six times faster than the rest of the population.
    D. is largely responsible for the high cost of medical care.
    E. on average has an annual income between $20,000 and $50,000.

15. The passage states that by the year 2030, there will be

    A. no money left in the Social Security fund.
    B. only 81 men for every 100 women in the United States.
    C. 51 million elderly Americans.
    D. only two workers for every American over the age of 65.
    E. a new U.S. health care system.

16. Which of the following statements about the U.S. elderly population is TRUE?

    A. It is largely responsible for the nation's current housing shortage.
    B. It is expected to double within the next 40 years.
    C. It is the wealthiest segment of the U.S. population.
    D. It represents almost 30 percent of the U.S. population.
    E. It constitutes the population majority in the Sunbelt states.

17. According to the passage, the "baby boom" generation

    A. has the highest life expectancy of any generation in U.S. history.
    B. has a median age of 33.
    C. includes approximately 75 million people born between 1946 and 1964.
    D. perceives its aging parents as a financial burden.
    E. is starting to enter the ranks of America's elderly.

GO TO THE NEXT PAGE

18. According to demographic experts, the southward migration of retirees in the past three decades is

    A. one cause of their relatively low incomes.

    B. responsible for the shrinking of the U.S. workforce.

    C. due to the availability of low-cost housing in the Sunbelt states.

    D. attributed to overcrowded conditions in the north.

    E. expected to diminish in the future.

19. According to the passage, the current divorce rate is

    A. approximately 50 percent.

    B. rising rapidly.

    C. less than 40 percent.

    D. slowly declining.

    E. not affecting family structure.

20. The author states that over the next few decades, increasing numbers of "baby boomers" will

    A. migrate west in search of employment.

    B. benefit from early retirement opportunities.

    C. join the elderly segment of the U.S. population.

    D. fail to qualify for health insurance.

    E. experience an increased birthrate.

21. All of the following are mentioned as having contributed to increased life expectancy EXCEPT

    A. the availability of better medical care.

    B. increased subsidies for the elderly.

    C. improved sanitation techniques.

    D. a decline in the birth rate.

    E. the growing popularity of physical fitness.

22. According to the passage, the majority of elderly people in the United States

    A. currently earn less than $20,000 per year.

    B. will suffer some sort of disability between the ages of 65 and 75.

    C. have been unable to purchase their own homes.

    D. continue to work at least 20 hours per week.

    E. do not depend on subsidies.

GO TO THE NEXT PAGE

23. The fact that health care costs for disabled elderly Americans are expected to double in the next ten years suggests that

    A. the federal government will be unable to finance a national health care system.

    B. the Medicaid/Medicare system will probably become even more expensive in the future.

    C. money will have to be borrowed from the Social Security fund in order to finance the Medicaid/Medicare system.

    D. "baby boomers" will be unable to receive federal health benefits as they grow older.

    E. the elderly received poor preventive care in the past.

24. Which of the following correctly describes the policy of early retirement?

    A. It will transform the U.S. workforce over the next several decades.

    B. It is a relatively recent phenomenon in U.S. history.

    C. It is thought to have been a major cause in the decline of the U.S. economy.

    D. It will become more popular in the 21st century.

    E. It restructured the U.S. workforce prior to World War II.

25. According to the U.S. Census Bureau, today's elderly population is

    A. larger than the current population of teenagers.

    B. larger than the current population of "boomers."

    C. smaller than the number of elderly people in 1950.

    D. smaller than the number of elderly people in 1970.

    E. larger than the projected elderly population in 2030.

26. The author speculates that in future decades, the typical U.S. family will probably be

    A. divorce-free.

    B. subsidized by Social Security.

    C. multigenerational.

    D. wealthier than today's family.

    E. youth-oriented.

27. The author suggests that over the past three decades, many of today's elderly people

    A. supplemented their incomes by working past the age of retirement.

    B. lost their Social Security benefits.

    C. suffered a serious physical disability.

    D. relocated to a warmer climate.

    E. lost their homes.

GO TO THE NEXT PAGE

28. According to the author, the federal government has not yet instituted a program mandating health care for all U.S. citizens because

    A. the federal deficit must first be eliminated.
    B. such a program would be too expensive.
    C. legislative lobbies have prevented it.
    D. Medicaid and Medicare have made it unnecessary.
    E. most U.S. citizens have private insurance.

Radioisotopes have been in use in scientific research for the last 50 years. Understanding radioisotopes first requires a grasp of basic atomic structure.

The atom is composed of two parts: a nucleus, consisting of protons and neutrons, and a series of electron shells surrounding the nucleus. The mass of an atom is concentrated in the nucleus. *Mass number* refers to the mass of an atom and is defined as the number of protons plus the number of neutrons in the nucleus of that atom. Protons and neutrons have approximately the same mass. The *atomic number* of an atom is defined as the number of protons in the nucleus of that atom. In a neutral atom, the number of electrons in the shells surrounding the nucleus must be equal to the number of protons in the nucleus. Two atoms that have the same atomic number belong to the same *element*. Though they must have the same number of protons, atoms of the same element may contain different numbers of neutrons. Such atoms are called *isotopes*. In other words, isotopes of the same element have identical atomic numbers but different mass numbers. For example, oxygen-15 and oxygen-16 have mass numbers of 15 and 16, respectively; however, both have the same atomic number, 8.

Isotopes whose nuclear structures are unstable undergo radioactive decay. All elements with atomic numbers higher than 83 have only unstable isotopes. Nuclear decay manifests itself in the emission of one of three possible types of particle or ray: alpha, beta, or gamma. Alpha particles are helium nuclei containing 2 protons and 2 neutrons. Emission of such particles results in a decrease of mass number by 4 and a decrease of atomic number by 2. Beta particles are high-speed electrons, produced when neutrons are converted into protons. The result of this type of emission is an increase in the atomic number by 1 while the mass number remains the same. The third type of emission, the gamma ray, is a high-energy X-ray emitted by the nucleus.

GO TO THE NEXT PAGE

The rate at which nuclei in a given radioactive substance decay is directly proportional to the number of nuclei in that substance. The half-life of an isotope is the amount of time required for one-half of the nuclei in any given radioactive sample to disintegrate.

Radioisotopes can be produced in cyclotrons and fission nuclear reactors. Cyclotrons accelerate rather than produce electrons and protons, which are then used as "bullets" to bombard non-radioactive targets. Electron and proton bullets must have a very high speed in order to overcome the repulsive forces of the electrons and protons of the targets. Fission reactors produce neutron bullets. Since neutrons are uncharged particles, they are not repelled by any part of the target atom and are therefore able to penetrate an atom much more easily than either protons or electrons. The use of neutrons thus allows a much wider variety of radioactive particles to be produced than when protons or electrons are used.

Radioactive emissions can be detected through the use of photographic film. Photographic film will darken upon exposure to radiation, indicating both the distribution and the total number of radioactive particles emitted by the sample being studied while it was in contact with the film. In a study of the uptake of radioactive material by a thin leaf, a photographic plate is pressed firmly against the leaf and kept in a totally darkened place. The more intense the radiation and the longer the exposure to it, the more the film will darken. Another means of detecting radiation, one more sensitive than film, is to use a Geiger counter. A Geiger counter operates by means of two electrodes sealed within a tube containing argon gas. The electrodes are held at a potential difference slightly less than the potential difference necessary for a charged particle to cross the gap between them. High-energy radioactive particles ionize the argon gas, allowing charge to bridge the gap between the electrodes, thereby producing a clicking noise in the instrument.

Geiger counters are not capable of detecting neutrons. Since neutrons are not charged, they are incapable of ionizing the argon gas and therefore cannot cause a current between the electrodes. Geiger counters will only indicate the presence of a radioactive material when they are receiving significantly more radiation than that normally present in the atmosphere. This atmospheric baseline is about 20 counts per second. The minimum number of atoms (N) that must be present in a radioactive sample for a Geiger counter to detect radiation is given by the formula $N = RT/0.693$, where T is the half-life of the radioactive material in seconds and R is a constant. R depends on both the atmospheric baseline and on the geometries of the Geiger counter and the sample. For a standard Geiger counter and an ordinary lab sample, about 10 percent of the radiation registers in the Geiger counter's tube. Based on this percentage, R can be calculated to be approximately 30.

The use of radioisotopes in research is based upon the fact that radioisotopes have the same chemical properties as their nonradioactive counterparts. In biological systems, radioactive substances will localize themselves in the same area as nonradioactive isotopes of the same element. Radioisotopes are introduced into an organism by mixing them with large quantities of nonradioactive substances in the diet.

In choosing a radioactive tracer, the half-life of the substance must be considered. Isotopes with very short half-lives will disintegrate too quickly to be detected. In addition, the shorter the half-life, the higher the intensity of the radiation. Too much radiation can damage the tissue it comes in contact with. It is for these reasons that carbon-14, which has a half-life of 5,730 years, is used rather than carbon-11, which has a half-life of only 20 minutes. Isotopes with very long half-lives emit radiation at a rate too small to be detected.

GO TO THE NEXT PAGE

In the past, radioactive tracers have been used in experiments which disprove the notion that all ingested food is used as a supply of energy and then excreted from the body. Studies of the mouth utilizing radioactive phosphorus have shown that ions are constantly exchanged between the saliva and the teeth. Exchange is not limited to the outer surface of the teeth but includes the inner pulp. When the salivary glands are removed from an organism, the teeth are found to decay rapidly. In a similar experiment utilizing radioactive calcium, replacement of atoms in bone was shown to take place in the same manner. The only exception to this constant replacement of ions occurs in the case of the iron found in hemoglobin. In healthy organisms, ingested iron is not incorporated into the hemoglobin but rather stored in the form of a protein complex or excreted. These experiments, then, show that the body is in a state of dynamic equilibrium: atoms are constantly being replaced in the body.

Radioactive substances are also used in experiments involving blood. Blood with radioactivity of known intensity is injected into an organism, and after a suitable period of time, a sample of blood is taken and the radiation intensity is determined. This makes it possible to determine the amount of blood present in an organism.

29. What is the advantage of using carbon-14 rather than carbon-11 in a biological experiment?

    A. It is easier to convert carbon-14 to carbon-12 than carbon-11 to carbon-12 by alpha emission.
    B. It is easier to convert carbon-14 to carbon-12 than carbon-11 to carbon-12 by beta emission.
    C. The half-life of carbon-14 is too short.
    D. The half-life of carbon-11 is too long.
    E. The radiation emitted by carbon-11 is too intense.

30. The advantage of photographic film over the Geiger counter in determining radioactivity is that

    A. film can discriminate between types of radiation.
    B. film indicates the area where the radiation is absorbed.
    C. atmospheric radiation does not interfere in film absorption.
    D. the Geiger counter cannot determine the intensity of radiation.
    E. film requires the use of an isotope.

31. Phosphorus-32 emits a beta particle. It will become

    A. aluminum-28.
    B. phosphorus-32.
    C. sulfur-32.
    D. nickel-53.
    E. antimony-51.

32. Photographic film badges are worn by workers in plants where radiation is present. The degree to which the film darkens indicates the

    A. lowest level of radiation for the day.
    B. type of radioactive emission.
    C. normal atmospheric radiation.
    D. total radiation absorbed over the period of time for which the badge is worn.
    E. total level of gamete damage suffered by the worker.

GO TO THE NEXT PAGE

33. What is the reason that neutrons CANNOT be detected by a Geiger counter?

   A. Neutral particles cannot ionize argon gas and therefore cannot cause a current to flow.
   B. Neutrons are too heavy to move and cause a current between the electrodes.
   C. Neutrons disintegrate at a rate equal to atmospheric radiation, and this rate is too slow to be detected by a Geiger counter.
   D. Neutron emission is impossible.
   E. Neutrons have too weak a charge.

34. The difference among isotopes of one element is in

   A. the charge of the nucleus.
   B. the electron configuration.
   C. the number of neutrons.
   D. the number of electrons.
   E. the number of protons.

35. In what respect is a Geiger counter more useful than photographic film in detecting radiation?

   A. A Geiger counter can detect the presence of neutrons.
   B. A Geiger counter is more sensitive than photographic film.
   C. A Geiger counter can measure atmospheric radiation, whereas photographic film cannot.
   D. A Geiger counter is less portable.
   E. A Geiger counter is more efficient than photographic film.

36. What disadvantage is there in using isotopes with very long half-lives as tracers as opposed to isotopes with shorter half-lives?

   A. Such isotopes can only be used in the treatment of hyperthyroidism.
   B. Such isotopes are cancerous.
   C. Such isotopes would not be able to enter the organism's bloodstream.
   D. The rate of emission from such isotopes is too small to be measured.
   E. Such isotopes are difficult to isolate.

GO TO THE NEXT PAGE

37. Which of the following is an advantage nuclear reactors have over cyclotrons in producing radioisotopes?

    A. Neutrons are capable of producing a larger variety of radioactive substances.

    B. A proton or an electron can penetrate an atom more easily than can a neutron.

    C. A cyclotron cannot accelerate protons and electrons to high enough speeds to bombard atoms.

    D. Neutron bullets are repelled by target atoms.

    E. Nuclear reactors are more energy-efficient than cyclotrons.

38. What would be the BEST title for the first two paragraphs?

    A. The Detection of Radioactive Emissions

    B. A History of the Study of Atoms

    C. The Production of Radioisotopes

    D. Dangers of Radioactive Experimentation

    E. The Structure of the Atom

39. What characteristic of radioisotopes allows them to be used in biological experiments?

    A. They have no side effects.

    B. They have the same chemical properties as their nonradioactive counterparts.

    C. They are inert.

    D. They are not harmful to the organism.

    E. They have extremely long half-lives.

40. All of the following statements concerning radioactive experiments with blood are true EXCEPT

    A. the amount of blood in an organism can be detected.

    B. radioactive blood is injected into an organism.

    C. there needs to be a waiting period before measuring the results.

    D. blood does not need to be drawn to obtain results.

    E. to determine accurate data, radiation intensity must be measured.

STOP. IF YOU FINISH BEFORE TIME IS CALLED, YOU MAY CHECK YOUR WORK ON THIS SECTION ONLY. DO NOT TURN TO ANY OTHER SECTION IN THE TEST.

Physics

40 questions – 50 minutes

Directions: Choose the best answer for each question from the five choices provided.

The values for the physical constants below are to be used as needed:

Gravitational acceleration at the surface of the Earth: $g = 10 \text{ m/s}^2$

Speed of light in a vacuum: $c = 3 \times 10^8 \text{ m/s}$

Charge of an electron: $e = 2.0 \times 10^{-19}$ Coulomb

1. Which vector represents the force exerted on q^+ by Q^+ and Q^-, which are equidistant from q^+?

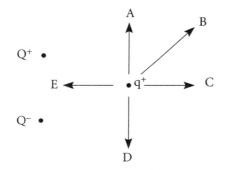

A. A
B. B
C. C
D. D
E. E

2. If light is shone on a mirror as shown below, at which surfaces will the light be reflected?

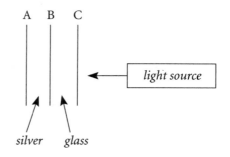

A. A
B. B
C. C
D. A and C
E. A, B, and C

GO TO THE NEXT PAGE

3. If 2 A pass through the 3-ohm resistor, what is the current passing through the 2-ohm resistor?

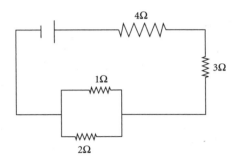

A. $\frac{3}{2}$A

B. 1 A

C. $\frac{4}{3}$A

D. $\frac{2}{3}$A

E. 2 A

4. How do the frequency and wavelength of light change when it passes from air to water?

A. The frequency decreases, and the wavelength remains the same.

B. The wavelength decreases, and the frequency remains the same.

C. Both the frequency and the wavelength decrease.

D. Both the wavelength and the frequency remain the same.

E. The wavelength increases, and the frequency decreases.

5. The operating temperature of a tungsten filament in an incandescent lamp is 2,450 K. If it were possible for this lamp to operate at a much higher temperature than 2,450 K, what would be the expected effect on the relative intensity values for the emitted electromagnetic wavelengths?

A. Shorter wavelengths would increase in relative intensity.

B. Longer wavelengths would increase in relative intensity.

C. Shorter wavelengths would decrease in relative intensity.

D. There would be no change in relative intensity.

E. Cannot be determined from the given information.

6. A stick of wood bobs up and down in the water as shown below. Which diagram represents the stick at minimum acceleration?

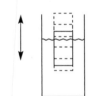

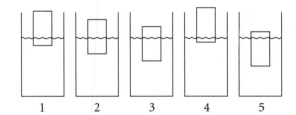

A. 1

B. 2

C. 3

D. 4

E. 5

GO TO THE NEXT PAGE

7. Light is traveling through a medium whose index of refraction is n_1 and is incident on a medium whose index of refraction is n_2. What must be the minimal angle of incidence such that total internal reflection is achieved?

A. $\sin^{-1}\left(\dfrac{n_2}{n_1}\right)$

B. $\tan^{-1}\left(\dfrac{n_1}{n_2}\right)$

C. $\sin^{-1}\left(\dfrac{n_1}{n_2}\right)$

D. $\sin\theta_2\left(\dfrac{n_2}{n_1}\right)$

E. None of the above

8. An element undergoes the following reaction:
$X + \alpha \rightarrow {}^1_0n + Y \rightarrow {}^{30}_{14}Si + \beta^+$ (α is an alpha particle and β^+ is a positron, i.e., e.)
What is the atomic number of X ?

A. 11

B. 12

C. 10

D. 14

E. 13

9. A bat locates insects through reflection of soundwaves (echo) off objects, a process known as echolocation. A sound is emitted ahead of the bat in the same direction as the bat travels. Assuming that the bat's velocity and the frequency of the emitted sonar are constant, what is the character of the frequency received by the bat? (Consider locating a stationary object.)

A. It is higher than that emitted by the bat.

B. It is lower than that emitted by the bat.

C. It is the same as that emitted by the bat.

D. It is out of the range of the bat's detection.

E. Its character cannot be determined from the above information.

10. A cubic block, with sides of length 5 cm, is floating partially submerged in water. The block is composed of an unknown substance. A second liquid of specific gravity 0.5, which is immiscible in water, is added to an additional depth of 6 cm. The block will

A. completely sink into the water.

B. remain partially submerged in water.

C. float upward but remain below the surface of the upper liquid.

D. float to the surface of the upper liquid.

E. Cannot be determined from the information given.

GO TO THE NEXT PAGE

11. Which of the following statements about steady fluid flow is TRUE in the pipe of constant cross section shown below?

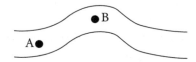

A. The pressure at A is greater than the pressure at B.

B. The pressure at B is greater than the pressure at A.

C. The volume flow per unit time at A is greater than the volume flow per unit time at B.

D. The volume flow per unit time at B is greater than the volume flow per unit time at A.

E. Two of the above

12. When a solid cube is submerged upright in a liquid, the liquid exerts a pressure on

A. the top of the cube.

B. the top and bottom of the cube.

C. the bottom of the cube.

D. the bottom and sides of the cube.

E. the top, bottom, and sides of the cube.

13. An electric heater is adding 1,000 BTU/hour of heat to the water in a perfectly insulated swimming pool. If there are 186,000 L of water in the pool, if the water is initially at 20°C, and if all of the added heat is used to warm the water, what will the water temperature be after 2 hours?
(1 BTU = 934 kcal)

A. 21°C

B. 25°C

C. 29°C

D. 30°C

E. 35°C

Questions 14 and 15 refer to the following:

There are two massless, open-topped circular tubes, each of which rests on a scale. (The scales are identical.) The tubes are filled to a height H with a liquid of density ρ. One tube has a radius D, whereas the other has a radius 4D.

14. The ratio of the pressure at the bottom of the narrow tube to the pressure at the bottom of the wide tube is

A. 1:1.

B. 1:4.

C. 4:1.

D. 1:16.

E. 16:1.

15. The ratio of the reading on the scale under the narrow tube to the reading on the scale under the wide tube is

A. 1:1.

B. 1:4.

C. 4:1.

D. 1:16.

E. 16:1.

GO TO THE NEXT PAGE

16. An electric dipole consists of two opposite charges of equal magnitude separated by a distance d. What is the direction of the electric field midway between the charges on a straight line joining the charges?

    A. The electric field is zero so it really has no direction.
    B. Toward the positive charge
    C. Toward the negative charge
    D. Perpendicular to the line joining the charges
    E. The direction of the field can't be determined without knowing the charge magnitudes.

17. A particle moves across the page from left to right in the presence of a uniform electric field directed toward the top of the page. Determine the type of charge and the direction of a uniform magnetic field that could result in zero net force on the particle.

    I. A positive charge and magnetic field directed out of the page
    II. A positive charge and magnetic field directed into the page
    III. An uncharged particle and magnetic field directed into the page

    A. I only
    B. II only
    C. III only
    D. I and III
    E. I and II

18. A 5-kg mass of water is cooled until it freezes at 0°C. What additional information is sufficient to determine the heat lost by this system?

    A. The specific heat of water
    B. The specific heat of water and the latent heat of fusion of water
    C. The initial temperature of the water and the specific heat of water
    D. The specific heat of water, the initial temperature of the water, and the latent heat of fusion of water
    E. The specific heat of ice, the initial temperature of the water, and the latent heat of fusion of water

19. A converging lens is used as the lens of a movie projector, forming a greatly magnified image on a large screen. Which of the following must be TRUE, assuming that the film acts as a real object?

    A. The image distance equals the object distance.
    B. The image is real and upright.
    C. The image is virtual and inverted.
    D. The image distance is greater than the object distance.
    E. The image is located at the focal point.

20. A real object is placed in front of a diverging mirror. Which of the following is always TRUE?

    A. The image distance is positive.
    B. The image distance is the same as the object distance.
    C. The image is upright.
    D. The image is inverted.
    E. The image is real.

GO TO THE NEXT PAGE

21. A microwave photon has a wavelength of 20 cm. A photon with a wavelength of 40 cm has

    A. the same energy.
    B. twice the energy.
    C. half the energy.
    D. one-quarter the energy.
    E. four times the energy.

22. A nucleus emits a gamma ray. Which of the following is TRUE?

    A. The nucleus gains energy.
    B. The nucleus loses energy.
    C. The atomic number decreases by one.
    D. The atomic number decreases by two.
    E. The number of electrons decreases by one.

23. A wave traveling along a string is described by the function $y = A\sin(kx - wt)$, where y is the displacement of the string from equilibrium and is measured in meters. What is the maximum displacement?

    A. 1 meter
    B. $\frac{\pi}{2}$ meters
    C. 2π meters
    D. A meters
    E. A^2 meters

24. A long, straight wire carries a current that is directed into the page. The magnetic field due to this current is

    A. directed into the page.
    B. directed out of the page.
    C. directed in a counterclockwise manner.
    D. directed in a clockwise manner.
    E. directed radially outward from the wire.

25. Two sound waves of amplitudes A_1 and A_2 meet at a point where they are 180° out of phase. Assume the wave with amplitude A_1 exhibits a crest and the wave with amplitude A_2 exhibits a valley at this point. The displacement of the resulting wave is

    A. 0.
    B. $A_1 - A_2$.
    C. $A_1 + A_2$.
    D. $A_2 - A_1$.
    E. $\frac{(A_1 + A_2)}{2}$.

26. A vessel used for deep-sea diving maintains an inside pressure equal to atmospheric pressure P_0. What maximum pressure must the hull be capable of withstanding at a depth of 1,000 m? Assume the density of seawater is ρ_s.

    A. P_0
    B. $P_0 + 1{,}000\rho_s g$
    C. $2P_0 + 1{,}000\rho_s g$
    D. $1{,}000\rho_s g$
    E. $\rho_s g$

27. For a pond to freeze over on a hot day, which law would have to be violated?

    A. The first law of thermodynamics
    B. The second law of thermodynamics
    C. Newton's first law
    D. Newton's second law
    E. Newton's third law

GO TO THE NEXT PAGE

28. Two blocks of mass m and 2m and of equal volume are submerged in water. The ratio of their respective apparent weights while underwater is

   A. 2:1.
   B. 1:2.
   C. 1:1.
   D. 3:2.
   E. Cannot be determined from the information given.

29. A cube of aluminum has been heated to its melting point but is still completely solid. If a little more heat is added

   A. some of the aluminum will melt, and the temperature will increase.
   B. some of the aluminum will melt, and the temperature will remain the same.
   C. some of the aluminum will melt, and the temperature will decrease.
   D. none of the aluminum will melt, but the temperature will increase.
   E. none of the aluminum will melt, and the temperature will remain the same.

30. A car rolls off a horizontal cliff 125 m high, and lands 100 m from the base of the cliff. How fast was the car moving when it rolled off the cliff?

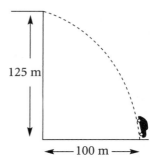

   A. 8 m/s
   B. 10 m/s
   C. 16 m/s
   D. 20 m/s
   E. 33 m/s

31. A 5-kg block moving with velocity v approaches a plane that is inclined at 30° to the horizontal and proceeds to slide up the plane. If the plane is 20 m long, the coefficient of kinetic friction, μ_k, is $\frac{1}{\sqrt{3}}$ and the block just reaches the top of the plane before coming to a stop, what must be the value of v ?

   A. $\frac{\sqrt{50}}{3}$ m/s

   B. 10 m/s

   C. 20 m/s

   D. $10\sqrt{3}$ m/s

   E. $\frac{20}{\sqrt{3}}$ m/s

GO TO THE NEXT PAGE

32. A mass m_1 slides down a frictionless plane that is inclined at an angle θ_1 to the horizontal. A mass m_2 slides down a second frictionless plane that is inclined at an angle θ_2 to the horizontal. The ratio of the acceleration of m_1 to that of m_2 is

   A. $\dfrac{m_1\sin\theta_1}{m_1\sin\theta_2}$

   B. $\dfrac{\sin\theta_1}{\sin\theta_2}$

   C. $\dfrac{\cos\theta_1}{\cos\theta_2}$

   D. $\dfrac{\theta_1}{\theta_2}$

   E. None of the above

33. A ball is thrown on the Earth with an initial speed y and angle θ and travels a horizontal distance x meters. How far would it have traveled if the experiment were repeated on the moon where gravitational acceleration is $\dfrac{1}{6}$ that of the Earth?

   A. x meters
   B. 2x meters
   C. 6x meters
   D. 12x meters
   E. 36x meters

34. A bomber flying at 900 mph and an altitude of 6,400 ft drops a 2-ton bomb above point A on the ground. How far from point A will the bomb land?

   A. 3,200 ft
   B. 6,400 ft
   C. 2.5 miles
   D. 5.0 miles
   E. 7.5 miles

35. When blue light of wavelength 470 nm travels from a medium with index of refraction 1.5 to a medium with index of refraction 1.0

   A. its wavelength increases.
   B. its frequency increases.
   C. its speed decreases.
   D. its energy decreases.
   E. its energy increases.

36. What is the effective resistance of the circuit below?

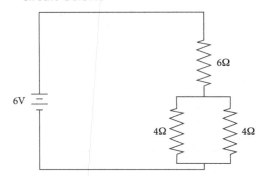

   A. 6 Ω
   B. 6.5 Ω
   C. 8 Ω
   D. 10 Ω
   E. 14 Ω

GO TO THE NEXT PAGE

37. The circuit shown below consists of two capacitors C_1 and C_2 and a voltage supply V. The electric potential at point a is equal to the electric potential at point

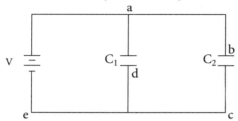

A. b.

B. c.

C. d.

D. e.

E. None of the above

38. An object travels at 30 m/s for 5 s, then accelerates uniformly at 15 m/s² for 4 s. How far does the object travel?

A. 120 m

B. 240 m

C. 390 m

D. 480 m

E. 510 m

39. Object A of mass M is released from height H, whereas object B of mass 0.5M is released from height 2H. What is the ratio of the velocity of object A to that of object B immediately before they hit the ground?

A. 1:1

B. $1:\sqrt{2}$

C. 1:2

D. 1:4

E. $\sqrt{2}:1$

40. A projectile is launched at an angle of 60° to the horizontal with an initial speed of 5 m/s. What is the speed of the projectile at its highest point?

A. 0 m/s

B. 5 m/s

C. 2.5 m/s

D. $\frac{5}{2}\sqrt{3}$ m/s

E. 9.8 m/s

STOP. IF YOU FINISH BEFORE TIME IS CALLED, YOU MAY CHECK YOUR WORK ON THIS SECTION ONLY. DO NOT TURN TO ANY OTHER SECTION IN THE TEST.

Quantitative Reasoning

50 questions—45 minutes

Directions: Choose the best answer for each question from the five choices provided.

1. An aquarium is filled with water. The aquarium has a base of $1\frac{1}{2}$ feet by 2 feet and a depth of $1\frac{1}{2}$ feet. If 1 gallon of water equals 231 cubic inches, how many gallons will it take to fill the aquarium?

   A. 1,039.5
   B. 51.3
   C. 33.7
   D. 29.9
   E. 28.0

2. $1\frac{7}{8} \times 2\frac{1}{10} \times \frac{6}{7} = ?$

   A. $3\frac{513}{280}$
   B. $2\frac{3}{40}$
   C. $3\frac{3}{8}$
   D. 12
   E. $1\frac{17}{24}$

3. Kate and Jim take a trip together. Jim drives half the distance at 40 miles per hour, and Kate drives the other half at 60 miles per hour. What is their average speed for the trip in miles per hour?

   A. 45
   B. 48
   C. 50
   D. 52
   E. 54

4. A machine has two meshed gears, one with 24 teeth and the other with 40 teeth. If the smaller gear revolves 15 times, how many times does the larger gear revolve?

   A. 3
   B. 6
   C. 9
   D. 20
   E. 25

5. If 23% of $\frac{2}{5}\left(\frac{190}{3x}\right) = 8$, what is x?

   A. $\frac{11}{6}$
   B. $\frac{57}{6}$
   C. $\frac{437}{200}$
   D. $\frac{437}{600}$
   E. $\frac{19}{6}$

6. If a heart beats 72 times every minute, how many times does it beat every second?

   A. 0.83
   B. 0.6
   C. 1.5
   D. 1.67
   E. 1.2

GO TO THE NEXT PAGE

7. $\dfrac{6534}{\frac{3}{4}} = ?$

A. $544\frac{1}{2}$

B. $4{,}900\frac{1}{2}$

C. $7{,}218$

D. $8{,}712$

E. $9{,}112$

8. $a = \pi r^2 h$, $\pi = \dfrac{22}{7}$, $h = 14$, $a = 396$, $r > 0$, $2r = ?$

A. 3

B. 6

C. 9

D. $2\sqrt{3}$

E. $2\sqrt{2}$

9. A number is larger than 5 by the same amount that it is smaller than 3 more than 14. What is the number?

A. 14

B. 12

C. 10

D. 11

E. 13

10. A circle passes through the point (0, 0) and the point (10, 0). Which of the following could NOT be a third point on the circle?

A. (2, 4)

B. (8, 4)

C. (2, –4)

D. (5, 0)

E. (1, –3)

11. If a is 25% of b and b is 60% of c, then $\dfrac{c}{a} = ?$

A. $\dfrac{5}{12}$

B. $\dfrac{20}{3}$

C. $\dfrac{48}{5}$

D. $\dfrac{12}{5}$

E. $\dfrac{5}{3}$

12. A chemist needs to make a solution that is 60% alcohol. If she has 4 liters of a solution that is 35% alcohol, how many liters of 80% solution will she need to add?

A. 2.5

B. 3.75

C. 4

D. 5

E. 5.5

13. $\dfrac{9}{8} - \dfrac{5}{12} + \dfrac{1}{2} - (?) = 1$

A. 5

B. $\dfrac{5}{24}$

C. $\dfrac{29}{24}$

D. $\dfrac{5}{12}$

E. $\dfrac{7}{12}$

14. What is the approximate area of the largest circle that can be drawn inside of a square with an area of 1,000 square inches? $\left(\pi = \dfrac{22}{7}\right)$

A. 785.7 square inches

B. 873.0 square inches

C. 99.4 square inches

D. 990.1 square inches

E. 314.1 square inches

GO TO THE NEXT PAGE

15. $\dfrac{a}{b} - \dfrac{b}{a} = ?$

    A. $\dfrac{ab}{a-b}$

    B. $\dfrac{ab}{b^2} - \dfrac{a^2}{ab}$

    C. $\dfrac{a^2 - b^2}{ab}$

    D. 0

    E. None of these

16. If 55% of $\dfrac{9z}{5} = 33$, $z = ?$

    A. $\dfrac{11}{5}$

    B. $\dfrac{165}{9}$

    C. $\dfrac{52}{99}$

    D. $\dfrac{363}{20}$

    E. $\dfrac{100}{3}$

17. What is the average of $\dfrac{1}{2}$, $\dfrac{2}{3}$, and $\dfrac{3}{4}$?

    A. $\dfrac{6}{36}$

    B. $\dfrac{23}{12}$

    C. $\dfrac{7}{12}$

    D. $\dfrac{23}{36}$

    E. $\dfrac{1}{4}$

18. 14 is to 35 as $2x$ is to 40. What is x ?

    A. 4

    B. 7

    C. 8

    D. 2

    E. $\dfrac{40}{7}$

19. Diane and Sandy want to paint their room. Diane could paint the room by herself in 6 hours. Sandy could paint it by herself in 4 hours. If they work together, how many hours will it take them to paint the room?

    A. $2\dfrac{2}{5}$

    B. $2\dfrac{1}{2}$

    C. 3

    D. 5

    E. 10

20. If 8 mL of water are added to 32 mL of a 5% sugar solution, what % of the resulting solution is sugar?

    A. 2.5

    B. 4

    C. 4.5

    D. 5

    E. 6

21. The average of 5 scores is 9.6. If the highest and lowest scores are dropped, the average rises to 9.7. Compute the average of the highest and lowest scores.

    A. 9.35

    B. 9.45

    C. 9.55

    D. 9.65

    E. 9.75

22. $\dfrac{10\text{ feet }(x)\text{ inches}}{9\text{ feet }(3)\text{ inches}}$ approximates 1.2. $x = ?$

    A. 3

    B. 13.2

    C. 10

    D. 1.2

    E. 8

GO TO THE NEXT PAGE

23. Arrange the following numbers from the greatest to least.

a. $\frac{2}{3}$ b. $\frac{5}{11}$ c. $\frac{7}{9}$ d. $\frac{3}{4}$ e. $\frac{5}{8}$

A. a, d, c, b, e
B. b, d, e, a, c
C. e, c, a, d, b
D. c, b, e, d, a
E. c, d, a, e, b

24. In a class, 70% of the students are girls. If the girls have an average height of 5 feet 4 inches and the boys have an average height of 5 feet 8 inches, approximately what is the average height of the entire class?

A. 5 feet $4\frac{1}{2}$ inches
B. 5 feet 5 inches
C. 5 feet $5\frac{1}{2}$ inches
D. 5 feet 6 inches
E. 5 feet $6\frac{1}{2}$ inches

25. The cost if a ride at an amusement park rises from 75¢ to 90¢. After the rise, the number of riders decreases by 20%. What is the percent decrease in total revenues from the ride?

A. 4%
B. 5%
C. 8.5%
D. 16.67%
E. 20%

26. $\frac{4a - 7a + 6a}{6ab} = ?$

A. $\frac{-3}{b}$
B. $\frac{3a}{b}$
C. $\frac{5}{2a}$
D. $\frac{1}{2b}$
E. $\frac{a}{2b}$

27. Which is the largest?

A. 0.636
B. 0.163
C. 0.36
D. 0.136
E. 0.3

28. On 150 flips of a coin, 48% of the time it landed heads. If the coin is flipped another 100 times, on what percent of those flips must it land heads to raise the percent of heads to 50%?

A. 51%
B. 53%
C. 57%
D. 52%
E. 55%

29. Which is the smallest?

A. 0.3
B. $(0.3)^2$
C. $\sqrt{0.03}$
D. 0.03
E. $\sqrt{0.3}$

GO TO THE NEXT PAGE

30. What is the number of degrees in the angle formed by the minute and hour hands of a clock at 4:50?

    A. 155
    B. 180
    C. 150
    D. 165
    E. 175

31. $10.5 \div 0.35 =$

    A. 0.3
    B. 0.03
    C. 300
    D. 30
    E. 3

32. The lock above is at the correct setting when each of the three sections contains the correct digit from 1 to 5. How many of the possible settings will NOT open the lock?

    A. 63
    B. 24
    C. 124
    D. 215
    E. 14

33. A woman receives $286 gross pay for 48 hours work. This pay includes 8 hours of overtime at $1\frac{1}{2}$ times her normal hourly rate. Determine her normal hourly rate.

    A. $4.50
    B. $5.40
    C. $5.50
    D. $5.80
    E. $5.95

34. A fence 33 feet 4 inches long costs $99. What was the cost per foot of the fence?

    A. $3.33
    B. $3.03
    C. $2.97
    D. $3.00
    E. $2.47

35. If 1 ounce = 28 grams, $3\frac{1}{5}$ grams = (?) ounces.

    A. $\frac{1}{7}$
    B. $\frac{20}{7}$
    C. 8
    D. $\frac{4}{35}$
    E. $\frac{448}{5}$

36. $\frac{63}{3x} = 4\frac{2}{7}$. $x = ?$

    A. 0.1
    B. 4.29
    C. 5.3
    D. 2.1
    E. 4.9

37. An empty bottle weighs one-tenth of its filled weight. If the bottled is partially filled so that it weighs one-half of its filled weight, what fraction of the bottle is filled?

    A. $\frac{4}{9}$
    B. $\frac{4}{10}$
    C. $\frac{6}{10}$
    D. $\frac{45}{100}$
    E. $\frac{3}{4}$

GO TO THE NEXT PAGE

38. $x - y = 0.2z$

    $x + z = 1.6y$

    What % of $y = 0.4x$?

    A. 32%
    B. 33%
    C. 36%
    D. 40%
    E. 44%

39. $\dfrac{3y + 14 - y}{2y + 1} = 2.$ $y = ?$

    A. 0
    B. $5\frac{1}{2}$
    C. 6
    D. 11
    E. 12

40. A 39-ounce box of cereal costs 91¢, and an 18-ounce box of the same cereal costs 48¢. What is the ratio of the cost per pound of the larger box to the cost per pound of the smaller box?

    A. 0.875:1
    B. 0.9:1
    C. 0.93:1
    D. 1.14:1
    E. 2:3

41. ( ) is to 8 as $\frac{x}{6}$ is to ( ).

    A. 16 ... $\frac{x}{3}$
    B. 4 ... $\frac{x}{12}$
    C. 12 ... $\frac{x}{9}$
    D. 2 ... $2x$
    E. $6x$ ... 8

42. If a car dealer buys a car at 75% of the list price and sells it for 93% of the list price, what will the percent profit be?

    A. 18%
    B. 57%
    C. 13%
    D. 24%
    E. 21.2%

43. The volume of liquid in a container doubles every half hour. What is the percent increase in volume from 11:30 AM to 2:00 PM of the same day?

    A. 1,600%
    B. 160%
    C. 320%
    D. 3,100%
    E. 3,200%

44. Last year the ratio of teachers to students in a school was 1:8. This year the number of teachers increased by 10%, and the number of students also increased by 10%. What is the ratio of teachers to students this year?

    A. 1.1:8
    B. 2:9
    C. 1:8
    D. 1:8.8
    E. 11:18

45. $\sqrt{0.4761} = ?$

    A. 0.065
    B. 0.7
    C. 0.07
    D. 0.69
    E. 0.08

GO TO THE NEXT PAGE

46. If $\frac{8a}{9} = \frac{2b}{3}$ and $0.5b = \frac{4c}{5}$ how many $a = 24c$?

    A. 20
    B. 23
    C. 15
    D. $\frac{144}{5}$
    E. 18

47. In September a dentist saw $\frac{1}{3}$ more patients than he saw in August. In October, he saw $\frac{1}{5}$ more patients than he saw in September. If he saw 240 patients in October, how many did he see in August?

    A. 180
    B. 150
    C. 142
    D. 160
    E. 172

48. 90% of 40 = $\frac{5}{6}$ of (?)

    A. 36
    B. 33.33
    C. 43.2
    D. 45.6
    E. 75

49. Rebecca has twice as many toys as Jennifer. If Jennifer gives Rebecca four of her toys, then she will have one-fourth as many as Rebecca. How many toys does Rebecca have now?

    A. 6
    B. 10
    C. 16
    D. 20
    E. 24

50. If $c = \frac{2}{5}$, $\frac{1}{b} = 4$, and $a = 10$, what is $(b \bullet a) + \frac{1}{c}$?

    A. $2\frac{9}{10}$
    B. $40\frac{2}{5}$
    C. $42\frac{1}{5}$
    D. $42\frac{1}{2}$
    E. 5

STOP. IF YOU FINISH BEFORE TIME IS CALLED, YOU MAY CHECK YOUR WORK ON THIS SECTION ONLY. DO NOT TURN TO ANY OTHER SECTION IN THE TEST.

Full-Length Practice Test
ANSWER KEY

Survey of the Natural Sciences

1. C
2. B
3. B
4. D
5. A
6. D
7. B
8. B
9. B
10. E
11. D
12. B
13. C
14. B
15. B
16. C
17. A
18. E
19. D
20. B
21. B
22. D
23. B
24. B
25. A
26. C
27. E
28. A
29. C
30. B
31. C
32. A
33. D
34. C
35. D
36. E
37. B
38. D
39. C
40. D
41. D
42. E
43. B
44. D
45. A
46. C
47. C
48. D
49. C
50. D
51. D
52. C
53. C
54. D
55. A
56. B
57. D
58. D
59. C
60. E
61. C
62. E
63. E
64. C
65. A
66. D
67. B
68. A
69. D
70. C
71. E
72. C
73. C
74. D
75. E
76. E
77. D
78. C
79. A
80. A
81. D
82. E
83. C
84. B
85. C
86. E
87. A
88. D
89. C
90. E
91. D
92. A
93. B
94. C
95. B
96. B
97. A
98. A
99. B
100. A

Reading Comprehension

1. A
2. B
3. E
4. D
5. B
6. D
7. A
8. B
9. D
10. E
11. C
12. D
13. C
14. C
15. B
16. E
17. C
18. D
19. B
20. C
21. E
22. A
23. C
24. B
25. D
26. A
27. D
28. B
29. B
30. A
31. C
32. D
33. C
34. A
35. E
36. B
37. A
38. C
39. D
40. E
41. B
42. A
43. C
44. B
45. D
46. A
47. E
48. D
49. B
50. D

Physics

1. D
2. E
3. D
4. B
5. A
6. B
7. A
8. E
9. A
10. E
11. A
12. E
13. D
14. A
15. D
16. C
17. D
18. D
19. D
20. C
21. C
22. B
23. D
24. D
25. B
26. D
27. B
28. E
29. B
30. D
31. C
32. B
33. C
34. D
35. A
36. C
37. A
38. C
39. B
40. C

Quantitative Reasoning

1. C
2. C
3. B
4. C
5. D
6. E
7. D
8. B
9. D
10. D
11. B
12. D
13. B
14. A
15. C
16. E
17. D
18. C
19. A
20. B
21. B
22. B
23. E
24. B
25. A
26. D
27. A
28. B
29. D
30. A
31. D
32. C
33. C
34. C
35. D
36. E
37. A
38. E
39. C
40. A
41. C
42. D
43. D
44. C
45. D
46. A
47. B
48. C
49. D
50. E

Full-Length Practice OAT CONVERSION CHART

To use this chart, find the number of correct answers you had in each section to determine your scaled score for that section. To calculate your Total Score, take the average of your six Scaled Scores and round to the nearest whole number.

SCALED SCORE	Biology	General Chemistry	Organic Chemistry	Reading Comprehension	Physics	Quantitative Reasoning
400	36–40	30	27–30	40	37–40	35–40
390	35	29	26	37–39	36	33–34
380	33–34	28	25	35–36	34–35	32
370	32	27	24	34	33	31
360	31	26	23	33	31–32	29–30
350	30	25	21–22	31–32	30	27–28
340	28–29	23–24	20	29–30	29	24–26
330	27	22	18–19	28	27–28	22–23
320	25–26	20–21	16–17	27	25–26	21
310	23–24	18–19	15	26	24	20
300	22	16–17	13–14	25	22–23	18–19
290	20–21	15	12	23–24	21	17
280	19	13–14	11	21–22	20	16
270	17–18	12	10	20	18–19	14–15
260	14–16	10–11	9	19	17	13
250	13	9	8	17–18	16	12
240	12	8	7	16	15	10–11
230	11	7	6	14–15	14	8–9
220	10	6	5	11–13	13	7
210	8–9	5	4	6–10	12	6
200	0–7	0–4	0–3	0–5	0–11	0–5

Survey of the Natural Sciences
ANSWERS AND EXPLANATIONS

ANSWER KEY

1. C	21. B	41. D	61. C	81. D
2. B	22. D	42. E	62. E	82. E
3. B	23. B	43. B	63. E	83. C
4. D	24. B	44. D	64. C	84. B
5. A	25. A	45. A	65. A	85. C
6. D	26. C	46. C	66. D	86. E
7. B	27. E	47. C	67. B	87. A
8. B	28. A	48. D	68. A	88. D
9. B	29. C	49. C	69. D	89. C
10. E	30. B	50. D	70. C	90. E
11. D	31. C	51. D	71. E	91. D
12. B	32. A	52. C	72. C	92. A
13. C	33. D	53. C	73. C	93. B
14. B	34. C	54. D	74. D	94. C
15. B	35. D	55. A	75. E	95. B
16. C	36. E	56. B	76. E	96. B
17. A	37. B	57. D	77. D	97. A
18. E	38. D	58. D	78. C	98. A
19. D	39. C	59. C	79. A	99. B
20. B	40. D	60. E	80. A	100. A

1. C

In a BB × bb cross, the F_1 generation genotype will be entirely heterozygous (Bb) and express the dominant phenotype. Therefore, (A) and (B) would appear in the F_1 generation. In the F_2 generation formed by crossing Bb × Bb, BB, Bb, and bb would be formed in a 1:2:1 ratio. Because the recessive could not appear in the F_1 generation but could appear in the F_2 generation (Bb × Bb cross), (C) is the only correct answer.

2. B

Distinctions between plants and animals include the following: (1) animals generally go through a larval stage—a developmental stage between the fertilized egg and the adult (i.e., the metamorphosis of tadpoles and caterpillars), whereas plants do not pass through intermediate larval stages; (2) plants are typically photosynthetic and sessile, and animals are generally heterotrophic and motile; (3) plant structure is adapted for maximum exposure to light, air, and soil by extensive branching, whereas animals are adapted for minimum surface exposure in that they are extremely compact; and (4) plant cells contain cell walls composed of cellulose.

3. B

The ectoderm primarily forms the skin, nervous system, and eyes, whereas the endoderm forms the digestive tract, the liver and the pancreas, the bladder, and the respiratory system. The mesoderm forms the musculoskeletal system and all other internal organs, such as the kidneys and the reproductive organs. (B) is the only answer that correctly associates those two with the retina and the lungs. (A) is incorrect because the heart is developed from mesoderm, and (C) is incorrect because the skeletal muscles are developed from the mesoderm. (D) and (E) are incorrect because the stomach muscle and uterus are also developed from the mesoderm.

4. D

The number of gametes can be calculated 2^n, where n = the number of heterozygous genes. In this case, n = 3, so the number of gametes = $2^3 \Rightarrow 8$.

5. A

Inbreeding occurs when one breeds animals that are closely related. (B) is incorrect; hybridization occurs when one breeds animals that are phylogenetically distinct to develop an animal that has characteristics of both parents. (C) is incorrect because cross-breeding is the crossing of two animals and can be used to determine phenotype when the genotype is known; or to determine genotype when the phenotype is known; or to investigate codominance, expressivity, or penetrance. (D) is incorrect; selective breeding is the creation of certain strains of specific traits by controlled breeding. (E) is incorrect; test breeding is breeding of an organism with a homozygous recessive to determine whether an organism is homozygous dominant or heterozygous dominant for a given trait.

6. D

Chlorophyll is a green pigment essential as an electron donor, and for light capture in photosynthesis. When photons of light strike chlorophyll molecules, those molecules transfer the energy of the light to their electrons. This energy (1) is then transferred to ADP to form ATP, (2) is transferred to NADP to form NADPH, and (3) splits H_2O into

$2H^+$ and $\frac{1}{2}O_2$.

7. B

The allantois is found in the eggs of birds and reptiles and is used as a receptacle for nitrogenous wastes. The vessels of this structure also lie close enough to the surface of the shell to enable the exchange of gases. (A) is incorrect because the amnion is the innermost fluid-filled embryonic membrane; it forms a protective sac surrounding the embryos of birds, reptiles, and mammals. (C) is incorrect because the chorion is the outermost extra-embryonic membrane of reptiles and birds that separates the embryo from the albumin. (D) is incorrect because the umbilical cord connects the embryo to the placenta. Gas exchange occurs in the placenta. (E) is incorrect because the yolk sac contains food for the developing embryo.

8. B

A cell that is n (haploid) cannot undergo meiosis to become $\frac{1}{2}$n. (A), (C), and (D) are incorrect because there are a number of organisms that are haploid and these organisms undergo mitosis and divide and grow. An example of such an organism is a braconid wasp. These animals in the haploid form are males (n), and females (2n) are formed only when a female mates. (E) is incorrect because an organism, diploid or haploid, must be able to digest to maintain life.

9. B

(A) is incorrect because NADH$_2$ is formed from NAD during the Krebs cycle, and (C) and (D) have nothing to do with the Krebs cycle. Answer (E) is false because glycogen formation occurs only in hepatic cells and does not occur in every cell.

10. E

RNA is made up of a ribose sugar bound to a phosphate group, which is then bound to one of the four bases. (A) is incorrect because RNA is characterized by having uracil as one of its bases rather than thymine, and (B) is incorrect because DNA utilizes thymine rather than uracil. (C) is incorrect because RNA doesn't replicate in eukaryotic cells. Although in some retroviruses RNA will synthesize DNA, this is not known as the replication of DNA. (D) is incorrect because tRNA actually picks up the amino acids and brings them to the ribosome and the mRNA carries to the ribosome the message of the protein that is to be produced.

11. D

Enzymes are necessary to catalyze the reactions that allow the breakdown of glucose into ATP. (A) is incorrect because enzymes are typically proteins. (B) is incorrect because enzymes typically act most effectively at a physiological pH of 7–7.4, except for the enzymes that break down protein in the stomach, which act most effectively in an acidic environment. (C) is incorrect because enzymes do not always require a coenzyme to function. (E) is incorrect because enzymes are never irreversibly changed during a reaction. They just increase the rate of the reaction.

12. B

Homologous recombination occurs during metaphase I after tetrad formation. The farther apart two genes are, the more likely a homologous recombination will occur between them. Therefore, the genes that are farthest apart are most likely to cross over. Also, genes are more likely to recombine the farther away from the centromere they are.

13. C

A point or frameshift mutation in a gene may be evidenced by a corresponding mutation in the protein. (A) has nothing to do with how DNA might control the synthesis of a protein, and (B) is false because DNA actually directs amino acid synthesis by serving as the template that determines the sequence of the mRNA. (D) and (E) are both true but are not the best answers. Each of these answers could be merely coincidental and do not fully support the statement.

14. B
Ribosomes, the site of protein production, give the rough endoplasmic reticulum (ER) its characteristic appearance. The function of the ER is to transport proteins around the cells or for export out of the cell. Sections of the ER are lined with ribosomes where proteins are produced and then transported to the appropriate areas. (A) is incorrect because lysosomes are membrane-bound organelles in the cytoplasm that have very low pH, are filled with proteolytic enzymes, and are the site of degradation in the cell. (C) is incorrect because mitochondria are also membrane-bound organelles and are the site of cellular respiration. (D) is incorrect because the Golgi apparatus is also a membrane-bound organelle and follows the ER in the production of proteins. It is here that proteins are glycosylated and further post-translationally modified and packaged. (E) is incorrect because histones are proteins in the nucleus that bind to DNA like "beads on a string."

15. B
The eggs are released from the ovaries and are picked up by the fallopian tubes. In the case of fertilization, a haploid sperm will swim to the egg and fertilize it. The fertilized egg will then continue down the fallopian tube until it reaches the uterus, where it will implant. (C) is incorrect because fertilization in the uterus can occur but is rare and sometimes associated with complications such as cervical implantation. (D) and (E) would both disallow implantation of the fertilized egg into the uterus.

16. C
A characteristic difference between eukaryotes and prokaryotes is the presence of membrane-bound organelles in eukaryotes. (A), (B), and (D) are incorrect because both of these cell types have ribosomal RNA, plasma membranes, and ribosomes.

17. A
A totipotent cell is one that has the ability to differentiate and mature into any cell type.

(B) and (C) are the opposite of totipotent. (D) is incorrect because the DNA of any cell is species-specific, so a totipotent cell will only be able to develop into a cell of that organism, and (E) is incorrect because these cells are usually unspecialized cells of multicellular organisms and are not found in unicellular organisms.

18. E
The endosymbiotic hypothesis states that blue-green algae entered into a symbiotic arrangement with early eukaryotic plants to develop into chloroplasts and bacteria entered into a similar arrangement with eukaryotic animal cells to become mitochondria. Chloroplasts and mitochondria have a plasma membrane (their inner membrane) and the ability to produce their own proteins without utilizing the cell's machinery. In addition, they have circular DNA, and their rRNA subunits are characteristic of prokaryotes.

19. D
Spermatogenesis occurs in the seminiferous tubule, and the sperm mature over a period of 2–4 days, in the epididymis. The epididymis leads to the vas deferens, which connects to the urethra to allow for ejaculation. The seminal vesicle, prostate gland, and Cowper's gland all contribute seminal fluid to lubricate, nourish, and buffer the sperm.

20. B
The electron transport chain is a complex carrier mechanism located on the inside of the inner mitochondrial membrane. During oxidative phosphorylation, ATP is produced when high-energy potential electrons are transferred from NADH and $FADH_2$ to oxygen by a series of carriers located in the inner mitochondrial membrane. As the electrons are transferred from carrier to carrier, free energy is released, which is then used to form ATP. The last carrier of the electron transport chain, cytochrome a3, passes its electron to the final electron acceptor, O_2. In addition to the electrons, O_2 picks up a pair of hydrogen ions from the surrounding medium, forming water.

21. B

Mesoderm produces the musculoskeletal system as well as the internal organs and the reproductive system. Ectoderm develops into the epidermis, the neural tissue, and the eyes. Endoderm develops into the digestive and respiratory tracts and the bladder.

22. D

Gastrulation begins with the blastula forming an inpocket into the pre-existing blastocoel. This invagination forms the archenteron, which will develop into the digestive tract. The hole that forms from the blastocoel is known as the blastopore and becomes the anus. Therefore, gastrulation forms the archenteron and the blastopore, but the blastocoel was already present.

23. B

Neurulation is the process of neural tube formation. The neural plate invaginates and forms a tube. A chemokine from an underlying mesodermal structure called the notochord (B) induces neurulation. The neural ectoderm (D) is formed during neurulation, and the neural crest (E) is formed after the neural tube. The endodermal layer (C) plays no role in neurulation, and neither does the archenteron (A), an endodermal structure that becomes the digestive tract.

24. B

Photosynthesis occurs in two steps. Step one is the light reaction in which visible light, especially that in the red/blue wavelengths, produces ATP and $NADPH_2$ through the splitting of CO_2 and H_2O. O_2 is produced during the splitting of water. During the dark cycle, carbohydrates such as glucose are synthesized when you have $NADPH_2$, ATP, and CO_2, and this will occur anytime these three compounds are present, regardless of the presence of light.

25. A

The blastula is the hollow-ball stage of embryonic development. It develops from the morula, a solid cluster of cells. The center of the blastula is termed the blastocoel. This invaginates during gastrulation to form the gastrula. At this stage, mesoderm is formed, and the archenteron and blastopore are formed. The next stage is called the neurula, and

in this stage the ectoderm forms the nerve cord. Therefore (B), (C), (D), and (E) all correctly represent the stages of the embryonic development, and (A) is incorrect as the blastula is a hollow ball of cells.

26. C

Fat contains approximately 9 calories/gram while carbohydrates and proteins contain only 4 calories/gram. Sugar and starch are two forms of carbohydrates. Vitamins are coenzymes, which are typically not metabolized.

27. E

mRNA includes a coded base sequence called a codon. tRNA, which carries the amino acids to the mRNA and the ribosome, has a complementary strand called the anti-codon. Therefore, a tRNA with an anti-codon of AAC should match the mRNA codon UUG. Remember that in RNA, adenine bonds with uracil and guanine bonds with cytosine.

28. A

In the light reaction, light splits H_2O into excited electrons, H^+ and O_2. The excited electrons go on to form ATP, and H^+ is incorporated in the carbohydrates produced during the dark reaction. The O_2 is released into the environment as a waste product of this reaction. (B) is incorrect because CO_2 donates the carbon and the oxygen required for carbohydrate formation in the dark reaction. (C) and (D) are end products of photosynthesis, and answer (E) is incorrect because chlorophyll is involved in the initial capture of sunlight.

29. C

The number of genetically distinct offspring is found by multiplying the number of distinct gametes each parent can produce. The number of gametes can be calculated from the formula 2^n, where n = the number of heterozygous genes. The AaBbCc parent can produce 8 unique gametes ($2^3 = 8$), and the AaBBCc parent can produce 4 ($2^2 = 4$). Therefore, the possible number of different offspring is $8 \times 4 = 32$.

30. B

Identical twins are produced when a zygote produced by one egg and one sperm splits during the four- or eight-cell stage to develop into two genetically identical organisms. (A) is incorrect because identical twins will be the same gender but fraternal twins can also be the same gender. (D) is incorrect because these are termed fraternal twins and are no more genetically alike than siblings. (C) and (E) are impossible events.

31. C

In the light reaction, chlorophyll absorbs energy to split water into excited electrons, H^+ and O_2. The excited electrons make ATP through photophosphorylation. In the dark reaction, carbohydrates are produced, without the need for sunlight, by CO_2, the H^+ ions in the form of $NADPH_2$, and ATP. (B) is incorrect because that describes cellular respiration. (D) is incorrect because that does not occur; and (E) is incorrect because H_2O is split, not CO_2.

32. A

Multiple alleles describe more than two allele possibilities. In the ABO blood group, there are three alleles: A and B, which are codominant over the recessive allele O. There are four possible phenotypes, A, B, AB, and O, and six possible genotypes, AA, AO, BB, BO, AB, and OO. (B) refers to crossing organisms heterozygous for two traits such as AaBb × AaBb. This cross will have the characteristic 9:3:3:1 ratio of offspring. (C) refers to recessive alleles, which are not expressed unless they are homozygous. (D) refers to the fact that two genes will be inherited independently of each other if they are not linked physically on the chromosome. (E) refers to changes in genes through spontaneous changes in base sequence.

33. D

In the nucleus, DNA is produced during cell division, and RNA is transcribed. mRNA travels from the nucleus into the endoplasmic reticulum where it is translated on the ribosomes into polypeptides.

34. C

If a male is affected with red-green color blindness, his genotype would be $X^{cb}Y$. If he mated with a normal female, XX, their female offspring would be all $X^{cb}X$, receiving one good copy of the X chromosome from their mother and the color blindness gene from their father. Because this is a recessive trait, all the offspring (100%) would be carriers.

The male offspring of this mating would all be XY (100% normal), receiving one good copy of the X chromosome from their mother and receiving their Y chromosome from their father.

35. D

Mutations in somatic cells affect only the individuals involved and no progeny, because they cannot be passed on to the next generation and will not affect gamete formation. These mutations are typically recessive although there are some instances of dominant negative mutations. The major concern about mutations in somatic cells is the development of tumors as a result of a protein that has lost its function due to a somatic mutation. This is the basis for tumors such as malignant melanomas caused by mutations to the DNA as a result of UV irradiation.

36. E

Nondisjunction is a failure of homologous pairs to separate after synapsis. The result is an extra chromosome or a missing chromosome for a given pair. For example, Down syndrome is due to an extra chromosome 21. The number of chromosomes in a case of single nondisjunction is $2n + 1$ or $2n - 1$. In Down syndrome, it is 47. Most of these embryos are aborted early in their development, and only a few, like Down syndrome trisomy 21, trisomy 13, and trisomy 18, are viable, albeit with developmental disorders. Breakage near the centromere might be induced by environmental factors such as mutagens, but would not be caused by nondisjunction.

37. B

DNA replication occurs during the S phase so that each daughter cell will receive a complete copy of the genome. DNA replication is semiconservative: half of the original DNA (one strand) is present in each of the new, or daughter, double-stranded DNA molecules. As always, purines bind to pyrimidines; more specifically, adenine binds to thymine whereas cytosine binds to guanine. Okazaki fragments are formed on the lagging strand so that although DNA is synthesized in the 5' to 3' direction in short segments, overall it is synthesized in the 3' to 5' direction.

38. D

Let R = dominant red color and r = recessive white color. There are two possible red genotypes for the unknown offspring: RR (pure homozygous red) and Rr (heterozygous red). The unknown offspring will be referred to as R_. If the cross in (A) were performed, crossing R_ with Rr (red plant with a white parent), then you would be able to determine the unknown genotype. If there were any white offspring, the unknown genotype must be Rr. If only red offspring resulted, then the genotype must be RR. If the cross in (B) were performed, crossing R_ with RR, you would not be able to determine the genotype. If the unknown allele was recessive, it would be masked by the homozygous dominant red genotype. The only phenotype that can result from a parent that is RR is red, so any white allele would never be exposed. If the cross in (C) were performed, crossing R_ with rr, you would be able to determine the unknown genotype of the offspring. If there were any white offspring, the unknown genotype must be Rr. If only red offspring resulted, then the genotype must be RR. Therefore (D), two of the above, is the correct answer.

39. C

AO × AB potentially will result in offspring with the genotypes AA, AB, AO, or BO. As you can see, OO homozygous blood type O is impossible in this mating.

40. D

Given that males have a frequency of color blindness of 1 in 12, you know that the gene frequency of the color-blindness allele is 1 in 12. Because females would require both copies of the color-blindness allele to be color blind, the frequency of color-blind females is $\frac{1}{12} \times \frac{1}{12}$, or $\frac{1}{144}$.

41. D

The density of a gas is the mass of the gas divided by the volume it occupies. For simplicity, we can assume a 1-mole sample of the gas, which occupies 22.4 L at STP. If XY_2 were in fact the molecular formula, then the mass of one mole would be 14 grams and the density would be

$$\frac{14 \text{ g}}{22.4 \text{ L}} = \frac{0.63 \text{ g}}{\text{L}}$$

Because the density is given to be approximately twice as much, it follows that the molecular weight must be twice as much and, therefore, that the molecular formula must be twice the empirical formula, or X_2Y_4.

As for the wrong choices, (A) and (C) can be dismissed for not being integral multiples of the empirical formula, XY_2. The calculation done above could have been repeated on each of the remaining choices, or avoided by a rough approximation on the remaining choices:

$$\frac{14 \text{ g}}{22.4 \text{ L}} < \frac{1 \text{ g}}{\text{L}}, \frac{28 \text{ g}}{22.4 \text{ L}} > \frac{1 \text{ g}}{\text{L}}, \frac{56 \text{ g}}{22.4 \text{ L}} > \frac{2 \text{ g}}{\text{L}}$$

42. E

To answer this question correctly, first write and balance the equation for the combustion described:

$$C_3H_8 + 5 O_2 \rightarrow 3 CO_2 + 4 H_2O$$

For every mole of propane, 5 mol of oxygen will be required. The formula weight of propane is 44 g/mol $(3 \times 12 + 8 \times 1)$, so 88 g will be 2 mol and, therefore, 10 mol of oxygen will be required. At 32 g/mol, 10 mol of O_2 is 320 g.

43. B

According to the periodic table provided with the test, the atomic weight of bromine is 79.9 g/mol. Because 1.204×10^{24} is twice Avogadro's number, 1.204×10^{24} atoms correspond to 2 mol, and the total mass of this number of bromine atoms will be 2 x 79.9 g/mol, or 159.8 g. Note that a rough approximation allows you to dismiss (A), (D), and (E). The question then becomes "more or less than 160?"

44. D

The element has an atomic number of 16, corresponding to 16 protons in its nucleus. A neutral atom of X would thus have 16 electrons surrounding its nucleus. To acquire a –2 charge, an atom of X must acquire two extra electrons, bringing the total number of electrons on the X^{2-} ion to 18. Note that wrong answer (A) corresponds to the number of electrons that must be added to produce the –2 charge, rather than the total number of electrons as requested. (B) and (C) would be correct if we had been asked for the number of electrons in a

4+ or 2+ cation, respectively, rather than the 2– anion. (E) might have been correct if the question had asked for the total number of nucleons rather than for the number of electrons. Note that the atomic weight of the element is an extraneous piece of information that is not necessary for the problem.

45. A
Given that Mg is 2.4312% of the chlorophyll, a 100-g sample of chlorophyll will contain 2.4312 g of magnesium. Because the atomic weight of magnesium is close to 24.312 g/mol, this 2.4312 g will correspond to about one-tenth of a mole, or 6.022×10^{22} atoms. The wrong answers here result from errors in the placement of the decimal point.

46. C
This is a limiting reactant problem, recognizable as such because the quantities of both reactants are given. As occasionally happens, we can recycle some scratch-work from an earlier question. The reaction is the same as that used in question 42, and the same balanced equation applies:

$$C_3H_8 + 5\ O_2 \rightarrow 3\ CO_2 + 4\ H_2O$$

Having found that 320 g of oxygen were required for complete combustion of 88 g of propane in the earlier question, it follows that oxygen will be the limiting reactant here, with only 160 g available. This corresponds to 5 mol of oxygen (molecular weight = 32 g), which in turn implies that 3 mol of carbon dioxide are produced. After determining the formula weight of CO_2 to be 44 g/mol, an answer of 132 g, or (C), is reached.

47. C
The valence, or outermost, electrons are those involved in bonding; it is these same electrons that will determine the chemical properties of an element, simply defined as its ability to combine with other elements or compounds. The number of valence electrons, as offered in (C), is then what most affects the general behavior of an element in the presence of another substance. Elements with a large number of valence electrons (i.e., those found toward the right side of the periodic table), are nonmetallic, with large ionization

energies and electronegativities, for instance, and are thus likely to combine with metals (with a relatively small number of valence electrons) to form ionic compounds.

(A) is incorrect because the electrons in an *s* orbital will affect chemical behavior only if the *s* orbital in question is part of the valence shell; inner *s* orbitals, however, house core electrons which are not involved in bonding. (B) is wrong in that it refers to the protons contained in the nucleus of the atom; the nucleus itself is not involved directly in bond formation, i.e., it does not directly influence chemical interactions, or behavior. (D), although correctly identifying electrons as the influential factor, distorts the truth in saying that it is the total number of electrons, rather than the number in the valence shell. Finally, (E) refers to atomic mass, which, like the number of protons in (B), is wrong in that nuclear rather than chemical properties will be affected by this factor.

48. D
Atomic radii are greatest toward the lower left-hand corner of the periodic table, with cesium, Cs, the largest naturally occurring atom. Atomic radius decreases as one moves from left to right across the table, disqualifying (A), (C), and (E). (B) can be eliminated because atomic size increases, along with principal quantum number, as one moves downward in the periodic table, leaving us with (D), the credited choice.

49. C
This question on VSEPR theory and molecular geometries can be answered by drawing the proper Lewis structure and applying the theory or, more conveniently, by comparing the given compound to a more familiar reference compound. The former approach requires that the Lewis structure be correctly composed of a central nitrogen atom bonded to three surrounding fluorine atoms, with one lone pair of electrons remaining on the nitrogen atom.

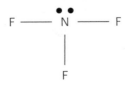

Because four regions of electron density surround the central atom, the electronic geometry is tetrahedral, but because only three of these regions are composed of bonded electrons, the molecular geometry is trigonal pyramidal. In short, the nitrogen trifluoride molecule is of the general formula AB_3U and, thus, has the electronic and molecular geometries associated with this general formula. To approach this problem by comparison to a reference compound, NF_3 is just like NH_3, except that the H atoms have been replaced by F atoms. Because ammonia is a trigonal pyramid, it follows that NF_3 will be as well.

50. D

In general, a cation is smaller than a neutral atom of the same element because the removal of an electron or electrons to form the cation leaves fewer electrons to shield each other from the attractive force of the nucleus. The remaining electrons on the cation are thus drawn in closer to the nucleus, resulting in a reduction in size. Conversely, anions are generally larger than the corresponding neutral atoms due to an increased number of electrons shielding the attractive nuclear force and repelling each other. When attempting to compare the sizes of ions of different elements, it is generally most convenient to compare them to an intermediate species. In this example, each answer choice offers an isoelectronic series of atoms and ions—i.e., each entry in (A), (B), (C), and (D) has 54 electrons, the xenon configuration. With the same number of electrons being attracted to a different nuclear charge, it follows that size will decrease in the same order as atomic number and, therefore, the positive charge of the nucleus increases. Only (D) provides the elements in increasing atomic number order from Te, number 52, through La, number 57.

51. D

This question is testing some basic concepts of quantum mechanics, the relationship between the principal and azimuthal quantum numbers n and l. The secondary, or azimuthal, quantum number l can take on any value from zero to $(n-1)$; when $n = 4$, l can thus have the values 0, 1, 2, 3, as stated in (D).

52. C

This question on reaction stoichiometry requires us to recognize which of the two reactants is the limiting reactant. The equation is provided in its fully balanced form, and we can see that magnesium nitride reacts with water in a 1:6 ratio. Thus 2 mol of magnesium nitride would require 12 mol of water to react fully, which is more than is available in this case. Water is therefore the limiting reactant. Because 2 mol of ammonia are produced for every 6 mol of water, 9 mol of water should yield 3 mol of ammonia. (D), which is incorrect, most likely results from ignoring the limiting reactant aspect of the problem.

53. C

This question may appear to be testing bonding, but it can be answered based on periodic trends. Metallic character increases toward the left side of the periodic table. Sodium and magnesium are both active metals and thus combine with hydrogen to form ionic hydrides. (This is true for any Group IA or IIA metal.) Nitrogen, on the other hand, is a nonmetal and thus combines with hydrogen to form a molecular compound held together by covalent bonding.

54. D

Because 8.0 grams of hydrogen correspond to 4 moles, and they undergo combustion completely, the heat released will be twice that of the reaction as written, which describes the combustion of 2 moles of hydrogen gas: $\Delta H = 2 \times 115.60$ kcal $= 231.2$ kcal.

55. A

This question requires you to interpret the given electron configuration. Adding the superscripts first, we can see that there are 20 electrons all together. This finding is sufficient to dispose of (C), (D), and (E) because they have 21, 19, and 18 electrons, respectively. Calcium does have 20 electrons when neutral; to distinguish between (A) and (B), we will thus need to inspect the order of orbital occupancy. According to the Aufbau principle, 20 electrons should result in the electron configuration $1s^2 2s^2 2p^6 3s^2 3p^6 4s^2$. By occupying the $3d$ subshell instead of the 4s subshell, the given configuration indicates an excited state, and (A) is correct.

56. B

This question can be answered by applying the relationship $\Delta H_{rxn} = \Delta H^{\circ}_{f}$(products) − ΔH°_{f}(reactants). Recalling that ΔH°_{f} for any element is zero, we can substitute values as follows:

$$\Delta H_{rxn} = H^{\circ}_{f}(CO_2) - \frac{1}{2} H_f(O_2) - H^{\circ}_{f}(CO)$$

$$= (-94.05) - (0) - (-26.41)$$

$$= -94.05 + 26.41 = -67.64$$

Note the potential for approximation: −100 + 25 = −75 is close enough for the choices offered. (A) and (D) result if you add the values instead of subtracting them, whereas (C) and (D) come from losing track of the minus sign.

57. D

Increasing pressure would be the result of a decrease in volume (V), an increase in temperature (T), or an increase in the number of moles of gas (n) in the container. Because we are asked about the number of molecules of gas B in an identical container at the same temperature, we can focus on this last variable. To raise the pressure from 25 to 125 torr, or five times as much, we need five times as many moles, or equivalently, five times as many molecules. Because we began with one mole of gas A, we need five moles of gas B; converting moles to molecules, we get (5 mol) × (6.02 × 10²³ molecules/mol) = 3 × 10²⁴ molecules, as stated in (D). (A) results if we misread the question stem and solved for the number of moles instead of the number of molecules, (B) if we forgot to multiply by five, (C) if we messed up the exponent in our calculation, and (E) if we gave up too soon. Note that (B) and (C) could have been eliminated upon the realization that if the pressure is higher, the number of molecules must be greater than that contained in the original sample of gas A.

58. D

Gas volume is proportional to the number of moles of gas present in the sample, all other things being equal. As such, we can predict the required volume by finding the number of moles, or vice versa. Given that 1.0 mL of blood produces 0.15 mL of oxygen, we can extrapolate that 100 mL of the same blood will produce 15 mL of the gas under the same conditions of temperature and pressure. Because one mole of an ideal gas occupies 22.4 L at STP, it follows that 1 mmol of the gas will occupy 22.4 mL, also at STP. The following calculation is therefore valid:

$$15 \text{ mL} \times \frac{1 \text{ mmol}}{22.4 \text{ mL}} = \frac{15}{22.4} \text{ mmol}$$

59. C

This question asks us to apply Le Châtelier's principle to determine which of the choices offered will increase the yield of iodine or, in other words, shift the equilibrium to the right. Because the reaction shown has oxygen as a reactant, addition of oxygen should produce the desired result. (A) is incorrect because the reaction has heat shown as a product; raising the temperature would thus shift the equilibrium to the left. (B) is wrong because addition of a catalyst has no effect on the ultimate position of the equilibrium but only on its rate of attainment. (D) is incorrect because water is a product; adding H_2O would thus shift the equilibrium toward the reactant side, decreasing the yield of iodine. Finally, (E) is wrong because there are more moles of gas shown on the reactant side of the given reaction; an increase in pressure would thus shift toward production of product, while a decrease in pressure would shift the equilibrium to the left.

60. E

This question on periodic trends can be translated to "Which of the following is closest to the upper right-hand corner of the periodic table?", excluding the last column of the table. Chlorine, (E), is above bromine, (D), and far to the right of lithium and sodium, (B) and (C), respectively. Although helium, (A), is furthest in the upper right direction, it is an inert gas and thus does not have a propensity to accept electrons. Remember that the periodic trend of electron affinity, as well as that of electronegativity, does not apply to the rare gases.

61. C

An exothermic reaction is one for which heat is emitted (i.e., one for which ΔH is negative). The sign of ΔH is not directly transferred to ΔG, which also depends partially on the sign and magnitude of ΔS (the entropy change) and on the value of T (the absolute temperature), because $\Delta G = \Delta H - T\Delta S$.

62. E

The balanced equation is:

$$8\,KMnO_4 + 3\,NH_3 \rightarrow 3\,KNO_3 + 8\,MnO_2 + 5\,KOH + 2\,H_2O$$

Adding up the coefficients on the reactant and product sides, then subtracting as the question dictates, yields $(3 + 8 + 5 + 2) - (8 + 3) = 18 - 11 = 7$.

63. E

This question requires us to determine an empirical formula from a given mass ratio. Because the ratio is given as 6 g of carbon for 1 g of hydrogen, and because the atomic weight of carbon is 12 g/mol, it would probably be most convenient just to double the whole ratio. The ratio then becomes 12 g of C for every 2 g of H, or 1 mol C for every 2 mol H. (A) and (B) can be eliminated because they do not contain the correct ratio of carbon to hydrogen content. One may also question whether (A) is a valid empirical formula because it conveys structural information—the presence of a hydroxyl group making it a methanol molecule—that should not be present in an empirical formula, which merely gives the simplest whole number ratio of the atoms present in the compound. (C) and (D) can also be eliminated because the subscripts can be reduced further, making them invalid as empirical formulas. Note that one may easily jump erroneously to (C) as the answer if one does not keep in mind the definition of an empirical formula. (E) lists the atoms in the simplest whole number ratio possible and has the correct proportion of carbon to hydrogen, making it the correct choice. Notice that it was never claimed that the compound contains only carbon and hydrogen!

64. C

This thermodynamics question can be answered by applying the fundamental relationship $\Delta H_{rxn} = \Delta H_f(\text{products}) - \Delta H_f(\text{reactants})$. Recalling that ΔH_f for any element is zero, we can substitute values as follows:

$$\Delta H_{rxn} = 3\,\Delta H^\circ_f(H_2O,\,g) + \Delta H^\circ_f(W,\,s) - \Delta H^\circ_f(WO_3,\,s)$$

$$- 3\,\Delta H^\circ_f(H_2,\,g) = 3(-57.798) + (0) - (-200.84) - 3(0)$$

$$= -173.39 + 200.84 = 27.45$$

Note that the approximation $-180 + 200 = 20$ is quite sufficient to distinguish among the choices offered.

65. A

The magnetic number, m_l, can take on any of the integral values from negative l to positive l inclusive. When $l = 3$, m_l can thus have the values $-3, -2, -1, 0, 1, 2, 3$, as are listed in (A).

66. D

As one descends the column in the periodic table, the principal quantum numbers of the valence shells, and hence the atomic and ionic radii, increase. (D), beryllium, located at the top of Group IIA, is thus the smallest of the ions listed. The increasing order of ionic radius is $Be^{2+} < Mg^{2+} < Ca^{2+} < Sr^{2+}$; the remaining choices are thus incorrect, because each of the other ions is larger than Be^{2+}.

67. B

The value of the equilibrium constant is dependent on temperature. (A), (C), and (E) may change the relative concentrations of the species at equilibrium but would not change the numerical value of K; thus these three choices are incorrect. (D) doesn't affect the position of equilibrium at all, making it incorrect as well.

68. A

It is a general and very nonquantitative rule that many reactions will double their rates for each 10° increase in temperature. This somewhat oddball question can probably best be answered by dismissing the incorrect choices because the stem gives little hint as to what to predict for an answer. (B) is incorrect because, although velocity of particles does increase with increasing temperature, it is unlikely to double for a small temperature rise. (C) can be dismissed because increasing temperature will usually expand a substance; with an increase in volume, the concentration actually decreases. (D) is wrong because the pressure of a gas is proportional to its absolute temperature; a 10°C rise in temperature will thus only double the pressure if the initial temperature was 10 K, a very unlikely temperature for a gas. (The ideal gas law is unlikely to apply at such a low temperature anyway.) Finally, (E) is wrong because in an endothermic reaction, as the question stem indicated, heat is absorbed and not evolved.

69. D

This question requires that you calculate the formula weight of quinine from the given formula and then convert the given mass, in grams, to the number of molecules via Avogadro's number. The formula weight is the sum of the atomic weights of the atoms in the formula, thus, the formula weight of quinine is

$$20 (12) + 24 (1) + 2 (14) + 2 (16)$$

$$= 240 + 24 + 28 + 32 = 324 \text{ g/mol}.$$

There are thus $\frac{16.2}{324}$ moles of quinine in the sample. We can observe that $\frac{16.2}{324}$ is $\frac{1}{20}$; the answer should therefore be about $\frac{1}{20}$ of Avogadro's number, 6×10^{23}.

70. C

Metallic character is the result of the combination of low ionization energy, electron affinity, and electronegativity that increase toward the lower left-hand corner of the periodic table. (Remember that cesium, Cs, is the most metallic naturally occurring element!) The question can thus be translated as, "which of the following lists elements, in order, from upper-right to lower-left on the periodic table?" The four elements listed in the choices are all in the same column of the table, Group IVA, and so we need only to check the vertical arrangement of these elements, which should then be from top to bottom. Descending the column now, the order is Si, Ge, Sn, Pb, the same as that in (C).

71. E

The key here is that bond length decreases as bond order increases (single > double > triple). Thus, reduction of the bond to a lower bond order will result in a longer bond, which is given only in (E). However, even if you did not remember this fact about bonding, there still is a hint here that could help you guess the correct answer. No one would expect you to memorize the exact bond lengths in question, because this is really mindless trivia. However, you could guess that you need to see the trend. There are three choices that are reductions in bond length (none of which you are expected to know!), so you could discount (A), (B), and (C). The only unique answers are (D), no change, and (E), elongation. Because the student might imagine that there should be some difference between the two bond lengths, (E) is the logical choice. The form of the question itself often suggests an answer.

72. C

The slowest and, hence, rate-determining step in an S_N1 reaction is the formation of the carbocation. Molecules that form stable carbocations are therefore more likely to undergo S_N1 reactions. Remember, carbocation stability decreases in this order: tertiary > secondary > primary > methyl. (A) is a primary bromide and would not be expected to react via the S_N1 mechanism at all. (B), (D), and (E) are secondary and will also not be expected to react as readily as (C), the most substituted (tertiary) bromide.

73. C

Obviously, rotation must occur for configuration A to transform into configuration B. However, double bonds, composed of a σ and a π bond, are not free to rotate (hence eliminating (E)), whereas single bonds composed of one π bond have rotational freedom. Therefore, the π bond must be broken, and rotated around the central carbon-carbon σ bond to yield configuration B after reforming the π bond. (A) and (D) are incorrect because breaking the σ bond alone does not alter the stable geometry of the molecule: unlike σ orbitals, π bonds do not have cylindrical symmetry, and rotation about one would disrupt the favorable overlap. (B) is incorrect because the σ bond does not need to be broken.

74.   D

The *sp* hybridization is found only on atoms that are bonded to two other species (each bonded group can be replaced by a lone pair of electrons). With more substituents, more atomic orbitals must be deployed for hybridization to accommodate the expanded valency. (A), (B), and (C) are all *sp²* hybridized (three different bonding partners), whereas (E) is *sp³* hybridized (four bonding partners).

75.   E

The first step in identifying the compound with the most stereoisomers is to determine the number of chiral centers in each molecule. (A) and (D) have three chiral centers each, while choices (B), (C), and (E) have four, as asterisked below:

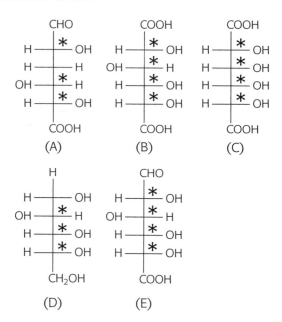

(A) and (D) are thus eliminated. The presence of four chiral centers generally implies the existence of $2^4 = 16$ stereoisomers, except in the cases of *meso* structures, which despite possessing chiral centers are nonetheless superimposable upon their mirror images. The presence of *meso* compounds means that certain enantiomeric pairs are actually identical structures and, thus, the number of stereoisomers

would be lowered. (C) in fact is a *meso* compound, as it is seen easily that it possesses a plane of symmetry and is therefore superimposable upon its mirror image. (B), being itself a stereoisomer of (C), will likewise possess fewer than 16 stereoisomers. (E), in contrast, has different groups attached on each end (an aldehyde on one and a carboxylic acid on the other), and there is no possibility that any of its stereoisomers will be a *meso* compound. It will therefore possess the full 16 stereoisomers allowed by its four chiral centers and is the correct choice.

76.   E

Methyl acetate is an ester composed of acetate (the acid half) and methanol (the alcohol part). (A) is incorrect; it is acetic acid. (B) is simply sodium acetate, a common buffering salt. (C) is dimethyl ether. (D) and (E) are both esters. However, the name should give the clue that one methyl group is present. (D) is incorrect because ethyl acetate (or ethyl ethanoate), a common solvent, does not have a methyl group. Only (E) corresponds to methyl acetate.

77.   D

Properties that stabilize the S_N1 carbocation intermediate or destabilize the S_N2 transition state will favor S_N1 reactions. (A) is incorrect because polar rather than nonpolar solvents will help stabilize the ionic (charged) intermediate, favoring S_N1 mechanisms. (B) is incorrect because temperature does not specifically affect either reaction type one way or the other (although high temperature tends to favor elimination reactions over substitutions in general). (D) is correct because a higher concentration of nucleophile will affect only S_N2 reaction kinetics, whereas S_N1 kinetics is independent of nucleophile concentration. (C) is incorrect because weak nucleophiles will have a hard time displacing the leaving group. This will favor the formation of the carbocation intermediate *before* nucleophilic attack, which is an S_N1 reaction. Obviously, (E) must be incorrect due to the discussion above.

78.   C

Atoms in the ground state have their electrons in the lowest energy configuration. Upon absorbing energy, one or more of the electrons will get promoted into an orbital of higher energy, increasing the energy of the electronic configuration. This does not involve the necessary loss of the electron in question (although it could), which eliminates (A), (B), and (E). In principle, the number of core electrons could also decrease if a core electron is excited to the valence level, but again, this is not a requirement for excitation. The energy is increased and not decreased, so (D) is also incorrect.

79. A

As an uncharged organic molecule, dimethylpropylamine could dissolve at least partially in most organic solvents, eliminating (C) and (D). In aqueous solutions, the amine moiety could act as a base by accepting a proton and acquiring a positive charge, making an ammonium ion, which would be soluble to some extent in water. For this to happen, there must be a supply of protons, whether from the water itself or from an acid. Either dilute or concentrated acid would suffice, thus eliminating (B) and (E). A KOH solution would be very proton-poor, which would leave the amine unprotonated and uncharged. When uncharged, organic molecules are not very soluble in water, so (A) is correct.

80. A

Both cyclohexane and benzene have six carbons. Cyclohexane and other saturated six-member ring structures are found predominantly in the chair formation, but benzene is an unsaturated ring that has a planar geometry. This eliminates (B) and therefore (E) as well. (C) and (D) are also incorrect because benzene is not as stable as cyclohexane thermodynamically. Note that one often says that benzene is stabilized by the resonance delocalization of the π electrons. This does not mean, however, that it is more stable than its fully hydrogenated analog cyclohexane; the extra stability is in reference to nonconjugated trienes.

81. D

The first step in arriving at the correct IUPAC name for an alkane is the identification of the longest unbranched carbon chain in the molecule. In this case, there are many possible choices for the carbon skeleton (because of the equivalence of the four methyl groups), but they all contain three carbon atoms, so the root name for this molecule would be propane.

The only possible candidates then become (C) and (D). Prefixes like *iso*, *neo*, and *sec-* are used in the IUPAC system to label substituents but are not used in naming the backbone; therefore, (D) is correct. One can verify that after singling out a carbon skeleton, the two remaining methyl groups will be attached to the middle carbon atom of the three (i.e., the one numbered two), so 2,2-dimethyl propane is indeed the IUPAC name for the molecule. It should be pointed out that none of the other choices is a valid IUPAC name for *any* compound. Incidentally, the compound is more commonly known as neopentane, and this common name is also recognized by the IUPAC.

82. E

Enantiomers are nonsuperimposable mirror-image isomers of chiral compounds. As mirror images, they occur in pairs, so (D) cannot be correct. The Fischer projections can be rotated in the page, or both pairs of substituents can be exchanged, without changing the chirality of the compound. If compound I is rotated 180° in the page, it gives compound II. These two compounds are therefore identical and are not enantiomers. Compound I is the mirror image of compound III (imagine holding a mirror between compounds I and III), so they are enantiomers. Because I and II are identical, II and III must also be enantiomers.

83. C

The Lewis structure of benzene shows a ring structure with three double bonds and three single bonds. However, this is one case where the inadequacy of the Lewis dot structure approach is revealed. The alternating double bonds drawn are actually π bonds occupied by electrons delocalized about the ring. All six bonds in benzene are equivalent and possess characteristics intermediate between those of single and double bonds. (A) and (B) are therefore incorrect. (D) is incorrect because although benzene is often drawn as two resonant structures where the positions of the single and double bonds have been exchanged, this is merely an attempt to fix the inadequacy of the Lewis structures. No one resonant structure is an accurate depiction of benzene at any one instant of time, and in particular resonant structures should never be thought of as mixtures of different species.

84. B

The oxygen atom has six valence electrons and needs to form two bonds to share two extra electrons to form a stable octet. Therefore, oxygen usually has two unshared electron pairs and two bonds (two single bonds, as in the water molecule, or a double bond, as in the carbonyl group). Oxygen has three bonds here but has done so at the expense of its other unshared electron pair. According to the rule of assigning formal charges to atoms in a molecule, formal charge = valency – half the number of bonding electrons – number of unshared electrons. Thus, in the case of oxygen here, the formal charge

$$= 6 - \left(\frac{1}{2} \times 6\right) - 2 = 1.$$ (A) is incorrect because carbon,

with a valency of four, here participates in four bonds and does not possess any lone pairs. Its formal charge is therefore zero. (C) is incorrect because this type of structure is common for six-ringed structures with oxygen, notably the anomeric carbon of monosaccharides undergoing glycosidic reactions. (D) and (E) are incorrect for the reasons given above.

85. C

The first step toward naming alkanes is to identify the longest carbon chain, which in this case contains nine carbon atoms. This eliminates (B) and (D). The substituents should then be named alphabetically, keeping the numbers of the substituents as small as possible. Here, the substituents are 1,2 dimethylpropyl (using the same rules again to identify the longest chain) and a methyl group. The compound is named 5-(1,2-dimethylpropyl)-2-methylnonane, which is (C).

86. E

Aromatic compounds are cyclic, planar compounds with $(4n + 2)$ π electrons (where n is any non-negative integer). This is known as Hückel's rule. Compound I is benzene with 6 π electrons ($n = 1$) and is therefore aromatic. Compound II, naphthalene, has 10 or ($4 \times 2 + 2$) π electrons and is also aromatic. Compounds III (furan) and IV (pyrrole) are both examples of heterocyclic compounds (cyclic compounds having elements other than carbon in the ring backbone). The oxygen in furan has two lone pairs of electrons. One of the two pairs would participate in the delocalized π cloud, which together with the two double bonds drawn would yield a total of 6 π electrons, thus making furan aromatic. (The other lone pair will occupy an sp^2 orbital orthogonal to the π system.) The nitrogen in pyrrole has a lone pair of electrons that is part of the π system, and thus pyrrole is also aromatic with 6 π electrons. The correct answer must then be all of the above, or (E).

87. A

Boiling points for similar compounds are determined by the amount of hydrogen bonding, dipole moment, and molecular weight, in that order. Hydrogen-bonding and dipole moments increase the attraction molecules have among themselves, which raises the boiling point. Compounds I and III, as carboxylic acids, contain both polar carbonyl groups and hydroxyl groups that are capable of hydrogen bonding. They will thus have the strongest intermolecular interactions and, consequently, the highest boiling points. Because compound III is one methylene unit larger than compound I, it should have the higher boiling point of the two. After these two comes compound IV, which, as an alcohol with a hydroxyl group, is also capable of hydrogen bonding. Compound V is next. It is slightly heavier than compound II but, more importantly, will have a dipole moment because of the high electronegativity of the bromine atom, which will give bromine a slight negative charge. Compound II, a straight chain alkane, has the lowest boiling point. Arranging this information from lowest to highest, we have II, V, IV, I, and III, which is (A). Note that a rudimentary knowledge of what governs boiling points is sufficient to rule out other choices without the need to arrange the five compounds precisely. Straight-chain unbranched alkanes do not possess strong polarity and will be expected to have the lowest boiling points among the compounds, thus eliminating (D) and (E). Compound III is expected to have a higher boiling point than compound I because of its additional methylene group (but otherwise similar chemical functionality). With these two pieces of information alone, one can arrive at the correct answer of (A).

88. D

Amides are amine groups directly bonded to a carbonyl carbon. (A) is a primary amine, with the alkyl group attached to it being an ether. (B) is a secondary amine. Neither of these choices contains a carbonyl group, which is necessary. (C) is a ketone with a tertiary amine substituent: it would be an amide if the intervening methylene group between the carbonyl carbon and the nitrogen were removed.

89. C

Stereoisomers are isomers that arise from the different spatial arrangements of groups attached to double bonds or chiral centers. In this case, the compound has two carbon atoms that are stereocenters (second and third). Each will have either *R* or *S* designations. The possible isomers are then *S,S*, *S,R*, *R,S*, or *R,R*, which is (C). Note that if the two halogens are the same, then the number of stereoisomers will be 3, because then *R,S* would be identical to *S,R*, known as a *meso* compound.

90. E

Overlapping orbitals that are perpendicular to the axis of the bond are features of π bonds. Because the overlap is not cylindrically symmetric, rotation about the interatomic axis would break such bonds. Double bonds consist of one σ and one π bond, whereas triple bonds consist of one σ and two π bonds. (The two π bonds in a triple bond are perpendicular to each other.) (A) and (B) are incorrect because σ bonds, found in single bonds, are formed when the overlap is along the axis joining the atoms. (C) and (D) are incorrect because double and triple bonds differ only in the number of π bonds, not in their nature.

91. D

The compound in question has the common name neopentyl chloride (A) but also has a name assigned under the IUPAC guidelines. (You are expected to know certain common names.) To identify the IUPAC name, one first observes that the longest unbranched chain contains three carbon atoms, and thus the compound is a propane. In numbering the carbon atoms, one tries to minimize the numbers of those with substituents. In this case, we have a chlorine attached to one end and two methyl groups attached to the middle carbon atom,

and given a choice between 1,2 and 2,3, we opt for the former. Alphabetizing the substituents, one arrives at the IUPAC name 1-chloro-2,2-dimethylpropane, which is (B). Both (A) and (B) can be names for the compound shown, and so (D) is correct.

92. A

A secondary amine consists of a nitrogen attached to one hydrogen atom and two alkyl groups. (B) is a tertiary, (C) a primary, and (D) a quaternary amine. (E) is ammonia, which is technically not an amine at all.

93. B

The greater the number of alkyl groups attached to the sp^2 hybridized carbons (i.e., the more substituted they are), the more stable the alkene. Molecule IV has two methyl groups on each side of the double bond and will thus be the most stable among the five, followed by molecule II, which has two methyl groups on one side and one on the other. Next comes molecule I, which has one methyl group on each side. (It is worthwhile to point out that the *trans* configuration would be more stable then the *cis* one, but this aspect is irrelevant here.) Molecule V has only one methyl group on one side, whereas molecule III has none and will therefore be the least stable. Thus, stability in increasing order would go III, V, I, II, IV, which is indicated in (B). Note once again that one can pick out the correct answer without having to determine the entire sequence: knowing that III is the least stable and IV is the most stable would be sufficient.

94. C

The complete oxidation of any hydrocarbon (or carbohydrate) composed solely of carbon, hydrogen, and oxygen is a combustion reaction leading to the products CO_2 and H_2O. (A) is incorrect because combustion reactions such as this are always exothermic. This is the basis of energy sources such as natural gas, propane, octane, etc. (B) is incorrect because the compound listed is an alkane, not an alkene. (D) and (E) do not have the right products.

95. B

Because each carbon of acetylene has two bonding partners (one carbon and one hydrogen), it is *sp* hybridized. The rest of the choices are all true and therefore incorrect. Acetylene, or ethyne, has the molecular formula C_2H_2 (alkynes in general have the molecular formula C_nH_n), and is a linear molecule with a triple bond (one σ and two π bonds). Because it is also symmetric, the (already weak) polarity of the C–H bonds cancel each other vectorially, so the molecule does not have a net dipole moment, making it relatively nonpolar: it is only slightly soluble in water. (A), (C), (D), and (E) are therefore all true.

96. B
Resonance is a mechanism by which molecules are stabilized by delocalization of charges. (A) and (D) are incorrect because all aromatic compounds owe their stability (compared with nonconjugated alkenes and alkynes) to resonance of their conjugated, or alternating, double bonds. (C) is incorrect because organic acid anions, such as the acetate ion depicted here, stabilize their negative charge between the two oxygen atoms of the acid moiety. Finally, (E) is incorrect because one can draw an equivalent resonance structure in which the positive charge of the molecule switches to the other end and the double bond jumps to the other carbons. The π electrons of the double bond are thus delocalized over all three carbon atoms. Only (B), having no double bonds or charges to delocalize, is without stabilizing resonance forms.

97. A
The ion in (A), an allyl cation, is the only one of the choices that has a resonance form that can delocalize the positive charge and thereby stabilize the cation:

$$CH_3 - CH = CH - \overset{\oplus}{CH_2}$$

$$CH_3 - \overset{\oplus}{CH} - CH = CH_2$$

In (B) and (C), the double bond is unable to participate in charge delocalization because of the intervening sp^3 hybridized carbon, which disrupts the π system. In (C), the phenyl group and the double bond are conjugated but do not affect the positive charge. The same is true for the phenyl group in (D). (If the intervening methylene group were removed

we would have the very stable benzyl cation.) (E), a vinyl cation, is also incorrect because the π bond is perpendicular to the empty p orbital of the carbon atom bearing the positive charge; stabilization through delocalization thus cannot take place.

98. A
Of the compounds listed, only alcohols are capable of hydrogen bonding, which is the most important factor when discussing the melting/boiling points of organic compounds. (B), (C), and (D) all may possess dipole moments that will cause them to boil at higher temperatures than that of an alkane (E) of similar molecular weight. However, the dipole interactions are much weaker than are hydrogen-bonding interactions.

99. B
This is a simple matter of evaluating the effects of steric hindrance upon molecule stability. The two phenyl groups are very bulky substituents (much larger than the bromine atoms) and will strive to be as far away from each other as possible. (A) and (C) both will have more steric repulsion than (B), because the phenyl groups will be fighting to occupy the same space. The phenyl rings can, of course, relieve part of the steric repulsion by rotating out of the plane of the double-bonded carbons, but then this means we will have to give up the favorable delocalization of the π electron system that we have in (B).

100. A
This is a textbook S_N2 reaction in which the oxygen atom on the ethoxide ion acts as a nucleophile and displaces the iodine. The iodide ion is a good leaving group, and ethoxide is a good nucleophile. The methyl species is sterically unhindered, and the ethoxide is not a very bulky base (which would have favored E2 over S_N2). The resultant products are $C_2H_5OCH_3$ (ethyl methyl ether) and iodide ion that may complex with the positive sodium ion, depending on the solvent. This reaction is, in fact, a Williamson ether synthesis.

Reading Comprehension
ANSWERS AND EXPLANATIONS

ANSWER KEY

1. A	9. E	17. C	25. A	33. A
2. B	10. C	18. E	26. C	34. C
3. E	11. C	19. A	27. D	35. B
4. D	12. C	20. C	28. C	36. D
5. B	13. E	21. D	29. E	37. A
6. D	14. C	22. A	30. B	38. E
7. B	15. D	23. B	31. C	39. B
8. D	16. B	24. B	32. D	40. D

1. A

The passage states clearly that the speech pathologist and the orthodontist deal with problems of improper speech in different contexts, one functional and the other structural. While it may be argued that orthodontists need more training than speech pathologists, the passage does not address this issue. In addition, the passage does not indicate that orthodontics and speech therapists are contraindicated in cases of lisping or that one works better on adolescents. Orthodontics corrects structural anomalies, not functional disorders. Therefore, choice (A) is the correct answer.

2. B

The author of the passage states that the purpose of passive methods of speech therapy is to direct the child's articulatory organs into the proper position for making a correct sound. Speech therapy itself supposes the development of new sounds, and passive therapy methods involve close personal contact between therapist and child. However, passive methods of speech therapy are not effective in cases of severe malocclusion.

3. E

One of the main benefits of speech therapy is that it takes what is already there—the child's vocal anatomy—and teaches the child to utilize it effectively.

As a result, surgery is often unnecessary, as described in choice (E). Choice (A) is incorrect because many patients do achieve desired results, especially with problems of sibilant articulation. Choice (B) is wrong because in many cases speech defects can be treated without the use of orthodontic equipment. Choice (C) is also incorrect because the passage does not mention lack of emotional support as a cause of speech defects. The correlation of speech problems and learning disabilities (D) is not addressed in the passage and has little foundation.

4. D

The author states that the cardinal rule of speech therapy is that the patient must learn an entirely new sound to compensate for the one he or she is incapable of articulating. It is quite possible that the child with a speech disorder may be better served if orthodontic treatment is completed before speech therapy is initiated, thereby preserving the anatomy during the therapeutic process. While active methods of speech therapy are important, the passive methods of speech therapy are equally critical. Therefore, choice (D) is correct.

5. B

The author states that the active methods of speech therapy are deductive in nature, as they begin with sounds that the child can already make, and work toward the sound that is to be learned. Passive methods retrain the articulatory organs. While the use of mirrors for speech therapy is often associated with passive methods, it is not this characteristic that is essential to active speech therapy. The use of active therapy does not obviate the use of passive therapy. Thus, choice (B) is correct.

6. D

It can be inferred from the passage that problems with the articulation of sibilants generally appear late in the child's language development because the *s* sounds are the last to appear in the course of development. The correction of sibilants can be performed using active speech therapy, but not always easily, and can be completed without the use of surgery. Usually, the sibilant mispronunciations lie in the manner in which the child verbalizes the *s* sound, not in the anatomy. Therefore, choice (D) is correct.

7. B

During the description of active speech therapy, the author provides the caveat that the speech therapists must avoid the demonstration of perfect pronunciation because it is of no use to the patient and predisposes the patient to tension and nervousness. While it may be argued that choice (A) is a viable option, the speech therapist should be more aware of the proper pronunciation shortcoming rather than the treatment of a class III malocclusion with the subsequent referral of the patient to a surgeon. Speech therapists often associate articulative mechanisms with particular sounds and more often than not can correct lisps without the help of orthodontists. Therefore, choice (B) is correct.

8. D

The author states that the recommended attitude of therapy is the combined use of orthodontists and speech therapists, rendering results faster and more positive. The author believes that the benefit from speech therapy can often come when orthodontic work is not performed; however, in many cases orthodontics aid in the process of speech therapy. While orthodontic treatment is sometimes detrimental to the progress speech therapy alone has made, it is never contraindicated to the treatment of structural vocal defects. The passage does not mention the use of modern advances in dental surgery for the treatment of speech disorders. Therefore, choice (D) is correct.

9. E

The passage states that an appliance for class II malocclusion must be worn for at least 13 hours a day. To save the child more emotional embarrassment, this appliance is worn at night. The night brace is also worn in class III malocclusion, but this was not presented as an answer choice. Treatment of problems with sibilant articulation involving night braces is not discussed in the passage. Therefore, choice (E) is correct.

10. C

The passage states that as a form of preventive dentistry, orthodontics is concerned with the correction of dental anomalies for the purpose of heading off future difficulties. It is not speech pathology, or functional therapy, or sibilant modification; these therapies are initiated by speech therapists. Therefore, choice (C) is correct.

11. C

Active methods of speech therapy, which begin with sounds that the child can already make, are often desired in lisping because the child is usually able to pronounce some of the *s* sounds. Usually, these children do not need orthodontic treatment; active speech therapy is sufficient. Therefore, choice (C) is correct.

12. C

An example the author gives of initiating passive speech therapy is for a therapist to show a child how to approximate the position of the front teeth. This is in accordance with learning the proper alignment of the front teeth. Listening to recordings and performing exercises to increase tongue flexibility are not passive processes, nor is recognizing that changing one's speech habits is an emotional process as well as a physical one. Wearing a night brace would be a treatment prescribed by a orthodontist, not a speech therapist.

13. E

In the description of class I malocclusions, the author argues against the use of removable appliances. Removable appliances, he claims, may be neglected, which can bring progress to a halt. Class II malocclusive patients often suffer from "buck teeth." In addition, the passage does not mention the irritation of removal devices to gums or the age of patients with fixed appliances. Therefore, choice (E) is correct.

14. C

The passage states the number of U.S. citizens 85 years old and older is growing six times as fast as the rest of the population. It makes no mention of these citizens being predominantly male; instead, it argues that the majority of these individuals are female. The author does note that hundreds of thousands of senior citizens have migrated to the Sunbelt states over the last 30 years. Yet he never delineates what percentage of these seniors is over 85. Further, there is no indication in the passage that those 85 and older primarily live in the Sunbelt states. In addition, the 85-year-old and older population is not solely responsible for the high cost of medical care. The passage indicates that it is the disabled elderly (hence, not just those 85 and older) and people without insurance of all ages who are contributing to high costs. Finally, there is no indication in the passage that those 85 and older on average garner an annual income between $20,000 and $50,000. The facts that "77 percent of elderly Americans have annual incomes of less than $20,000" and that "most elderly Americans come to depend heavily on federal and state subsidies...as their earning power declines and their need for health care increases" seem to imply that, if anything, those 85 and older most likely do not earn average annual incomes between $20,000 and $50,000.

15. D

The author indicates in lines 84–86 that "by the year 2030, there'll only be two workers for every person 65 and older." While the passage mentions the threat to Social Security by constant borrowing to pay interest on the national debt, the author never indicates that there will be no money left in Social Security by 2030. The passage never indicates that there will be a ratio of 81 men for every 100 women in the U.S. by 2030; rather, it reveals that by the age of 65, there are only 81 men left for every 100 women. Choice (C) is simply incorrect. The passage reveals that by the year 2030, there will be 65 million senior citizens (not 51 million). Finally, while the last paragraph of the passage indicates that in the next few decades the U.S. population may demand a less expensive health care system, it never specifically says that there will be a new system in place in 2030.

16. B

The author states in lines 131–133 that "the elderly population will double within the next 40 years." There is no indication in the passage that there is a current housing shortage (much less that the elderly are responsible for such a shortage) or that the elderly are the wealthiest segment of the U.S. population (in fact, the passage reveals that most elderly come to rely heavily on federal and state subsidies). In addition, the passage never mentions that the elderly account for 30 percent of the U.S. population; rather, it reflects that by 1990 "spending on the elderly accounted for 30 percent of the annual federal budget." Finally, although there has been a large flux of senior citizens into Sunbelt states over the last 30 years, there is no evidence in the passage that seniors constitute the majority of the population in these states.

17. C

The passage defines the "baby boom" generation as the generation born after World War II. It goes on to state that between 1946 and 1964 (the baby boom period), more than 75 million Americans were born. The baby boom generation does not have the highest life expectancy of any generation; rather, the newest generation does, owing to medical advances, etc. The median age of the U.S. population (in general) at the start of the 1990s was 33; there is no indication in the passage of the median age of the baby boom generation. In addition, there is no evidence that the baby boom generation regards its parents as a financial burden. In fact, the passage seems to imply that many of the baby boom generation's parents are taking care of them. As the author indicates, "today's elders often find themselves acting as family bankers," and most own their homes while their children encounter difficulty in financing a home. Finally, baby boomers have not yet reached the ranks of the elderly; as the passage indicates, "in less than two decades, they will join the ranks of America's elderly."

18. E

According to the author, demographic experts predict that the southward migration of the elderly will diminish in the future, since surveys have found that the great majority of people 55 and older would prefer not to relocate. The passage does not correlate southward migration with relatively low incomes or with the shrinking of the U.S. workforce. This shrinking, rather, has been attributed to the fact that the number of available young workers is decreasing. In addition, there is no indication that seniors migrated south because of the availability of low-cost housing. Finally, there is no evidence in the passage that seniors migrated to the south because of overcrowded conditions in the north.

19. A

The author states that presently one out of every two marriages ends in divorce; thus, the current divorce rate is approximately 50 percent (not less than 40 percent). In addition, there is no indication in the passage that the divorce rate is rising rapidly or slowly declining. Finally, the current divorce rate is affecting family structures, as the author states that with the present occurrence of divorce, "a significant number of today's grandparents are suddenly faced with the task of raising or helping to raise their grandchildren."

20. C

The passage specifically indicates that "in less than two decades, they [the baby boom generation] will join the ranks of America's elderly." There is no evidence that baby boomers will migrate west in search of employment or that baby boomers (specifically) will fail to qualify for health insurance. The passage clearly states that early retirement will probably "become a thing of the past" and that "[a]s the number of available younger workers shrinks, elderly people will become more attractive as prospective employees." Finally, an increased birthrate for this generation in the future is wrong, as the passage reveals that millions of baby boomers have already entered middle age and that in the next two decades they will join the ranks of the elderly.

21. D

The author lists a myriad of factors that contribute to increased life expectancy, including improved public sanitation, the ever-increasing popularity of physical fitness, federal and state aid for the poor and senior

citizens, and advances in medicine. No mention is made of a decline in birth rate.

22. A

According to the passage, 77 percent of the elderly earn less than $20,000 per year. While the passage notes that the cost of providing care for disabled elderly will double in the next decade, there is no indication that a majority of the elderly suffer a disability between the ages of 65 and 75. In addition, the author states that approximately 75 percent of today's elderly own their own homes. It can also be construed that a majority of the elderly no longer work. The passage states that at present, only 15 percent of 65-year-old men work, that the median retirement age is now 61, and that early retirement flourished over the last four decades. Finally, the elderly do depend on subsidies, and in large numbers. According to the passage, "[a]s their earning power declines and their need for health care increases, most elderly Americans come to depend heavily on federal and state subsidies."

23. B

The author states that the cost of caring for disabled elderly Americans is expected to double in the next decade alone. This cost will add to the continuous upward spiral of medical costs that threaten the Medicaid/Medicare system. In all likelihood, then, these systems will become increasingly expensive. There is no indication in the passage that the government will be unable to finance a national health care system; in fact, the only obstacles that the author notes to such a system are the medical establishment and various special interest groups. In addition, there is no evidence that the government will have to (or be able to) borrow from Social Security to finance Medicaid/Medicare. It may be argued that baby boomers will be unable to receive federal health benefits as they grow older if costs continue to escalate. Yet, according to the passage, this group will not be without federal health benefits, as it will probably demand a national health care system over the next few decades. Finally, while the passage does note the improvement of medicine in the recent past, there is no indication that the ensuing increase in health care costs of the elderly can be correlated with poor care in the past.

24. B

It can be inferred from the passage that the process of early retirement is a relatively recent phenomenon. The author supports this inference by stating that in 1950, about 50 percent of all 65-year-old men still worked; today, only 15 percent of them do. Early retirement will not transform the workforce of the future; rather, it is said to have transformed the workforce of the past 40 years. In addition, it will most likely not become more popular in the next century, as the passage states that it will soon become a thing of the past. There is no indication that early retirement is correlated with a decline in the U.S. economy. Finally, there is no proof in the passage that early retirement restructured the U.S. workforce prior to World War II; instead, the passage reflects that early retirement transformed the workforce after WW II.

25. A

The passage states that elders—those people 65 and older—now outnumber teenagers for the first time in American history. It can be inferred that today's elderly population is not larger than the current population of baby boomers, as the passage notes that the reason the elderly population will be even larger in the future is that the baby boom generation will be entering the ranks of senior citizens. The elderly population of today is larger than that of 1950 or 1970; the passage states that "the population of elders has doubled in just 40 years." Finally, the elderly population of today will not be larger than the projected elderly population of the year 2030. As the passage indicates, "the elderly population will double within the next 40 years."

26. C

The author of the passage states that one offshoot of the aging of America will be a gradual restructuring of the family unit away from the traditional nuclear family and toward a multigenerational family dominated by elders, not by their adult children. Thus, the typical U.S. family will not be youth-oriented. In addition, there is no specific indication that this family type will be wealthier than today's family structure or that this family unit will be subsidized by Social Security. Finally, the passage never mentions that the typical future family structure will be free from divorce (in fact, the opposite could be argued, as the author states that one of every two marriages today ends in divorce).

27. D

The author states that over the past 30 years, hundreds of thousands of senior citizens migrated south to Sunbelt states. There is no indication in the passage that many seniors worked past the age of retirement, lost their Social Security benefits, or suffered a serious physical disability. Finally, there is no evidence that many of the elderly lost their homes over the past 30 years; on the contrary, the passage notes that 75 percent of today's elderly own their own homes.

28. C

The author argues that a nationalized health care system has not been implemented in the United States because the medical establishment and various special interest groups have so far blocked legislation aimed at creating one. There is no indication in the passage that the federal deficit, the efficacy of Medicare/Medicaid, or expense is the impediment to a national health care system. Finally, according to the passage, millions of U.S. citizens cannot afford private health insurance (which is an argument for nationalizing health care).

29. E

The paragraph states that carbon-14 rather than carbon-11 is used in biological experiments because carbon-14 has a half-life of 5,730 years while carbon-11 has a half-life of only 20 minutes. The short half-life causes it to disintegrate too quickly to be detected and emit too intense a radiation, which may be detrimental to tissue with which it comes into contact.

30. B

As the passage describes, the Geiger counter merely indicates the presence of a radioactive material when it receives significantly more radiation than that normally present in the atmosphere. In contrast, radioactive emissions detected via photographic film are indicated both with respect to the total number of radioactive particles emitted by the sample as well as by the distribution. Therefore, choice (B) is correct because the film can indicate the area where the radiation is absorbed.

31. C

The passage describes a beta particle as a high-speed electron that is produced when neutrons are converted to protons. While this type of emission will raise the atomic number by 1, the mass number will remain the same. Therefore, phosphorus-32 emitting a beta particle will result in the formation of an atom with 1 higher proton number but the same mass number. This would be sulfur-32 (proton number of 33, mass number of 32).

32. D

The passage states that photographic films will darken when exposed to radiation of higher intensity or for longer duration. Therefore, the degree to which photographic film badges worn by workers in plants where radiation is present darken represents the total radiation absorbed over the period of time for which the badge is worn.

33. A

Geiger counters are composed of two electrodes sealed in a tube containing argon gas. High-energy radioactive particles ionize the argon gas and allow charges to bridge the gap between the electrodes. The result of this process is the clicking noise of a Geiger counter. The passage states that Geiger counters are incapable of detecting neutrons because neutrons are not charged. This is because uncharged atomic components cannot ionize argon gas and, therefore, cannot cause a current between the electrodes of a Geiger counter. Therefore, choice (A) is correct.

34. C

Isotopes, as defined in the passage, are elements with the same number of protons and different numbers of neutrons. The distinction of an isotope has nothing to do with the charge of the nucleus, the electron configuration, or the number of electrons.

35. B

Although the photographic film can detect location of radiation (something the Geiger counter cannot), it is less sensitive than the Geiger counter. Choice (A) is incorrect, as a Geiger counter cannot detect the presence of neutrons, and Geiger counters are not able to detect atmospheric radiation (choice C). The Geiger counter

is more portable than photographic film. The efficiency of the Geiger counter and the film is not discussed.

36. D

The passage states the disadvantages of using isotopes with short half-lives: 1) short half-lives result in disintegration of isotopes that cannot be detected, and 2) the intensity of radiation emitted by isotopes with short half-lives is more damaging to tissue. However, in contrast, the disadvantage of the isotopes with long half-lives is that they often emit radiation at a rate too small to be detected.

37. A

Cyclotrons accelerate electrons and protons, while fission reactors produce neutron bullets. Because neutrons are uncharged particles, they are not repelled by any part of a target atom and can therefore penetrate an atom much more easily than either protons or electrons. It follows that the use of neutrons allows for a much wider variety of radioactive particles to be produced than when protons or electrons are used.

38. E

The first two paragraphs of the passage describe the general structure and nomenclature used when describing an atom. Therefore, choice (E) is the most logical answer. The history of the study of atoms is not delineated within the passage, and the detection of radioactive emissions and the production of radioisotopes, while addressed in the passage, are not discussed within the first two paragraphs. Dangers of radioactive experiments are also not touched upon in the first two paragraphs of this passage.

39. B

The passage states that the use of radioisotopes in research is based upon the fact that radioisotopes have the same chemical properties as their nonradioactive counterparts. For example, in biological systems, radioactive substances will localize themselves in the same area as nonradioactive isotopes of the same element. Therefore, choice (B) is correct. Choice (A) is a poor possibility because isotopes with short half-lives have significant side effects stemming from tissue damage. Additionally, these isotopes are not inert; they emit radiation. Often, they can be harmful to the organism being studied. Isotopes with very long half-lives emit radiation at a rate too small to be detected.

40. D

Look for the false statement in these choices. In the final paragraph, the author discusses the use of radioisotopes in experiments that involve blood. Choice (D) is incorrect because blood does need to be taken in this type of experimentation to determine the radiation intensity. Since radiation intensity must be measured, choice (E) is a true statement. Choice (A) is correct—this is the purpose of the experiment. The second sentence states that radioactive blood is injected into the organism, making choice (B) a correct statement. Choice (C) is a true statement because blood must be drawn after "a suitable period of time."

Physics
ANSWERS AND EXPLANATIONS

ANSWER KEY

1. D	9. A	17. D	25. B	33. C
2. E	10. E	18. D	26. D	34. D
3. D	11. A	19. D	27. B	35. A
4. B	12. E	20. C	28. E	36. C
5. A	13. D	21. C	29. B	37. A
6. B	14. A	22. B	30. D	38. C
7. A	15. D	23. D	31. C	39. B
8. E	16. C	24. D	32. B	40. C

1. D

The force on q^+ due to Q^+ is directed along the line joining the two and also directed away from Q^+ because the two charges repel. The force on q^+ due to Q^- is directed along the line joining the two and toward Q^- because the two charges attract. The net force due to the two charges is the vector sum of the force due to each. So we have to sum two vectors, one of which is directed toward the bottom right part of the page and the other toward the bottom left part of the page. Clearly the net vector will be directed generally downward.

2. E

The system is a simple schematic of a mirror, which consists of a piece of glass and a silver backing. In general, whenever light reaches an interface, some of it is reflected and the rest of it is transmitted (and refracted). The proportion of light that is reflected depends on such factors as the relative indices of refraction of the two media, the angle of incidence, and the wavelength of the light. Reflection, then, occurs at all three interfaces, although with different intensities.

3. D

From Kirchhoff's first law, we know that if 2 A pass through the 3Ω resistor, then 2 A must also pass through the combination of the 2Ω and 1Ω resistors.

We then have $2 = I_1 + I_2$, where I_1 is the current through the 1Ω resistor and I_2 is the current through the 2Ω resistor. Because the resistors are in parallel, we also know that the voltage drop across each is the same, so $I_1(1) = I_2(2)$ (i.e., the voltage drop is IR). Substituting for I_1 in the first equation we have $2 = 2I_2 + I_2 = 3I_2 \Rightarrow I_2 = \frac{2}{3}$ A.

4. B

When light passes from one medium to another, its frequency remains the same and its wavelength changes. The only answer choice consistent with this is (B). For completeness, let's see just how the wavelength changes. We should remember that the index of refraction of water is greater than that of air. Also recall that $v = \frac{c}{n}$, where n is the index of refraction and v is the speed of light in the medium. But it's also true that $v = \lambda f$, so we have $\lambda f = \frac{c}{n} \Rightarrow \lambda = \frac{c}{nf}$. Thus, given constant frequency, we see that wavelength decreases when index of refraction increases. Another way to think about this is to remember that speed always decreases when going through a medium with greater index of refraction. Given fixed frequency, speed can only decrease when wavelength decreases.

5. A

All objects radiate electromagnetic radiation because of their nonzero absolute temperature. Also, the intensity of radiation is proportional to the temperature. Given that the energy of radiation, E, is related to frequency by $E = hf$, higher temperature means higher frequency of radiation. Because the speed of the radiation is simply the speed of light, c, we also have that $c = \lambda f$. So higher frequency means shorter wavelength. Thus, higher temperature means a greater intensity of shorter wavelength radiation.

6. B

From the top figure, we see that the equilibrium configuration of the stick is such that approximately half the stick is submerged. In this case, equilibrium means that the downward force of gravity is exactly balanced by the upward buoyant force, resulting in zero acceleration. Consider figure 1. Because less of the stick is submerged than at equilibrium, we know that the upward buoyant force is smaller than the downward gravitational force, so there will be a net downward force and thus a nonzero acceleration. In figure 2, the stick has the same configuration as at equilibrium, which means no net force and, thus, zero acceleration. (B) is then the correct answer choice. For completeness, consider the other choices. Figure 3 shows a scenario where a greater portion of the stick is submerged than at equilibrium. This means the buoyant force will be greater than the force of gravity and there will be a net upward force and, thus, nonzero acceleration. Figure 4 is essentially the same general case as figure 1, and figure 5 is the same general case as figure 3.

7. A

Total internal reflection occurs when the angle of refraction equals 90°. From Snell's law, we have $n_1\sin\theta_1 = n_2\sin\theta_2$. Total internal reflection means $\sin\theta_2 = \sin 90° = 1$. Thus, the minimal angle of incidence for total internal reflection is found from $n_1\sin\theta_1 = n_2$, which implies $\theta_1 = \sin^{-1}\left(\frac{n_2}{n_1}\right)$.

8. E

Notice that the end products of the given reaction are a nucleus with atomic number 14 and a positron, which is a particle with atomic number 1. Because atomic number must balance on both sides of a reaction, we know that the atomic number of nucleus Y is 15. Now notice that Y is produced from nucleus X and an alpha particle. Recall that an alpha particle is just a helium nucleus. So the atomic number of X plus 2 must equal 15 (the atomic number of the neutron, n, is 0), which means the atomic number of X is 13.

9. A

Consider what must occur for the bat to receive an echo. The sound emitted by the bat must reflect off an object and then be received by the bat. Reflection occurs because the incident soundwave causes the molecules at the surface of the object to oscillate, giving rise to a reflected sound wave. Consider the frequency of the sound received at the position of the stationary object. According to the Doppler effect, this frequency will be greater than the frequency produced by the bat because the bat is moving toward the stationary object. The reflected frequency (echo) is then higher than the frequency emitted by the bat. Because the bat is moving toward this reflected sound wave, the frequency perceived by the bat is even higher than the frequency of the echo. The net effect is that the bat receives a frequency higher than the original frequency emitted.

10. E

We're given that a certain block floats in water but not given any information that would allow us to determine the density of the block, other than to know that the density of the block is less than the density of water (because the block floats). The second liquid mentioned has a specific gravity of 0.5, which means that its density is $\frac{1}{2}$ the density of water. Without any information to determine the density of the block, we don't know if the block's density is greater or less than that of the second liquid. In other words, if the block's density is less than that of the liquid, it will float to the top. If the block's density is greater than that of the liquid, the block will sink to the bottom of the liquid and be partially submerged in the water. We conclude that we have insufficient information to determine what happens to the block.

11. A

Recall that pressures in flowing fluids are described by Bernoulli's equation and volume flow rates by the continuity equation. Specifically, the continuity equation states that the volume flow rate is a constant; thus, we can eliminate (C) and (D). Now recall that Bernoulli's equation states

$P_1 + \frac{1}{2}\rho v_1^2 + \rho g y_1 = P_2 + \frac{1}{2}\rho v_2^2 + \rho g y_2$, where 1 and 2

refer to any two points in the fluid flow. Let's consider 1 and 2 to be A and B, respectively. Because the cross section is constant, we know the velocity at A is the same as the velocity at B (this follows from the continuity equation). Thus, we have $P_A + \rho g y_A = P_B +$

$\rho g y_B$. Now notice that $y_B > y_A$, which implies (from the equation) $P_A > P_B$.

12. E

The pressure in a liquid exists in all directions, so there will be pressure on the top, the bottom, and the sides of the cube.

13. D

Heat added to a substance is related to the change in temperature of the substance via the equation $\Delta Q = mc\Delta T$, where m is the mass of the substance, c is the specific heat, ΔQ is the heat added, and ΔT is the change in temperature (final minus initial). The specific heat of water is 1 cal/(gm·°C), 1 L = 1,000 cm^3, and the density of water is 1 g/cm^3. The volume of the pool is then 1.86×10^8 cm^3, which corresponds to a mass of $m = \rho V = (1)(1.86 \times 10^8) = 1.86 \times 10^8$ g. The total amount of heat added is 1,000 BTU/hour $\times$ 2 hour = 2,000 BTU = (2,000)(934 kcal) = 1.868×10^6 kcal = 1.868×10^9 cal. So our equation becomes $1.868 \times 10^9 = (1.86 \times 10^8)(1)\Delta T$; $\Delta T = 10$. Given an initial temperature of 20°C, we have a final temperature of 30°C.

14. A

The pressure at a depth H below the surface of a liquid is given by $P = P_o + \rho g H$, where P_o is the pressure at the surface, and ρ is the density of the liquid. Notice that this expression has no reference to the dimensions of the container holding the liquid. Because both tubes are filled to the same height, the pressure at the bottom of each will be the same.

15. D

To determine the scale reading, we'll have to compute the weight of the liquid in each tube. The weight of the liquid is simply mg, where m is the mass of the liquid. Expressing mass in terms of density by $m = \rho V$, we have weight equals $\rho g V$. So given equal liquid densities, weight is simply proportional to volume of liquid. Now recall that the volume of a cylinder is base $\times$ height = $\pi r^2 H$, where r is the radius of the cylinder (tube). The narrower tube has volume $V_1 = \pi D^2 H$, and the wider tube has volume $V_2 = \pi(4D)^2 H = 16\pi D^2 H$. The ratio of V_1 to V_2 is then 1:16, which is also the ratio of the weights.

16. C

The electric field of a collection of charges is the vector sum of the electric fields due to each of the separate charges. Recall that electric fields point away from positive charges and toward negative charges. Consider any point along the line joining the positive and negative charge. The electric field due to the positive charge is directed away from the positive charge, which means it's directed toward the negative charge. Likewise, the electric field due to the negative charge is directed toward the negative charge. Thus, the total electric field is the sum of two vectors, both directed toward the negative charge. The result is clearly a vector directed at the negative charge.

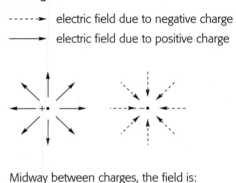

Midway between charges, the field is:

17. D

To solve this problem, we have to consider the combined effect of an electric and a magnetic field. The total force on a given particle will be the vector sum of the forces due to the electric and magnetic fields. Uncharged particles, of course, experience no force from either field; thus, we immediately determine that III is a true statement. We then eliminate (A), (B), and (E). Consider choice I. A positive charge will experience a force in the direction of an electric field (i.e., toward the top of the page). If this charge moves across the page from left to right and a magnetic field is directed out of the page, then the right-hand rule gives a magnetic force down the page. The sum of the electric and magnetic fields, in this case, can equal zero, resulting in no net force. Choice I is correct, which means (D) is correct. For completeness, choice II will give an electric force toward the top of the page and a magnetic force toward the top of the page. The net force will then be toward the top of the page, which means the net force isn't zero.

18. D
When an object loses heat, its temperature changes according to $Q = mc\Delta T$, where c is the specific heat and ΔT is the change in temperature. We're given the mass and final temperature but not the specific heat of water or the initial temperature. From this information we can rule out (A), (B), and (E). We're told, however, that the water turns to ice. Thus, in addition to the heat lost in cooling the water to 0°C, the water loses latent heat as it turns to ice. The latent heat is given by mL, where L is the latent heat of fusion of water. Thus we require the initial temperature, the specific heat of water, and the latent heat of fusion of water.

19. D
Consider (A), which states that the image distance equals the object distance. If this is true, then the magnification has magnitude 1, because $m = -\dfrac{i}{o}$, where i is the image distance and o is the object distance. Because we're told the image is greatly magnified we can safely rule out this choice. (B) says the image is real and upright. A real image means that i > 0. Given o > 0, we have m < 0, which gives an inverted image. So we rule out (B). (C) can be ruled out because a virtual image wouldn't be projected on a screen. (D) is correct because i > o will give a magnification. For completeness, we rule out (E) because an image at the focal point implies o is infinity, which implies m = 0 (i.e., the image is a point).

20. C
Image formation by a diverging mirror is governed by the equation $\dfrac{1}{o} + \dfrac{1}{i} = \dfrac{1}{f}$ where o is the object distance, i is the image distance and f is the focal length and is negative. A real object means o > 0, which then implies (via the above equation) i < 0. Consider the answer choices. (A) is clearly false because we've found i < 0. In general the image distance is different than the object distance, so we can rule out (B). From the equation $m = -\dfrac{i}{o}$, and the fact that i < 0, we determine that m > 0, which means the image is

upright. Thus (C) is true. (E) is ruled out because it's actually the same as (A).

21. C
Because all the answer choices deal with the energy of a photon, we need an expression that relates energy and wavelength. Recall E = hf is the equation relating energy and frequency. For a photon, frequency and wavelength are related via $c = \lambda f$. Substituting for frequency in the energy equation, we have $E = hc/\lambda$. Thus, energy is inversely proportional to wavelength. Doubling the wavelength will result in halving the energy.

22. B
A gamma ray is simply a ray of energy. Thus, when a nucleus emits a gamma ray, the atomic number and the mass number remain the same, but the gamma ray carries away energy. The result is that the nucleus loses energy and becomes more stable.

23. D
The maximum displacement is given by the maximum of the function Asin(kx-wt). The maximum of any sine function is always 1. Thus, the maximum of the given function is simply A, which means that the maximum displacement is A meters.

24. D
This problem requires a direct application of the right-hand rule for determining the direction of magnetic fields produced by currents. The rule says to put the thumb of the right hand along the direction of the current and then the fingers of the right hand curl in the direction of the field. For a current directed into the page, this gives a magnetic field that curls in a clockwise sense.

25. B
When two waves are 180° out of phase and meet, they exhibit destructive interference. This means that one wave has a crest and the other a valley at this point. For an amplitude of A, a crest means a displacement of A, and a valley means a displacement of –A. The displacement of the superposition of the two waves is then the sum of the displacements of each wave. The wave with amplitude A_1 exhibits a crest so it contributes a

displacement of A_1. The wave with amplitude A_2 exhibits a valley, so it contributes a displacement of $-A_2$. The resulting displacement is $A_1 - A_2$. Note that (A) is correct only if the two interfering waves have the same amplitude. If the amplitudes are different, as is the case here, the destructive interference is not total.

26. D

The absolute pressure at a depth of 1,000 m is $P_o + 1,000\rho_s g$. This pressure must be balanced by an equal and opposite pressure to avoid a breach of the hull of the vessel. Given that the inside cabin pressure is P_o, the hull must be capable of withstanding the remaining pressure of $1,000\rho_s g$.

27. B

According to the second law of thermodynamics, heat spontaneously flows from a hot body to a cold body but not the other way around. For the pond to freeze it must lose heat. Regardless of the initial water temperature, at some point in the freezing process heat will be flowing spontaneously (without outside intervention) from a colder body (the pond) to a warmer body (the air). This violates the second law of thermodynamics.

28. E

The apparent weight of an object is the difference between the downward gravitational force on the object (mg) and the upward buoyant force on the object. Recall that the upward buoyant force is given by ρgV, where ρ is the density of the liquid and V is the volume of the liquid displaced. Because both blocks are of equal volume and are completely submerged, they will both experience the same upward buoyant force F_B. The apparent weight of the mass m block is then $W_1 = mg - F_B$, and the apparent weight of the mass 2m block is then $W_2 = 2mg - F_B$. The ratio of the apparent weights is $\dfrac{mg - F_B}{2mg - F_B}$ and thus can't be determined without knowledge of F_B.

29. B

Recall that when a solid melts into a liquid, the phase transition occurs at a constant temperature; and that heat must be added at this constant temperature simply to cause this transition to occur. Physically,

this latent heat is used to break the interatomic bonds that form the structure of the solid. So adding a bit more heat to the block will cause some of the aluminum to melt, but the temperature will remain at the melting point.

30. D

To determine the initial speed of the car, we can use the equation describing the horizontal motion of the car (i.e., $x = v_{ox}t$, where v_{ox} is the initial speed). We're given a horizontal range of $x = 100$ m, so to find speed, we simply need to know the amount of time required to hit the ground. To summarize, $v_{ox} = 100/t$, where t is the time to hit the ground. To find t, we'll use the equation describing the vertical motion of the car. The equation is $y = 125 - \frac{1}{2}gt^2$, where we take the ground as $y = 0$. We have $t = 5$ s. We then find $v_{ox} = \dfrac{100}{5} = 20$ m/s.

31. C

A fairly simple way to solve this problem is to use the equation $v^2 = v_o^2 + 2ad$. We know that when the block has gone a distance of 20 m, its speed is zero. So we have $0 = v_o^2 - 40a \rightarrow v_o = \sqrt{40a}$. Note that we have used a minus sign in front of acceleration because we know the acceleration up the plane is negative (deceleration). To find the acceleration we'll use Newton's second law, $F = ma$. The two forces on the object are the component of gravity down the plane and the frictional force, which is also down the plane. The gravitational force is given by $mg\sin30° = (5)(10)(0.5) = 25$ N. The frictional force is given by $\mu N = \mu mg\cos30° = \left(\dfrac{1}{\sqrt{3}}\right)(5)(10)\left(\dfrac{\sqrt{3}}{2}\right) = 25$ N. Thus, the total force down the plane is 50 N. So the acceleration is $a = 50/5 = 10$ m/s². We then have $v_o = \sqrt{400} = 20$ m/s.

32. B

To determine acceleration, we'll use Newton's second law, $a = F/m$. The acceleration experienced by a mass sliding down an inclined plane is directed down the plane and due to the component of the object's weight down the plane. This component is given by $mg\sin\theta$, where θ is the angle of the incline. We then have $a = mg\sin\theta/m = g\sin\theta$. The ratio of the accelerations is then given by $g\sin\theta_1/g\sin\theta_2 = \sin\theta_1/\sin\theta_2$.

33. C

First let's see what determines the range of a projectile. Recall the equation for horizontal motion of a projectile is $x = v_{ox}t$, where v_{ox} is the initial horizontal velocity. The range in the x direction is simply $x = v_{ox}T$, where T is the amount of time the projectile is in the air. The amount of time in the air is determined by the equations for the vertical motion. Specifically, the vertical velocity is given by $v_y = v_{oy} - gt$, where v_{oy} is the initial vertical velocity. We should recall that in the absence of air resistance, a projectile takes as much time to fall from its maximum height as it does to reach the maximum height. The time to reach the maximum height is found by setting $v_y = 0$ and solving for t, which gives a time of v_{oy}/g. Thus, the total time of flight is twice this, or $T = 2v_{oy}/g$, so we see that range in the x direction is proportional to T and, thus, inversely proportional to g. Thus, if g is reduced by a factor of $\frac{1}{6}$, the range is increased by a factor of 6.

34. D

We'll treat the bomb as a two-dimensional projectile whose initial velocity is only in the horizontal direction and of magnitude 900 mph. We're asked for the horizontal range of the projectile, which is obtained from $x = v_{ox}T$, where T is the time the projectile is in the air and $v_{ox} = 900$ mph. To find the time in the air, we use the equation for vertical motion.

In the present case this becomes $y = 6{,}400 - \frac{1}{2}gt^2$, where we take the ground as $y = 0$ and where the initial vertical velocity is zero. Recalling that $g = 32$ ft/s^2, and setting $y = 0$, we have $0 = 6{,}400 - 16T^2 \Rightarrow$ T = 20 s. The horizontal range is then $x = 20v_{ox}$ To convert from mph to ft/s use 1 mph = 5,280 ft/3,600 s, so 900 mph $= \dfrac{(900)(5280)}{3600}$ ft/s.

The horizontal range is then $x = \dfrac{(20)(900)(5280)}{3600}$ ft $= \dfrac{(20)(900)}{3600}$ miles = 5 miles.

35. A

The light is traveling from a medium with a higher refractive index to one with a lower refractive index. The speed of light is therefore increased. (The lower the index of refraction, the higher the speed of light in that medium.) $v = f\lambda$, where v is the speed, f the frequency, and λ the wavelength. Because v increases, either f or λ (or both) must increase. Frequency does not change upon entering a new medium, as this is a property characteristic of the source of light and is independent of the medium. Therefore the wavelength must increase.

36. C

The two parallel 4-ohm resistors give an effective resistance of $\dfrac{1}{\left(\frac{1}{4}+\frac{1}{4}\right)} = \dfrac{1}{\left(\frac{2}{4}\right)} = 2$ ohms. This is in series with the 6-ohm resistor, giving an effective resistance of $6 + 2 = 8$ ohms for the circuit.

37. A

Point b is connected to point a without any circuit element in between. The electrical potential energy must therefore be the same at these two points, so they are at the same potential.

38. C

Calculate the distance traveled over the constant velocity and uniform acceleration stretches separately and then combine them to get the total distance traveled:

$$x = v\Delta t_1 + (v_i\Delta t_2 + \frac{1}{2} a\Delta t_2{}^2)$$

$$\downarrow \qquad\qquad \downarrow$$

constant v   constant a

Thus v is the constant velocity of 30 m/s; Δt_1 is the time over which this constant speed applies (i.e., 5 s), and v_i is the initial speed when the object first starts to accelerate and is therefore the same as the constant speed of 30 m/s, Δt_2 is 4 s, and a is 15 m/s^2. Putting this all together

$$x = (30 \times 5) + (30 \times 4 + 0.5 \times 15 \times 16)$$

$$= 150 + (120 + 120) = 390$$
m

Don't be fooled by (B), which is the distance traveled over the uniform acceleration stretch.

39. B
Immediately before it hits the ground, an object has zero potential energy. All of its initial energy has been converted into kinetic energy, and this application of energy conservation allows us to determine the correct answer choice. Object A has an initial gravitational potential energy of MgH. It is released (rather than thrown down or tossed up), so its initial kinetic energy is zero. Immediately before it hits the ground, its kinetic energy is

$$\frac{1}{2} M v_A^2 = MgH$$

$$v_A = 2\sqrt{gH}$$

As for object B, its initial potential energy is $(0.5M)g(2H) = MgH$ as well. Its velocity immediately before it hits the ground is

$$\frac{1}{2} \left(\frac{1}{2}M\right) v_B^2 = MgH$$

$$v_B = 2\sqrt{gH}$$

The ratio of v_A to v_B is therefore

$$\sqrt{2gH} : 2\sqrt{gH} = \sqrt{2} : 2 = 1 : \sqrt{2}$$

40. C
The key to this problem is to realize that at its highest point, the velocity of the projectile is completely in the horizontal direction. Recall that for projectile motion, the horizontal velocity is actually constant because there is no force acting along the horizontal direction. Thus, the velocity at the highest point equals the horizontal component of the initial velocity. From the information given, the initial horizontal velocity is $5\cos60°$ m/s. Thus, the speed at the highest point is $5\cos60°$ m/s = $(5 \times \frac{1}{2})$ m/s = 2.5 m/s.

Quantitative Reasoning
ANSWERS AND EXPLANATIONS

ANSWER KEY

1. C	11. B	21. B	31. D	41. C
2. C	12. D	22. B	32. C	42. D
3. B	13. B	23. E	33. C	43. D
4. C	14. A	24. B	34. C	44. C
5. D	15. C	25. A	35. D	45. D
6. E	16. E	26. D	36. E	46. A
7. D	17. D	27. A	37. A	47. B
8. B	18. C	28. B	38. E	48. C
9. D	19. A	29. D	39. C	49. D
10. D	20. B	30. A	40. A	50. E

1. C

Because the dimensions of the aquarium are in feet whereas the unit gallon is defined in terms of cubic inches, we want either to convert the number of feet in each dimension of the aquarium to inches or convert the number of cubic inches in a gallon to the number of cubic feet in a gallon. Because converting the number of cubic inches in a gallon to the number of cubic feet in a gallon involves fractions, we'll convert the dimensions of the aquarium from feet to inches instead.

The base of the aquarium has dimensions of $1\frac{1}{2}$ feet by 2 feet, and the depth is $1\frac{1}{2}$ feet. There are 12 inches in a foot, so the dimensions of the base are $1\frac{1}{2} \times 12$, or 18 inches, and 2×12, or 24 inches. The depth is $1\frac{1}{2} \times 12$, or 18 inches. The volume of a rectangular box is length×width×height, so the volume of the aquarium in cubic inches is $18 \times 24 \times 18 = 432 \times 18 = 7,776$. Because the volume of the aquarium is 7,776 cubic inches and there are 231 cubic inches in a gallon, the number of gallons needed to fill the aquarium is $\frac{7776}{231} = \frac{2592}{77}$. You can tell by estimation that this is a little more than 30, and the only answer choice that is a little more than 30 is (C). Therefore

(C), 33.7, must be correct. If you work accurately with $\frac{2592}{77}$, you'll find that $\frac{2592}{77} = 33\frac{51}{77}$, and $33\frac{51}{77}$ to the nearest tenth is 33.7.

2. C

Here you want to find the value of $1\frac{7}{8} \times 2\frac{1}{10} \times \frac{6}{7}$. Notice that $1\frac{7}{8}$ is about 2 and $2\frac{1}{10}$ is also about 2. So $1\frac{7}{8} \times 2\frac{1}{10} \times \frac{6}{7}$ is approximately $2 \times 2 \times \frac{6}{7} = 4 \times \frac{6}{7} = \frac{24}{7} = 3\frac{3}{7}$. Notice that choice (A), $3\frac{513}{280}$ is greater than 4 because the fractional part of this number, $\frac{513}{280}$, is greater than 1. The only answer choice that is close to $3\frac{3}{7}$ is (C), $3\frac{3}{8}$, so (C) must be correct.

You can also solve this question by converting the mixed numbers $1\frac{7}{8}$ and $2\frac{1}{10}$ to improper fractions and then doing the multiplication. To convert a mixed number to an improper fraction, multiply the whole number part by the denominator and then add the numerator. The result is the new numerator over the same denominator. So to convert $1\frac{7}{8}$ to an improper fraction, first multiply 1 by 8 and then add 7 to get the new numerator 15. The denominator is the denominator 8 of the original mixed number, so $1\frac{7}{8} = \frac{15}{8}$. Similarly, $2\frac{1}{10} = \frac{2 \times 10 + 1}{10} = \frac{20 + 1}{10} = \frac{21}{10}$. Now we're ready to find the product.

$$1\frac{7}{8} \times 2\frac{1}{10} \times \frac{6}{7}$$
$$= \frac{15}{8} \times \frac{21}{10} \times \frac{6}{7}$$

Cancel the factors of 7 in 7 and in 21:

$$= \frac{15}{8} \times \frac{3}{10} \times \frac{6}{1}$$

Cancel the factors of 5 in 15 and in 10:

$$= \frac{3}{8} \times \frac{3}{2} \times \frac{6}{1}$$

Cancel the factors of 2 in 2 and in 6:

$$= \frac{3}{8} \times \frac{3}{1} \times \frac{3}{1}$$
$$= \frac{27}{8}$$
$$= 3\frac{3}{8}$$

3. B

Because there are no actual distances specified in the question, you can pick a value for the distance and work with it. Be sure to pick a number that's easy to work with. Here, you want half of the distance to be a multiple of 40 and 60. Because the smallest common multiple of 40 and 60 is 120, let each half-distance be 120 miles, i.e., we're letting the distances that Jim and Kate each drive be 120 miles. Use the formula Distance = Rate × Time. Because Jim drove for 120 miles at 40 miles per hour, the time he spent driving was $\frac{\text{Distance}}{\text{Rate}} = \frac{120}{40} = 3$ hours. Because Kate drove for 120 miles at 60 miles per hour, the time she spent driving was $\frac{\text{Distance}}{\text{Rate}} = \frac{120}{60} = 2$ hours. The total distance driven was 120 + 120 = 240 miles, and the total time driving was 3 + 2 = 5 hours, so the average speed for the trip was $\frac{\text{Total Distance}}{\text{Total Time}} = \frac{240}{5} = 48$ miles per hour.

4. C

Because a tooth of one gear always touches a tooth of the other gear, the number of teeth of one gear multiplied by the number of times it revolves always equals the number of teeth of the other gear multiplied by the number of times it revolves. Let N be the number of times the larger gear revolves. Then 40 × N = 24 × 15, so

$$N = \frac{24 \times 15}{40} = \frac{6 \times 15}{10} = \frac{3 \times 15}{5} = 3 \times 3 = 9.$$

5. D

First convert 23% to a fraction. Whenever you convert a percent to a fraction (and also whenever you convert a percent to a decimal), you divide the percent by 100%, having the percent symbols drop out. So 23% $= \frac{23\%}{100\%} = \frac{23}{100}$. The word *of* immediately after 23% means "times." We have the equation $\frac{23}{100} \times \frac{2}{5}\left(\frac{190}{3x}\right)$ = 8. Now solve this equation for x.

$$\frac{23}{100} \times \frac{2}{5}\left(\frac{190}{3x}\right) = 8$$
$$\frac{23}{100} \times \frac{2}{5} \times \frac{190}{3x} = 8$$
$$x = \frac{23}{100} \times \frac{2}{5} \times \frac{190}{3 \times 8}$$
$$= \frac{23}{100} \times \frac{2}{5} \times \frac{190}{24}$$

Now find what this value of x equals.

$$x = \frac{23}{100} \times \frac{2}{5} \times \frac{190}{24}$$

Cancel a factor of 10 from the 100 and the 190:

$$= \frac{23}{10} \times \frac{2}{5} \times \frac{19}{24}$$

Cancel a factor of 2 from the 10 and the 2:

$$= \frac{23}{5} \times \frac{1}{5} \times \frac{19}{24}$$
$$= \frac{23 \times 19}{5 \times 5 \times 24} = \frac{437}{600}$$

6. E

There are 60 seconds in a minute, so if a heart beats 72 times in 1 minute, it beats 72 times in 60 seconds. Thus in 1 second, the heart beats $\frac{72}{60} = \frac{12}{10} = 1.2$ times.

7. D

To divide by a fraction, you invert the fraction and multiply.

To divide by $\frac{3}{4}$, you invert the $\frac{3}{4}$, getting $\frac{4}{3}$, and then multiply by $\frac{4}{3}$. Thus, $\frac{6,534}{\frac{3}{4}} = 6,534 \times \frac{4}{3} = 2,178 \times 4 = 8,712$.

8. B

Plug the values of π, h, and a into the equation and solve for the value of r. (This formula is actually a geometric formula, however if you don't recognize it, it doesn't matter. In geometry, π, with its usual meaning, is often approximated by $\frac{22}{7}$; however, in the solution, π can just be considered to be replaced by $\frac{22}{7}$.) Be careful to answer what the question requires; find the value of 2r and choose the answer choice that indicates the value of 2r.

$$a = r^2 h$$
$$396 = \frac{22}{7} r^2 (14)$$
$$22(2) r^2 = 396$$

$$44r^2 = 396$$
$$r^2 = \frac{396}{44}$$
$$r^2 = 9$$
$$r = 3 \text{ or } r = -3$$

Because $r > 0$, $r = 3$, So $2r = 2(3) = 6$. The value of $2r$ is 6 and (B) is correct.

9. D

Translate the English of the question stem into math. You will obtain an equation that can be solved for the value of the number. Call the number N. "A number is larger than 5 by" means "N – 5." Next, "the same" means "=", so now we have "N – 5 =." There are several steps in translating "amount that it is smaller than 3 more than 14." The word "it" refers to the number N, so "amount that it is smaller than 3 more than 14" means "amount that N is smaller than 3 more than 14." "3 more than 14" means "3 + 14." So "amount that it is smaller than 3 more than 14" means "(3 + 14) – N." So "A NUMBER is larger than 5 by the same amount that it is smaller than 3 more than 14" means that N – 5 = (3 + 14) – N. Now solve this equation for N.

$$N - 5 = (3 + 14) - N$$
$$N - 5 = 17 - N$$
$$2N - 5 = 17$$
$$2N = 22$$
$$N = \frac{22}{2}$$
$$N = 11$$

10. D

A circle can be drawn that goes through any three points that do not all lie on a straight line. If three points do lie on a straight line, no circle can be drawn that goes through all three of these points. The points (0, 0) and (10, 0) both have a y-coordinate of 0, so these two points are on the x-axis, which is the line with the equation y = 0. Look for a point among the answer choice, that is on the x-axis. Look for this point by looking for a point with a y-coordinate of 0. (D), (5, 0), has a y-coordinate

of 0. Thus (5, 0) could not be a point on a circle passing through the two points (0, 0) and (10, 0).

11. B

Translate the information in the question stem into math and then try to find the value of $\frac{c}{a}$. "is" means "equals," so "a is" means "a =". The fractional equivalent of 25% is $\frac{1}{4}$. Now, "of" means "times," so "25% of b" means "$\frac{1}{4} \times b$" or "$\frac{1}{4}b$" and "a is 25% of b" means that $a = \frac{1}{4}b$. The translation of "b is 60% of c" is similar. The fractional equivalent of 60% is $\frac{3}{5}$, so "b is 60% of c" means that $b = \frac{3}{5}$ c. Now we have the two equations $a = \frac{1}{4}b$ and $b = \frac{3}{5}c$. Because we want to find the value of $\frac{c}{a}$, use the equation $b = \frac{3}{5}c$ and substitute $\frac{3}{5}c$ for b into the equation $a = \frac{1}{4}b$. When we do this we'll be left with an equation that only contains the variables a and c. We can then try to solve this equation for the value of $\frac{c}{a}$. Substituting $\frac{3}{5}c$ for b into the equation $a = \frac{1}{4}b$ gives us $a = \frac{1}{4}(\frac{3}{5}c)$. Now solve this equation for the value of $\frac{c}{a}$.

$$a = \frac{1}{4}\left(\frac{3}{5}c\right)$$
$$a = \frac{1}{4} \times \frac{3}{5} \times c$$
$$a = \frac{3}{20} \times c$$
$$1 = \frac{3}{20} \times \frac{c}{a}$$
$$20 = 3 \times \frac{c}{a}$$
$$\frac{20}{3} = \frac{c}{a}$$

Therefore, $\frac{c}{a} = \frac{20}{3}$ and (B) is correct.

12. D

Call the number of liters of an 80% solution that are needed x. The new solution will then contain 4 + x liters. The 4 liters of solution that are 35% alcohol contain (35% of 4) liters of alcohol. Because the answer choices are all decimals, convert 35% to a decimal. Whenever you convert a percent to a decimal (also whenever you convert a percent to a fraction), you divide the percent by 100%, and the percent symbols cancel.

Therefore, $35\% = \dfrac{35\%}{100\%} = \dfrac{35}{100} = \dfrac{7}{20} = 0.35$ and the 4 liters of solution that are 35% alcohol contain 0.35(4), or 1.4 liters of alcohol. The x liters of solution that are added are 80% alcohol. The decimal equivalent of 80% is 0.8, so the x liters of solution that are 80% alcohol contain 0.8x liters of alcohol. Therefore, the 4 + x liters of solution will contain 1.4 + 0.8x liters of alcohol. Now these 4 + x liters of solution are to be 60% alcohol, and the decimal equivalent of 60% is 0.6, so we can write down this equation:

$\dfrac{1.4 + 0.8x}{4 + x} = 0.6$. Now solve this equation for x.

$$\dfrac{1.4 + 0.8x}{4 + x} = 0.6$$
$$1.4 + 0.8x = 0.6(4 + x)$$
$$1.4 + 0.8x = 2.4 + 0.6x$$
$$0.8x = 1.0 + 0.6x$$
$$0.2x = 1$$
$$x = \dfrac{1}{0.2} = \dfrac{10}{2} = 5$$

Therefore, 5 liters must be added, and (D) is correct.

13.   B

The value represented by the question mark must be found. First, add and subtract the fractions on the left side. To add and subtract fractions, find a common denominator. Let's try to find the least common multiple of 12, 8, and 2. (Actually, because 8 is a multiple of 2, the least common multiple of 12 and 8 must be the least common multiple of 12, 8, and 2.) We could find the least common denominator here by taking multiples of the largest denominator, 12, until we get multiples of the other denominators, 8 and 2. Of course, 12 itself, which is 12 times 1, is not a multiple of 8. Try 12 times 2: 12 times 2 is 24, and 24 is a multiple of both $8 (24 = 8 \times 3)$ and $2 (24 = 2 \times 12)$. Now convert each of the fractions to an equivalent fraction with a denominator of 24:

$$\dfrac{9}{8} = \dfrac{9}{8} \times \dfrac{3}{3} = \dfrac{9 \times 3}{8 \times 3} = \dfrac{27}{24}$$

$$\dfrac{5}{12} = \dfrac{5}{12} \times \dfrac{2}{2} = \dfrac{5 \times 2}{12 \times 2} = \dfrac{10}{24}$$

$$\dfrac{1}{2} = \dfrac{1}{2} \times \dfrac{12}{12} = \dfrac{1 \times 12}{2 \times 12} = \dfrac{12}{24}$$

and then

$$\dfrac{9}{8} - \dfrac{5}{12} + \dfrac{1}{2} = \dfrac{27}{24} - \dfrac{10}{24} + \dfrac{12}{24} = \dfrac{27 - 10 + 12}{24} = \dfrac{29}{24}$$

Therefore, $\dfrac{29}{24} - (?) = 1$ and

$$? = \dfrac{29}{24} - 1 = \dfrac{29}{24} - \dfrac{24}{24} = \dfrac{29 - 24}{24} = \dfrac{5}{24}.$$

(B) is correct.

14.   A

The area of a square is equal to the length of its side squared, and the area of this square is 1,000 square inches. If we call the length of a side of this square x, then $x^2 = 1{,}000$. Therefore, $x = \sqrt{1{,}000}$. We could simplify this radical by finding a perfect square that is a factor of the quantity 1,000 under the radical sign, but there is no need to because we will be squaring a quantity closely related to $\sqrt{1000}$ when we find the area of the circle, so the radical symbols will drop out. The diameter of the largest circle that can be drawn inside this square is equal to the length of the side of the square. The diameter of this circle is $\sqrt{1000}$. The diameter of a circle is always twice its radius, and equivalently, the radius of a circle is always $\dfrac{1}{2}$ of its diameter. The radius of the largest possible circle here is therefore $\dfrac{1}{2}\sqrt{1000}$. The area of a circle with a radius r is πr^2, so the area of this circle is $\pi\left(\dfrac{1}{2}\sqrt{1000}\right)^2$. Use the approximation $\dfrac{22}{7}$ for π. Then $\pi\left(\dfrac{1}{2}\sqrt{1000}\right)^2$ is approximately

$$\dfrac{22}{7}\left(\dfrac{1}{2}\sqrt{1000}\right)^2 = \dfrac{22}{7} \times \dfrac{1}{2} \times \sqrt{1000} \times \dfrac{1}{2} \times \sqrt{1000}$$
$$= \dfrac{22}{7} \times \dfrac{1}{2} \times \dfrac{1}{2} \times \sqrt{1000} \times \sqrt{1000}$$
$$= \dfrac{22}{7} \times \dfrac{1}{4} \times 1{,}000$$
$$= \dfrac{5{,}500}{7}$$
$$= 785\dfrac{5}{7}$$

Clearly, $785\dfrac{5}{7}$ is much closer to (A), 785.7, than to any other choice, so (A) must be correct. (When you're taking the test, you should not spend time converting $785\dfrac{5}{7}$ to a decimal and round the result to the nearest tenth. However, if you did convert $785\dfrac{5}{7}$ to a decimal and round the result to the nearest tenth, you would get 785.7. Never do such computations unless they are necessary.)

15. C

To subtract the algebraic expressions, find a common denominator for the two fractions. The fraction $\frac{a}{b}$ has the denominator b and the fraction $\frac{b}{a}$ has the denominator a. The common denominator to use here is the lowest common denominator, which is the product of the denominators, ab. Now convert each fraction to an equivalent fraction having a denominator ab and then do the subtraction.

$$\frac{a}{b} - \frac{b}{a} = \left(\frac{a}{b} \times \frac{a}{a}\right) - \left(\frac{b}{a} \times \frac{b}{b}\right)$$
$$= \frac{a^2}{ab} - \frac{b^2}{ab}$$
$$= \frac{a^2 - b^2}{ab}$$

(C) is correct.

16. E

First, convert 55% to a fraction. Whenever you convert a percent to a fraction (also whenever you convert a percent to a decimal), you divide the percent by 100%, thus the percent symbols cancel. $55\% = \frac{55\%}{100\%} = \frac{55}{100} = \frac{11}{20}$. The word "of" means "times," so "55% of" means "55% times," which is "$\frac{11}{20}$ times"; thus, you have the equation $\frac{11}{20}\left(\frac{9z}{5}\right) = 33$, which you can solve for z.

$$\frac{11}{20}\left(\frac{9z}{5}\right) = 33$$

Multiply the fractions on the left side:

$$\frac{11(9z)}{20(5)} = 33$$
$$\frac{99z}{100} = 33$$

Divide both sides by 33: $\frac{3z}{100} = 1$

Multiply both sides by 100: $3z = 100$

Divide both sides by 3: $z = \frac{100}{3}$

17. D

The average formula is Average $= \frac{\text{Sum of the Terms}}{\text{Number of Terms}}$ (i.e., the average of a group of terms is the sum of the terms divided by the number of terms). The average of the numbers $\frac{1}{2}$, $\frac{2}{3}$, and $\frac{3}{4}$ is the sum of these

three fractions divided by 3, so the average of these numbers is $\frac{\frac{1}{2} + \frac{2}{3} + \frac{3}{4}}{3}$. To find the sum of the fractions in the numerator, $\frac{1}{2} + \frac{2}{3} + \frac{3}{4}$, find a common denominator for the fractions $\frac{1}{2}$, $\frac{2}{3}$, and $\frac{3}{4}$. You could find the lowest common denominator by taking multiples of the largest denominator, 4, until you get multiples of the other denominators, 3 and 2: 4 times 1 is 4, and 4 is not a multiple of 3. Try 4 times 2. 4 times 2 is 8, and 8 is not a multiple of 3. Now try 4 times 3: 4 times 3 is 12, and 12 is a multiple of both 2 ($12 = 2 \times 6$) and 3 ($12 = 3 \times 4$). Now convert each of the fractions to an equivalent fraction with a denominator of 12.

$$\frac{1}{2} = \frac{1}{2} \times \frac{6}{6} = \frac{1 \times 6}{2 \times 6} = \frac{6}{12}$$
$$\frac{2}{3} = \frac{2}{3} \times \frac{4}{4} = \frac{2 \times 4}{3 \times 4} = \frac{8}{12}$$
$$\frac{3}{4} = \frac{3}{4} \times \frac{3}{3} = \frac{3 \times 3}{4 \times 3} = \frac{9}{12}$$

So $\frac{1}{2} + \frac{2}{3} + \frac{3}{4} = \frac{6}{12} + \frac{8}{12} + \frac{9}{12} = \frac{6 + 8 + 9}{12} = \frac{23}{12}$.

Finally, the average is

$$\frac{\frac{1}{2} + \frac{2}{3} + \frac{3}{4}}{3} = \frac{\left(\frac{23}{12}\right)}{3} = \frac{23}{12} \times \frac{1}{3} = \frac{23 \times 1}{12 \times 3}$$
$$= \frac{23}{36}$$

(D) is correct.

18. C

This is a proportion question. "14 is to 35" just means the ratio of 14 to 35, "2x is to 40" just means the ratio of 2x to 40, and "14 is to 35 as 2x is to 40" means that the ratio of 14 to 35 is equal to the ratio of 2x to 40. Now write the corresponding equation with the ratios replaced by fractions.

$$\frac{14}{35} = \frac{2x}{40}$$

Now solve this equation for x.

$$\frac{14}{35} = \frac{2x}{40}$$

On the right side, divide the numerator and denominator by 2:

$$\frac{14}{35} = \frac{x}{20}$$

On the left side, divide the numerator and denominator by 7:

$$\frac{2}{5} = \frac{x}{20}$$

Cross multiply: $\qquad 2(20) = 5x$

Simplify the left side. $\qquad 40 = 5x$

Divide both sides by 5: $\qquad \dfrac{40}{5} = x$

$\qquad\qquad\qquad\qquad\qquad 8 = x$

Therefore, $x = 8$ and (C) is correct.

19. A

Write the rate of each person in terms of rooms painted per hour, add these rates, and then find how long it would take working at this combined rate to paint 1 room. Diane can paint 1 room in 6 hours, so her rate of painting rooms is $\dfrac{1}{6}$ rooms per hour. Sandy can paint one room in 4 hours, so her rate of painting rooms is $\dfrac{1}{4}$ rooms per hour. The rate at which both of them paint when they work together is $\dfrac{1}{6} + \dfrac{1}{4}$ rooms per hour. Now $\dfrac{1}{6} + \dfrac{1}{4} = \dfrac{2}{12} + \dfrac{3}{12} = \dfrac{2+3}{12} = \dfrac{5}{12}$, so their rate when they work together is $\dfrac{5}{12}$ rooms per hour. The number of hours it takes them to paint one room is the reciprocal of $\dfrac{5}{12}$, which is $\dfrac{12}{5}$. None of the answer choices is $\dfrac{12}{5}$; however, $\dfrac{12}{5} = 2\dfrac{2}{5}$. (A) is correct. If it was not immediately clear to you why if the combined rate is $\dfrac{5}{12}$ rooms per hour, then the time needed to paint 1 room, in hours, is the reciprocal of $\dfrac{5}{12}$, you can use the formula Work = Rate × Time, and here, work = 1 room, rate = $\dfrac{5}{12}$ rooms per hour, and the time in hours is unknown. Therefore,

1 room = $\left(\dfrac{5}{12}\text{ rooms per hour}\right)$ × time,

time = $\dfrac{1}{\left(\frac{5}{12}\right)}$ hours, and the number of hours is indeed the reciprocal of $\dfrac{5}{12}$.

20. B

To find the percent of the resulting solution that is sugar, we need the number of milliliters of sugar in the resulting solution and the total number of milliliters of the resulting solution. The number of milliliters of sugar in the resulting solution is the number of milliliters in the original solution, because the 8 milliliters of water that are added contain just water and no sugar. Therefore, the number of milliliters of sugar in the resulting solution is 5% of 32. To find 5% of 32, convert 5% to a decimal. Whenever you convert a percent to a decimal (and also whenever you convert a percent to a fraction), you divide the percent by 100%, having the percent symbols cancel. Therefore,

$5\% = \dfrac{5\%}{100\%} = \dfrac{5}{100} = \dfrac{1}{20} = 0.05$, and 5% of 32 is $0.05(32)$, which is 1.6. The total number of milliliters in the resulting solution is the original 32 plus the added 8, so the total number of milliliters of resulting solution is 40. The fraction of the resulting solution that is sugar is $\dfrac{1.6}{40}$. The percent of the resulting solution that is sugar is the fraction of the resulting solution that is sugar, $\dfrac{1.6}{40}$, converted to a percent. To convert a fraction (or a decimal) to a percent, multiply that fraction (or decimal) by 100%. The percent of the resulting solution that is sugar is $\dfrac{1.6}{40} \times 100\% = \dfrac{1.6}{4} \times 10\% = \dfrac{1.6}{2} \times 5\% = 0.8 \times 5\% = 4\%$.

21. B

You need to know the average formula: Average = $\dfrac{\text{Sum of the terms}}{\text{Number of terms}}$. In this question, it is convenient to work with the sums of the scores, so you should therefore work with the average formula in the rearranged form Sum of the terms = Average × Number of terms. The average of the five scores is 9.6, and the sum of the five scores is 9.6 × 5, or 48. When the highest and lowest scores are dropped, the average rises to 9.7 and the sum of the remaining three scores is 9.7 × 3, or 29.1. The sum of the highest and lowest scores can be found by subtracting from the sum of all five scores the sum of the three scores that remain when the highest and lowest scores are removed. The sum of the highest and lowest scores is 48 − 29.1, which equals 18.9. The average of the highest and lowest scores is $\dfrac{18.9}{2}$, which equals 9.45.

22. B

If $\dfrac{10\text{ feet }(x)\text{ inches}}{9\text{ feet 3 inches}}$ approximates 1.2, then 10 feet (x) inches is approximately 1.2(9 feet 3 inches). The first thing we will do is rewrite 1.2(9 feet 3 inches)

more simply in terms of feet and inches. Now 1.2(9 feet 3 inches) is 1.2(9 feet) plus 1.2(3 inches). 1.2(9 feet) = 10.8 feet. There are 12 inches in a foot, so in 0.8 feet there are 0.8(12), or 9.6 inches, and thus 1.2(9 feet) = 10 feet plus 9.6 inches. 1.2(3 inches) = 3.6 inches. So 1.2(9 feet 3 inches) equals 10 feet plus 9.6 inches plus 3.6 inches, which equals 10 feet plus 13.2 inches. Because 10 feet (x) inches is approximately 1.2(9 feet 3 inches), we can say that 10 feet (x) inches is approximately 10 feet plus 13.2 inches. There is no need to rewrite 10 feet plus 13.2 inches as an integer number of feet plus some number N of inches where N is less than 12. Notice that 10 feet (x) inches is approximately equal to 10 feet plus 13.2 inches, so among the answer choices, (B) is clearly closest to 13.2.

23. E

One way to solve this is by looking for pairs of fractions that are relatively easier to compare, then making these less difficult comparisons of fractions, and then eliminating answer choices as soon as you can. First, $\frac{2}{3}$ is $\frac{1}{3}$ less than 1 whereas $\frac{3}{4}$ is $\frac{1}{4}$ less than 1. Because $\frac{1}{4}$ is less than $\frac{1}{3}$, $\frac{3}{4}$ is closer to 1 than $\frac{2}{3}$, i.e., $\frac{3}{4}$ is greater than $\frac{2}{3}$. So d, representing $\frac{3}{4}$, must be on the list before a, representing $\frac{2}{3}$. (A) and (C) have a occurring before d, i.e., they incorrectly say that $\frac{2}{3}$ is greater than $\frac{3}{4}$. Eliminate (A) and (C). Next, $\frac{5}{8}$ and $\frac{5}{11}$ both have the same numerator. Whenever you have two fractions (that both have positive numerators and positive denominators) that have the same numerator, the fraction with the smaller denominator is the larger fraction. So $\frac{5}{8}$ is greater than $\frac{5}{11}$. So e, representing $\frac{5}{8}$, must be on the list before b, representing $\frac{5}{11}$. (B) and (D) have b on their lists before e; that is, they incorrectly say that $\frac{5}{11}$ is greater than $\frac{5}{8}$. Eliminate (B) and (D). Now that all four incorrect answer choices have been eliminated, you know that (E) must be correct.

This question could have been solved with other comparisons. For example, $\frac{5}{11}$ is the only fraction less than $\frac{1}{2}$ because it is the only fraction whose denominator is greater than twice its numerator.

Therefore $\frac{5}{11}$ is the smallest fraction, and b, representing $\frac{5}{11}$, must be last on the list. You can eliminate (A), (B), and (D), which do not have b for the last entry on their lists. Next, $\frac{3}{4}$ is greater than $\frac{5}{8}$ because $\frac{3}{4} = \frac{6}{8}$, and $\frac{6}{8}$ is greater than $\frac{5}{8}$, so d, representing $\frac{3}{4}$, must be on the list before e, representing $\frac{5}{8}$. (C) has e on the list before d, i.e, this choice incorrectly says that $\frac{5}{8}$ is greater than $\frac{3}{4}$. Therefore eliminate (C). Now that all four incorrect choices have been eliminated, you know that (E) must be correct.

24. B

Because 70% of the students are girls, the other 30% of the students are boys. The average height of the girls has 70% of the total average, whereas the average height of the boys has the other 30% of the total average. Because the average height of the girls contributes so much more to the total, you know that the average of the entire class will have to be closer to the average height of the girls than to the average height of the boys. You therefore know that the average of the entire class will have to be less than 5 feet 6 inches, which is midway between 5 feet 4 inches and 5 feet 8 inches. You can eliminate choices (D) and (E). Now let's find the overall average. The decimal equivalent of 70% is 0.7, and the decimal equivalent of 30% is 0.3. The average height is

0.7(5 feet 4 inches) + 0.3(5 feet 8 inches)

= 0.7(5 feet) + 0.7(4 inches) + 0.3(5 feet) + 0.3(8 inches)

= [0.7(5 feet) + 0.3(5 feet)] + [0.7(4 inches) + 0.3(8 inches)]

= (0.7 + 0.3)(5 feet) + (2.8 inches + 2.4 inches)

= (5 feet) + (5.2 inches)

This is closest to (B), 5 feet 5 inches, so (B) must be correct.

25. A

This question can be solved by picking a number appropriately. The number to pick here is for the number of riders. Always pick a number that is easy to work with. Say that the original number of riders was 10. Then because the original cost of the ride was 75¢, the original total revenue was 75(10), or 750¢. There is no need to convert this to dollars. After the price rose to 90¢, the number of riders decreased by 20%. The fractional equivalent of 20% is $\frac{1}{5}$, so the number of riders decreased by $\frac{1}{5}$. The new number of riders was $10 - \frac{1}{5}(10) = 10 - 2 = 8$. The new total revenue was 90(8), or 720¢. The total revenue decreased from 750¢ to 720¢. The decrease in total revenues was 750 − 720 = 30¢. The fractional decrease is always found by dividing the amount of decrease by the *original whole*.

The fractional decrease is $\frac{30}{750} = \frac{1}{25}$. The percent decrease is just the fractional decrease converted to a percent. To convert a fraction (or decimal) to a percent, multiply that fraction (or decimal) by 100%. The fractional decrease is $\frac{1}{25} \times 100\%$, which is 4%. Notice that you could find the percent decrease from 750 to 720 in one step according to the formula

Percent decrease =

$$\frac{\text{Original value} - \text{New value}}{\text{Original value}} \times 100\%.$$

Used here, percent decrease

$$= \frac{750 - 720}{750} \times 100\% = \frac{30}{750} \times 100\%$$

$$= \frac{1}{25} \times 100\% = 4\%.$$

26. D
The expression $\frac{4a - 7a + 6a}{6ab}$ is to be simplified.

First combine the terms in the numerator.
$$\frac{4a - 7a + 6a}{6ab} = \frac{3a}{6ab}$$

Now cancel a factor of 3 from the numerator and denominator. $\frac{3a}{6ab} = \frac{a}{2ab}$

Now cancel a factor of a from the numerator and denominator: $\frac{a}{2ab} = \frac{1}{2b}$

(D) is correct.

27. A
To compare two decimal numbers that are between 0 and 1, look at the tenths digit first. If the tenths

digit in one number is larger, that number is larger. If the tenths digit is the same in both numbers, look at the hundredths digit next. If the hundredths digit in one number is larger, that number is larger. If the hundredths digit is the same in both numbers, look at the thousandths digits. If the thousandths digit in one number is larger that number is larger. If the thousandths digits are the same, look at the ten-thousandths digits. Continue this way until a comparison has been made. Looking at the numbers of the answer choices, the tenths digit of choice (A) is 6, whereas the tenths digits of the other choices are all less than 6. Therefore (A), 0.636, is largest.

28. B
Of the first 150 flips, 48% were heads: 48% of 150 is $\frac{48}{100} \times 150 = \frac{24}{50} \times 150 = 24 \times 3 = 72$. If the coin is flipped another 100 times, it will have been flipped a total of 150 + 100 = 250 times. If the overall percent of heads is to be 50%, then 50% of all the 250 tosses must be heads. The fractional equivalent of 50% is $\frac{1}{2}$, so $\frac{1}{2}$ of 250, or 125 heads, must have been tossed. Because 72 heads were tossed in the first 150 flips, 125 − 72 or 53 heads must be tossed in the next 100 flips. Of the next 100 tosses, 53 (i.e., 53%) must be heads. (B) is correct.

29. D
The easiest to compare are (A) and (D), so let's compare these first. Because 0.03 is less than 0.3, eliminate (A). (C) and (E) are relatively easy to compare: 0.03 is less than 0.3, and $\sqrt{0.03}$ is less than $\sqrt{0.3}$ because there is a smaller number under the radical sign of $\sqrt{0.03}$ than under the radical sign of $\sqrt{0.3}$. We can eliminate (E). Now (D) can be compared with (B) if the value of (B) is found: $(0.3)^2 = 0.3 \times 0.3 = 0.09$, so 0.03 is less than $(0.3)^2 = 0.09$. Eliminate (B). We're down to just (C) and (D). Now (D), 0.03, can be compared to (C), $\sqrt{0.03}$, if you know about the properties of numbers between 0 and 1. The number 0.03 is less than $\sqrt{0.03}$ because a positive number

between 0 and 1 is less than the positive square root of that number. (For example, $\frac{1}{4}$ is less than $\sqrt{\frac{1}{4}} = \frac{1}{2}$.) Eliminate (C). Now that all four incorrect choices have been eliminated, we know that (D) must be correct.

30. A

In this solution, the positions of the minute hand and the hour hand at different times will be described in terms of the number of degrees they have moved clockwise away from a vertical line drawn from the center of the clock to the 12 on top. At 4:00, the minute hand points to the 12 on top whereas the hour hand points to the 4. The hour hand is $\frac{4}{12}$ of $360°$, or $\frac{1}{3}(360) = 120°$ clockwise from the vertical line described. Now let's see where the minute and hour hands wind up after 50 minutes. In 1 hour (60 minutes), the minute hand will move $360°$, and 50 minutes is $\frac{50}{60}$ of an hour, which is $\frac{5}{6}$ of an hour. Therefore, in 50 minutes, the minute hand will move $\frac{5}{6}$ of $360°$, which is $300°$. At 4:50, the minute hand has moved clockwise $300°$ from the vertical line described. In 1 hour, the hour hand moves clockwise from one number on the clock to the next number. There are 12 numbers on the clock, so in 1 hour, the hour hand moves $\frac{1}{12}$ of $360°$, which is $30°$. We have seen that 50 minutes is $\frac{5}{6}$ of an hour, so in 50 minutes, the hour hand will have moved clockwise $\frac{5}{6}$ of $30°$, or $25°$. At 4:00, the hour hand, which was pointing at the 4, was $120°$ clockwise away from the vertical line described; therefore at 4:50, the hour hand will be $120 + 25$, or $145°$ clockwise away from the vertical line described. The minute hand is $300°$ away from this vertical line, so the minute hand and the hour hand form an angle of measure $300 - 145$, or $155°$. Because this $155°$ angle is less than $180°$, we have found the smaller of the two angles formed by the hour and minute hand, and (A) is correct.

31. D

Because you're dividing 10.5 by a positive number less than 1, the result must be greater than 10.5, so you can eliminate (A), (B), and (E). Using a little estimation, 10.5 is about 10 and 0.35 is about $\frac{1}{3}$, so $10.5 \div 0.35$ is approximately $10 \div \frac{1}{3}$, which equals $10 \times \frac{3}{1}$, or 30. Choice (C), 300, is much too large,

so eliminate (C). Now that all four incorrect choices have been eliminated, we know that (D) must be correct. Note that our approximation, $10 \div \frac{1}{3}$, of $10.5 \div 0.35$, happened to be the exact value of $10.5 \div 0.35$, but this was just a coincidence.

You could also actually do the division in $10.5 \div 0.35$. Multiply both numbers by a power with a base of 10 to get rid of all the decimal points. Because 10.5 has one digit to the right of the decimal point whereas 0.35 has two digits to the right of the decimal point, multiply both numbers by 10^2, or 100.

Then, $10.5 \div 0.35 = (10.5 \times 100) \div (0.35 \times 100)$ $= 1{,}050 \div 35 = 30$.

32. C

There is only one correct setting. To find the number of possible settings that will not open the lock, find the total number of possible settings and subtract 1 from that number. In the section furthest to the left, any integer from 1 through 5 can be placed. Similarly, in the middle and right sections, any integer from 1 through 5 can be placed in each section. Therefore, the total number of settings is $5 \times 5 \times 5 = 25 \times 5 = 125$, and the number of settings that will not work is $125 - 1$, or 124.

33. C

Let R be her normal hourly rate, in dollars per hour. The pay is in two types. The first $48 - 8$ or 40 hours are at the normal rate of R dollars per hour. The final 8 hours are paid at a rate of $1\frac{1}{2}R$ dollars per hour. In the first 40 hours, she earns $R \times 40$, or 40R dollars. In the final 8 hours, she earns $1\frac{1}{2}R \times 8$, or 12R dollars. Altogether she earns $40R + 12R$ or 52R dollars. She earned 286 dollars, so $52R = 286$ and $R = \frac{286}{52} = 5\frac{26}{52} = 5\frac{1}{2} = 5.50$. (C) is correct.

34. C

First, convert 33 feet and 4 inches to feet. There are 12 inches in a foot, so in 1 inch there is $\frac{1}{12}$ of a foot and in 4 inches there is $4 \times \frac{1}{12} = \frac{1}{3}$ of a foot. Therefore, 33 feet and 4 inches is 33 feet and $\frac{1}{3}$ of a foot, which is $33\frac{1}{3}$ feet. To find the cost in dollars per foot of a $99 fence that is $33\frac{1}{3}$ feet long, divide $99 by $33\frac{1}{3}$ feet. It is easier to divide 99 by the simplest improper fraction equal to $33\frac{1}{3}$, so first convert $33\frac{1}{3}$ to that improper fraction. $33\frac{1}{3} = \frac{3 \times 33 + 1}{3}$ $= \frac{99 + 1}{3} = \frac{100}{3}$. Finally, the cost in dollars per foot is $\frac{99}{\left(\frac{100}{3}\right)} = 99 \times \frac{3}{100} = \frac{297}{100} = 2.97$. (C) is correct.

35. D

To find out how many ounces there are in $3\frac{1}{5}$ grams, first find the number of ounces that there are in 1 gram and then multiply this number by $3\frac{1}{5}$. Because 1 ounce = 28 grams, dividing both sides by 28 gives $\frac{1}{28}$ ounce = 1 gram (i.e., in 1 gram there is $\frac{1}{28}$ of an ounce, in $3\frac{1}{5}$ grams there is $3\frac{1}{5} \times \frac{1}{28}$ of an ounce). All that remains to be done is work out the value of $3\frac{1}{5} \times \frac{1}{28}$. First, convert $3\frac{1}{5}$ to an improper fraction. $3\frac{1}{5} = \frac{3 \times 5 + 1}{5} = \frac{15 + 1}{5} = \frac{16}{5}$. Then, $3\frac{1}{5} \times \frac{1}{28} = \frac{16}{5} \times \frac{1}{28} = \frac{4}{5} \times \frac{1}{7} = \frac{4}{35}$. Therefore, there is $\frac{4}{35}$ of an ounce in $3\frac{1}{5}$ grams, and (D) is correct.

It is often helpful to check and see if the answer you got looks reasonable, and our answer of $\frac{4}{35}$ here certainly does look reasonable. Notice that if 1 ounce = 28 grams, then $3\frac{1}{5}$ grams, which is much less than 28 grams, must be less than 1 ounce and our answer does look reasonable. Notice that (B), (C), and (E), which are all greater than 1, can be eliminated just from knowing that $3\frac{1}{5}$ grams must be less than 1 ounce.

36. E

Solve the equation $\frac{63}{3x} = 4\frac{2}{7}$ for x.

$$\frac{63}{3x} = 4\frac{2}{7}$$

Cancel a factor of 3 from the 63 and the 3 on the left:

$$\frac{21}{x} = 4\frac{2}{7}$$

Convert $4\frac{2}{7}$ on the right to an improper fraction:

$$\frac{21}{x} = \frac{4 \times 7 + 2}{7}$$

$$\frac{21}{x} = \frac{30}{7}$$

Cross multiply: $\quad 21(7) = (x)(30)$

Multiply each side: $\quad 147 = 30x$

Divide both sides by 30: $\quad \frac{147}{30} = x$

Cancel a factor of 3 from the 147 and the 30:

$$\frac{49}{10} = x$$

Convert $\frac{49}{10}$ to a decimal: $\quad 4.9 = x$

37. A

This is a good question to solve by picking numbers. Always pick numbers that are easy to work with. Let the empty bottle weigh 10 units. This weight of 10 is $\frac{1}{10}$ of the weight of the bottle when it is full, so when the bottle is full the weight of the bottle is 100 units. This weight of 100 is the sum of the weight of 10 of the empty bottle and the weight of the contents that fill the bottle. So the weight of the contents that fill the bottle is 100 – 10, or 90 units.

If the bottle is filled so that it weighs $\frac{1}{2}$ of its full weight, the bottle is filled so that it weighs $\frac{1}{2}$ of 100, or 50. To find the actual weight of the amount put in the bottle, subtract the weight 10 of the empty bottle from the weight 50 of the partially filled bottle, and the weight of the amount in the partially filled bottle is 50 – 10, or 40. The weight of the contents in a completely filled bottle is 90, and the weight of the contents in this partially filled bottle is 40.

Therefore, the fraction of the bottle that is filled is $\frac{40}{90}$, which is equal to $\frac{4}{9}$. (A) is correct.

38. E

It's important that we understand what the question requires. We have to determine what percent 0.4x is of y. Let's begin with an easier question. What fraction of y is 0.4x? Well, $\frac{0.4x}{y}$ is the fraction of y that 0.4x is. To find the percent that 0.4x is of y, convert $\frac{0.4x}{y}$ to a percent. Let's use the equations to find the value of the fraction $\dfrac{0.4x}{y}$, and then we'll convert this fraction to a percent.

There are two equations with the three variables x, y, and z. Because we are trying to find the value of the expression $\dfrac{0.4x}{y}$ (and then convert this to a percent), let's try to manipulate the equations to get a new equation which does not contain the variable z. Let's solve the first equation, $x - y = 0.2z$, for z. All we must do to solve the first equation, $x - y = 0.2z$, for z is divide both sides of this equation by 0.2, and then $\dfrac{x-y}{0.2} = z$. Now $0.2 = \dfrac{1}{5}$, so $\dfrac{x-y}{\left(\frac{1}{5}\right)} = z$, $(x - y) \times \dfrac{5}{1} = z$, and $z = 5(x - y)$. Now substitute $5(x - y)$ for z into the other equation, $x + z = 1.6y$, and then $x + 5(x - y) = 1.6y$. We would like to solve this equation for the value of $\dfrac{0.4x}{y}$ and then convert this to a percent. Let's first try to solve this equation for the value of $\dfrac{x}{y}$. If we can do this, then we can find the value of $\dfrac{0.4x}{y}$, and finally we can convert this to a percent.

$$x + 5(x - y) = 1.6y$$

$$x + 5x - 5y = 1.6y$$

$$6x - 5y = 1.6y$$

$$6x = 6.6y$$

$$\frac{6x}{y} = 6.6$$

$$\frac{x}{y} = \frac{6.6}{6}$$

$$\frac{x}{y} = 1.1$$

Because $\dfrac{x}{y} = 1.1$, $\dfrac{0.4x}{y} = 0.4\left(\dfrac{x}{y}\right) = 0.4(1.1) = 0.44$. All we must do is convert 0.44 to a percent. $0.44 = \dfrac{44}{100} = 44\%$. (E) is correct.

39. C
Solve the equation $\dfrac{3y + 14 - y}{2y + 1} = 2$ for the value of y.

$$\frac{3y + 14 - y}{2y + 1} = 2$$

Combine the y-terms in the numerator of the left side:

$$\frac{2y + 14}{2y + 1} = 2$$

Multiply both sides by $2y + 1$:

$$2y + 14 = 2(2y + 1)$$

Multiply out the right side: $2y + 14 = 4y + 2$

Subtract 2y from both sides: $14 = 2y + 2$

Subtract 2 from both sides: $12 = 2y$

Divide both sides by 2: $\dfrac{12}{2} = y$

$$6 = y$$

40. A
There are 16 ounces in a pound, so in an ounce there is $\dfrac{1}{16}$ of a pound. The 39-ounce box weighs $39\left(\dfrac{1}{16}\right)$ pounds. This larger box costs 91¢, so the cost per pound of this 39-ounce box is $\dfrac{91}{39\left(\frac{1}{16}\right)}$, or $\dfrac{91}{39} \times 16$¢ per pound. The 18-ounce box weighs $18\left(\dfrac{1}{16}\right)$ pounds. The cost per pound of the smaller 18-ounce box is $\dfrac{48}{18\left(\frac{1}{16}\right)}$, $\dfrac{48}{18} \times 16$¢ per pound. The ratio of the cost per pound of the larger box to the cost per pound of the smaller box is $\dfrac{\left(\frac{91}{39} \times 16\right)}{\left(\frac{48}{18} \times 16\right)}$.

Now find the value of $\dfrac{\left(\frac{91}{39} \times 16\right)}{\left(\frac{48}{18} \times 16\right)}$.

$$\frac{\left(\frac{91}{39} \times 16\right)}{\left(\frac{48}{18} \times 16\right)}$$

Divide the numerator and the denominator of this fraction by 16:

$$= \frac{\left(\frac{91}{39}\right)}{\left(\frac{48}{18}\right)}$$

To divide by a fraction, invert that fraction and multiply:

$$= \frac{91}{39} \times \frac{18}{48}$$

Divide the numerator and denominator of $\frac{91}{39}$ by 13 and the numerator and denominator of $\frac{18}{48}$ by 6:

$$= \frac{7}{3} \times \frac{3}{8}$$

Cancel a factor of 3 from the denominator of $\frac{7}{3}$ and the numerator of $\frac{3}{8}$:

$$= \frac{7}{8}$$

The ratio is $\frac{7}{8}$. The decimal equivalent of $\frac{7}{8}$ is 0.875. The ratio is 0.875:1.

41. C

The phrase "is to" appearing in this question is related to the meaning of the word ratio. For example, the phrase "4 is to 17" means the ratio of 4 to 17. The sentence "3 is to 12 as 7 is to 28" says (correctly) that the ratio of 3 to 12 is equal to the ratio of 7 to 28.

Run through the answer choices until you find the correct one that works.

(A): The ratio of 16 to 8 is $\frac{16}{8}$, or 2. The ratio of $\frac{x}{6}$ to $\frac{x}{3}$ is $\frac{\left(\frac{x}{6}\right)}{\left(\frac{x}{3}\right)} = \frac{x}{6} \times \frac{3}{x} = \frac{1}{2}$. The ratios are not the same, so (A) is not correct.

(B): The ratio of 4 to 8 is $\frac{4}{8}$, or $\frac{1}{2}$. The ratio of $\frac{x}{6}$ to $\frac{x}{12}$ is $\frac{\left(\frac{x}{6}\right)}{\left(\frac{x}{12}\right)} = \frac{x}{6} \times \frac{12}{x} = \frac{12}{6} = 2$. The ratios are not the same, so (B) is not correct.

(C): The ratio of 12 to 8 is $\frac{12}{8}$, or $\frac{3}{2}$. The ratio of $\frac{x}{6}$ to $\frac{x}{9}$ is $\frac{\left(\frac{x}{6}\right)}{\left(\frac{x}{9}\right)} = \frac{x}{6} \times \frac{9}{x} = \frac{9}{6} = \frac{3}{2}$. The ratio of 12 to 8 is equal to the ratio of $\frac{x}{6}$ to $\frac{x}{9}$, and (C) is correct.

42. D

This is a good question to solve by picking a number. Always pick numbers that are easy to work with. In percent questions, it is often good to pick 100, and this is the case with this question. It does not matter if the numbers you pick are not what you would expect from everyday life. What matters is that the

numbers you pick are easy to work with and consistent with everything the question says. Let the list price of the car be $100. The dealer bought the car at 75% of the list price, so he bought the car for 75% of $100, which is $75. The dealer sold the car for 93% of $100, which is $93. His profit was $93 − 75, or $18. The percent profit is the percent that the profit is of the amount the dealer spent to buy the car, so the percent profit is the percent that 18 is of 75. Expressed as a fraction, we have $\frac{18}{75}$, and we just have to convert this fraction to a percent:

$$\frac{18}{75} = \frac{18}{75} \times 100\% = \frac{6}{25} \times 100\% = 6 \times 4\% = 24\%.$$

43. D

This question can be solved by picking a number for the original volume of the container or letting a variable represent the original volume. Let's solve this question by letting the original volume be represented by the variable x. From 11:30 AM to 2:00 PM of the same day there are $2\frac{1}{2}$ hours. The number of half-hours in $2\frac{1}{2}$ hours is $2\frac{1}{2} \times 2$, or 5.

From 11:30 AM to 12 noon, the volume doubles from x to 2x.

From 12 noon to 12:30 PM, the volume doubles from 2x to 4x.

From 12:30 PM to 1:00 PM, the volume doubles from 4x to 8x.

From 1:00 PM to 1:30 PM, the volume doubles from 8x to 16x.

From 1:30 p.m. to 2:00 p.m., the volume doubles from 16x to 32x.

So the volume increased from x at 11:30 AM to 32x at 2:00 PM.

In general, the percent increase is equal to $\frac{\text{Amount of increase}}{\text{Original amount}} \times 100\%$.

Here, the percent increase is $\frac{32x - x}{x} \times 100\% = \frac{31x}{x} \times 100\% = \frac{31}{1} \times 100\% = 31 \times 100\% = 3,100\%$.

44. C

Call the number of teachers N. Because the ratio of teachers to students is 1:8, or 1 to 8, the number of students is 8N. The number of teachers increased by 10%. The fractional equivalent of 10% is 0.1, so this year the number of teachers is N + 0.1N = 1.1N. The number of students also increased by 10%, so the new number of students is 8N + 0.1(8N) = 8N + 0.8N = 8.8N. The ratio of the teachers to students this year is the ratio 1.1N to 8.8N, which in fractional form is $\frac{1.1N}{8.8N}$. Simplify this fraction. $\frac{1.1N}{8.8N}$ $= \frac{1.1}{8.8} = \frac{11}{88} = \frac{1}{8}$. The ratio this year is $\frac{1}{8}$, which is a ratio of 1:8, or 1 to 8.

45. D

Rearrange $\sqrt{.4761}$ using the law of radicals, which says that $\sqrt{\frac{a}{b}} = \frac{\sqrt{a}}{\sqrt{b}}$.

$$\sqrt{.4761} = \sqrt{\frac{4,761}{10,000}} = \frac{\sqrt{4,761}}{\sqrt{10,000}} = \frac{\sqrt{4,761}}{100}$$

Now use a little guesswork to find what $\sqrt{.4761}$ is equal to. The number 4,761 under the radical sign is, for our purposes here, relatively close to 4,900, which is 70^2, so $\sqrt{4,900} = 70$ and $\sqrt{4,761}$ is close to and a little bit less than $\sqrt{4,900}$, which is 70. If we test 69 by squaring it to see if we get 4,761, we find that $69^2 = 69 \times 69 = 4,761$, so it works, and $\sqrt{4,761} = 69$. Getting back to our work with $\sqrt{.4761}$, we then find that

$$\sqrt{.4761} = \frac{\sqrt{4,761}}{100} = \frac{69}{100} = 0.69$$

46. A

This question can be solved by picking a value for one of the variables in the equations $\frac{8a}{9} = \frac{2b}{3}$ and $0.5b = \frac{4c}{5}$, finding the values of all variables, and then finding out how many a's will equal 24 c's. Because a and c are the variables of interest, let's pick a value for one of these variables that is easy to work with. Because c is in the equation $0.5b = \frac{4c}{5}$, let's let c = 5 so that the 5 in the denominator of the fraction on the right can cancel with the 5 in the numerator of that fraction when c is replaced with 5.

Plug 5 for c into the equation $0.5b = \frac{4c}{5}$ and find the value of b that results. $0.5b = \frac{4(5)}{5}$, $\frac{1}{2}b = 4$,

and b = 8. Now substitute 8 for b into the equation $\frac{8a}{9} = \frac{2b}{3}$ and find the corresponding value of a. Therefore $\frac{8a}{9} = \frac{2b}{3}$, $\frac{8a}{9} = \frac{2(8)}{3}$, and dividing both sides of this last equation by 8 gives $\frac{a}{9} = \frac{2}{3}$, so a = $\frac{2}{3}$, 9 = 2 × 3 = 6, and thus a = 6 and c = 5. We want to know how many a's equal 24 c's. Well, 24 c's is 24(5), or 120. We want to figure out how many a's equal 120, where a = 6; i.e., we want to figure out what number multiplied by 6 equals 120. That number is 120 divided by 6, which is 20. So 20 a's equal 24 c's. (A), or 20, is correct.

47. B

Call the number of patients the dentist saw in August N.

In September, he saw $\frac{1}{3}$ more patients than he did in August, so in September he saw $N + \frac{1}{3}N = 1\frac{1}{3}N$ patients. Because the increase from September to October will require multiplying $1\frac{1}{3}N$ by another fraction, it is more convenient to work with $\frac{4}{3}N$ rather than $1\frac{1}{3}N$, and so the number of patients he saw in September was $\frac{4}{3}N$. In October, he saw $\frac{1}{5}$ more patients than he did in September, so the number of patients he saw in October was

$$\left(\frac{4}{3}N\right) + \frac{1}{5}\left(\frac{4}{3}N\right) = \left(\frac{4}{3}N\right)\left(1 + \frac{1}{5}\right) = \frac{4}{3}N\left(\frac{6}{5}\right) = \frac{24}{15}N = \frac{8}{5}N.$$

The number of patients he saw in October was $\frac{8}{5}N$, and the question tells us that he saw 240 patients in October. Therefore, $\frac{8}{5}N = 240$, 8N = 240(5), and N = $\frac{240(5)}{8}$ = 30(5) = 150. He saw 150 patients in August, and (B) is correct.

This answer can be checked in not a lot of time. Suppose that he saw 150 patients in August. In September he saw $\frac{1}{3}$ patients more than the 150 he saw in August, so in September he saw 150 + $\frac{1}{3}$(150) = 150 + 50 = 200 patients. In October, he saw $\frac{1}{5}$ patients more than the 200 he saw in September, so in October he saw 200 + $\frac{1}{5}$(200) = 200 + 40 = 240 patients. Now 240 is the right number of patients seen in October, so we know that 150 is the correct number of patients seen in August, and we have now checked that (B) is indeed correct.

48. C

Let's use the variable x in place of the question mark (and the parentheses that contain it). Then we want to find x where 90% of $40 = \frac{5}{6}$ of x. The fractional equivalent of 90% is $\frac{9}{10}$, and the word *of* means "times," so $\frac{9}{10}(40) = \frac{5}{6}x$. Solve this equation for x.

$$\frac{9}{10}(40) = \frac{5}{6}x$$

$$9(4) = \frac{5}{6}x$$

$$36 = \frac{5}{6}x$$

$$36(6) = 5x$$

$$216 = 5x$$

$$x = \frac{216}{5} = 43.2$$

49. D

Translate the information in the question stem into math. Let R be the number of toys that Rebecca has and let J be the number of toys that Jennifer has. The first sentence says that Rebecca has twice as many toys as Jennifer does. This means that R = 2J. The second sentence says that if Jennifer gives Rebecca four of her toys, Jennifer will have one-fourth the number of toys that Rebecca has. We're letting J be the number of toys that Jennifer has and we're letting R be the number of toys that Rebecca has. If Jennifer gives Rebecca four toys, then Jennifer will have four fewer toys, or J − 4 toys, whereas Rebecca will have four more toys, or R + 4 toys, so $J - 4 = \frac{1}{4}(R + 4)$. Now we have the two equations R = 2J and $J - 4 = \frac{1}{4}(R + 4)$, which we can solve for the value of R. There are various ways these two equations can be solved. To solve for R directly, let's solve the equation R = 2J for J in terms of R, and then plug the value of J, which is in terms of R, into the equation $J - 4 = \frac{1}{4}(R + 4)$. Dividing both sides of the equation R = 2J by 2 gives $J = \frac{R}{2}$. Now plug $\frac{R}{2}$ for J into the equation $J - 4 = \frac{1}{4}(R + 4)$, and we get

the equation $\frac{R}{2} - 4 = \frac{1}{4}(R + 4)$. Solve this equation for the value of R.

$$\frac{R}{2} - 4 = \frac{1}{4}(R + 4)$$

Multiply both sides by 4 to get rid of both denominators:

$$4\left(\frac{R}{2} - 4\right) = 4\left[\frac{1}{4}(R + 4)\right]$$

Multiply out each side: $2R - 16 = R + 4$

Subtract R from both sides: $R - 16 = 4$

Add 16 to each side: $R = 20$

Therefore, Rebecca has 20 toys, and (D) is correct.

50. E

Substitute the values of a, b, and c into the expression $(b \times a) + \frac{1}{c}$. The question stem gives us the values of c and a. We'll have to do just a little work to find the value of b. Because $\frac{1}{b} = 4$, 1 = 4b, and $b = \frac{1}{4}$. You could also have found the value of b if you realized that $\frac{1}{b} = 4$ says that the reciprocal of b is 4, so b must be $\frac{1}{4}$. Now substitute 10 for a, $\frac{1}{4}$ for b, and $\frac{2}{5}$ for c into the expression $(b \times a) + \frac{1}{c}$, and then $(b \times a) + \frac{1}{c} = \left(\frac{1}{4} \times 10\right) + \frac{1}{\left(\frac{2}{5}\right)} = \frac{5}{2} + \frac{5}{2} = \frac{10}{2} = 5$.

Index

Tear-Out, Quick Reference Study Sheets for Biology, General Chemistry, Physics and Organic Chemistry

The following OAT Study Sheets are your one-stop resource for the key diagrams, charts, equations, and formulas that you are sure to see on the exam. This color-coded guide is separated into four OAT subtopics: Biology, General Chemistry, Physics and Organic Chemistry. Each topic features the most important highlights you will want to review in between study sessions and before your test day. Carefully tear out the pages to create a light and portable on-the-go resource that you can use to study anytime, anywhere.